NANOBIOMATERIALS
DEVELOPMENT AND APPLICATIONS

Advances in Materials Science and Engineering

Series Editor

Sam Zhang

Aerospace Materials Handbook, *edited by Sam Zhang and Dongliang Zhao*

Biological and Biomedical Coatings Handbook: Applications, *edited by Sam Zhang*

Biological and Biomedical Coatings Handbook: Processing and Characterization, *edited by Sam Zhang*

Hydroxyapatite Coatings for Biomedical Applications, *edited by Sam Zhang*

Nanobiomaterials: Development and Applications, *Dong Kee Yi and Georgia C. Papaefthymiou*

Micro- and Macromechanical Properties of Materials, *Yichun Zhou, Li Yang, and Yongli Huang*

NANOBIOMATERIALS
DEVELOPMENT AND APPLICATIONS

Edited by

DONG KEE YI
GEORGIA C. PAPAEFTHYMIOU

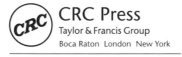

CRC Press
Taylor & Francis Group
Boca Raton London New York

CRC Press is an imprint of the
Taylor & Francis Group, an **informa** business

CRC Press
Taylor & Francis Group
6000 Broken Sound Parkway NW, Suite 300
Boca Raton, FL 33487-2742

Printed on acid-free paper
Version Date: 20130701

International Standard Book Number-13: 978-1-4398-7641-1 (Hardback)

Library of Congress Cataloging-in-Publication Data

Nanobiomaterials : development and applications / edited by Dong Kee Yi and Georgia
    C. Papaefthymiou.
      p. ; cm. -- (Advances in materials science and engineering)
    Includes bibliographical references.
    ISBN 978-1-4398-7641-1 (hardcover)
    I. Yi, Dong Kee. II. Papaefthymiou, Georgia C. III. Series: Advances in materials
science and engineering.
    [DNLM: 1. Nanostructures. 2. Biocompatible Materials. QT 36.5]

R857.N34
610.28--dc23   2013014257

Visit the Taylor & Francis Web site at
http://www.taylorandfrancis.com

and the CRC Press Web site at
http://www.crcpress.com

Contents

PART I Nanomaterials in Nanobiotechnologies: Preparation, Characterization, and Applications

PART II Soft Block Nanobuilding: New Preparation Routes of Soft Nanomaterials Using Biomolecules

PART III Nanomaterials and Bio-MEMS: Nano- and Microscale Hybridization of Materials and Applications

PART IV Nanotoxicity Studies and Applications in Eco-Biosystems

Series Preface

ADVANCES IN MATERIALS SCIENCE AND ENGINEERING

SERIES STATEMENT

Materials form the foundation of technologies that govern our everyday life, from housing and household appliances to handheld phones, drug delivery systems, airplanes, and satellites. Development of new and increasingly tailored materials is key to further advance important applications with the potential to dramatically enhance and enrich our experiences.

The *Advances in Materials Science and Engineering* series by CRC Press/ Taylor & Francis Group is designed to help meet new and exciting challenges in materials science and engineering disciplines.

The books and monographs in the series are based on cutting edge research and development, and thus are up to date with new discoveries, new understanding, and new insights in all aspects of materials development, including processing and characterization and applications in metallurgy, bulk or surface engineering, interfaces, thin films, coatings, and composites, just to name a few.

The series aims at delivering an authoritative information source to readers in academia, research institutes, and industry. The publisher and its series editor are fully aware of the importance of materials science and engineering as the foundation for many other disciplines of knowledge. As such, the team is committed to making this series the most comprehensive and accurate literary source to serve the whole materials world and the associated fields.

As series editor, I thank all authors and editors of the books in this series for their noble contributions to the advancement of materials science and engineering and to the advancement of humankind.

Sam Zhang

Preface

Nanobiotechnology is a recently activated term describing the convergence of molecular biology and engineering. The combination of these disciplines over the last decade has realized a new class of smart devices or systems for biological and chemical analysis defined by improved specificity and sensitivity as well as higher rates of molecular recognition compared with previous solutions. Advances have been made in nanobiochip materials, biomimetic materials, nanocomposite materials, interface biomaterials, photocatalytic materials, nanomotors, nanobiosensors, and nano drug delivery systems, with enormous prospect in industrial, defense, and medical applications of great societal impact. Such technological advances are the direct outcome of the continuous exchange of ideas, which is taking place across the border between the biological and physical sciences in many areas of nanoscience. This interdisciplinary exchange is based on the premise that nanotechnology offers biology new tools, while biology offers nanotechnology new types of functional materials. The ability to observe intracellular structures with high selectivity and follow their dynamic behavior is the greatest challenge of biology to nanoscience that drives the nanotechnological development of a variety of bioimaging probes. Understanding the rotatory flagellar motor of bacteria and adapting it to biotechnological needs is another challenge. Nanotechnology makes use of biomimetic or bio-inspired processes for the production of nanosized materials for applications not only in biology but also in a variety of seemingly unrelated fields including nanoelectronics. On the other hand, the fruits of nanotechnology are increasingly being applied to expanding areas of biomedical and therapeutic processes. Nanotechnology is affording biomedicine new nanostructures and scaffolds for tissue engineering, nanoparticle probes for magnetic resonance imaging (MRI), targeted drug delivery and hyperthermia cancer therapy, photonic band structures, new optical imaging probes, and carbon nanotube–based technological advances for drug and gene delivery, to name a few. Thus, nanobiotechnology constitutes "a bridge between nano and bio," with nanoscale materials providing the building blocks for the construction of the "bridge."

The present volume of the *Advances in Materials Science and Engineering* series provides an update on developments, and new findings and applications on many of the topics mentioned above that comprise active areas of multidisciplinary bionanomaterials research. It presents 12 chapters contributed by an international team of investigators, who are actively engaged in the forefront of research in their respective disciplines. These 12 chapters fall under 4 broad themes, and thus the book is internally organized into 4 parts: Part I, "Nanomaterials in Nanobiotechnologies: Preparation, Characterization, and Applications"; Part II, "Soft Block Nanobuilding: New Preparation Routes of Soft Nanomaterials Using Biomolecules"; Part III, "Nanomaterials and Bio-MEMS: Nano- and Microscale Hybridization of Materials and Applications"; and Part IV, "Nanotoxicity Studies and Applications in Eco-Biosystems." Potential readers who will benefit from this volume include advanced undergraduate and graduate students engaged in nanobiomaterials research, industrial researchers, pharmaceutical innovators, medical and public health personnel as well as environmental scientists and engineers. The reader will come away with a better appreciation of the importance of this interdisciplinary field to biotechnology, biomedicine, and environmental remediation—all subjects of importance to society at large. A brief description of the contents of each chapter follows.

In Part I, Chapter 1, "Bio-Inspired Magnetic Nanoparticles," reviews the biomineralization of iron in biological processes and the biomimetic synthesis of magnetic nanoparticles within protein cages and viral capsids, block copolymers, microemulsions, and silica shells, as well as the magnetic characterization of the thus-derived magnetic nanosystems. Chapter 2, "Nanoparticles for Bioimaging," introduces semiconductor nanocrystals or quantum dots (QDs) and their photonic properties and reviews their synthesis, surface modification, and applications in cell labeling and targeting for medical applications in cancer diagnosis and therapy as well as other novel applications. Chapter 3, "Biomedical Applications of Dendrimer Porphyrin or Phthalocyanine," discusses the design of dendritic materials and their use in photodynamic therapy, the development of dendritic photosensitizer-loaded micelles for photochemical delivery and as drug carriers, as well as diagnostic applications of the dendrimer porphyrin. Chapter 4, "Polymeric Nanoparticles in Cancer Therapy," focuses on the use of natural and synthetic polymer-based nanoparticles for cancer therapy. Chapter 5, "Carbon Nanotube Bioconjugates," presents an in-depth discussion of the rapidly advancing area of carbon nanotube bioconjugation, reactivity, and functionalization for applications in cell imaging, pharmacokinetics, protein and antigen transfection, nucleic acid delivery, tumor targeting, and cancer therapy. Chapter 6, "Biocatalytic Nanosystems," addresses the subject of enzyme immobilization using nanomaterials, nanoparticle and nanoporous supports, novel nanosystems for biocatalysis, nanoentrapment, single-enzyme nanoparticles, and biocatalytic nanosystems for biosensing. Chapter 7, "Magnetically Induced Hyperthermia for Biomedical Applications," presents a lucid discussion of the physics of heat dissipation mechanisms of magnetic ferrofluids and magnetic hyperthermia instrumentation for *in vitro* and *in vivo* studies in animal models.

In Part II, Chapter 8, "Engineered Biomolecules as Nanomaterials," discusses the manufacturing of functional nanomaterials using rod-shaped filamentous and spherical or nearly spherical viruses.

In Part III, Chapter 9, "Microfluidic-Based Polymer Scaffold Design for Tissue Engineering," presents the design of polymeric scaffolds, microfluidic cell culture systems, and bioreactors for tissue engineering. Chapter 10, "Fabrication of Mobile Hybrid Microswimmers Using Micro/Nanoparticles and Bacterial Flagella," gives a fascinating discussion of biomimetic device fabrication and bio-inspired engineering and locomotion, using micro- and nano-sized particles and bacterial flagella.

In Part IV, Chapter 11, "Environmental Applications of Nanomaterials," introduces the area of nanotechnology for environmental remediation and decontamination using nanomaterials and environmental biosensors, and discusses the environmental impact of nanomaterials in terms of toxicity and impact on ecosystems. Chapter 12, "Cytotoxicity of Biosynthesized Nanomaterials and Functionalized Nanomaterials: Use in Therapy," discusses the intra- and extracellular biosynthesis of nanoparticles by bacteria and their functionalization, cytotoxicity mechanisms, and potential use in therapy.

We thank all the authors and coauthors of these chapters for their valuable contributions to this volume and for their patience and dedication during all stages of the preparation and production of this book. We especially thank Dr. Sam Zhang, the editor of the *Advances in Materials Science and Engineering* series, for inviting and encouraging us to edit the present volume on nanoscale materials applications in bionanotechnologies. Last, but not least, special thanks are due to the staff at CRC Press for their professional support, patience, and dedication in all phases of the preparation of the book.

Dong Kee Yi
Department of Bionanotechnology
Gachon University
Sungnam City, Republic of Korea

Georgia C. Papaefthymiou
Department of Physics
Villanova University
Villanova, Pennsylvania

Editors

Dong Kee Yi received his BS in 1996 from the Seoul National University, MS in 1998 from POSTECH, and PhD in materials science and engineering in 2003 from Gwangju Institute of Science and Technology (GIST), Korea. He was a post-doctoral fellow at Brown University and at the Institute of Bioengineering and Nanotechnology in Singapore from 2003 to 2005. He worked as a senior scientist in Samsung Advanced Institute of Technology from 2005 to 2007. Since 2007, he has been working as a faculty member at the Department of Bionanotechnology, Gachon University, Korea.

Professor Yi serves on the editorial board of *ISRN Nanotechnology* and writes reviews for journals from leading scientific societies including American Chemical Society, Royal Society of Chemistry, and American Institute of Physics. He has been involved in the fields of nanomaterial preparation and application, bioimaging, and colloid science for the past 12 years. He has authored and coauthored more than 60 peer-reviewed international journal articles and worked as an inventor for 32 international patents.

Professor Yi works on research/technology evaluation and advisory panels for the governments of China, Korea, and Romania. He has also worked as a consultant to industrial organizations in Korea. He was featured in the first edition of *Who's Who in Asia* and *Who's Who of Emerging Leaders* (2007). Since 2004, he has been featured in *Who's Who in the World* and *2000 Outstanding Intellectuals of the Twenty-First Century*.

Georgia C. Papaefthymiou, a graduate of Columbia University in New York, is a professor of physics at Villanova University, Villanova, Pennsylvania, and is a visiting research professor at the National Centre for Scientific Research (NCSR) Demokritos, Athens, Greece. She is the recipient of a Marie Curie Chair of Excellence award from the European Union with the Institute of Materials Science of Demokritos and a CAPES award from the Ministry of Education of Brazil with the Brazilian Center for Research in Physics in Rio de Janeiro. Her research interests are in condensed matter physics encompassing areas in (1) cluster science and the transition from molecular to bulk behavior with increasing cluster size; (2) nanoscale magnetism and fundamental studies and applications to nanotechnology and nanomedicine; (3) multiferroic materials; and (4) iron-containing proteins. She is the author or coauthor of over 150 publications that include peer-reviewed articles, book chapters, reviews, conference proceedings, and opinion pieces. She is on the board of editors of the *Journal of Materials*; peer reviewer for multiple physics, chemistry, and materials journals; and grant reviewer for the National Science Foundation and the Department of Energy of the United States and for Aristeia of Greece.

Contributors

U. Kei Cheang
Department of Mechanical
    Engineering & Mechanics
Drexel University
Philadelphia, Pennsylvania

Hun Je Cho
Water Environmental Center
Korea Institute of Science and
    Technology
Seoul, Republic of Korea

Eamonn Devlin
Institute of Advanced Materials,
    Physicochemical Processes,
    Nanotechnology & Microsystems
National Centre for Scientific Research
    "Demokritos"
Attiki, Greece

Georgios Diamantopoulos
Institute of Advanced Materials,
    Physicochemical Processes,
    Nanotechnology & Microsystems
National Centre for Scientific Research
    "Demokritos"
Attiki, Greece

Michael Fardis
Institute of Advanced Materials,
    Physicochemical Processes,
    Nanotechnology & Microsystems
National Centre for Scientific Research
    "Demokritos"
Attiki, Greece

Woo-Dong Jang
Department of Chemistry
Yonsei University
Seoul, Republic of Korea

Eleni Karakosta
Institute of Advanced Materials,
    Physicochemical Processes,
    Nanotechnology &
    Microsystems
National Centre for Scientific Research
    "Demokritos"
Attiki, Greece

Byoung Chan Kim
Water Environmental Center
Korea Institute of Science and
    Technology
Seoul, Republic of Korea

Kwangmeyung Kim
Biomedical Research Institute
Korea Institute of Science and
    Technology
Seoul, Republic of Korea

Min Jun Kim
Department of Mechanical
    Engineering & Mechanics
and
School of Biomedical Engineering,
    Science & Health Systems
Drexel University
Philadelphia, Pennsylvania

Sanghyo Kim
Department of Bionanotechnology
Gachon University
Gyeonggi-do, Republic of Korea

Won-Gun Koh
Department of Chemical and
    Biomolecular Engineering
Yonsei University Seoul
Seoul, Republic of Korea

Heebeom Koo
Biomedical Research Institute
Korea Institute of Science and
    Technology
Seoul, Republic of Korea

Ick Chan Kwon
Biomedical Research Institute
Korea Institute of Science and
    Technology
Seoul, Republic of Korea

Changha Lee
School of Urban and Environmental
    Engineering
Ulsan National Institute of Science and
    Technology
Ulsan, Republic of Korea

Jaesang Lee
Water Environmental Center
Korea Institute of Science and
    Technology
Seoul, Republic of Korea

Min-Ho Lee
Medical IT Technology
Korea Electronics Technology
    Institute
Seongnam, Republic of Korea

Su Seong Lee
Institute of Bioengineering and
    Nanotechnology
The Nanos
Singapore

Yun Jung Lee
Department of Energy Engineering
Hanyang University
Seoul, Republic of Korea

Jaehong Lim
Institute of Bioengineering and
    Nanotechnology
The Nanos
Singapore

Yong Taik Lim
Department of Analytical Science
    and Technology
Chungnam National University
Daejeon, Republic of Korea

Mohana Marimuthu
Department of Bionanotechnology
Gachon University
Gyeonggi-do, Republic of Korea

Ki Tae Nam
Department of Materials Science
    and Engineering
Seoul National University
Seoul, Republic of Korea

Georgia C. Papaefthymiou
Department of Physics
Villanova University
Villanova, Pennsylvania

Georgios Papavassiliou
Institute of Advanced Materials,
    Physicochemical Processes,
    Nanotechnology & Microsystems
National Centre for Scientific Research
    "Demokritos"
Attiki, Greece

Hye Sun Park
Department of Analytical Science and
    Technology
Chungnam National University
Daejeon, Republic of Korea

Ioannis Rabias
Institute of Advanced Materials,
    Physicochemical Processes,
    Nanotechnology & Microsystems
National Centre for Scientific Research
    "Demokritos"
Attiki, Greece

Monica Samal
Department of Bionanotechnology
Gachon University
Seoul, Republic of Korea

Shashadhar Samal
Department of Chemistry
S.B.R. Govt. (Autonomous) Women's
    College
Berhampur, India

Ramesh Subbiah
University of Science
    and Technology
Daejeon, Republic of Korea
and
Center for Biomaterials
and
Nanomaterials Center
Korea Institute of Science
    and Technology
Seoul, Republic of Korea

Danai Tsitrouli
Institute of Advanced Materials,
    Physicochemical Processes,
    Nanotechnology & Microsystems
National Centre for Scientific Research
    "Demokritos"
Attiki, Greece

Vassilios Tzitzios
Institute of Advanced
    Materials, Physicochemical
    Processes, Nanotechnology &
    Microsystems
National Centre for Scientific
    Research "Demokritos"
Attiki, Greece

Murugan Veerapandian
Department of Bionanotechnology
Gachon University
Gyeonggi-do, Republic of Korea

Ji Young Yhee
Biomedical Research Institute
Korea Institute of Science
    and Technology
Seoul, Republic of Korea

Dong Kee Yi
Department of Bionanotechnology
Gachon University
Seoul, Republic of Korea

Kyusik Yun
Department of Bionanotechnology
Gachon University
Gyeonggi-do, Republic of Korea

Part I

Nanomaterials in
Nanobiotechnologies:
Preparation, Characterization,
and Applications

1 Bio-Inspired Magnetic Nanoparticles

Georgia C. Papaefthymiou
Villanova University

Eamonn Devlin
National Center of Scientific Research "Demokritos"

CONTENTS

1.1 INTRODUCTION

Materials science explores the relationship between the structure and properties of materials. Borrowing techniques and practices from solid-state chemistry and physics for the synthesis and characterization of materials, it has developed as a separate scientific area. Originally, it had no affinity with biology, but the advent and integration of nanoscience and nanotechnology into materials science has changed this dramatically [1,2]. Nanotechnology deals with the manipulation of matter at the atomic and molecular levels for the bottom-up synthesis of materials. The synthesis of supramolecular structures in nature is the archetypical example of such processes. Today materials science draws inspiration from biology and strives to reproduce or mimic biological processes in the synthesis of materials. In the specific case of magnetic nanoparticles, the subject of this chapter, it is the ubiquitous process of biomineralization that has been particularly inspiring [3,4].

Through the process of biomineralization nature integrates hard inorganic materials with the soft organic world of biology. Living organisms can provide chemical environments that control the nucleation and growth of unique mineral phases, forming exceptional nanocomposite materials, such as bone or seashell. Bone is the archetypical biological nanocomposite, consisting of hard apatite, a form of calcium phosphate, and soft organic tissue, the protein collagen—the nanoscale plate-like crystals of apatite being dispersed within the collagen fiber matrix [5,6]. The outstanding mechanical properties of bone do not derive simply from those of the component materials, but depend on how they are arranged and how this arrangement is altered under stress. For example, bone is twice as strong in compression as in tension or torsion. This is due to the fact that collagen does not act as glue, but more like a net in which the apatite particles are trapped and allowed to move against each other. In the biomineralization of bone, end-use functionality dictates the formation of a nanostructured material, as the mechanical properties of bone cannot be reproduced by bulk apatite, that is, its nanocomposite structure is essential to its function. There exists a growing interest in the processes by which such complex and intricate hierarchical biomineral architectures can be reproduced in the laboratory for the production of functional materials, without the harsh high-temperature and high-pressure requirements of solid-state chemistry.

In the case of magnetite biomineralization of magnetotactic bacteria, the formation of a chain of single-domain magnetic particles (MPs) within membrane vesicles is essential for the construction of a biomagnetic compass [7,8]. Nano-ferrihydrite biomineralization in the ferritins derives from the metabolic need for iron [9–12]. Time and again biological examples show that nature produces unique structures with end-use functionality in mind. This is also the goal of materials science today.

In this chapter we explore bio-inspired routes to iron-based magnetic nanoparticle formation. To appreciate this rapidly growing field, we must first review some general basic principles encountered in the biogenesis of magnetic nanoparticles.

1.2 BIOMINERALIZATION OF IRON IN BIOLOGICAL PROCESSES

Biomineralization of iron in biological processes is encountered in two major areas: the biomineralization of ferrihydrite in the ferritins for iron metabolic purposes and the biomineralization of magnetite in magnetosomes for magnetoreception and navigation in microbial and higher living organisms.

1.2.1 FERRIHYDRITE GROWN WITHIN APOFERRITIN

The availability of iron for metabolic purposes requires a mechanism for the efficient and reversible storage of iron. Nature has solved this problem by forming a dense solid particle within the ferritin molecule, shown in Figure 1.1, where a large number of Fe atoms are stored [9–12].

Iron stored
as mineral
inside ferritin

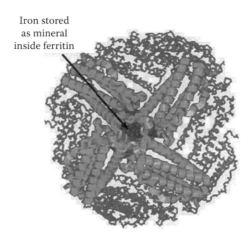

FIGURE 1.1 Ribbon representation of the ferritin molecule. A polymeric shell consisting of 24 polypeptide subunits encapsulates a particle of biomineralized ferrihydrite. Shell dimensions: inner diameter 7 nm; outer diameter 12 nm.

Ferritins represent a family of proteins that are widespread in biological systems. Although there are differences among them, their overall similarities are more important than their differences. They are all large multicomponent proteins that self-assemble to form molecular cages, within which a hydrated ferric oxide is mineralized. The mammalian ferritin cage, also known as apoferritin, is a heteropolymer consisting of 24 amino acid chains of two types: H (heavy) and L (light). It has an inner diameter of ~7 nm and an outer diameter of ~12 nm. In the interior cavity of the protein cage it forms a micellar core of hydrated iron(III) oxide (ferrihydrite), with various amounts of phosphate inclusions. It was first described by V. Laufberger in 1937 [13] as a protein isolated from horse spleen, which contains about 20% iron. The nanocomposite state of ferrihydrite in ferritin affords a high surface-area-to-volume ratio, that is, an increased proportion of surface iron sites enhancing the iron storage and release processes. The formation of ferritin is a classic example of nature's response to the challenging problem of the nucleation and growth of nanoparticles for the efficient packing of iron atoms.

1.2.1.1 The Challenge of Nanoparticle Nucleation and Growth

In a homogeneous medium, particle nucleation is generally hindered due to the energetically demanding process of interface formation at the boundary of the nucleated phase, the nascent particle surface. The nucleation energy barrier can be overcome kinetically in supersaturated solutions where encounters or collisions between atoms or molecules are frequent. One must consider the change in Gibbs free energy, ΔG, that results from nucleation [14], as in all types of phase transitions. Bonding is energetically favored, as particle formation liberates ΔG_v of energy per unit volume. However, the creation of an interfacial boundary consumes ΔG_s free energy per unit interfacial area. For the formation of a spherical cluster of radius r, the overall change in Gibbs free energy is given by

$$\Delta G = -\frac{4\pi}{3}r^3\Delta G_v + 4\pi r^2\Delta G_s. \tag{1.1}$$

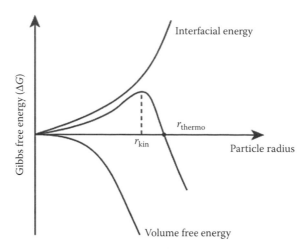

FIGURE 1.2 Particle nucleation and growth: change in volume, surface, and total Gibbs free energy, ΔG, as a function of particle radius. The kinetic and thermodynamic critical radii are indicated.

The first term gives the energy gained in creating the volume of the particle, thus this is the term that drives nucleation, while the second term gives the energy lost due to surface tension at the interface, and thus is the term that hinders nucleation. Figure 1.2 gives a sketch of the dependence of various terms on r.

For very small particles, ΔG is positive, due to the high surface-area-to-volume ratio, making nucleation thermodynamically unfavorable. The graph of ΔG as a function of r reaches a maximum when $d(\Delta G)/dr = 0$. The maximum occurs at

$$r_{kin} = \frac{2\Delta G_s}{\Delta G_v}, \tag{1.2}$$

which defines the kinetic critical radius for nucleation. For $r > r_{kin}$, further growth of the nucleated cluster is kinetically favored as ΔG decreases with increasing particle size. The radius r_{thermo} above which ΔG becomes negative defines the thermodynamic critical radius. The particle, once nucleated, is thermodynamically driven to continuous growth and the formation of bulk material. Surface passivation with terminal ligation is needed to arrest the growth at the nanoscale.

In heterogeneous nucleation, the positive energy associated with surface tension at phase boundaries is greatly reduced since the presence of nucleation sites eliminates the particle/solution interface in the process of particle nucleation. Thus, energetic considerations for heterogeneous nucleation are less demanding, and nucleation can be more readily initiated.

1.2.1.2 Particle Nucleation and Growth in the Ferritins

Ferritin provides (1) the nucleation sites for iron polymerization, (2) the means to promote supersaturation conditions within the confined space of the protein cage, and (3) the terminal ligation needed to stabilize the nanoparticles. The molecular properties of the amino acid cage are designed to induce ferrihydrite formation in the interior of the protein rather than in the bulk solution. This is achieved by the presence of negatively charged glutamic acid residues, the nucleation sites, which line the interior wall of apoferritin with COO^- ions that attract Fe^{2+} ions and lead to double-layer formation with an increased density of iron ions at the interior protein surface [15]. The molecular cage also functions as a catalyst for the oxidation of $Fe^{2+} \rightarrow Fe^{3+}$ at a binuclear iron-binding site known as the ferroxidase center [16], using O_2 or H_2O_2 as the oxidant [17], and induces the hydrolytic polymerization of iron to form the ferrihydrite core, according to reactions as follows:

$$2Fe^{2+} + O_2 + 4H_2O \rightarrow 2Fe(O)OH_{(core)} + H_2O_2 + 4H^+, \qquad (1.3)$$

$$2Fe^{2+} + H_2O_2 + 2H_2O \rightarrow 2Fe(O)OH_{(core)} + 4H^+, \qquad (1.4)$$

$$4Fe^{2+} + O_2 + 6H_2O \rightarrow 4Fe(O)OH_{(core)} + 8H^+. \qquad (1.5)$$

X-ray crystal structure determination of ferritin by Pauline Harrison and coworkers in 1991 [18] indicated that between amino acid chains or subunits there are small pores, or channels, of about 0.3 nm diameter, through which ions and small molecules can travel. These channels play a crucial role in ferritin's ability to uptake and release iron in a controlled fashion. They are of two types: fourfold channels are formed at the intersection of four subunits, while threefold channels are formed at the intersection of three subunits. The two types of channels have different properties, and thus perform different functions. The walls of the threefold channels are lined with charged, polar (hydrophilic) amino acids such as aspartate and glutamate, while the walls of a four-fold channel are lined with nonpolar (hydrophobic) amino acids, such as alanine and leucine. The polarity of the threefold channels facilitates interaction with the Fe^{2+} ions. In contrast, the nonpolar nature of the fourfold channels cannot facilitate ion passage between the interior and the exterior of the protein. It is believed that the function of the fourfold channels is the transport of electrons into and out of the cavity, allowing oxidation or reduction of iron to take place on the mineral core surface.

Ferrihydrite, or hydrous ferric oxide, can be precipitated directly from oxygenated iron-rich aqueous solutions as a fine-grained, defective nanomaterial with varying degrees of crystallinity. Its powder x-ray diffraction (XRD) pattern can change from two broad scattered bands, in its most disordered state, to a maximum of six strong lines, in its most crystalline state [19], as shown in Figure 1.3. The six-line form corresponds to the nominal chemical formula $FeOOH \cdot 0.4H_2O$; however, the exact structure is fundamentally indeterminate as the water content is variable.

In native ferritin, the iron is stored as ferrihydrite with the inclusion of various amounts of phosphate with the general chemical formula $[FeO(OH)]_8[FeO(H_2PO_4)]$. One of the most readily (commercially) available source of ferritin for experimentation is that which is extracted from equine spleen, or horse spleen ferritin (HoSF). Figure 1.4 shows a transmission electron microscopy (TEM) micrograph of an *in vivo* produced HoSF sample. The dark spots correspond to the electron-rich iron ferritin core with a diameter of ~7 nm, consistent with the internal size of the protein shell, which maintains the hydrous iron oxide particles isolated from each other,

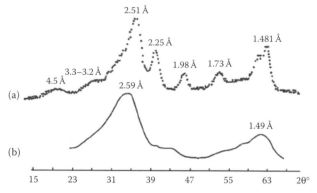

FIGURE 1.3 Six-line (a) and two-line (b) ferrihydrite XRD patterns, CuKα radiation. (Reproduced with kind permission of the Mineralogical Society of Great Britain and Ireland from the paper by Drits, V. A., et al., Structural model for ferrihydrite, *Clay Miner.*, 28, 185–207, 1993.)

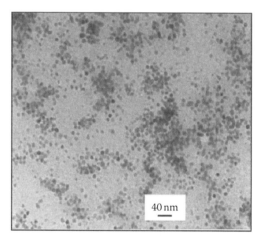

FIGURE 1.4 TEM micrograph of native *in vivo* produced HoSF ferritin. (Sample purchased from Sigma-Aldrich.)

preventing coagulation. The *in vivo* produced biomineral core may be removed from the protein to obtain apoferritin, allowing subsequent *in vitro* reconstitution of the core under controlled laboratory conditions in the absence of phosphates. Through this process, "reconstituted ferritins" with differing degrees of iron loading can be prepared. The XRD spectra of the derived cores indicate the formation of ferrihydrite, with the degree of crystallinity increasing with particle size [20].

1.2.2 Magnetite Grown within Membrane Vesicles

Magnetite is the most common of the known iron oxide biominerals. Biologically precipitated magnetite was first identified by H. Lowenstam in 1962 [21] in the denticle capping of chitons (primitive marine mollusks) in which magnetite precipitation and tooth formation [22] proceed through the biochemically controlled reduction of ferrihydrite. The mineral hardens the major lateral teeth of chitons, enabling them to scrape surface and embedded algae from hard marine rocks for food. Unlike ferrihydrite, which is a common product of both biological and inorganic processes, magnetite is naturally formed inorganically only at elevated temperatures and pressures in igneous and metamorphic rocks. Yet, organisms ranging from bacteria to vertebrates are capable of forming magnetite under ambient conditions. By natural selection, the chitons have found a route to biochemically mediate the transformation of ferrihydrite to magnetite at atmospheric temperatures and pressures. Biological magnetite deposits have also been identified with another entirely different biological function, "magnetoreception," which is the ability of living organisms to sense the polarity and inclination of the Earth's magnetic field [23]. Some bacteria, honey bees, homing pigeons, and migratory fish are known to possess this sense.

Magnetotactic bacteria [7,8] synthesize membrane-enclosed intracellular crystalline MPs, called magnetosomes, comprised primarily of iron oxides or, in rare cases, iron sulfides. Magnetosomes are nanometer-sized, magnetic mineral crystal deposits enveloped by a stable membrane that contains some lipids and proteins, often referred to as the membrane vesicle. They are aligned to form chains within the bacterium, creating a biomagnetic compass that enables the bacterium to orient in the Earth's magnetic field, a phenomenon known as "magnetotaxis." These are microaerobic bacteria, endowed with flagella that allow them to swim and migrate along oxygen gradients in aquatic environments. They were first reported in 1975 by the microbiologist Richard P. Blakemore [24]. Studies have revealed that magnetic bacteria tightly control the synthesis of their own magnetite, mediated by the magnetosome membrane that has a distinct biochemical composition and contains specific magnetosome membrane proteins (MMPs) [25,26]. Since 1975, a variety of strains have been found to exist in marine and freshwater habitats. Figure 1.5 shows TEM micrographs of magnetosomes and bacteria representing three different strains of typical magnetotactic bacteria. Note that magnetosomes can be isolated from bacteria with intact magnetosome membranes surrounding the MPs, as indicated in Figure 1.5c, where the magnetosome membranes, indicated by the arrow, are clearly visible.

Detailed studies of the crystal structure of the magnetite particles within the magnetosomes indicate that they contain highly crystalline magnetite nanoparticles of cubo-octahedral shape, yielding superior magnetic properties. Overall, magnetosome crystals have high chemical purity, narrow size distribution, and species-specific morphologies, unattainable in inorganically precipitated magnetite. These features point to magnetosome formation under strict biological control [25], a process known as "biologically controlled mineralization."

The archetypical core/shell architectural model of the ferritin molecule and bacterial magnetosomes is presently widely being used in materials science in bio-inspired routes for the formation and application of magnetic nanoparticles. Recent efforts focus on the use of protein cages and viral capsids as space-confined reaction vesicles for the formation of magnetic nanoparticles, but various other polymeric and inorganic shells are also being explored in core/shell nanoarchitectures. In the case of

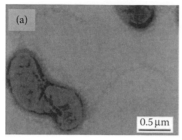

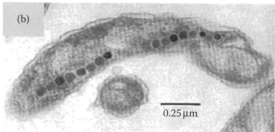

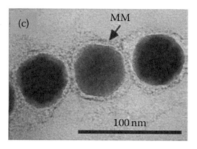

FIGURE 1.5 TEM micrographs of typical magnetotactic bacteria and magnetosomes. (a) *Magnetotactic spirillum* (MV-4) with a flagellum at each end of the cell and a chain of electron-dense, magnetite-containing magnetosomes along the long axis of the cell. (From Bazylinski, D. A. and R. B. Frankel, Magnetosome formation in prokaryotes, *Nat. Rev. Microbiol.*, 2004. 2: pp. 217–230. Reprinted with permission from Nature Publishing Group *Nature Reviews Microbiology*, copyright 2004.) (b) TEM micrograph of thin-sectioned magnetic cells of *Magnetotactic spirillum* (MS-1). The chains of crystals within the cell are clearly visible. (From Frankel, R. B., et al., Magnetite in freshwater magnetotactic bacteria, *Science*, 1979. 203: pp. 1355–1356. Reprinted with permission of AAAS.) (c) Isolated magnetosomes from *Magnetospirillum gryphiswaldense*. Arrow indicates the magnetosome membrane (MM). (From Schüler, D., Molecular analysis of a subcellular compartment: The magnetosome membrane in *Magnetospirillum gryphiswaldense*, *Arch. Microbiol.*, 2004. 181: pp. 1–7. With kind permission from Springer Science+Business Media.)

magnetic nanoparticles, the shell carries out the additional function of steric isolation of the magnetic nanoparticles to minimize magnetic interactions between particles and thus prevent particle agglomeration, an important issue in ferrofluid preparations for biomedical applications [27].

1.3 BIOMIMETIC MAGNETIC NANOPARTICLES

Broadly, we define "biomimetic," as any synthesis procedure in which hard inorganic nanoparticles are incorporated within soft polymeric matrices, surfactants, or polypeptide cages, in order to address the critical issues of size confinement, surface terminal ligation, and dispersion. We then expand our definition of "biomimetic" to include other biocompatible core/shell magnetic nanoparticles such as those encapsulated in silica.

1.3.1 FERRITE NANOPARTICLES GROWN WITHIN BLOCK COPOLYMER NANOREACTORS

The rich magnetic behavior of spinel ferrites stems from the presence of two magnetic sublattices that originate from the magnetic interaction between cations, with magnetic moments situated in tetrahedral and octahedral coordination sites, strongly exchange-coupled to produce ferrimagnetic ground states. Theoretically, they can be obtained from magnetite Fe_3O_4 by the substitution of Fe^{2+} by another transition metal. Solid solutions of the form $T_xFe_{3-x}O_4$ (where $T = Cu^{2+}$, Co^{2+}, Mg^{2+}, Zn^{2+}, Ni^{2+}, etc.) can be prepared [28,29]. Such substitutions into the parent structure of Fe_3O_4 modify the incipient magnetic exchange interactions between and within sublattices and, therefore, the overall magnetic behavior of the system. Microphase separation of diblock copolymers results in heterogeneous structures with lamellar, cylindrical, or spherical microdomains, as shown in Figure 1.6 [30,31]. These microdomains can serve as nanoreactors, or space-constrained reaction vesicles, analogous to protein cages and membrane vesicles, for the nucleation and growth of magnetic nanoparticles.

Figure 1.7 shows a schematic diagram of $CoFe_2O_4$ nanoparticle formation by self-assembly within a diblock copolymer matrix consisting of polynorbornene (NOR) and polynorbornene-dicarboxylic acid (NORCOOH), with a repeat unit ratio of 400/50, synthesized using ring-opening metathesis polymerization (ROMP) [32]. $FeCl_3$ and $CoCl_2$ were used as precursors (polymer:$FeCl_3$:$CoCl_2$ = 1:25.0:12.5 mol). The metal salts were introduced while the polymer was in solution, before the microphase separation of the two blocks could occur. Rapid diffusion and attachment of the metal salts to the polymer, due to their high affinity for the COOH groups, resulted in the dispersion of the metal salts within the copolymer matrix [28].

A solid film was subsequently formed via static casting over a period of 3 days. The films were then washed with NaOH and H_2O. The $FeCl_3$ and $CoCl_2$ salts reacted with NaOH and water within the NORCOOH nanoreactors. As a result, $CoFe_2O_4$ nanocrystals were formed within the self-assembled NORCOOH nanospheres of the diblock copolymer matrix. Figure 1.8 shows the TEM micrograph of the resulting

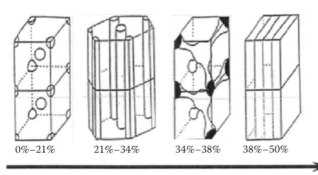

| 0%–21% | 21%–34% | 34%–38% | 38%–50% |

Increasing volume fraction of minority component

FIGURE 1.6 Microphase separation of diblock copolymers into heterogeneous structures with lamellar, cylindrical, or spherical microdomains.

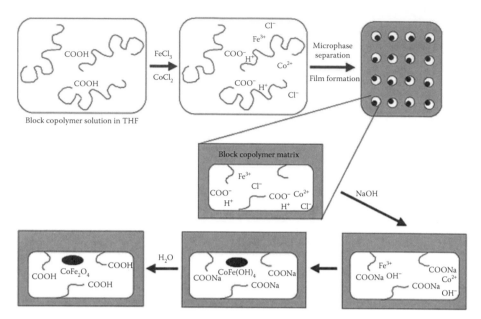

FIGURE 1.7 Schematic of formation of $CoFe_2O_4$ nanoparticles within the diblock copolymer. (Reproduced from Papaefthymiou, G. C., et al., Magnetic and structural characterization of $CoFe_2O_4$ nanoparticles encapsulated within block copolymer films, *Rev. Adv. Mater. Sci.*, 10, 306–313, 2005, with kind permission of Advanced Study Center Co. Ltd.)

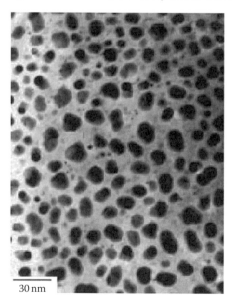

FIGURE 1.8 Morphology of block copolymer films: highly dispersed $CoFe_2O_4$ nanoparticles, oval in shape and of average diameter d of 9.6 ± 2.8 nm, are observed. (Reprinted with permission from Ahmed, S. R., et al., Magnetic properties of $CoFe_2O_4$ nanoparticles synthesized through a block co-polymer nanoreactor route, *Appl. Phys. Lett.*, 2002. 80(9): pp. 1616–1618. Copyright 2002, American Institute of Physics.)

cobalt ferrite nanoparticles [28]. The particles are well separated by the intervening polymer, but they are not of uniform size or shape, with an effective average diameter of 9.6 nm and a standard deviation of ±2.8 nm.

1.3.2 PREPARATION OF MAGNETIC NANOPARTICLES USING MICROEMULSIONS

Emulsions are mixtures of two immiscible or unblendable liquids, such as polar and nonpolar solvents, usually referred to as "water and oil" mixtures, depicted in Figure 1.9. Such mixtures form colloidal systems in which both the dispersed and continuous phases are liquid. For the emulsion to be formed, rigorous shaking of the mixture is necessary (Figure 1.9b). Due to high interfacial tension, the colloidal phase is unstable, and, over time, phase separation occurs, as depicted in Figure 1.9c. If surfactants are added to the mixture, the surfactant molecules self-assemble at the interface between the two immiscible phases, where they introduce a degree of continuity, reducing the interfacial tension and, thus, stabilizing the colloid (Figure 1.9d).

Microemulsions are clear, stable, isotropic liquid mixtures of oil, water, and surfactant. In contrast to ordinary emulsions, due to the presence of surfactants, microemulsions form upon simple mixing of the components and do not require the high shear conditions generally used in the formation of ordinary emulsions. The two basic types of microemulsions are (1) direct, oil dispersed in water (o/w), and (2) reversed, water dispersed in oil (w/o), determined by the relative amounts of the two phases present in the mixture. Figure 1.10 depicts the interface structure in

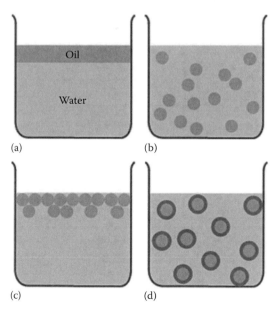

(a)   (b)

(c)   (d)

FIGURE 1.9   (a) Mixture of two immiscible liquids, (b) formation of emulsion through rigorous shaking, (c) subsequent phase separation after cessation of shaking, and (d) stable microemulsion in the presence of surfactants indicated by the solid circle drawn at the interface of the two phases.

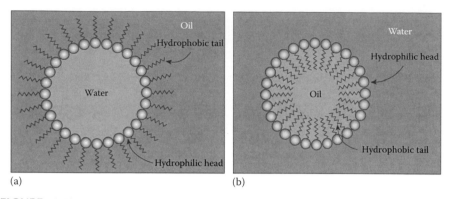

FIGURE 1.10 Depiction of interface characteristics in (a) reversed and (b) direct microemulsions.

a water–oil–surfactant mixture in a microemulsion. It is oil in water or water in oil droplets stabilized by just a monolayer of surfactant. Thus, even in small quantities, surfactants markedly affect the surface characteristics of the dispersed phase.

Relative to bulk solutions, microemulsions can be used to add extra control over chemical reactions. Chemical reactions to produce magnetic nanoparticles can be carried out within the microscopic pools of water confined in reversed microemulsions. Both metallic and metal oxide nanoparticles have been prepared through this method. The uniform nanoreactors impose kinetic and hydrodynamic constraints on particle formation, limit particle size, and lead to the production of monodispersed nanoparticles, in ways that mimic the protein cage of ferritin. Due to Brownian motion the droplets undergo frequent collisions, during which they have the ability to exchange the content of their water pools. Afterward, the droplets separate back into independent droplets of the same size. This makes it possible for chemical reactions to take place between the compounds solubilized in the different droplets. In addition, chemical reactants may be exchanged between the exterior and interior of the droplets, similarly to ferritin and lipid bilayer function in biological cells. Metal magnetic nanoparticles can be formed by mixing two reversed microemulsions with the same water content, one containing the metal salt to be reduced and the other the reducing agent, such that the reduction reaction takes place exclusively within the droplets as they exchange solute molecules.

As an example, we mention the synthesis of cobalt magnetic nanoparticles in reversed microemulsions done by Pileni and coworkers [33]. They mixed two Na(AOT) [sodium bis(2-ethylhexyl) sulfosuccinate] microemulsion solutions of similar water content. The first contained $Co(AOT)_2$ (derived from $CoCl_2$) within its water pool, while the second contained the reducing agent $NaBH_4$ (sodium borohydride) within its water pool. The mixing resulted in the formation of colloidal particles of metallic cobalt. Figure 1.11 shows the TEM patterns obtained and the histogram of the diameter size distribution. Spherical nanoparticles, well separated from each other by the enclosed surfactant layer, are seen. The particles spontaneously form hexagonally packed 2D networks, or superlattices, due to their narrow size distribution. The surfactant coating mimics the protein shell of ferritin in constraining the particles to

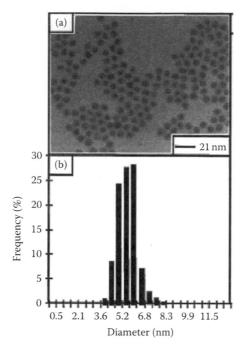

FIGURE 1.11 Monodispersed Co nanoparticles produced in a reversed microemulsion solution: (a) TEM micrograph and (b) particle size distribution, $d = (5.8 \pm 0.5)$ nm. (Reprinted with permission from Petit, C., et al., Cobalt nanosized particles organized in a 2D superlattice: Synthesis, characterization, and magnetic properties, *J. Phys. Chem. B*, 1999, 103: pp. 1805–1810. Copyright 1999 American Chemical Society.)

a well-defined size and providing terminal ligation to passivate the surface. Assuming a log-normal distribution, analysis of the histogram in Figure 1.11b indicates particles of mean diameter $d = (5.8 \pm 0.5)$ nm.

While microemulsions are obtained from three-component mixtures of water, organic solvents, and surfactants, two-component mixtures of just water and surfactants result in the formation of surfactant aggregates, or micelles, with the polar heads pointing outward toward the water and the hydrophobic tails inward. Mixtures of organic solvents and surfactants also produce surfactant aggregates or inverse micelles. In many synthetic processes involving magnetic nanoparticles, surfactants are simply added to the reaction mixture in order to provide surface passivation, biocompatibility, and steric separation of the encapsulated nanoparticles. The resulting core/shell structures replicate those of ferritin, in the sense that an inorganic solid particle is encapsulated within an organic coat. Thus, such structures are generally considered to be biomimetic.

1.3.3 Magnetic Nanoparticles Grown within Protein Cages

Under reducing conditions and in the presence of iron chelators, ferritin can be depleted of its ferrihydrite biomineral core and reconstituted under conditions favoring the synthesis of magnetic iron oxide phases, magnetite or maghemite. In 1992,

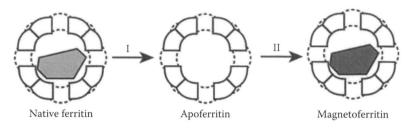

Native ferritin   Apoferritin   Magnetoferritin

FIGURE 1.12 Schematic depicting the synthesis route for the formation of magnetoferritin. (See text.) (From Meldrum, F. C., et al., Magnetoferritin: In vitro synthesis of a novel magnetic protein, *Science*, 1992. 257: pp. 522–523. Reprinted with permission of AAAS.)

Stephen Mann and coworkers [34] demonstrated for the first time the synthesis of such ferrimagnetic phases within ferritin via this process, schematically depicted in Figure 1.12.

In their experiment, the iron was removed from native HoSF by dialysis, under a nitrogen atmosphere, against thioglycolic acid ($HSCH_2COOH$) in sodium acetate (CH_3COONa) buffer at pH 4.5 (step I in Figure 1.12). The resulting apoferritin solution was buffered at pH 8.5 and maintained at a temperature of 55–60°C under argon in a water bath. Fe^{2+} solution, prepared by the dissolution of ferrous ammonium sulfate, $(NH_4)_2Fe(SO_4)_2 \bullet 6H_2O$ in deaerated water, was added slowly in small increments along with small amounts of air to produce slow oxidation (step II in Figure 1.12). The data confirmed that the protein cage remained intact and that the MPs were formed within the protein shell [34].

This seminal experiment established the use of apoferritin as a confined reaction vesicle, or nanoreactor, for the production of iron oxide nanoparticles. The process takes advantage of the unusual stability of the apoferritin shell at elevated temperatures (60°C) and pH (8.5) needed for the synthesis of magnetite, as low-temperature methods failed to produce magnetite in the presence of the protein shell. It is believed that magnetite production within the ferritin cage proceeds in an analogous way to that of ferrihydrite, that is, through the controlled oxidation of Fe^{2+} ions at the ferroxidase center and subsequent migration and nucleation at the COO^--lined interior surface of the protein cage. Just as in the case of ferritin biomineralization *in vivo*, this process is presumably favored over the competing reaction in bulk solution because of the catalytic oxidation of Fe^{2+} by ferritin and the increased iron-ion concentration within the protein interior cavity. This differentiation between "inside" and "outside" is essential to the effective *in vivo* functioning of the protein and is also central to the ferritin nanotemplating approach for the synthesis of nanophase materials within the apoferritin shell.

The synthesis of magnetoferritin is now well established, having been reproduced by other investigators at various degrees of iron loading, and its magnetic properties have been widely studied [35]. Fitting of superparamagnetic data for ferritin and magnetoferritin to the Langevin function indicates roughly a core with a magnetic moment of $\mu_c \sim 300\ \mu_B$ for ferritin [36], as opposed to $\mu_c \sim 13{,}100\ \mu_B$ for magnetoferritin, corresponding to a magnetoferritin particle core containing of the order of 12,000 Fe atoms [35]. The large difference in magnetic moment is due primarily to the fact that the ferrihydrite core is antiferromagnetic, with the particle moment arising only from noncompensated spins at its surface. In contrast, the core of magnetoferritin comprises magnetite and/or maghemite, both structures being ferrimagnetic with noncompensated spin sublattices throughout the particle volume.

To date, many other magnetic phases have been synthesized within apoferritin, further supporting the notion that the reactions are not specific to iron and that the electrostatic properties of the protein play a significant role in the process of mineralization. In addition to metal oxide and hydroxide phases [35], metallic magnetic nanoparticles of Ni and Co have been produced within horse spleen apoferritin [37], as indicated schematically in Figure 1.13. Once the Ni^{2+} and Co^{2+} ions have entered the protein cavity, they can react with $NaBH_4$, which is small enough to pass through the threefold channels and enter the apoferritin interior. Thus, the divalent metal ions, attached to the interior wall of the apoferritin cage, undergo reduction to zero valence to produce metallic magnetic nanoparticles. Metal–alloy nanoparticles have also been produced within apoferritin, such as FePt or CoPt [38] as well as binary phase Fe/Co oxides [39].

Mammalian ferritin belongs to a "ferritin superfamily" of similar but distinct protein cages occurring in bacterial life forms that are capable of sequestering iron. These afford additional supramolecular templates for bio-inspired materials synthesis. Among these, Dps [deoxyribonucleic acid (DNA)-binding proteins from starved cells] proteins have been extensively investigated and used in the biomimetic synthesis of magnetic nanoparticles. Dps proteins possess a shell structure of 12 identical amino acid subunits, as opposed to the 24 heteropolymer subunits of the canonical ferritins. They are smaller than mammalian ferritins possessing an

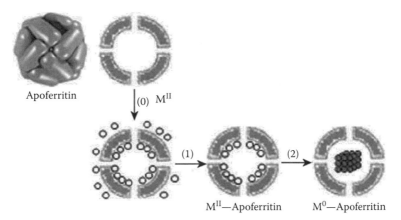

Apoferritin

(0) M^{II}

(1)

(2)

M^{II}—Apoferritin M^0—Apoferritin

FIGURE 1.13 Schematic representation of apoferritin-encapsulated Ni and Co metal nanoparticles: M^{II} = Ni^{2+} or Co^{2+}, M^0 = Co or Ni. (0) Addition of M^{II}, (1) Dialysis and chromatography. (2) Addition of $NaBH_4$. (From Galvez, N., et al., Apoferritin-encapsulated Ni and Co superparamagnetic nanoparticles, *J. Mat. Chem.*, 2006, 16: pp. 2757–2761. Copyright 2006 The Royal Society of Chemistry, reproduced with permission.)

Exterior surface   Interior cavity

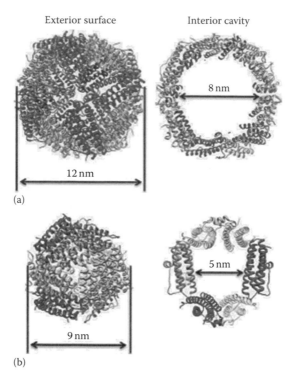

(a)

(b)

FIGURE 1.14 Ribbon representation of the exterior surface and the interior cavity of HuHF (a) and Dps protein from *Listeria innocua* (b). (Reprinted from *Biochim. Biophys. Acta*, 1800, Uchida, M., et al., The ferritin superfamily: Supramolecular templates for materials synthesis, 834–845, Copyright 2010, with permission from Elsevier.)

exterior diameter of ~9 nm and a central cavity with diameter of ~5 nm. Figure 1.14 gives a ribbon representation of *in vitro* produced homopolymer, recombinant human apoferritin consisting of 24 H-chains (HuHF) and that of Dps protein [40]. Dps proteins were first identified in the bacterium *Escherichia coli* in 1992, and since their discovery homologous structures have been found in other bacteria and archaea.

The 3D crystal structure of Dps proteins exhibits two types of threefold symmetry channels, one of which is lined with hydrophilic amino acids that can facilitate the entrance of cations to the interior cavity of the protein. As in the case of mammalian ferritin, once the iron ions are inside the cavity, they are electrostatically attracted to the negatively charged surface of the interior wall where the mineralization reactions can be initiated. The electrostatic surface of *Listeria innocua* Dps is similar to that of canonical ferritins, with clusters of glutamic acid residues lining the surface with negatively charged COO^- ions that facilitate iron cluster nucleation. The oxyhydroxide mineral core formed within the Dps cavity can accommodate up to 500 Fe atoms, as opposed to 4500 Fe atoms in mammalian ferritin. Investigators have used the Dps cage to form mineralized γ-Fe_2O_3 nanoparticles. Treatment of the protein at pH 8.5 and 65°C with 400 Fe^{2+}

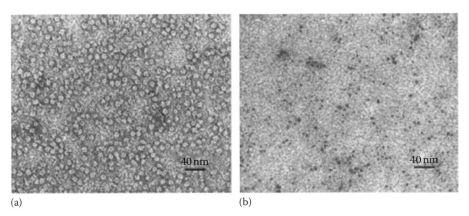

(a)   (b)

FIGURE 1.15 TEM micrograph of the *Listeria innocua* Dps cage mineralized with γ-Fe_2O_3 stained with uranyl acetate (a) and unstained (b). (From Allen, M., et al. Protein cage constrained synthesis of ferrimagnetic iron oxide nanoparticles. *Adv. Mater.*, 2002, 14, 1562–1565. Copyright Wiley-VCH Verlag GmbH & Co. KGaA. Reproduced with permission.)

per protein and stoichiometric amounts of H_2O_2 resulted in the formation of a homogeneous solution with deep brown coloration. TEM micrographs of negatively stained proteins with uranyl acetate, shown in Figure 1.15a, indicate that the mineralized iron oxide phase is contained within the *L. innocua* Dps cage. The iron oxide mineral particle diameter of 4.1 ± 1.1 nm for the unstained proteins, shown in Figure 1.15b, correlates well with the inner diameter of the Dps protein cage [41].

Furthermore, the reaction of Co^{2+}, instead of Fe^{2+}, with H_2O_2 at pH 8.5 at an elevated temperature of 65°C results in the formation of Co_3O_4 within the Dps protein cage, while the same reaction carried out at 23°C forms Co(O)OH within the cage, indicating that the temperature at which the reaction is performed can influence the nature of the mineralized phase within the protein [41]. As the formation of many inorganic phases requires reactions that take place at elevated temperatures, often higher than most proteins can tolerate, investigators have sought to isolate protein templates from thermophilic (heat-loving) and hyperthermophilic bacterial and archaeal organisms found in hot springs, in acidic soils, and near volcano vents. Such organisms were first discovered in the 1960s by Thomas Brock and have successfully expanded the temperature range of biomimetic magnetic nanoparticle synthesis. For example, a ferritin-like protein has been isolated from the anaerobic marine bacterium *Pyrococcus furiosus* [42], which lives in thermal springs where temperatures can reach 120°C. The structure of this protein is homologous to other ferritins and the synthesis of maghemite within this ferritin cage has been demonstrated [42]. Its wide temperature stability opens up the possibility of biomimetic synthesis at temperatures unattainable with other biomolecular templates. As the number of protein cages isolated from hyperthermophilic organisms increases, so too will the variety and size of magnetic nanoparticles that can be synthesized using biomimetic approaches.

1.3.4 MAGNETIC NANOPARTICLES GROWN WITHIN VIRAL CAPSIDS

In addition to the ferritins, nature provides us with a large selection of protein cages in the form of viral capsids, which can also function as nanoreactors for the biomimetic self-assembly of nanomaterials. Increasingly, genetic engineering techniques are being applied to the design of mutant protein cages, with electrostatic properties conducive to the self-assembly of magnetic nanomaterials. Figure 1.16 gives examples of space-filling images of viral capsids and protein and enzyme cages [43]. These include capsids of both plant and bacterial viruses. Non-viral protein cages include the canonical ferritins, Dps proteins, heat shock proteins (Hsps), and the enzyme lumazine synthase. In their biological functions, these architectures serve diverse roles from nucleic acid storage and transport in viruses, chaperon function to prevent protein misfolding and denaturation in Hsps, iron sequestration in the ferritins, and enzymatic action in lumazine synthase. However, they all share the same architectural principle in being assembled from a limited number of polypeptide subunits to form robust nanocages; they also share the ability to have their functionality altered through both chemical and genetic means.

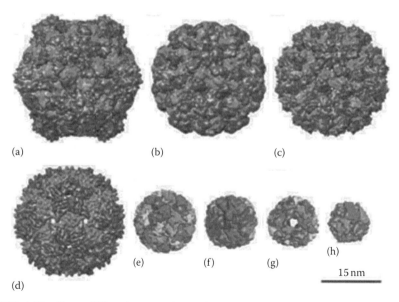

(a) (b) (c) (d) (e) (f) (g) (h)

15 nm

FIGURE 1.16 Space-filling images of protein cage architectures with various (exterior) diameters, d: (a) Cowpea mosaic virus ($d = 31$ nm); (b) Brome mosaic virus ($d = 28$ nm); (c) Cowpea chlorotic mottle virus ($d = 28$ nm); (d) MS2 bacteriophage ($d = 27$ nm); (e) lumazine synthase ($d = 15$ nm); (f) ferritin ($d = 12$ nm); (g) small heat shock protein ($d = 12$ nm); (h) Dps protein ($d = 9$ nm). Mosaic viruses are plant viruses that make the leaves of infected plants acquire a specked appearance, while the MS2 bacteriophage is a virus that infects the bacterium *Escherichia coli*. (From Uchida, M., et al. Biological containers: Protein cages as multifunctional platforms. *Adv. Mater.*, 2007, 19, 1025–1042. Copyright Wiley-VCH Verlag GmbH & Co. KGaA. Reproduced with permission.)

The discovery of viruses dates back to 1892, with Dmitri Ivanovsky's description of a nonbacterial pathogen infecting tobacco plants, leading to the discovery of the tobacco mosaic virus in 1898 by Martinus Beijerinck. Since then, over 5000 viruses have been described in detail; they are the most abundant type of biological entity. The viral capsids, once depleted of their genomic content, can be engineered to possess negatively charged interior walls, and thus electrostatically attract Fe^{2+} ions and induce the hydrolytic polymerization of iron within their interior cavities in a way analogous to that of the ferritin protein cage.

Viral capsids are presently among the most extensively studied biological templates in the biomimetic synthesis of inorganic nanoparticles. Due to their well-defined architectures and readily accessible genetic information, they afford unlimited possibilities for structural modification via genetic engineering. Their interior space is normally reserved for their genome, where in their native state the viral capsids act as host containers for nucleic acid storage and transport. However, purified viral coat protein subunits can be easily assembled *in vitro* into empty virions even in the absence of RNA or DNA, and can therefore be utilized as constrained reaction vesicles. In 1998, investigators Douglas and Young [44] pioneered the approach of using viral capsids for the synthesis of size-constrained inorganic and organic polymer species. In their experiments, they used Cowpea chlorotic mottle virus (CCMV) as a model system for reversibly gated entrapment of inorganic minerals. CCMV is an icosahedral virus composed of 180 identical subunits forming a protein cage with an inner diameter of 18 nm and an outer diameter of 28 nm (Figure 1.16a). This affords a cavity diameter approximately twice as large as that of ferritin, defining a new upper limit for the crystal size of entrapped minerals. The exact size of the capsid depends on the pH of the medium, as it undergoes a pH-dependent reversible swelling behavior. The capsid increases its dimensions by about 10% compared to the non-swollen form when the pH of the medium is raised to ≥ 6.5. In its swollen (open) state, the CCMV capsid provides 60 open pores of about 2-nm diameter each that allow small external guest molecules to diffuse into the internal space [44]. Such dynamic structural transitions induced by chemical switches are common in many virions providing unique molecular gating mechanisms to control the containment and release of entrapped materials—a property important in the design of targeted drug delivery agents in bionanotechnology.

X-ray structural analysis indicates that the basic arginine and lysine amino acids line the interior wall of the CCMV capsid, providing a large positive charge. The positive charge is necessary for the native virus to package and condense the anionic viral genome. This is opposite to the case of ferritin where the interior wall is lined with acidic glutamic acid, which provides a negative charge to the interior protein cage wall. Thus, the native capsid exhibits an electrostatic attraction for negatively charged species in the bulk solution, unlike ferritin. Indeed, the first material crystallized within the viral capsid was accomplished by the electrostatic attraction and subsequent oligomerization of aqueous molecular tungstate (WO_4^{2-}) ions to form macromolecular complexes of paratungstate ($H_2W_{12}O_{42}^{10-}$). Young and Douglas demonstrated, however, that it was possible to alter the chemical properties of the protein cage through rational design without disturbing the overall architecture of the capsid [45]. They accomplished this by genetically engineering the protein to replace the basic residues of the native capsid with glutamic acid, forming a mutant capsid, with the electrostatic characteristics of the interior wall changed from cationic to anionic. The altered electrostatic character of the interior of the protein favors strong interaction with ferrous ions, which promotes oxidative hydrolysis and formation of size-constrained iron oxide particles within the viral capsid in a fashion similar to that of apoferritin.

The electrostatically altered viral protein cage catalyzed the rapid oxidation of Fe^{2+}, leading to the formation of iron oxide magnetic nanoparticles. Specifically, the purified mutant proteins were treated with aliquots of Fe^{2+} at pH 6.5 and allowed to oxidize in air. Single and double mineralization processes, with loading factors of 2000 and 6000 Fe atoms per protein cage, were carried out, resulting in the formation of spherical particles with core diameters of (8.2 ± 1.6) nm and (24 ± 3.5) nm [45]. High-resolution TEM images indicated that the resulting nanoparticles were single-crystalline lepidocrocite.

Biotechnological processes borrowed from protein engineering techniques, such as screening combinatorial peptide libraries using phage display, are currently being explored for the identification of peptide sequences with high specificity toward particular inorganic materials and in some cases with high specificity toward unique crystal faces. Phage display, first described by George P. Smith in 1985, is a laboratory technique for the study of protein–protein, protein–peptide, and protein–DNA interactions that use bacteriophage (viruses that infect bacteria) to connect proteins with the genetic information that encodes them. One of the most common bacteriophage used in phage display is the filamentous M13 bacteriophage. Identification of peptide sequences that promote the nucleation of specific crystallographic phases is extremely useful in the direct synthesis of magnetic nanoparticles with desired properties and crystal structure, e.g., the hard magnetic FePt and CoPt nanoparticles in their high anisotropy face-centered tetragonal (fct) phase, also known as the $L1_0$ phase, without the need for postsynthesis high-temperature annealing. Unlike previous examples, in this approach, biological interactions control the nucleation of nanoparticles with no isomorphous complement in nature. For example, the identification of a specific peptide sequence from screening the M13 bacteriophage engineered into the protein cage of MjHsp from the thermophilic archaeon *Methanococcus jannaschii* directs the peptide-specific recognition synthesis of $L1_0$ CoPt nanoparticles, which exhibit room-temperature ferromagnetism [46]. Eliminating the high-temperature annealing step would greatly simplify the production of hard magnetic nanoparticles suitable for device applications.

1.3.5 Maghemite Core/Silica Shell Nanoarchitectures

Surfactant and protein coats render magnetic nanoparticles biocompatible. There are also biocompatible inorganic materials, further extending the scope and range of bio-inspired magnetic nanoparticle synthesis. Silica is just such a material, being nontoxic and water soluble. Yi et al. [47] produced γ-Fe_2O_3 magnetic nanoparticles encapsulated within silica shells of finely tuned thicknesses. Thermal decomposition

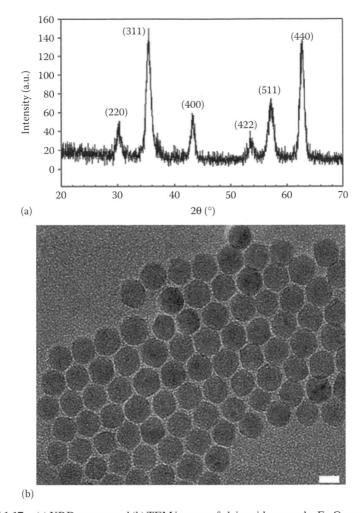

(a)

(b)

FIGURE 1.17 (a) XRD pattern and (b) TEM images of oleic acid-covered γ-Fe$_2$O$_3$ nanocrystals. Scale bar: 10 nm. (Reprinted with permission from Yi, D. K., et al., Nanoparticle architectures templated by SiO$_2$/Fe$_2$O$_3$ nanocomposites, *Chem. Mater.*, 2006, 18: pp. 614–619. Copyright 2006 American Chemical Society.)

of iron pentacarbonyl [Fe(CO)$_5$] in the presence of oleic acid produced monodispersed metal iron particles. Controlled oxidation using trimethylamine oxide [(CH$_3$)$_3$NO] as a mild oxidant produced highly crystalline γ-Fe$_2$O$_3$ particles. Figure 1.17 gives XRD and TEM characterization of the resulting highly uniform, oleic acid-covered, γ-Fe$_2$O$_3$ magnetic nanoparticles. XRD patterns confirm the presence of Fe$_2$O$_3$. The TEM characterization indicated monodispersed nanoparticles of average diameter d of (12.5 $\pm$ 0.2) nm, forming highly ordered 2D superlattices on the TEM grid, as seen in Figure 1.17b.

Uniform, silica-coated maghemite (Fe$_2$O$_3$/SiO$_2$) nanoparticles were then prepared using the oleic acid-covered monodispersed γ-Fe$_2$O$_3$ nanocrystals. Silica coating on the γ-Fe$_2$O$_3$ nanoparticles was performed through the formation of water-in-cyclohexane

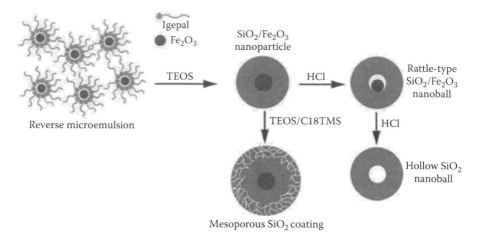

FIGURE 1.18 Schematic of the synthesis of MP/SiO₂/MS nanoarchitectures. C18TMS, octadecyltrimethoxysilane; MP, magnetic particle; MS, mesoporous silica; SiO₂, solid silica; TEOS, tetraethyl orthosilicate. (Reprinted with permission from Yi, D. K., et al., Nanoparticle architectures templated by SiO₂/Fe₂O₃ nanocomposites, *Chem. Mater.*, 2006, 18: pp. 614–619. Copyright 2006 American Chemical Society.)

reverse microemulsion, as schematically depicted in Figure 1.18. The Fe_2O_3/SiO_2 core–shell nanoparticles were then used as a platform for deriving higher nanoparticle architectures.

The silica coating was tunable between ~1.8 and ~30 nm, as shown in Figure 1.19a–d. Subsequently, a second layer of mesoporous silica (MS) of 10 and 21 nm thickness was applied to the 25-nm silica-coated nanoparticles to form MP/SiO₂/MS nanoarchitectures (Figure 1.20a and b).

Well-controlled particle size and morphology are important for the application of SiO_2-coated magnetic nanoparticles in biomedical applications, such as magnetic resonance imaging, magnetic relaxometry, magnetic cell separation, and drug delivery [47]. By introducing an MS coating and by creating rattle-type silica balls with magnetic nanoparticles, applications in catalysis and chemical sensing and separations may be explored [47]. For biomedical applications, we note that the MS coating could be loaded with pharmaceuticals or DNA for targeted drug delivery or gene transfection therapies, respectively.

1.4 MAGNETIC CHARACTERIZATION OF IRON-BASED MAGNETIC NANOPARTICLES

Detailed magnetic characterization of bio-inspired magnetic nanoparticles is of utmost importance in the development of biocompatible magnetic agents for various applications in biomedicine and biotechnology. The magnetic properties of nanometer-sized particles and their assemblies are dominated by finite-size effects [48] and superparamagnetism and interparticle interactions [49] that can affect their quality and suitability for various applications. Thus, in-depth magnetic characterization of prepared nanostructures and their assemblies is an essential component to their development.

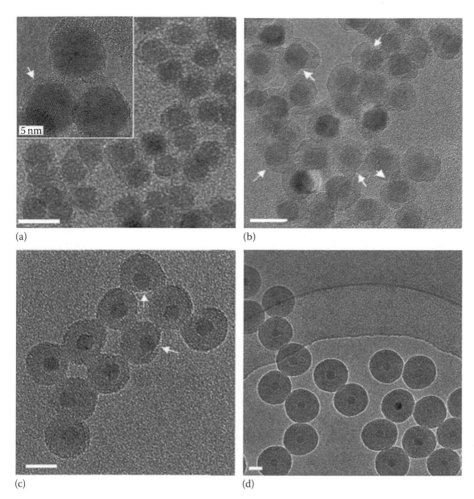

(a) (b)

(c) (d)

FIGURE 1.19 TEM micrographs of ~12.5 nm γ-Fe_2O_3 oleic acid-encapsulated particles covered with solid silica shell. Shell thicknesses from 1.8 to 30 nm were achieved: (a) ~1.8 nm, (b) ~4 nm, (c) ~9 nm, and (d) ~25 nm. Arrows indicate asymmetric silica coating. Scale bar: 20 nm. (Reprinted with permission from Yi, D. K., et al., Nanoparticle architectures templated by SiO_2/Fe_2O_3 nanocomposites, *Chem. Mater.*, 2006, 18: pp. 614–619. Copyright 2006 American Chemical Society.)

For iron-based superparamagnetic particles, the combination of two techniques, [57]Fe Mössbauer spectroscopy and superconducting quantum interference device (SQUID) magnetometry, has been proven especially powerful [50].

[57]Fe Mössbauer spectroscopy [51–53] probes specific atomic sites within the nanocrystalline lattice of the particles through the hyperfine interactions of the [57]Fe nucleus with its electronic surroundings and yields atomic detail on the particles' magnetic and electronic properties. SQUID magnetometry probes the total magnetic moment, or superspin, of the nanoparticle via its interaction with an applied magnetic field. Furthermore, for investigations of dynamic nanomagnetism, the

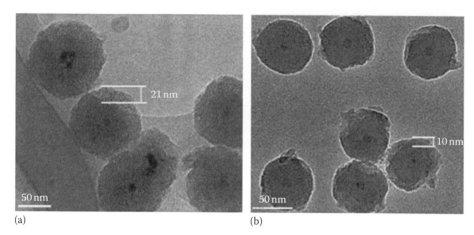

FIGURE 1.20 TEM micrographs of γ-Fe$_2$O$_3$ core (MP), solid silica shell (SiO$_2$), and mesoporous silica (MS) shell nanocomposites (MP/SiO$_2$/MS). The MS shell thicknesses of 21 nm (a) and 10 nm (b) are shown. (Reprinted with permission from Yi, D. K., et al., Nanoparticle architectures templated by SiO$_2$/Fe$_2$O$_3$ nanocomposites, *Chem. Mater.*, 2006, 18: pp. 614–619. Copyright 2006 American Chemical Society.)

complementarities of SQUID magnetization and Mössbauer measurements make their combination very desirable. Magnetization measurements give the *macro*scopic or bulk magnetism of the sample in the presence of an externally applied magnetic field, averaged over an experimental measurement time window of the order of 10 s. Mössbauer γ-ray resonance spectroscopy, on the other hand, provides *micro*magnetic characterization of the nanomaterial, that is, measures internal hyperfine magnetic fields (or local magnetic moments) within 10^{-8} s, and affords zero-applied field magnetic studies. A consequence of the relatively short Mössbauer spectroscopy measurement time are higher blocking temperatures, below which spin reversals are blocked, compared to magnetization measurements. This enables examination of the spin fluctuation dynamics over a convenient experimental temperature range.

We demonstrate the applicability of this approach in two separate cases: (1) assemblies of noninteracting, or magnetically isolated, magnetic nanoparticles and (2) nanoparticle assembly with various strengths of magnetostatic interparticle interactions. The specific systems we chose are (1) *in vitro* reconstituted HoSF and (2) maghemite/silica/MS nanoarchitectures with various silica coating thicknesses.

1.4.1 Isolated Magnetic Nanoparticles

The magnetic properties of isolated magnetic nanoparticles [54] are of interest in a broad spectrum of biomedical applications [55]. Superparamagnetism, characteristic of isolated small magnetically ordered structures, is due to thermally driven spin reversals over the anisotropy energy barrier $E_a = K_u V$, where V is the volume of the particle and K_u is its effective, uniaxial magnetic anisotropy density [56–60], schematically depicted in Figure 1.21. For isolated particles, the spin relaxation time, τ_s, for reversals along opposite directions of the anisotropy axis, or easy axis

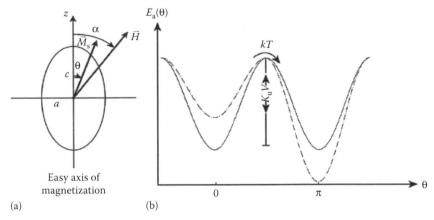

(a) (b)

FIGURE 1.21 (a) Representation of a uniaxial magnetic nanoparticle of total magnetic moment vector, $\vec{M}_s$, in an applied field, $\vec{H}$; the easy axis of magnetization is along the c-axis. (b) Magnetic, orientational potential energy as a function of the angle θ between the magnetic moment vector of the particle and its easy axis of magnetization, in the absence of a magnetic field (solid curve) and in the presence of a magnetic field (broken line) applied along the easy axis of magnetization.

of magnetization, follows the Arrhenius equation (Equation 1.6), first proposed by Néel [56], where τ_0 is a material constant, k is Boltzmann's constant, and T is the temperature [57–60].

In magnetization studies, the presence of the anisotropy barrier, E_a, produces a characteristic peak in the magnetization curve of zero-field-cooled (ZFC) samples, which determines the blocking temperature, T_B, in Equation 1.7, where $\tau_m \sim 10$ s is the characteristic measuring time:

$$\tau_s = \tau_0 \exp\left(\frac{K_u V}{kT}\right), \tag{1.6}$$

$$T_B = \frac{K_u V/k}{\ln\left(\tau_m/\tau_0\right)}. \tag{1.7}$$

In Mössbauer studies, the ^{57}Fe nuclear Zeeman splitting in the internal magnetic field, H_{hf}, is observed if τ_s is longer than $\tau_L \sim 10^{-8}$ s, the Larmor precession time of the ^{57}Fe excited state nuclear spin about H_{hf}. Thus, τ_L determines τ_m for Mössbauer [50]. Above and below T_B, collapsed quadrupolar spectra and six-line magnetic spectra are seen, respectively. For a distribution of particle volumes, a distribution in T_B is obtained. The temperature at which the quadrupolar and magnetic subspectra contribute equally to the overall absorption area of the spectrum defines T_B experimentally. T_B is not an intrinsic physical quantity of the nanoparticle, since it is technique dependent; K_u, though, is. Solving Equation 1.7 for K_u, we obtain

$$K_u = \left[\ln\left(\frac{\tau_L}{\tau_0}\right)\right]\left(\frac{k}{V}\right)T_B. \tag{1.8}$$

Equation 1.6 contains three unknowns: K_u, τ_0, and V. Measuring T_B with two techniques of widely different τ_m, combined with TEM measurements of V, can allow the determination of all three parameters. When thermal energies are not sufficient to induce spin reversals, a diminished hyperfine magnetic field may be observed in Mössbauer spectroscopy according to the collective magnetic excitations (CME) model of Mørup and Topsøe [61] given in Equation 1.9, where H_{hf}^0 is the saturation magnetic hyperfine field for $T \to 0$. Measurement of H_{hf} at two different temperatures can determine H_{hf}^0 and K_u independently of τ_0.

$$H_{hf}(T) = H_{hf}^0 \left(1 - \frac{kT}{2K_u V} \right). \tag{1.9}$$

Below T_B, magnetization measurements can determine the particle's coercivity, H_c; saturation magnetization, M_s; and remnant magnetization, M_r [62]. The temperature dependence of the coercivity is given to a first approximation by Equation 1.10 [63], where H_c^0 is the saturation coercive field as $T \to 0$:

$$H_c(T) = H_c^0 \left[1 - \left(\frac{T}{T_B} \right)^{1/2} \right]. \tag{1.10}$$

All the micromagnetic parameters introduced above (K_u, H_{hf}^0, H_c^0, M_s, M_r)—together with the electronic Mössbauer parameters of isomer shift, δ; quadrupole splitting, ΔE_Q; and internal hyperfine field, H_{hf}—uniquely characterize the micromagnetic structure of isolated MPs.

We illustrate the above theoretical framework with studies on *in vitro* reconstituted HoSF carried out by the authors [64]. The sample was prepared by reacting horse spleen apoferritin with Fe(II) and using O_2 as the oxidant. Specifically, the protein was diluted to 2 μM concentration at a pH = 7.5 buffer to give a volume of 6 mL. To this solution was added 15 increments of 24 μL 0.049 M ^{57}FeSO$_4$ at pH = 2 at intervals of at least 1.5 h over a period of 2 days, to a total iron loading of 1500 ^{57}Fe atoms per protein. The protein was subsequently freeze dried. Figure 1.22 gives the Mössbauer spectra obtained over a wide temperature range. We note the gradual transition of the Mössbauer spectral signature from fast relaxation ($\tau_s < \tau_L$), quadrupolar doublets, to slow relaxation ($\tau_s > \tau_L$), magnetic sextets, with decreasing T, determining T_B (Mössbauer) ~37 K for this sample. The energy difference between the two absorption peaks observed at high temperatures defines the quadrupole splitting, ΔE_Q, while the difference between the outer absorption peaks of the low-temperature spectrum gives a measure of the hyperfine magnetic field, H_{hf}, experienced by the ^{57}Fe nucleus.

The spectra have been fit to the superposition of two poorly resolved subsites (Table 1.1), which we associate with core, interior (smaller ΔE_Q, larger H_{hf}), and surface (larger ΔE_Q, smaller H_{hf}) iron sites, usually referred to as the core/shell model of ferritin, depicted in Figure 1.23 [65]. A crystalline, collinearly spin-ordered ferrihydrite core is envisioned surrounded by an amorphous, spin-disordered surface layer with distorted, low-iron coordination symmetry, all encapsulated within a protein shell. Figure 1.24 plots the reduced hyperfine fields $H_{hf}(T)/H_{hf}^0$ versus T for core and surface sites.

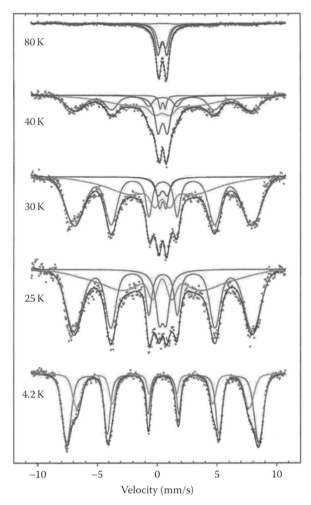

80 K

40 K

30 K

25 K

4.2 K

−10   −5   0   5   10
Velocity (mm/s)

FIGURE 1.22   (See color insert.) Mössbauer spectra of lyophilized *in vitro* reconstituted HoSF to 1500 [57]Fe atoms per protein. Solid lines through the experimental points are least square fits to a superposition of two types of iron subsites, including hyperfine field distributions. Subspectra are shown above the experimental data (see text and Table 1.1). (From Papaefthymiou, G. C., et al. Electronic and magnetic characterization of in vivo produced vs. in vitro reconstituted horse spleen ferritin. *Nanophase and Nanocomposite Materials V*, S. Komarneni, K. Kaneko, J. C. Parker, and P. O'Brien, eds., HH03-27, 2007. Copyright Materials Research Society. Reproduced with permission.)

The temperature dependence of the hyperfine magnetic field recorded at interior iron sites is consistent with the CME model [61] where no more than a 15% reduction of H_{hf} is observed before the spectrum collapses to a quadrupole doublet, corresponding to an antiferromagnetic core undergoing CME. However, the precipitous reduction of the hyperfine field at surface sites is inconsistent with superparamagnetism. It is rather indicative of a more complex energy landscape than

TABLE 1.1

Mössbauer Hyperfine Parameters for Lyophilized *In Vitro* Reconstituted HoSF to 1500 ^{57}Fe Atoms per Protein at Various Temperatures

T (K)	δ (mm/s)	ΔE_Q or ε (mm/s)	H_{hf} (kOe)	Fractional Area
80	0.48	0.56	0.0	0.40
	0.46	0.75	0.0	0.51
	0.47	0.0	456	0.09
40	0.48	0.42	0.0	0.03
	0.47	0.77	0.0	0.19
	0.47	0.0	456	0.38
	0.43	0.0	226	0.40
30	0.48	0.54	0.0	0.06
	0.46	0.78	0.0	0.05
	0.49	0.0	459	0.59
	0.43	0.0	231	0.30
25	0.47	0.57	0.0	0.12
	0.49	0.0	461	0.56
	0.43	0.0	304	0.32
4.2	0.48	−0.07	497	0.66
	0.48	0.02	444	0.34

Isomer shifts, δ, are referenced to metallic iron at room temperature.

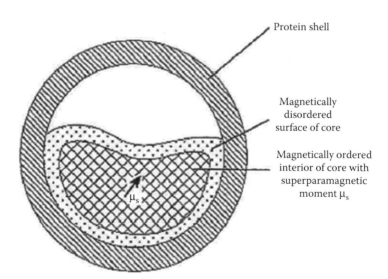

FIGURE 1.23 Core/shell model of ferritin. A highly crystalline core surrounded by an amorphous surface, all encapsulated within the protein coat. (From Brooks, R. A., et al. Relaxometry and magnetometry of ferritin. *Mag. Res. Med.*, 1998, 40, 227–235. Copyright Wiley-VCH Verlag GmbH & Co. KGaA. Reproduced with permission.)

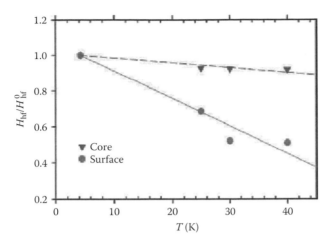

FIGURE 1.24 Temperature dependence of the reduced hyperfine fields at core (interior) and surface iron sites. The steeper slope of surface fields is indicative of a more complex energy landscape at the surface that supports spin wave excitations (see text). (From Papaefthymiou, G. C., et al. Electronic and magnetic characterization of in vivo produced vs. in vitro reconstituted horse spleen ferritin. *Nanophase and Nanocomposite Materials V*, S. Komarneni, K. Kaneko, J. C. Parker, and P. O'Brien, eds., HH03-27, 2007. Copyright Materials Research Society. Reproduced with permission.)

the double potential energy well of Figure 1.21 and points to the presence of spin canting, surface anisotropy, and spin wave excitation processes [66].

Figure 1.25 gives the ZFC/FC magnetization curves for a reconstituted sample of HoSF in an applied field of 500 Oe [65]. The maximum in the ZFC curve gives T_B (magnetization) = 13 K. The following features of the observed magnetization curves are hallmarks of isolated MPs: (1) the sharp peak at the maximum in the ZFC curve, (2) the T^{-1}-like dependence of the FC magnetization curve, and (3) the coincidence of the maximum in the ZFC curve, T_{max}, and the bifurcation or branching temperature, T_{br}, where the ZFC and FC curves separate. Below T_B, ferritin is hysteretic with the coercivity following Equation 1.10 [36] as seen in Figure 1.26.

The magnetic behavior of ferritin is archetypical of isolated MPs. The weak magnetic moment of the ferritin core, $\mu \sim 300 \ \mu_B$ [36], arising from uncompensated spins at defect and surface sites of an otherwise antiferromagnetic lattice, combined with the presence of the 2.5-nm protein coat, is responsible for this behavior. Thus, at a center-to-center distance of only 12 nm (ferritin core diameter = 7 nm; Figure 1.1), the ferritin cores are magnetically isolated and their relaxation properties are well represented by the above theory of isolated magnetic nanoparticles. The magnetic and Mössbauer properties of ferritin have recently been reviewed in detail [67].

1.4.2 INTERACTING MAGNETIC NANOPARTICLES

The magnetic properties of ferrimagnetic nanoparticle assemblies require determination of the intrinsic properties of the individual particles, but additionally, of the interparticle interactions as they can possess moments hundreds or thousands of

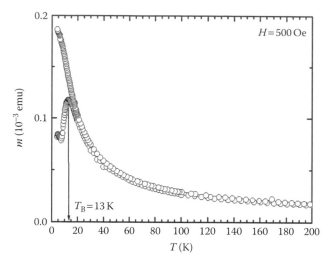

FIGURE 1.25 ZFC/FC magnetization curves for HoSF. (From Papaefthymiou, G. C., et al. Electronic and magnetic characterization of in vivo produced vs. in vitro reconstituted horse spleen ferritin. *Nanophase and Nanocomposite Materials V*, S. Komarneni, K. Kaneko, J. C. Parker, and P. O'Brien, eds., HH03-27, 2007. Copyright Materials Research Society. Reproduced with permission.)

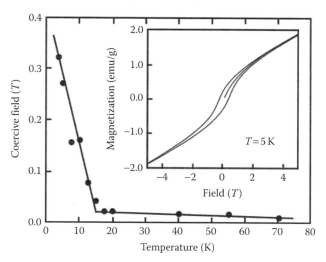

FIGURE 1.26 Temperature dependence of the coercivity, H_c, of ferritin, the inset shows the full hysteresis loop at $T = 5$ K. (Reprinted from Kilcoyne S. H. and R. Cywinski, Ferritin: A model superparamagnet, *J. Magn. Magn. Mater.*, 1995, 140: pp. 1466–1467, Copyright 1995 with permission from Elsevier.)

times stronger than those of antiferromagnetic particles. MPs in close proximity interact magnetically via two distinct mechanisms: magnetic exchange across contacting particle boundaries and magnetostatic, dipole–dipole (d–d) interactions [68–72]. The latter, being long range, are present in most ferrimagnetic particle assemblies. In assemblies of ferrimagnetic core/shell nanoparticles, such

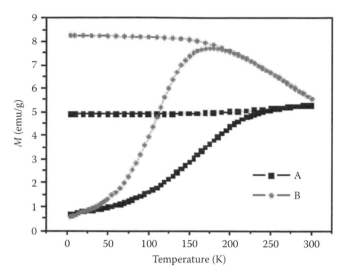

FIGURE 1.27 ZFC/FC magnetization data for 12.5-nm γ-Fe$_2$O$_3$ nanoparticles covered with a coat of 1-nm oleic acid (sample A) and 1-nm oleic acid + 4-nm silica shell (sample B). (Reprinted with permission from Papaefthymiou, G. C., et al., Interparticle interactions in magnetic core/shell nanoarchitectures, *Phys. Rev. B*, 80, 024406-1–024406-10, 2009. Copyright 2009 by the American Physical Society.)

as γ-Fe$_2$O$_3$ or Fe$_3$O$_4$, a thin nonmagnetic coat eliminates magnetic exchange across grain boundaries, but d–d interactions persist. The magnetic relaxation phenomena of the nanoparticle assembly no longer reflect the Néel-type fluctuations of individual particle moments of Equation 1.6, but rather the collective magnetic behavior of the assembly. In this case, Mössbauer and ZFC/FC magnetization measurements yield drastically different signatures than those observed in HoSF (see above). We demonstrate the difference with results on the γ-Fe$_2$O$_3$/SiO$_2$/MS nanoarchitectures described in Section 1.3.5.

Figure 1.27 shows the ZFC/FC data for the 12.5-nm oleic acid-coated maghemite particles (sample A) and the 1-nm oleic acid- and 4-nm silica-coated maghemite particles (sample B). The curve characteristics are very different from those of ferritin. The maximum in the ZFC curve is very broad, the FC M versus T curve is flat, and T_{max} does not coincide with T_{br}. This behavior is the hallmark of strongly interacting MPs.

The orientational magnetic interaction energy between the magnetic moments, $\vec{\mu}_i$ and $\vec{\mu}_j$, of two MPs within an assembly is given as follows [73]:

$$U_{ij} = \left(\frac{\mu_0}{4\pi}\right)\left[\frac{\vec{\mu}_i \cdot \vec{\mu}_j}{r_{ij}^3} - \frac{3(\vec{\mu}_i \cdot \vec{r}_{ij})(\vec{\mu}_j \cdot \vec{r}_{ij})}{r_{ij}^5}\right], \tag{1.11}$$

where $\vec{r}_{ij}$ gives the interparticle separation distance (center to center). For high magnetic dilution, the large distance separating the particles makes this interaction weak. For weakly interacting particles, the maximum in the ZFC curve would shift according to the following equation:

$$T_{max} = \frac{K_u V_m + U_{int}}{k \ln(\tau_m/\tau_0)},$$

(1.12)

where U_{int} is a measure of the average effective interparticle interaction energy within the nanoparticle assembly and V_m is the magnetic volume of the particle excluding the silica shell. For small values of the interaction energy compared to the uniaxial magnetic anisotropy energy of the particle ($U_{int} < K_u V_m$), T_{max} would fall close to the superparamagnetic blocking temperature, T_B, for the isolated MPs. However, for large particle moments and small separations between particles, U_{int} can become dominant. For randomly oriented single-domain MPs, and for $U_{int} > K_u V_m$, it can lead to collective magnetic phenomena and spin-glass-like magnetic ordering as the temperature is lowered and thermal energies become comparable to U_{int}. In such a case of strongly interacting particles, T_{max} gives a measure of the spin-glass freezing temperature of the system [70–75], $T_{max} = U_{int}/k$, rather than the superparamagnetic blocking temperature, T_B, of individual particles. This is the case for the data of samples A and B presented in Figure 1.27. With increasing silica coating thickness, the interparticle separation increases and T_{max} moves to lower temperatures as seen in Figure 1.28, tending to T_B.

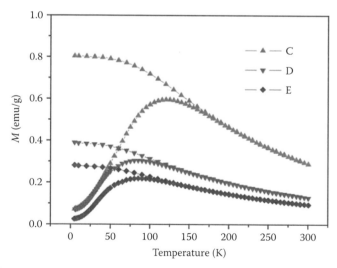

FIGURE 1.28 ZFC/FC magnetization data for 12.5-nm maghemite with 25-nm silica coating (sample C), 25-nm silica coating + 10-nm MS (sample D), and 25-nm silica coating + 21-nm MS (sample E). (Reprinted with permission from Papaefthymiou, G. C., et al., Interparticle interactions in magnetic core/shell nanoarchitectures, *Phys. Rev. B*, 80, 024406-1–024406-10, 2009. Copyright 2009 by the American Physical Society.)

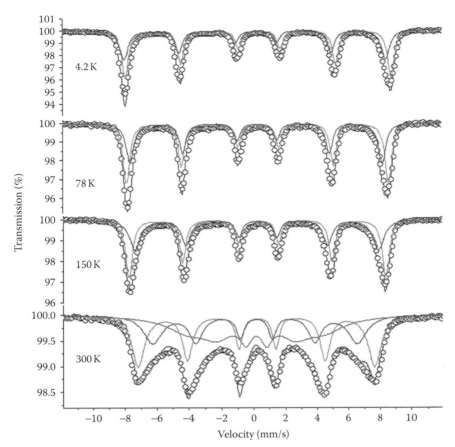

FIGURE 1.29 **(See color insert.)** Mössbauer spectra of sample A at various temperatures. The spectra are fit to the superposition of two iron sites, the tetrahedral and octahedral coordination sites of the spinel crystallographic structure, with an additional intermediate relaxation component at 300 K. (Reprinted with permission from Papaefthymiou, G. C., et al., Interparticle interactions in magnetic core/shell nanoarchitectures, *Phys. Rev. B*, 80, 024406-1–024406-10, 2009. Copyright 2009 by the American Physical Society.)

Figure 1.29 shows the Mössbauer spectra of sample A at various temperatures, $4.2 < T < 300$ K. Again two subsites are poorly resolved, associated in this case with the tetrahedral and octahedral iron sites of the spinel crystallographic structure. The spectra do not enter the superparamagnetic regime even at room temperature. Figure 1.30 shows the Mössbauer spectra of samples A, B, and C at room temperature. With increasing interparticle distance, faster spin relaxation is observed. With a silica coating of 25 nm, and thus a minimum center-to-center interparticle separation of 62.5 nm, the Mössbauer spectrum shows dynamic spin relaxation producing a diffuse broadened absorption with no sharp magnetic or quadrupolar absorption lines, indicating an intermediate spin relaxation time, $\tau_s \sim \tau_L$.

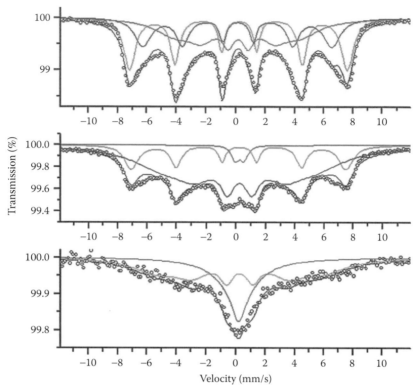

FIGURE 1.30 **(See color insert.)** Room-temperature Mössbauer spectra of samples A, B, and C. With increasing magnetic core separation, spin relaxation increases, collapsing the magnetic spectral signature. (Reprinted with permission from Papaefthymiou, G. C., et al., Interparticle interactions in magnetic core/shell nanoarchitectures, *Phys. Rev. B*, 80, 024406-1–024406-10, 2009. Copyright 2009 by the American Physical Society.)

Table 1.2 summarizes the results of the magnetic investigations of the $MP/SiO_2/MS$ nanoarchitectures and classifies the different nanoparticle assemblies in terms of strength of interparticle interactions. The data for the most magnetically dilute nanoparticles (sample E) yield an estimated value of the uniaxial magnetic anisotropy density $K_u = 2.37 \times 10^4$ J/m³, which is five times larger than the magnetocrystalline anisotropy of bulk maghemite, $K_{mc} = 0.47 \times 10^4$ J/m³. This increase is attributed to surface and strain effects that dominate the magnetic anisotropy density in small particles [76]. At an interparticle distance of 82.5 nm (sample D), the dipolar interaction energy has a value of $U_{int} = 2.6 \times 10^{-22}$ J. A distance larger than 105 nm is necessary for isolated particle behavior. With increasing magnetic volume fraction, U_{int} becomes increasingly dominant, leading to spin-glass-like magnetic ordering at T_{max} [49].

1.5 CONCLUSION

In this chapter, we explored the bio-inspired synthesis of iron oxide and ferrite magnetic nanoparticles within constrained reaction vehicles derived from block copolymers, bacterial membrane vesicles, surfactants, protein cages, and viral capsids

TABLE 1.2
Selected Magnetic Parameters from Magnetization Measurements of 12.5-nm
γ-Fe_2O_3 Nanoparticles with and without Silica Shell

Sample	Silica Shell Thickness (nm)	r (nm)	V_m/V	T_{max} (K)	T_{br} (K)	Classification
A	0	12.5	1.0	>300	250	Strong interaction (spin glass)
B	4	20.5	0.227	175	185	Strong interaction (spin glass)
C	25	62.5	0.008	120	160	Intermediate interaction
D	35 [25 (SiO_2) + 10 (MS)]	82.5	0.003	77	110	Weak interaction
E	46 [25 (SiO_2) + 21 (MS)]	104.5	0.002	75	100	Isolated (superparamagnetic)

as well as silica shells. We also explored the biomimetic synthesis of some metal and metal–alloy nanoparticles. We have taken a glimpse into the power of genetic engineering techniques in tailoring the electrostatic properties of the surfaces of protein nanotemplates in order to induce the nucleation and polymerization of a variety of phases, analogous to the iron biomineralization processes carried out by ferritin *in vivo*. Protein cages are amenable to molecular modifications by both chemical and genetic engineering means. The application of genetic engineering techniques in materials science holds great promise for the future of magnetic nanoparticle synthesis and their applications.

We also considered the magnetic characterization of Fe-based bio-inspired magnetic nanoparticles. In particular, the combination of Mössbauer and magnetometry measurements to probe local and total moments, static magnetic properties, and dynamic spin relaxation phenomena in magnetic nanoparticles was visited. The type and thickness of the encapsulating coat, whether polymeric or inorganic, can affect the magnetic properties of the particle assembly, and thus can be profitably utilized to tailor the magnetic properties to specific applications.

The exterior surface of protein nanotemplates and silica shells can be endowed with specific molecule recognition properties that can be used in (1) nanoparticle arraying, or nanopatterning, on flat substrates for applications in the magnetic recording industry [77,78], a process coined the "bio nano process" for the fabrication of nanoelectronic components, and (2) targeted drug delivery and bioimaging [79].

ACKNOWLEDGMENTS

This work was supported by the National Science Foundation at Villanova University and a European Commission Marie Curie Grant at NCSR "Demokritos."

REFERENCES

1. Niemeyer, C. M., Nanoparticles, proteins, and nucleic acids: Biotechnology meets materials science, *Angew. Chem. Int. Ed.*, 2001. 40: pp. 4128–4158.
2. Whitesides, G. M., Nanoscience, nanotechnology, and chemistry, *Small*, 2005. 1: pp. 172–179.

3. Mann, S., Mineralization in biological systems, inorganic elements in biology, *Struct. Bond.*, 1981. 54: pp. 125–174.

4. Mann, S., *Biomineralization: Principles and Concepts in Bioinorganic Materials Chemistry.* Oxford: Oxford University Press, 2001.

5. Weiner, S. and W. Traub, Bone structure: From angstroms to microns, *FASEB J.*, 1992. 6: pp. 879–885.

6. Olszta, M. J., et al., Bone structure and formation: A new perspective, *Mat. Sci. Eng. R.*, 2007. 58: pp. 77–116.

7. Bazylinski, D. A. and R. B. Frankel, Magnetosome formation in prokaryotes, *Nat. Rev. Microbiol.*, 2004. 2: pp. 217–230.

8. Frankel, R. B., et al., Magnetite in freshwater magnetotactic bacteria, *Science*, 1979. 203: pp. 1355–1356.

9. Chasteen, N. D. and P. M. Harrison, Mineralization in ferritin: An efficient means of iron storage, *J. Struct. Biol.*, 1999. 126: pp. 182–194.

10. Waldo G. S. and E. C. Theil, Ferritin and iron biomineralization, in *Comprehensive Supramolecular Chemistry*, K. S. Suslick, ed., Vol. 5. Oxford: Pergamon Press, 1996. pp. 65–89.

11. Harrison P. M. and P. Arosio, Ferritins: Molecular properties, iron storage function and cellular regulation, *Biochim. Biophys. Acta*, 1996. 1275: pp. 161–203.

12. Bou-Abdallah, F., guest ed., Ferritin: Structures, properties and applications, *Biochim. Biophys. Acta*, 2010. 1800(8): Special Issue.

13. Laufberger, V., Sur la cristallisation de la ferritine, *Bull. Soc. Chim. Biol.*, 1937. 19: pp. 1575–1582.

14. LaMer, V. K. and R. H. Dinegar, Theory, production and mechanism of formation of monodispersed hydrosols, *J. Am. Chem. Soc.*, 1950. 72: pp. 4847–4854.

15. Allen, M. A., et al., Constrained metal oxide mineralization: Lessons from ferritin applied to other protein cage architectures, in *Handbook of Biomineralization: Biomimentic and Bioinspired Chemistry*, P. Behrens and E. Baeuerlein, eds., Chap. 16, Weinheim, Germany: Wiley-VCH, 2007. p. 313.

16. Bou-Abdallah, F., et al., μ-1,2-Peroxobridged diiron (III) dimer formation in human H-chain ferritin, *Biochem. J.*, 2002. 364: pp. 57–63.

17. Bou-Abdallah, F., et al., A comparative Mössbauer study of the mineral cores of human H-chain ferritin employing dioxygen and hydrogen peroxide as iron oxidants, *Biophys. Chem.*, 2007. 130: pp. 114–121.

18. Harrison, P., et al., Solving the structure of human H ferritin by genetically engineering intermolecular crystal contacts, *Nature*, 1991. 349: pp. 541–544.

19. Drits, V. A., et al., Structural model for ferrihydrite, *Clay Miner.*, 1993. 28: pp. 185–207.

20. Michel, F. M., et al., Reactivity of ferritin and the structure of ferritin-derived ferrihydrite, *Biochim. Biophys. Acta*, 2010. 1800: pp. 871–885.

21. Lowenstam, H. A., Magnetite in the denticle capping in recent chitons (polyplacophora), *Geol. Soc. Am. Bul.*, 1962. 73: pp. 435–438.

22. Kirschvink, J. L. and H. A. Lowenstam, Mineralization and magnetization of chiton teeth: Paleomagnetism, sedimentologic and biologic implications of organic magnetite, *Earth Planet. Sci. Lett.*, 1979. 44: pp. 193–204.

23. Lindauer, M. and H. Martin, Magnetic effects in dancing bees, in *Animal Orientation and Navigation*, S. R. Galler et al., eds. Washington, DC: NASA, 1972. pp. 559–567.

24. Blakemore, R. P., Magnetotactic bacteria, *Science*, 1975. 190: pp. 377–379.

25. Tanaka, M., et al., MMS6 protein regulates crystal morphology during nano-sized magnetite biomineralization in vivo, *J. Biol. Chem.*, 2011. 286: pp. 6386–6392.

26. Schüler, D., Molecular analysis of a subcellular compartment: The magnetosome membrane in *Magnetospirillum gryphiswaldense*, *Arch. Microbiol.*, 2004. 181: pp. 1–7.

27. Papaefthymiou, G. C., et al., Gummic acid stabilized γ-Fe_2O_3 aqueous suspensions for biomedical applications, *Hyperfine Interact.*, 2009. 109: pp. 241–248.
28. Papaefthymiou, G. C., et al., Magnetic and structural characterization of $CoFe_2O_4$ nanoparticles encapsulated within block copolymer films, *Rev. Adv. Mater. Sci.*, 2005. 10: pp. 306–313.
29. Ahmed, S. R., et al., Magnetic properties of $CoFe_2O_4$ nanoparticles synthesized through a block co-polymer nanoreactor route, *Appl. Phys. Lett.*, 2002. 80(9): pp. 1616–1618.
30. Leibler, L., Theory of microphase separation in block copolymers, *Macromolecules*, 1980. 13: pp. 1602–1617.
31. Bates, F. S., Polymer-polymer phase behavior, *Science*, 1991. 251: pp. 898–905.
32. Sohn, B. H., et al., Magnetic properties of iron oxide nanoclusters within microdomains of block copolymers, *J. Magn. Magn. Mater.*, 1998. 182: pp. 216–224.
33. Petit, C., et al., Cobalt nanosized particles organized in a 2D superlattice: Synthesis, characterization, and magnetic properties, *J. Phys. Chem. B*, 1999. 103: pp. 1805–1810.
34. Meldrum, F. C., et al., Magnetoferritin: In vitro synthesis of a novel magnetic protein, *Science*, 1992. 257: pp. 522–523.
35. Klem, M. T., et al., Biomimetic magnetic nanoparticles, *Mater. Today*, 2005. 8(9): pp. 28–37.
36. Kilcoyne, S. H. and R. Cywinski, Ferritin: A model superparamagnet, *J. Magn. Magn. Mater.*, 1995. 140–144: pp. 1466–1467.
37. Gálvez, N., et al., Apoferritin-encapsulated Ni and Co superparamagnetic nanoparticles, *J. Mat. Chem.*, 2006. 16: pp. 2757–2761.
38. Warne, B., et al., Self assembled nanoparticulate Co:Pt for data storage applications, *IEEE Trans. Magn.*, 2000. 36: pp. 3009–3011.
39. Klem, M. T., et al., Synthetic control over magnetic moment and exchange bias in all-oxide materials encapsulated within spherical protein cage, *J. Am. Chem. Soc.*, 2007. 129: pp. 197–201.
40. Uchida, M., et al., The ferritin superfamily: Supramolecular templates for materials synthesis, *Biochim. Biophys. Acta*, 2010. 1800: pp. 834–845.
41. Allen, M., et al., Protein cage constrained synthesis of ferrimagnetic iron oxide nanoparticles, *Adv. Mater.*, 2002. 14: pp. 1562–1565.
42. Flenniken, M. D., et al., The small heat shock protein cage from *Methanococcus jannaschii* is a versatile nanoscale platform for genetic and chemical modification, *Nano Lett.*, 2003. 3: pp. 1573–1576.
43. Uchida, M., et al., Biological containers: Protein cages as multifunctional platforms, *Adv. Mater.*, 2007. 19: pp. 1025–1042.
44. Douglas, T. and M. Young, Host-guest encapsulation of materials by assembled virus protein cages, *Nature*, 1998. 393: pp. 152–155.
45. Douglas, T., et al., Protein engineering of a viral cage for constrained nanomaterials synthesis, *Adv. Mater.*, 2002. 14: pp. 415–418.
46. Reiss, B. D., et al., Biological routes to metal alloy ferromagnetic nanostructures, *Nano Lett.*, 2004. 4: pp. 1127–1132.
47. Yi, D. K., et al., Nanoparticle architectures templated by SiO_2/Fe_2O_3 nanocomposites, *Chem. Mater.*, 2006. 18: pp. 614–619 and references therein.
48. Papaefthymiou, G. C., Nanoparticle magnetism, *Nano Today*, 2009. 4: pp. 438–447 and references therein.
49. Papaefthymiou, G. C., et al., Interparticle interactions in magnetic core/shell nanoarchitectures, *Phys. Rev. B*, 2009. 80: pp. 024406-1–024406-10.
50. Papaefthymiou, G. C., Nanostructural studies by Mössbauer spectroscopy, in *Determining Nanoscale Properties of Materials by Microscopy and Spectroscopy*, M. Sarikaya, H. K. Wickramasinghe, and M. Isaacson, eds., MRS Symposium Proceedings, Vol. 332. Pittsburgh, PA: Materials Research Society, 1994. pp. 261–266.

51. Gütlich, P., et al., *Mössbauer Spectroscopy and Transition Metal Chemistry*. Berlin: Springer Verlag, 2010.
52. Long, G. J. and F. Grandjean, eds., *Mössbauer Spectroscopy Applied to Magnetism and Materials Science*, Vol. 2. New York: Plenum, 1996.
53. Long, G. J. and F. Grandjean, eds., *Mössbauer Spectroscopy Applied to Magnetism and Materials Science*, Vol. 2. New York: Plenum, 1993.
54. Dormann, J. L. and D. Fiorani, eds., *Magnetic Properties of Fine Particles*. North-Holland: Elsevier Science, 1991.
55. Pankhurst, Q. A., et al., Applications of magnetic nanoparticles in biomedicine, *J. Phys. D: Appl. Phys.*, 2003. 36: pp. R167–R181.
56. Néel, L., Theorie du trainage magnetique des ferromagnetiques en grains fins avec applications aux terres cuites, *Ann. Geophys.*, 1949. 5: pp. 99–136.
57. Brown, W. F., Thermal fluctuations of a single-domain particle, *Phys. Rev.*, 1963. 130: pp. 1677–1686.
58. Brown, W. F., Thermal fluctuations of a single-domain particle, *J. Appl. Phys.*, 1963. 34: pp. 1319–1320.
59. Brown, W. F., The fundamental theorem of fine ferromagnetic-particle theory. *J. Appl. Phys.*, 1968. 39: pp. 993–994.
60. Aharoni, A., Relaxation processes in small particles, in *Magnetic Properties of Fine Particles*, J. L. Dormann and D. Fiorani, eds. North-Holland: Elsevier Science, 1991. pp. 3–12.
61. Mørup, S. and H. Topsøe, Mössbauer studies of thermal excitations in magnetically ordered microcrystals, *Appl. Phys. (Berl.)*, 1976. 11: pp. 63–66.
62. O'Handley, R. C., *Modern Magnetic Materials*. New York: John Wiley & Sons, Inc., 2002.
63. Cullity, B. D. and C. D. Graham, *Introduction to Magnetic Materials*. Hoboken, NJ: IEEE Press, 2009.
64. Papaefthymiou, G. C., et al., Electronic and magnetic characterization of in vivo produced vs. in vitro reconstituted horse spleen ferritin, in *Nanophase and Nanocomposite Materials V*, S. Komarneni, K. Kaneko, J. C. Parker, and P. O'Brien, eds., Materials Research Society Symposia Proceedings, Vol. 1056E. Warrendale, PA: Materials Research Society, 2007, HH03-27.
65. Brooks, R. A., et al., Relaxometry and magnetometry of ferritin, *Mag. Res. Med.*, 1998. 40: pp. 227–235.
66. Kachkachi, H. and E. Bonet, Surface-induced cubic anisotropy in nanomagnets, *Phys. Rev. B*, 2006. 73: pp. 224402-1–224402-7.
67. Papaefthymiou, G. C., The Mössbauer and magnetic properties of ferritin cores, *Biochim. Biophys. Acta*, 2010. 1800: pp. 886–897.
68. Mørup, S., et al., Magnetic and mechanical coupling between ultrafine maghemite particles, *J. Magn. Magn. Mater.*, 1995. 140–144: pp. 409–410.
69. Mørup, S., et al., Experimental and theoretical studies of nanoparticles of antiferromagnetic materials, *J. Phys. Condens. Matter.*, 2007. 19: pp. 213202-1–213202-31.
70. Mørup, S., et al., Spin-glass-like ordering of the magnetic moments of interacting nanosized maghemite particles, *Phys. Rev. B*, 1995. 52: pp. 287–294.
71. Mørup, S., Superparamagnetism and spin glass ordering in magnetic nanocomposites, *Europhys. Lett.*, 1994. 28(9): pp. 671–676.
72. Rebbouh, L., et al., ^{57}Fe Mössbauer spectral and muon spin relaxation study of the magnetodynamics of monodispersed γ-Fe$_2$O$_3$ nanoparticles, *Phys. Rev. B*, 2007. 76: pp. 174422-1–174422-12.
73. Morrish, A. H., *The Physical Principles of Magnetism*, reprinted. New York: Institute of Electrical and Electronics Engineers, 2001. p. 476.
74. Luo, W., et al., Dipole interactions with random anisotropy in a frozen ferrofluids, *Phys. Rev. Lett.*, 1991. 67: pp. 2721–2724.

75. Binns, C., et al., Magnetic behavior of nanostructured films assembled from preformed Fe clusters embedded in Ag, *Phys. Rev. B*, 2002. 66: pp. 184413-1–184413-12.
76. Papaefthymiou, G. C., Strain anisotropies in core/shell magnetic nanostructures, in *Anisotropic Nanoparticles—Synthesis, Characterization and Applications*, S. J. Stranick, P. Searson, L. A. Lyon, and C. D. Keating, eds., Materials Research Society Symposium Proceedings, Vol. 635. Pittsburgh, PA: Materials Research Society, 2001. p. C2.4.1.
77. Matsui, T., et al., Realizing a two dimensional ordered array of ferritin molecules directly on a solid surface utilizing carbonaceous material affinity peptides, *Langmuir*, 2007. 23: pp. 1615–1618.
78. Yamazaki, G., et al., Nano-etching using nanodots mask fabricated by the bio-nano-process, *J. Polym. Sci. Technol.*, 2003. 16(3): pp. 439–444.
79. Koo, O. M., et al., Role of nanotechnology in targeted drug delivery and imaging: A concise review, *Nanomed. Nanotechnol. Biol. Med.*, 2005. 1(3): pp. 193–212.

2 Nanoparticles for Bioimaging

Hye Sun Park and Yong Taik Lim
Chungnam National University

CONTENTS

2.1 SEMICONDUCTOR NANOCRYSTALS

2.1.1 PHOTONIC PROPERTIES OF SEMICONDUCTOR NANOCRYSTALS

Quantum dots (QDs) are fluorescent semiconductor nanocrystals that have a diameter in the range of 1–10 nm [1]. Due to the nanoscale size, which is comparable to electron delocalization length, QDs have unique physical properties that are nonexistent in individual atoms or bulk semiconductor solids. The so-called quantum confinement effect is observed, when one or more dimensions of a semiconductor are reduced under the Bohr exciton radius, which is typically a few nanometers [2]. It is possible to systematically control the electronic energy-level spacings because of the quantum confinement effect, and the wavelength of light emission can also be controlled by adjusting the size of the semiconductor. The emission wavelength of QDs can be controlled over a wide range of spanning regions from the ultraviolet, through the visible, into the infrared, by selecting and adjusting the size and compositions [3–6]. Due to a radiative recombination of

43

an exciton, the emission of QDs is also characterized by a long lifetime (>10 ns), and a narrow and symmetric energy band [7]. Compared with the traditional fluorescent molecules that are characterized by red-tailed broad emission band and short lifetimes, QDs have several attractive optical features that are desirable for long-term, multitarget, and highly sensitive bioapplications. QDs have very large molar extinction coefficients, typically on the order of 0.5–5 × 10 M^{-1} cm^{-1}. This value is approximately 10–50-fold higher than those of organic dyes [8]. Due to the high molar extinction properties, QDs are attractive as highly sensitive fluorescent agents that can be used for the highly efficient fluorescence labeling of cells and tissues. With regard to the photostability, the photostability of QDs is typically several thousandfold more stable against photobleaching than organic dyes [9]. The unique and excellent photophysical properties of QDs allow the real-time monitoring of biological processes over long periods of time and have potentials for cancer biomarker assays and *in vivo* imaging where much longer times are needed. Another interesting photophysical properties is related to the longer excited state lifetime (20–50 ns), which is about 1 order of magnitude longer than that of organic dyes. Due to the longer lifetime, the effective separation of QD fluorescence from background fluorescence by a time-gated or time-delayed data acquisition mode is also possible [7,10]. Compared with those of organic dyes, the excitation and emission spectra of QDs are well separated and further improvement of detection sensitivity in imaging tissue biopsies is possible [11]. Finally, the size-dependent fluorescence of QDs provides the imaging and tracking of multiple targets simultaneously with single excitation source. This is of particular importance in cancer detection and diagnosis, since it has been realized that a panel of disease-specific molecular biomarkers can provide more accurate and reliable information with regard to the disease status and progression than any single biomarker [12].

2.1.2 SYNTHESIS OF QDs

In the periodic table, QD nanocrystals are composed of atoms that typically belong to group II and VI elements (e.g., CdSe, CdTe, ZnSe, etc.) or group III and V elements (e.g., InP, InAs, etc). Although various synthetic methods have been reported, two methods are most widely used. The first synthetic strategy is aqueous-phase synthesis in reverse micelles, which produces water-soluble QDs. However, the quality of QDs synthesized by this method is usually of low quality [13]. The second synthesis was conducted at an elevated temperature in an organic solvent in order to produce high-quality QDs. Also, it becomes the most widely used technique for the synthesis of highly homogeneous and highly crystalline QDs. The solvent is most commonly a mixture of trioctylphosphine, trioctylphosphine oxide, and hexadecylamine, all of which have long alkyl chains, and is nonpolar with high boiling point [14,15]. The QD nanocrystal core (e.g., CdSe) is often coated with a shell of a wider bandgap semiconductor material (e.g., ZnS or CdS). The so-called surface passivation process protects the core from oxidation and prevents the leaching of highly toxic Cd^{2+} ions. By reducing the surface defects and thus preventing nonradiative decay, it also drastically improves the quantum yield [16,17]. Through systematic study, it has been known that the higher bandgap semiconductor confines the charge carriers to the core QDs, resulting in the minimization of the surface recombination, that finally leads to a significant improvement in fluorescence quantum yields [17].

2.1.3 STRATEGY FOR AQUEOUS SOLUBLE QDS

As mentioned in Section 2.1.2, the surfactants used in the synthesis of QDs cause insolubility in water and prevent further functionalization [14,15]. For the application of the above-mentioned unique properties of QDs, water solubility, biocompatibility, and photostability are very important key technologies. So, flexible strategy of QD surface chemistry/functionality that will enable efficient coupling of these fluorescent inorganic probes to reagents capable of targeting and/or sensing ongoing biological processes is very important [18]. With regard to the synthesis and design of aqueous soluble QDs, several methods have been reported and the functionalization strategies summarized as follows: The first strategy is the direct encapsulation of hydrophobic QDs by hydrophilic polymers [19]; the second one is the ligand exchange of original surfactant with hydrophilic ligands, such as thiols [20,21]; and the third one is the formation of an interdigitated bilayer between amphiphilic molecules and the passivating surfactant layer on the QD surface [11,22,23]. The above-mentioned strategies exploit the hydrophobic nature of the nanoparticle surface by utilizing an amphiphilic poly(ethylene glycol) (PEG)-phospholipid [23]. Their hydrophobic portion interacts with the QD surface to create micelles, resulting in a self-assembled monolayer coating. In a typical synthesis, distearoylphosphatidyl ethanolamine (DSPE)-PEG 2000 amine was dissolved in chloroform, and tri-n-octylphosphine oxide (TOPO)-capped CdSe/ZnS QDs were added. QDs coated with DSPE-PEG 2000 amine was dried under argon gas and left in a vacuum desiccator to remove all traces of organic solvents. The PEG portion of the coating confers aqueous solubility and biocompatibility on them; at the same time, the use of modified PEG allows for bioconjugation [23]. To functionalize CdSe/ZnS QDs for bioconjugation and subsequent delivery and imaging studies, biomolecules (such as peptides) and heterobifunctional cross-linking reagent sulfosuccinimidyl-4-(N-maleimidomethyl)cyclohexane-1-carboxylate (Sulfo-SMCC) can be used.

2.1.4 SURFACE MODIFICATIONS OF QDS

For the successful conjugation of biomolecules onto QDs, appropriate surface modification strategy should be introduced. QDs can be functionalized with oligonucleotides, peptides, antibodies, and other molecules for cellular and *in vivo* imaging. There are several reasons why easy and robust bioconjugate chemistry strategies are needed [18,24]: (1) both the activity of the biomolecule and the functionality of the QD should be preserved; (2) the biomolecular orientation should be optimized such that the epitope point of the biomolecule should be in the outward direction; (3) the amount of biomolecules per QD should be predictable and reproducible; and (4) QD biomolecule conjugates should be stable in bioassay media (e.g., serum, plasma, blood, etc.). In a recent review, Algar et al. [25] suggested an interesting overview of the controlled display of biomolecules on nanoparticles toward the concept of

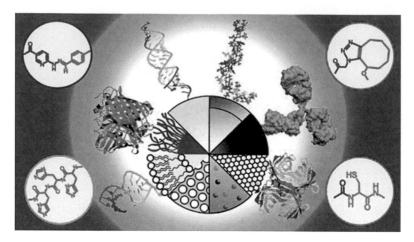

FIGURE 2.1 Schematic illustration for the bioconjugation of nanoparticles using various kinds of biomolecules. (Reprinted with permission from Algar, W.R., et al., 2011, 825–58. Copyright 2011 American Chemical Society.)

"bioorthogonal" chemistry (Figure 2.1). Because the size of QDs are of similar or larger size than biomolecules, it is extremely important that the binding sites point toward the target of interest and that the biomolecules do not hinder each other from efficiently binding to this target. So, the QD-labeling strategies require different approaches than bioconjugation with relatively small fluorescent dyes. Algar's conjugation strategy provides control over the orientations and positions of biomolecules on the QD surface, and therefore improves the performance of QD bioconjugates compared with that of QDs where biomolecules are randomly labeled on the surface of QDs [24,25].

2.2   BIOLOGICAL APPLICATIONS OF QDs

2.2.1   LABELING OF CELLS

Lei et al. [26] have demonstrated that PEG-coated QD–TAT (trans-activating transcriptional activator) peptide complexes were transported into living mesenchymal stem cells (MSCs) and assessed by fluorescent microscopy, laser confocal microscopy, and flow cytometry. The use of QD–TAT peptides in a multiplexing experiment, two color QDs (QD-520 and QD-645) are designed to bind to TAT peptides and introduced into the same stem cells simultaneously. In their research, both populations of bioconjugated QDs were identified in stem cells using confocal laser microscopy with a single 488-nm laser line. To get even a higher resolution than confocal microscopy, they observed the internalization of QD–TAT peptides by transmission electron microscopy (TEM). Figure 2.2 provides TEM images of intracellular QD–TAT peptides. In Figure 2.2a, the white arrowheads indicate endosomes and QD–TAT peptides are seen in the magnified image as black dots (Figure 2.2b), which surround the interior of the endosomes. The TEM images provide direct evidence that at least a portion of the internalized QD–TAT peptides was colocalized within the endosomes.

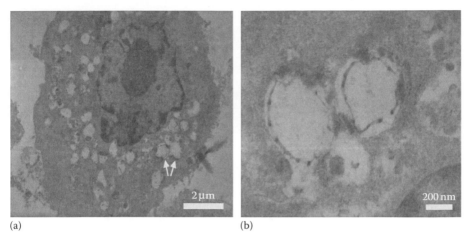

(a)   (b)

FIGURE 2.2   TEM analysis of the internalized QD–TAT peptides in MSCs. (a) TEM images of MSCs labeled by QD–TAT peptides, and the white arrowheads indicate endosomes. (b) A magnified view of endosomes in (a). QD–TAT peptides are seen as black dots surrounding the interior of the vesicles. (Reprinted with permission from Lei, Y., et al., 2008, 421–7. Copyright 2008 American Chemical Society.)

Yong et al. [27] reported the use of InP/ZnS QDs (as non-cadmium-based QDs) as targeted optical probes for labeling human pancreatic cancer cells, both immortalized and low-passage ones. For the synthesis of QD bioconjugates, they utilized antibodies such as anticlaudin 4 and anti-PSCA, whose corresponding antigen receptors are known to be overexpressed in both primary and metastatic pancreatic tumors [28–30]. In their research, to quantify the luminescence from the treated cells, flow cytometry was used as shown in Figure 2.3. The fluorescence intensity of untreated cells was in the range between 10^0 and 10^1, and the cells treated with unconjugated QDs exhibited luminescence intensity in the range between 10^1 and 10^2. Thus, the cells that exhibited luminescence intensity higher than 10^2 were taken as positively labeled with bioconjugates.

Le Gac et al. focused on an early and major event in the apoptotic cascade, the externalization of phosphatidylserine (PS) occurring through the "flipping" of the cell membrane [31,32]. Through specific recognition of PS moieties located on the outer membrane of the cells, they reported on QDs functionalized with Annexin V for detecting and staining apoptotic "living" cells. They exploited the well-known streptavidin–biotin interaction, by coupling biotinylated Annexin to QDs–streptavidin conjugates, because the coupling is known to be very strong and can be readily achieved starting from commercially available products (biotinylated Annexin V, QDs–streptavidin conjugates). Especially, they particularly demonstrated the superiority of QDs toward organic dyes with respect to bleaching issues [31]. They also emphasized that the photostability allowed for more frequent imaging, which enabled the visualization of fast events such as those occurring at the membrane level. In their research, two strategies were adopted (Figure 2.4): (1) QDs were first functionalized with Annexin V and subsequently added to apoptotic cells or (2) apoptotic cells were preincubated with Annexin V, and QDs were added later once Annexin V had bound to PS moieties [31].

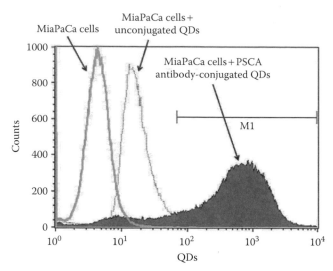

FIGURE 2.3 Flow cytometry data showing the relative uptake of unconjugated QDs and PSCA-conjugated QDs in MiaPaCa cells. The number of positively labeled cells was represented as the percentage of total cell counts. M1 indicates just gated region for analysis in cytometric curve, which is named by the instrument. (Reprinted with permission from Yong, K.-T., et al., 2009, 502–10. Copyright 2009 American Chemical Society.)

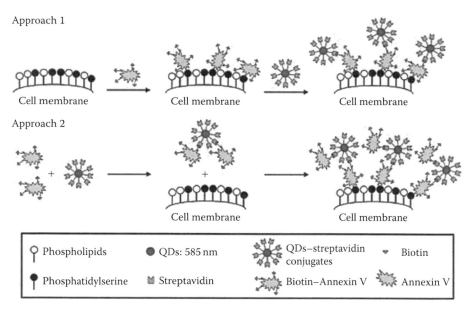

FIGURE 2.4 Two approaches used for staining apoptotic cells with Annexin V-coupled QDs. Approach 1: Preincubation of apoptotic cells with biotinylated Annexin V in a 2.5-mM CaCl$_2$ medium followed by addition of QDs–strepatvidin conjugates. Approach 2: Preparation of Annexin V-functionalized QDs subsequently added to cells. (Reprinted with permission from Le Gac, S., et al., 2006, 1863–9. Copyright 2006 American Chemical Society.)

2.2.2 TARGETING OF INTRACELLULAR ORGANELLES

To develop an efficient and general method for targeting QDs to the cytosol and subcellular organelles, Bayles et al. [33] have synthesized proton sponge-based core–shell polymer colloids that are able to bind QDs, transport them into the cell, and release them into the cytosol within a few hours of application (Figure 2.5a). In order to develop a more efficient and general method for the delivery of nanocrystals to the cytosol of nonphagocytic cells, they designed cationic core–shell polymer colloids containing a pH-buffering proton sponge using PEG dimethacrylate (PEGDMA, MW = 330 Da) cross-linked poly(2-(diethylamino)ethyl methacrylate) (PDEAEMA) for the core and poly(2-aminoethyl methacrylate) (PAEMA) for the shell (Figure 2.5b). Furthermore, they found that picomolar concentrations of QDs bound to polymer colloids are sufficient to give good cytosolic luminescence, with minimal evidence of residual endosomal staining patterns.

Through multivalent electrostatic interactions between the ammonium ions on the colloid shell and acidic streptavidin side chains (Figure 2.6), they showed that the addition of streptavidin-coated QDs [605-SA-QDs; diameter = 20 nm, λ_{em} = 605 nm, ζ = −9 mV in phosphate-buffered saline (PBS) at pH 7.4] to the colloids led to facile self-assembly. They also showed that the QD delivery efficiency to HeLa cells was markedly improved in the presence of polymer colloids. In the highest concentration tested (5 nM), the increase in the geometric mean fluorescence above background was approximately 20-fold [33].

Kim et al. [34] proposed the concept of cytosolic delivery of protein-conjugated QDs in live cells to label subcellular molecular targets using a carrier system that is environmentally responsive. Utilizing the surface of biodegradable polymers for cell penetration, the chemical and structural properties of protein-coated QDs can be preserved, thus enabling them to actively seek specific intracellular targets within the cytosol. They have designed a smart delivery system that undergoes endolysosomal to cytosolic translocation via pH-dependent reversal of nanocomposite surface charge polarity, by incorporating antibody-coated QDs within biodegradable polymeric nanospheres. Upon entering

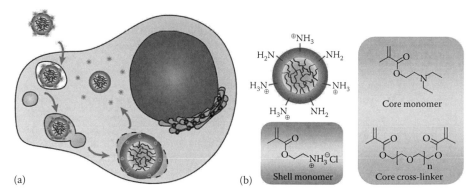

(a)   (b)

FIGURE 2.5 Delivery of nanocrystals to the cytosol of live cells with cationic core–shell polymer colloids. (a) Suggested mechanism of cellular uptake, trafficking, expansion, and endosomal rupture, leading to cytosolic delivery of nanocrystals. (b) Schematic depiction of cationic core–shell polymer colloids and their constituent monomers. (Reprinted with permission from Bayles, A.R., et al., 2010, 4086–92. Copyright 2010 American Chemical Society.)

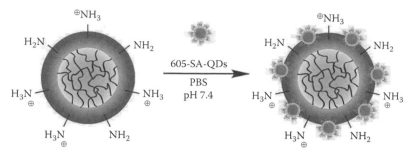

FIGURE 2.6 Adsorption of anionic streptavidin-coated QDs onto the surface of cationic core–shell polymer colloids via nonspecific electrostatic interactions. (Reprinted with permission from Bayles, A.R., et al., 2010, 4086–92. Copyright 2010 American Chemical Society.)

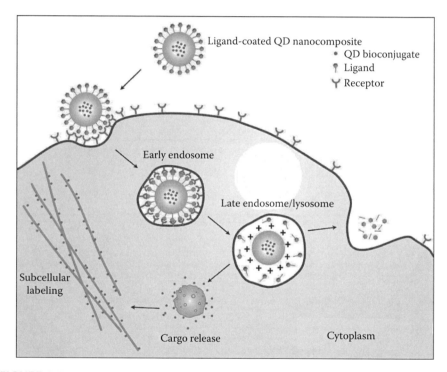

FIGURE 2.7 Mechanism of cytosolic delivery and subcellular targeting of QD nanocomposites. Schematic representation depicting QD nanocomposite escape from the endolysosomal compartment upon cellular internalization with cytosolic release of the encapsulated cargo. (Reprinted with permission from Kim, B.Y.S., et al., 2008, 3887–92. Copyright 2008 American Chemical Society.)

the cytosol, the polymer nanospheres undergo hydrolysis, thus releasing the QD bioconjugates (Figure 2.7) [35].The biocompatibility of the delivery system coupled with cell entry capabilities without disturbing the plasma membrane could extend the use of QD bioconjugates to selectively label subcellular structures, monitor and track cytoplasmic processes, and elucidate protein interactions in live cells [35].

Choi et al. [36] reported the study on the detection of the specific intracellular target protein in live cells based on TAT-conjugated QDs. In their research, they observed the PEG-polymer-coated QDs (pcQDs) modified with TAT and anti-green fluorescent protein (GFP) antibody specifically bound the intracellular target GFP in live cells. The anti-GFP-TAT-PEG-pcQD that initially colocalized with the GFP at the cellular membrane also translocated with the GFP after the endothelin-1 (ET-1) agonist treatment in agreement with the characteristic of the G-protein-coupled receptor (GPCR). They insisted that the results suggested that the controlled functionalization of PEGylated pcQD with both TAT and an antibody against a specific target protein could afford efficient cellular entry of QDs as well as specific detection of an intracellular target without significant nonspecific uptake or binding. As shown in Scheme 2.1, they conjugated

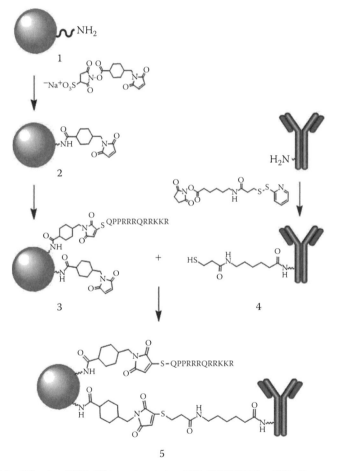

SCHEME 2.1 Diamino-PEG (5k) conjugated pcQD (NH2-PEG-pcQD, 1) was reacted with sulfo-SMCC to give SMCC-PEG-pcQD 2, followed by coupling reaction with cystein-modified TAT peptide. The partially modified TAT-PEG-pcQD 3 was further reacted with SPDP-modified anti-GFP 4 to yield anti-GFP-TAT-PEG-pcQD 5. As a control, anti-GFP-pcQD without TAT was synthesized by reacting 2 with 4 to yield anti-GFP-PEG-pcQD. (Reprinted with permission from Choi, Y., et al., 2011, 1576–86. Copyright 2011 American Chemical Society.)

anti-GFP antibody to TAT-PEG-pcQD using two different heterobifunctional linkers, sulfo-SMCC and sulfosuccinimidyl 6-(3′-[2-pyridyldithio]-propionamido)hexanoate (sulfo-LC-SPDP) [36].

They observed that anti-GFP-TAT-PEG-pcQDs were initially bound to the plasma membrane (white arrows) and some QDs were also observed in the cytoplasm (dark gray arrow) after 30-min incubation at 37°C (Figure 2.8a–c). Due to the presence of PEG molecules, the cellular uptake of anti-GFP-PEG-pcQD (without TAT) was negligible (Figure 2.8d). The nontargeted TAT-PEG-pcQD (without anti-GFP) showed punctate and even distribution mostly in the cytoplasm with no significant colocalization with GFP or membrane (Figure 2.8e). In this research, it was demonstrated that the localization of the anti-GFP-TAT-PEG-pcQD in the membrane region could be the result of the facilitated internalization of the QDs, owing to TAT conjugation and target binding due to the presence of anti-GFP antibody.

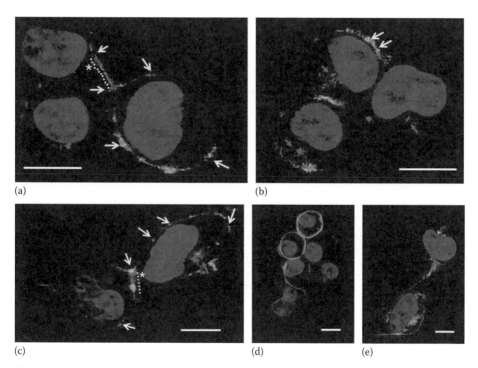

(a)

(b)

(c)

(d)

(e)

FIGURE 2.8 (a–c) After 30-min incubation, the red QD 5 were delivered to the plasma membrane (white arrows), preferentially localized with GFP signal as indicated by overlaid yellow color; QDs are often observed in the cytosol (dark gray arrow). QDs seemingly entrapped in the plasma membrane were moving rapidly along the membrane or traversing the filipodia of the cells (a; dotted line with asterisk) or along the cellular contacts (c; dotted line with asterisk). (d,e) Control cell images at the same conditions with the anti-GFP-PEG-pcQD (without TAT) showing nonsignificant endocytosis (d) and with the TAT-PEG-pcQD displaying punctuate and evenly distributed cellular uptake mostly in the cytoplasm (e). The images are shown as pseudo colors for overlays of blue channel (Hoechst33342 for nucleus), green channel (GFP), and red channel (pcQD). The scale bars correspond to 10 μm. (Reprinted with permission from Choi, Y., et al., 2011, 1576–86. Copyright 2011 American Chemical Society.)

2.2.3 Targeting of Specific Cells

Lee et al. [37] reported on the specific binding ability of the QD–cetuximab conjugates in live-cell experiments using a confocal microscope (Figure 2.9). Cetuximab (or Erbitux) is the first monoclonal antibody drug that targets the epidermal growth factor receptor (EGFR) overexpressed in most cancer cells [38]. They observed that the binding of QD–cetuximab conjugates to EGFR on the A549 cells occurred within 20 min (Figure 2.9c) and QD–cetuximab conjugate was found to bind competitively to the extracellular domain of EGFR showing exactly the same binding as cetuximab. Cetuximab binding has been known to inhibit the autophosphorylation of EGFR and induces its internalization [38]. After 1-h incubation, most QD–cetuximab conjugates were internalized into the cytoplasm (Figure 2.9d). The binding of QD–cetuximab conjugates to the cell membrane was completely blocked (Figure 2.9b), when the cells were pretreated with free cetuximab before adding the QD–cetuximab conjugates.

Liu et al. [39] reported a new class of imaging probes based on QDs with small molecular phenylboronic acid (PBA) tags, which allow highly specific and efficient labeling of sialic acids (SAs) on living cells. SAs with a nine-carbon backbone are commonly found at the terminal position of the glycan structures on cell membranes. The unique distribution and ubiquitous existence of SA on the cell membrane make them important mediators in various biological and pathological processes [40,41]. It is known that the stable complex of PBA with diols in a favorable configuration can only form in its dissociated state at pH close to its pK_a (Figure 2.10a). In their study, PBA-targeting ligand was linked on QDs with carboxylic acid surface functionality

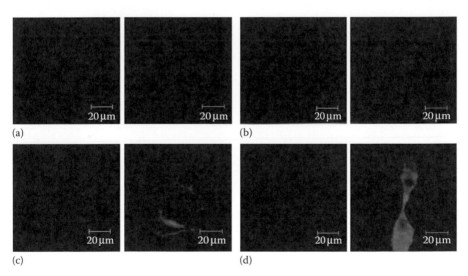

FIGURE 2.9 Competitive binding test of free cetuximab and QD–cetuximab conjugates: (a) A549 cell (control); (b) A549 cells incubated with QD–cetuximab conjugates after pretreatment of cetuximab (2-h incubation at 37°C); (c) QD–cetuximab conjugates for 20 min; and (d) A549 cells incubated with QD–cetuximab conjugates for 1 h. Bright field image is on the left side and fluorescence image on the right side. (Reprinted with permission from Lee, J., et al., 2010, 940–6. Copyright 2010 American Chemical Society.)

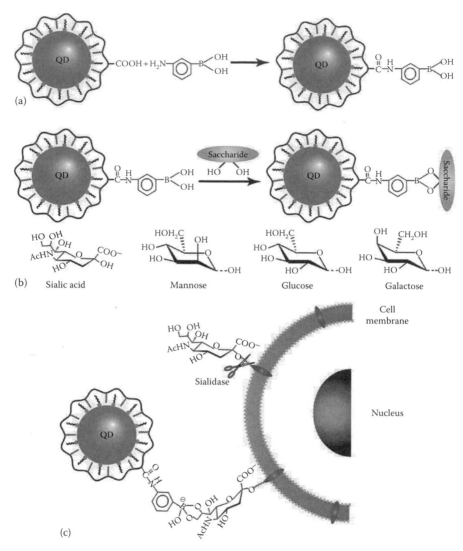

FIGURE 2.10 Schematic illustration of QD conjugation and the use of QD probes for specific labeling of SA on living cells. (a) Conjugation of carboxylic acid-functionalized QDs with 3-APBA by the 1-ethyl-3-(3-dimethylaminopropyl)carbodiimide (EDAC)-catalyzed reaction. (b) The reaction of PBA and diols in an aqueous solution. (c) Specific binding of QD with SA on living cells at the C-8,9-diol of SA. (Reprinted with permission from Liu, A., et al., 2011, 1124–30. Copyright 2011 American Chemical Society.)

by the carbodiimide-catalyzed reaction with 3-aminophenylboronic acid (APBA; Figure 2.10b). The specificity of QD binding was confirmed by the competitive assay with free SA and staining of cells treated with sialidase, which removes the SA moiety from glycans (Figure 2.10c). They also found that the labeled SAs undergo quick internalization shortly after surface binding via endocytosis and eventually distribute in the perinuclear region [39]. In the study, they demonstrated the potential of the

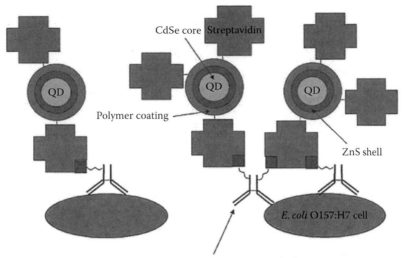

FIGURE 2.11 Labeling of *E. coli* O157:H7 cells with biotinylated anti-*E. coli* O157:H7 antibodies and streptavidin-conjugated CdSe/ZnS core/shell QDs. Drawing is not to scale. (Reprinted with permission from Hahn, M.A., et al., 2005, 4861–9. Copyright 2005 American Chemical Society.)

use of these QD probes to investigate diffusion dynamics of SA, which has been a significant challenge for glycan imaging.

Hahn et al. [42] presented fluorescent labeling and detection of intact bacterial cells with functionalized semiconductor QDs. They showed that the use of streptavidin-conjugated CdSe/ZnS core/shell QDs as sensitive, specific, and stable fluorometric labels for pathogenic *Escherichia coli* O157:H7. They used standard biochemical techniques utilizing the strong and well-known streptavidin–biotin interaction to selectively label heat-killed *E. coli* O157:H7 cells with biotinylated anti-*E. coli* O157:H7 antibodies and streptavidin-functionalized CdSe/ZnS core/ shell QDs (see Figure 2.11) [42].

In their research, they showed that the fluorescein isothiocyanate (FITC) fluorescence intensity quickly drops off to below the detectable limit within 20 s (Figure 2.12a), while the QD fluorescence remains quite high, even after 1 h of this continuous excitation (Figure 2.12b) [42].

2.2.4 MULTIPLEXED DETECTION AND IMAGING

Delehanty et al. [43] have shown an antibody-free, spaciotemporal strategy for the simultaneous, multicolor labeling of distinct intra- and extracellular compartments/structures in a live cellular system. They exploited multivalent peptide display on QDs and fluorescence resonance energy transfer (FRET), and incorporated both innate cellular processes (peptide- and polymer-mediated endocytoses and receptor–ligand interactions) along with physical microinjection as QD delivery platforms (Figure 2.13a). Multicolor fluorescent labeling of both intra- and extracellular structures is a powerful technique

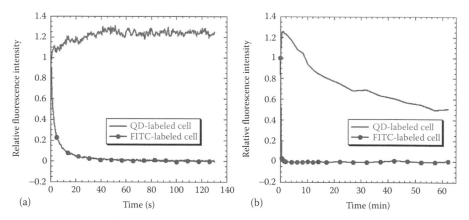

FIGURE 2.12 Relative fluorescence intensities from one *E. coli* O157:H7 cell labeled with anti-*E. coli* O157:H7 antibodies and streptavidin-modified CdSe/ZnS QDs and from one cell similarly labeled with FITC-conjugated streptavidin under continuous excitation. (a) Fluorescence monitored over the first 2 min of excitation. (b) Fluorescence monitored over the course of 1 h of excitation. (Reprinted with permission from Hahn, M.A., et al., 2005, 4861–9. Copyright 2005 American Chemical Society.)

for simultaneous monitoring of multiple complex biochemical processes [44–47]. They utilized CdSe/ZnS core/shell QDs with distinct photoluminescence (PL) emission arrayed across the visible spectrum. They also utilized a mixed ligand surface consisting of 1:1 dihydrolipoic acid (DHLA):DHLA-PEG (Figure 2.13b) for QDs requiring both pH stability and a net negative charge [43]. They have further demonstrated that QDs can be controllably assembled with ratios ranging from 1 to 50 peptides along with providing access to mixed surfaces displaying multiple peptide species; each of the latter can also differ in valence assembled per QD if so required.

Ghazani et al. [48] introduced a novel approach for profiling of protein expression of tumors in a quantitative manner. They employed QD bioconjugates in conjunction with an optical spectroscopy system with potential to detect single-molecule fluorescence, the ultimate in detection sensitivity, for high-throughput analysis of target antigens on tissue microarrays. In their study, a mask was derived from QD immunolabeling of the lung carcinoma tumor sections using pan-cytokeratin staining, a marker for epithelium cells. By using their normalizer algorithm, the mean signal intensity value from antigen-derived staining was obtained and divided by the cytokeratin signal, thereby normalizing each core to cellular content. Subsequently, the multiplexer algorithm combined the normalized values of all antigen expressions in each core to create a composite graph of expression profile across the entire array (Figure 2.14).

Klostranec et al. [49] demonstrated the successful convergence of nano- and micro-technologies with molecular diagnostics for high-throughput, multiplexed detection of infectious disease protein biomarkers. They have selected three diagnostic targets [hepatitis B virus (HBV), hepatitis C virus (HCV), and human immunodeficiency virus (HIV)] to demonstrate the utility of this integrated device for ID diagnostics. These three pathogens are the leading causes of global morbidity and mortality, and are all blood-borne viruses that use similar routes of transmission and are among

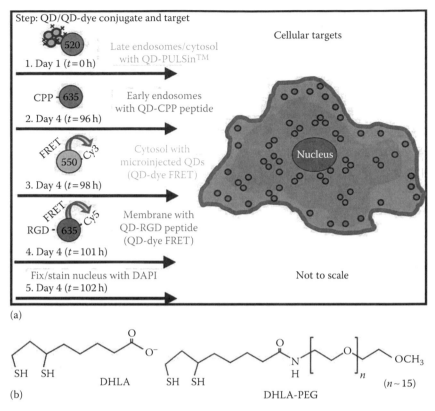

FIGURE 2.13 (a) Spatiotemporal strategy for multicolor QD labeling of A549 cells along with QD/QD-dye emissions utilized. (b) Structures of the QD capping ligands utilized to render the nanocrystals hydrophilic. CPP, cell-penetrating peptide. (Reprinted with permission from Delehanty, J.B., et al., 2011, 10482–9. Copyright 2011 American Chemical Society.)

the most prevalent IDs in the world [50–52]. Their detection system is composed of four parts (Figure 2.15a): (1) for selectivity and multiplexing capabilities, QD beads conjugated to targeting molecules; (2) sequential, high-throughput readout of single barcodes with no movable parts and portability potential enabled by electrokineti- cally driven microfluidics [53]; (3) real-time readout of flowing barcodes enabled by photon-counting detection systems; and (4) deconvolution of QD bead optical signals enabled by signal processing. QD beads were loaded into the sample well of a dispos- able polydimethylsiloxane (PDMS) microfluidic chip (Figure 2.15d). They have used electrokinetics, where electric fields propel fluids through small conduits, to trans- port QD beads in the microchannels. As a QD bead passed through a focused laser spot (488 nm, 25 mW), the fluorescence signal was collected by a 60× oil immersion objective (1.35 NA). In the experimental setup, the signal passed through an optical train of dichroic mirrors, bandpass filters, and focusing lenses before illuminating solid-state photodetectors. They reported that these detectors have response times several orders of magnitude less than the timescale of a flowing bead, allowing for discrimination of single versus aggregated beads in the flow [49].

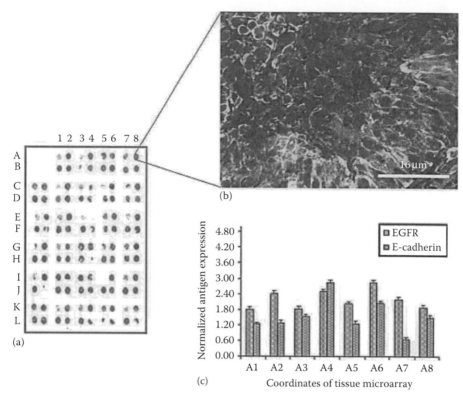

(a)

(b)

(c)

FIGURE 2.14 Quantification analysis of cancer-derived antigens in tissue microarray. Tissue cores on a tissue microarray (hematoxylin and eosin image, a) were stained for EGFR, cytokeratin, and E-cadherin. The fluorescent image is a composite picture of the antigens detected by individual QD immunostaining (of different color emission) for each of the targets. 4′,6-Diamidino-2-phenylindole (DAPI) staining is used to locate nuclei in blue (b). The normalizer algorithm normalizes tumor expression values (EGFR and E-cadherin) for epithelial content (cytokeratin). The multiplexer algorithm creates a composite profile of tumor antigen values in each core (c). Cores A1–A8 correspond to lung cancer xenografts RVH-6849, MGH8, MGH7, H520, H460, H157, H1264, and A549, respectively. (Reprinted with permission from Ghazani, A.A., et al., 2006, 2881–6. Copyright 2006 American Chemical Society.)

Giri et al. [54] demonstrated the capability of QD barcodes to detect nine different gene fragments stemming from five different infectious pathogens in a single sample volume and in a rapid fashion. In their study, they have examined the feasibility of using QD barcodes to detect genetic biomarkers of the blood-borne pathogens: HIV, malaria, HBV and HCV, and syphilis. Their study provided an important intermediate step in the translation of QD barcode technology for screening infectious disease agents in the developed and developing world [55–57]. QD barcodes were conjugated to single-stranded oligonucleotides (capture strands) that can hybridize to a target sequence. In their study, this target sequence was from a gene fragment from one of five pathogens [54]. This target sequence could also hybridize onto a secondary oligonucleotide that was conjugated with the dye Alexa Fluor 647 (λ_{ex} = 647 nm, λ_{em} = 667 nm) (Figure 2.16a). Since different capture strands

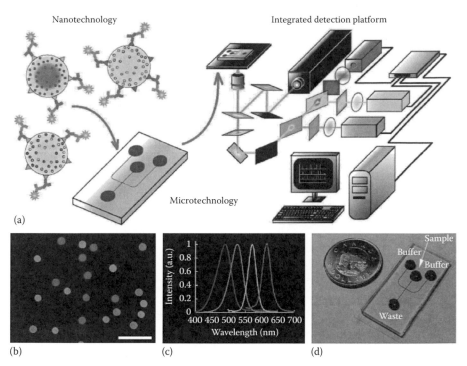

FIGURE 2.15 (a) Diagram illustrating the integration of QD beads, solution-based sandwich assay, microfluidics, and fluorescence detection with custom software for high-throughput, multiplexed blood-borne pathogen detection. (b) Fluorescence image of a collection of different color emitting, 5.0-μm-diameter polystyrene QD beads suitable for proteomic or genomic assays. (c) Normalized QD emission profiles corresponding to the QD used for the barcodes in (b), all excited using 365-nm light. (d) Sample microfluidic chip, fabricated in PDMS with wells labeled. (Reprinted with permission from Klostranec, J.M., et al., 2007, 2812–8. Copyright 2007 American Chemical Society.)

are coated onto different emitting QD barcodes, the optical signature of the barcode created by using two different emitting QDs (500 and 600 nm) identified the target sequence. After a library of QD barcodes conjugated to capture strands was placed into a vial along with the secondary oligonucleotide–Alexa Fluor 647 conjugate (denoted as SA), they introduced a target sequence into the vial. They showed that the target recognized both the QD barcodes and the SA, thereby assembling them together (Figure 2.16a and b). A positive detection was observed when a fluorescence signal arises from both the QDs inside the microbeads and Alexa Fluor 647 at the same time, by measuring the optical emission of this assembled complex in a flow cytometer.

2.2.5 NOVEL APPLICATIONS OF QDs

Wei et al. [58] studied surface plasmon-coupled emission (SPCE) of semiconductor QDs. They investigated the interaction between propagating surface plasmons (SPs) in silver nanowires (Ag NWs) and excitons generated in QDs [58]. In their study, they synthesized Ag NWs, which were about 100 nm in diameter and a few to tens of

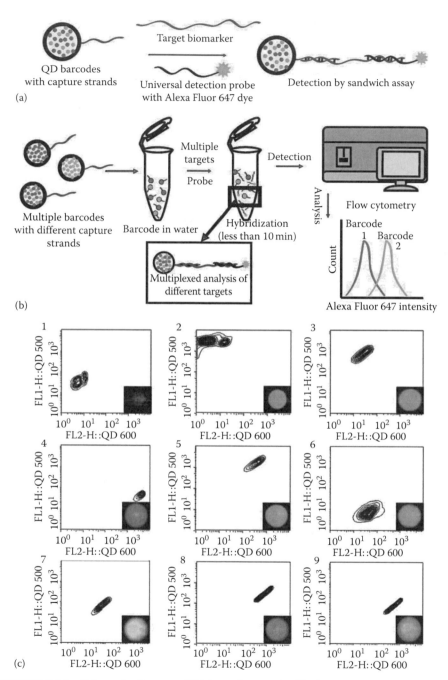

FIGURE 2.16 Schematic diagram of QD barcode assay. (a) The basic principles of detection in direct assay. (b) Flowchart shows the sequential steps involved in the assay. (c) Barcode library showing two-dimensional contour map plots obtained from flow cytometry study. (Reprinted with permission from Giri, S., et al., 2011, 1580–7. Copyright 2011 American Chemical Society.)

micrometers in length with single crystalline structure. Figure 2.17a showed a typical scanning electron microscope (SEM) image of the NWs. Figure 2.17b illustrates the schematics for experimental setup. White light was used as the illuminating source in transmission mode to find the Ag NWs on the sample. A continuous-wave laser at 532 nm was used for wide-field excitation of the QDs, while a mode-locked Ti:sapphire laser centered at 710 nm was used to launch propagating SPs in Ag NWs and excite QDs. The scattered light and fluorescence light from the sample were collected with the same objective and directed to a room-temperature charge-coupled device (CCD) camera for imaging or to a spectrometer with a liquid nitrogen-cooled CCD for spectral measurements. Figure 2.17c illustrated three processes: (1) In the first process (labeled as process I), the propagating SPs couple out as photons at the discontinuities of the NW; (2) the second process (labeled as process II) entails the excitation of QDs near the Ag NWs whose exciton decay can generate

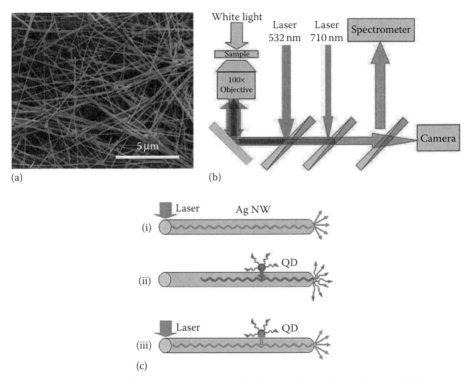

(a)   (b)

(c)

FIGURE 2.17   (a) SEM image of the Ag NWs. (b) Sketch of experimental setup. (c) Schematic illustration of the processes of the studied system. (i) When the 710 nm laser is focused on the NW end, the SPs are launched and propagate in the NW. At the discontinuities of the NW, the propagating SPs couple out as photons. (ii) The excitation of QDs near the Ag NWs whose exciton decay can generate propagating SPs in the NWs. (iii) The third process involves launching the SPs at the discontinuity of NWs, the interactions of the SPs with the QDs which generate excitons, and the radiative decay of excitons which are detected as photons. In the middle of this process, the exciton decay can also transfer its energy into generation of propagating SPs, thus reverting to process (ii). (Reprinted with permission from Wei, H., et al., 2009, 4168–71. Copyright 2009 American Chemical Society.)

propagating SPs in the NWs [59,60]; and (3) in the third process, the exciton decay can also transfer its energy into generation of propagating SPs, thus reverting to process II. Through the study, they showed that propagating SPs can excite excitons, which results in QD emission. They demonstrated that the energy was directly transferred from the propagating SPs to the excitons without converting to photons and the reverse process where the decay of excitons generates SPs [58].

2.3 MEDICAL APPLICATIONS OF QDs

2.3.1 Cancer Diagnosis

Barat et al. [61] demonstrated the biological modification of QDs for detection of target antigens using small bivalent engineered antibody fragments, cys-diabodies. They have devised novel type of bioconjugated QDs known as immunoQdots (iQDs) by thiol-specific oriented coupling of tumor-specific cys-diabodies, at a position away from the antigen-binding site to amino-PEG CdSe/ZnS QDs. They confirmed the specific receptor binding activity of anti-human epidermal growth receptor 2 (HER2) iQD 655 by flow cytometry on HER2-positive and HER2-negative cells. Through the immuno-fluorescence, they also showed the homogeneous surface labeling of the cell membrane with QD 655 conjugate. In addition, they successfully conjugated amino-PEG QD 800 to cys-diabodies specific for HER2, as well as prostate stem cell antigen (PSCA). They showed that simultaneous detection of two tumor antigens on lymph node carcinoma of the prostate (LNCaP)/PSCA prostate cancer cells (which express PSCA and HER2) in culture was possible using two iQDs: anti-HER2 iQD 655 and anti-PSCA iQD 800. Their study suggested that the thiol-specific conjugation method could be used as a general approach for site-specific oriented coupling of cys-diabodies to a wide variety of nanoparticles without disturbing the antigen-binding site and maintaining small size compared to intact antibody.

Because intact monoclonal antibodies are large (150 kDa), smaller antibody fragments would be preferable to intact IgGs (Figure 2.18a) for coupling to QDs [62,63]. It has been known that smaller antibody fragments are superior in their ability to extravasate and penetrate solid tumors *in vivo*, when compared with intact antibodies [64]. Genetically fusing the variable light (VL) and variable heavy (VH) chain domains of a parental antibody through a peptide linker results in the production of a single-chain variable fragment (scFv, 27 kDa), at about one-sixth the size of native antibody, with the same specificity as that of parental intact antibody [65]. As an approach to allow site-specific, thiol-reactive coupling at a site away from the antigen-binding site to a wide variety of agents, cysteine residues at the C-termini of scFv were introduced (Figure 2.18a) [66–69]. To determine whether the anti-HER2 iQD 655 could bind to HER2, HER2-expressing human breast carcinoma MCF7/HER2 cells were incubated with anti-HER2 iQD 655. Their results demonstrated homogeneous surface labeling of the cell membrane with minimal cytoplasmic labeling. With mock-conjugated QD 655, they also observed the minimal nonspecific binding to the cells (Figure 2.19).

Adopting QDs for their excellent brightness, photostability, monodispersity, and fluorescent yield, Gao et al. [70] linked arginine–glycine–aspartic acid (RGD) peptides

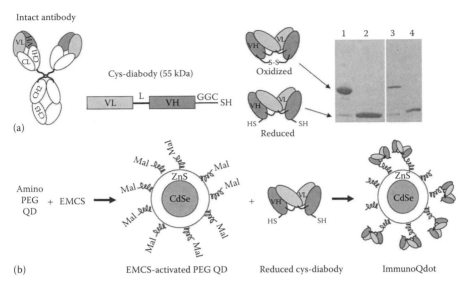

FIGURE 2.18　(a) Schematic drawing of an intact antibody showing variable light (VL) and heavy (VH) chain regions and constant light (CL) and heavy (CH) regions. CH1, CH2, and CH3 indicate three different constant heavy regions. Sodium dodecyl sulfate polyacrylamide gel electrophoresis (SDS-PAGE) of two cys-diabodies: lanes 1 and 2 are oxidized and reduced forms of anti-HER2 cys-diabody; 3 and 4 are oxidized and reduced forms of anti-PSCA cys-diabody. (b) Schematic illustration of the process of conjugating amino-PEG QDs with cys-diabody. EMCS, [*N*-ε-maleimidocaproyloxy] succinimide ester. (Reprinted with permission from Barat, B., et al., 2009, 1474–81. Copyright 2009 American Chemical Society.)

to target QDs specifically to newly formed/forming blood vessels expressing $\alpha v \beta 3$ integrins. They reported on a new type of stable and biocompatible dendron-coated InP/ZnS core/shell QDs as a clinically translatable nanoprobe for molecular imaging applications. Furthermore, the InP/ZnS core/shell QDs are highly interested as a type of promising near-infrared (NIR) fluorescent probes for biomedical applications [27,71]. After the surface coating of InP/ZnS QDs using dendron molecule and the DHLA conjugated to a short PEG ($n = 8$; DHLA-PEG8-COOH) [72], they conjugated RGD peptide dimers (RGD2) with QD710-Dendron through an amide bond to form QD710-Dendron–RGD2 conjugates (Figure 2.20) and tested the receptor-binding specificity. In their research, QD710-Dendron–RGD2 nanoprobe successfully imaged integrin $\alpha v \beta 3$-positive tumors (e.g., SKOV3 tumor) and tumor cells with high specificity.

Figure 2.21 showed that the fluorescent signals derived from both QD710-Dendron–RGD2 and QD710-Dendron appeared in tumors 1 h postinjection (p.i.), and tumors (arrows) were readily distinguished from surrounding tissues after 4 h in both groups. Although the tumor uptake of QD710-Dendron with visible contrast from surrounding tissues indicated the possibility of EPR effect for the suitably small-sized QD710-Dendron [11,73], the tumor fluorescence intensity dramatically decreased over time (Figure 2.21b). However, the tumor contrast was still apparent even after 24 h in the mice injected with QD710-Dendron–RGD2 (Figure 2.21a), suggesting that the highly specific targeting of QD710-Dendron–RGD2 to integrin $\alpha v \beta 3$-positive SKOV3 tumor induced the long-term retention of QDs in the tumor site [74,75].

QD 655   DAPI   Overlay

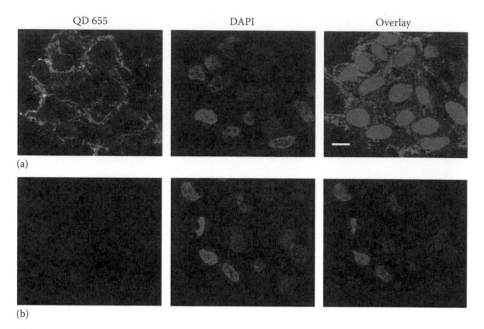

(a)

(b)

FIGURE 2.19 **(See color insert.)** Confocal microscopy images of MCF7/HER2 cells stained with anti-HER2 iQD 655 (a) and mock-conjugated QD 655 (b). Scale bar: 20 μm. (Reprinted with permission from Barat, B., et al., 2009, 1474–81. Copyright 2009 American Chemical Society.)

Kim et al. [76] have demonstrated the applicability of NIR-emitting core/shell/shell $InAs_xP_{1-x}$/InP/ZnSe QDs in a sentinel lymph node (SLN) mapping experiment. The $InAs_xP_{1-x}$-alloyed core has a graded internal composition with increasing arsenic content from the center to the edge of the dots. A first shell of InP leads to a redshift and an increase in quantum yield. The final shell of ZnSe serves to stabilize the dots for applications in aqueous environments, including NIR biomedical fluorescence imaging [77,78]. They used an intraoperative video imaging system that superimposes NIR fluorescence on a display of visible light anatomy. When injected intradermally into the paw of a mouse, the small amount and low concentration of NIR QDs injected could not be seen on the color video images (Figure 2.22a). However, the fluorescence image (Figure 2.22b and e) revealed the fine detail of lymphatic flow from the injection site to the SLN. In their research, injected QDs entered the lymphatics and migrated within 1 min to the sentinel node, which was easily detected through the skin using our intraoperative imaging system (Figure 2.22).

2.3.2 CANCER THERAPY

Weng et al. [79] describe the synthesis, biophysical characterization, tumor cell-selective internalization, and anticancer drug delivery of QD-conjugated immunoliposome (IL)-based nanoparticles. They have incorporated the unique optical properties of luminescent QDs into ILs for cancer diagnosis and treatment. Doxorubicin-loaded QD-ILs showed efficient anticancer activity, while no cytotoxicity was observed

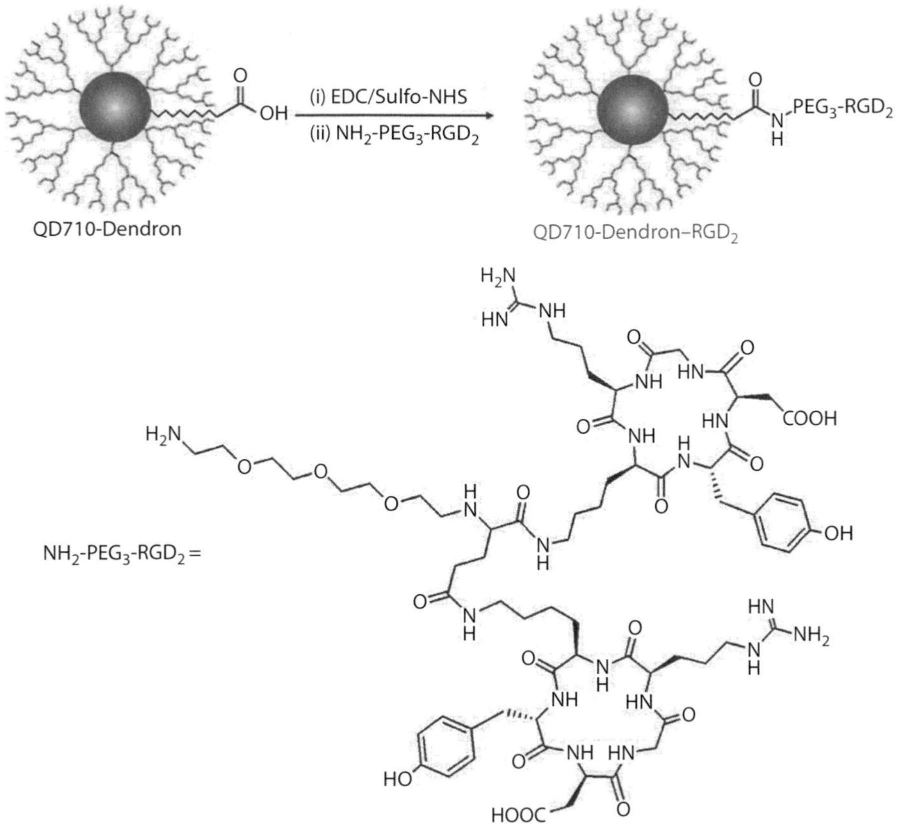

FIGURE 2.20 Structure and synthesis of QD710-Dendron–RGD2 conjugate. QD710-Dendron with carboxylate terminal group was conjugated with RGD dimer by carbodiimide coupling. (Reprinted with permission from Gao, J., et al., 2012, 281–6. Copyright 2012 American Chemical Society.)

for QD-ILs without chemotherapeutic payload [79]. Weng et al. hypothesized that conjugation of QDs to ILs would represent a feasible and novel strategy for QD-based cellular and *in vivo* tumor imaging, including integration of targeting, reporting, and drug delivery. Their design for QD-ILs was schematically illustrated in Figure 2.23. ILs against HER2(18, 19) and EGFR(20, 21) could efficiently deliver drugs to tumor cells and are in development for clinical testing [80–83].

Fluorescence signals were readily detected at the tumor site as well as in mononuclear phagocytic system (MPS) organs (24 h following injection) that were known to mediate liposome clearance (Figure 2.24a). Tumor fluorescence reached a plateau after 24 h, with up to 18% ± 5% of total body fluorescence localizing to the tumor region. When comparing tumor accumulation of targeted nanoparticles with nontargeted nanoparticles, both versions of nanoparticles showed highly efficient tumor accumulation, with 14.2% ± 3.7% and 13.7% ± 2.4%, respectively, of the total body fluorescence within the tumor being at 24 h. Thus, tumor accumulation was extremely high and comparable for both targeted and nontargeted nanoparticles.

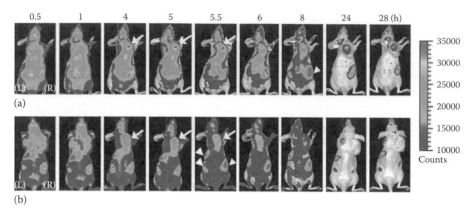

FIGURE 2.21   (See color insert.) *In vivo* NIR fluorescence imaging. The dorsal images of SKOV3 tumor-bearing (arrows) mice (L, left side; R, right side) injected with QD710-Dendorn–RGD2 (200 pmol) (a) and QD710-Dendron (200 pmol) (b) at 0.5, 1, 4, 5, 5.5, 6, 8, 24, and 28 h, respectively. The incidental high fluorescent signals in other body parts (arrowheads) might have originated from regular rodent food in stomach and feces in intestine. (Reprinted with permission from Gao, J., et al., 2012, 281–6. Copyright 2012 American Chemical Society.)

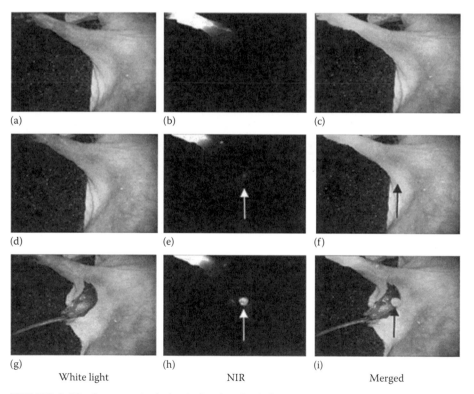

FIGURE 2.22   Images of p.i. (a–c), 3 min p.i. (d–f), and postresection (g–i) using white light, NIR fluorescence, and color/NIR merge, respectively. (Reprinted with permission from Kim, S.-W., et al., 2005, 10526–32. Copyright 2005 American Chemical Society.)

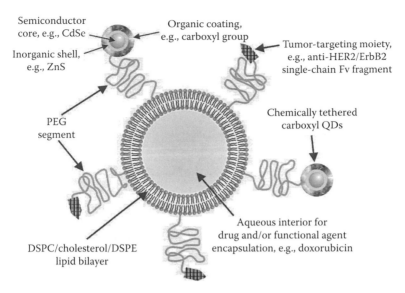

FIGURE 2.23 Schematic showing the structure of a QD-IL nanoparticle. DSPC, distearylphosphatidylcholine; DSPE, distearylphosphatidylethanolamine. (Reprinted with permission from Weng, K.C., et al., 2008, 2851–7. Copyright 2008 American Chemical Society.)

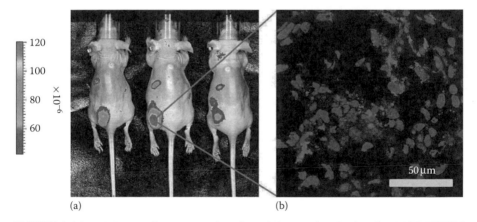

(a)   (b)

FIGURE 2.24 (a) *In vivo* fluorescence imaging of three nude mice bearing MCF-7/HER2 xenografts implanted in the lower back 30 h after intravenous injection with anti-HER2 QD-ILs. (b) A 5-μm section cut from frozen tumor tissues harvested at 48 h p.i. and examined by confocal microscopy by a 63× oil immersion objective (image size, 146 × 146 μm). QD-ILs are likely internalized to the cytosol of MCF-7/HER2 cells. (Reprinted with permission from Weng, K.C., et al., 2008, 2851–7. Copyright 2008 American Chemical Society.)

Tissue sections of tumors collected 48 h p.i. were examined by confocal microscopy (Figure 2.24b). In this research, QD-ILs showed extensive accumulation within tumor tissue and intracellularly within tumor cells [79].

Cho et al. [84] have developed a multifunctional nanocarrier system for medical diagnosis and treatment. Their unique system is composed of several key components,

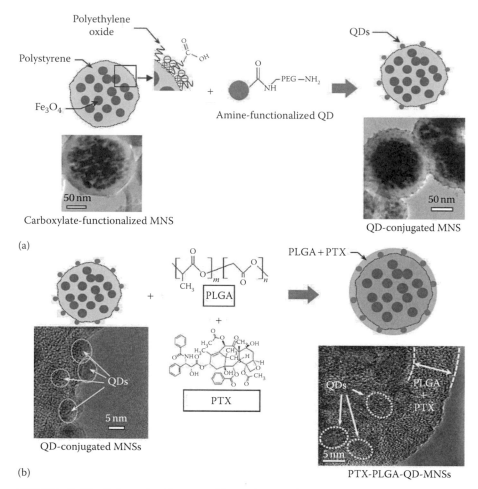

FIGURE 2.25 Schematic diagrams illustrating surface functionalization of MNSs: (a) conjugation of amine-functionalized QDs to the surface of carboxylate-functionalized MNSs using conventional *N*-hydroxysuccinimide (NHS)/EDC coupling method; (b) PTX loading using a thin PLGA coat on the surface of QD-MNSs. (Reprinted with permission from Cho, H.-S., et al., 2010, 5398–404. Copyright 2010 American Chemical Society.)

namely, fluorescent superparamagnetic nanoparticles for multimodal imaging and hyperthermia, tumor-specific antibodies for cell targeting, and anticancer drugs for localized treatment. The surface modification can be visualized in Figure 2.25a by a change in the smooth surface structure of the original magnetic nanospheres (MNSs) [transmission electron microscopy (TEM) image on the left] to a dark spotted, ruffled surface (TEM image on the right) after QD conjugation. Surface-immobilized QDs are more clearly identified by their distinctive lattice structures seen in the high-resolution TEM (HRTEM; Figure 2.25b) micrographs. In this study, they selected QDs with a visible emission wavelength of 655 nm for the *in vitro* cell imaging experiments, and QDs with an NIR emission wavelength of 800 nm for the *in vivo* and *ex vivo* imaging. After conjugation of QDs to MNSs, paclitaxel (PTX) was incorporated into the fluorescent nanocarrier using a drug-loaded poly(lactic-*co*-glycolic acid) (PLGA)-coating layer (PTX-PLGA-QD-MNSs).

Charron et al. [85] have found that the energy transfer between QDs and the molecular photosensitizer is the rate-determining step for the production of singlet oxygen and that the cell viabilities of the hybrid and free photosensitizer are comparable. Since QDs are inorganic nanocrystals, their optical properties are superior to organic fluorophores in regard to their absorption cross section, chemical and optical stability, and tenability, QDs are potentially interesting candidates as photosensitizers or "light antennas" for photodynamic therapy (PDT) [86]. PDT is a relatively new method for cancer treatment, in which tumor cells are destroyed by light-induced, local production of a reactive oxygen species (ROS), such as singlet oxygen ($^1O_2$) [87–90]. The ROS is generated by a photosensitizer, which has to be brought in close proximity to the tumor cells and is usually administered systemically. Several groups have found that QDs by themselves do not produce a detectable amount of singlet oxygen, while others reported that QDs produce singlet oxygen with low quantum yields of up to 0.05 [91,92]. Charron et al. [85] have coupled two types (sizes) of less-toxic InP/ZnS QDs to the photosensitizer chlorin e6. Figure 2.26 shows a diagram of the whole system with the different pathways for energy transfer being indicated. They have also assessed the PDT efficacy of the QD/chlorin e6 hybrids against a breast cancer (MDA-MB-231) cell line using a colorimetric 3-(4,5-dimethylthiazol-2yl)-2,5-diphenyltetrazolium bromide (MTT) assay. Through systematic analysis, they showed that the energy transfer between QDs and photosensitizers is a "bottleneck," which suggests that a better chemical design of the QD/photosensitizer hybrids in future embodiments is essential [85].

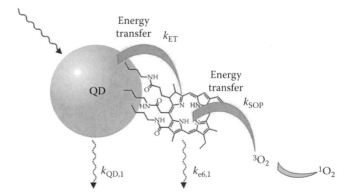

FIGURE 2.26 Energy transfer pathways in QD/chlorin e6 hybrids. (1) No energy transfer (QD luminescence). (2) Energy transfer from QD to chlorin e6 (chlorin e6 luminescence). (3) Energy transfer from QD to chlorin e6 to oxygen. k_{ET} denotes the rate constant for the energy transfer from QD to chlorin e6, k_{SOP} from chlorin e6 to oxygen, and $k_{QD,1}$ and $k_{e6,1}$ the luminescence of QD and chlorin e6. (Reprinted with permission from Charron, G., et al., 2012, 9334–42. Copyright 2012 American Chemical Society.)

2.3.3 OTHER APPLICATIONS (MULTIMODAL IMAGING)

Lim et al. [93] described the fabrication of multispectrally encoded nanoprobes, perfluorocarbon (PFC)/QD nanocomposite emulsions, which could provide both multispectral magnetic resonance (MR) and multicolor optical imaging modalities. They exploited the combination of the multispectral MR properties of four different PFC materials and the multicolor emission properties of three different colored CdSe/ZnS QDs. Scheme 2.2 shows a schematic illustration of the fabrication of the engineered PFC/QD nanocomposite emulsions comprising of PFC liquids containing fluorescent QDs and phospholipids. Multispectral MR signals were distinguishable by using different types of PFC materials with distinct MR spectra. As QD emissions are tunable for their sizes and chemical compositions, the multicolor QDs with minimum spectral overlaps could be incorporated into the PFC materials for wavelength tuning. To increase the compatibility of hydrophobic QDs with PFC, which have both hydrophobic and lipophobic properties, the coated QDs with hydrophobic ligands were exchanged with $1H,1H,2H,2H$-perfluorooctanethiol. Three different colored QDs were then dispersed into four different PFC materials to have distinguishable ^{19}F-based MR spectra. Finally, the PFC liquids containing QDs were emulsified into aqueous solutions using phospholipids and high shear force.

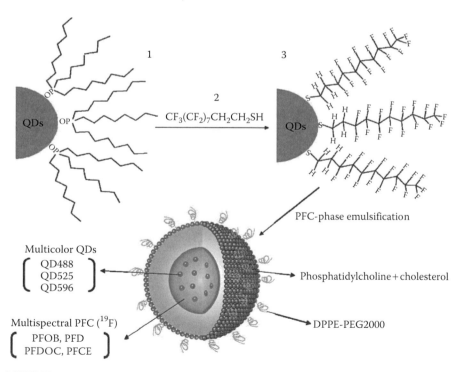

SCHEME 2.2 (See color insert.) Schematic illustration of the preparation of bimodal imaging nanoprobes having both ^{19}F-based multispectral MR and QD-based multicolor optical imaging capabilities. (Reprinted with permission from Lim, Y.T., et al., 2009, 17145–54. Copyright 2009 American Chemical Society.)

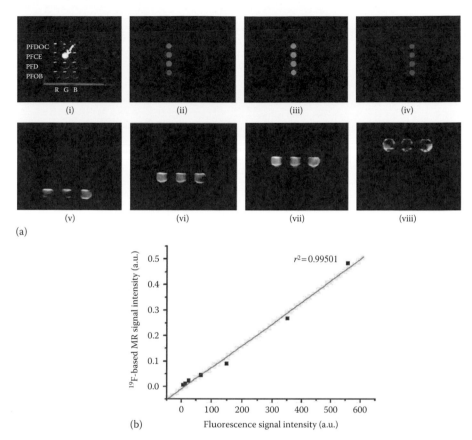

(a)

(b)

FIGURE 2.27 (a) Multicolor fluorescence (as pseudo black and white color by filter selection) (ii–iv) and resonance-selective ^{19}F MR (v–viii) detection of PFC/[CdSe/ZnS QDs] nanocomposite emulsions: (i) black and white image, pseudo color images obtained by using (ii) red, (iii) green, and (iv) blue filters, resonance-selective MR images for (v) PFOB, (vi) PFD, (vii) PFCE, and (viii) PFDOC. (b) Calibration curve representing the correlation between ^{19}F-based MR signals and fluorescence intensity. (Reprinted with permission from Lim, Y.T., et al., 2009, 17145–54. Copyright 2009 American Chemical Society.)

To determine whether the PFC/QD nanocomposite emulsions could be used for simultaneous detections using multispectral MR and multicolor optical imaging techniques, they prepared 12 spots corresponding to all of the permutations of the four different PFC liquids and three different colored QDs [Figure 2.27a(i)]. The pseudo color images (presented by black and white color) for blue, green, and red emissions of QDs dispersed in the four different PFCs [perfluorooctylbromide (PFOB), perfluoro-decalin (PFD), perfluoro-15-crown-5 ether (PFCE), and 1,8-dichloroperfluorooctane (PFDOC)] were selectively captured using appropriate wavelength optical filters; each independent fluorescence signal was shown as pseudo black and white images in Figure 2.27a (ii and iv). In each case, the desired emission was selectively acquired from the four different PFC/[CdSe/ZnS QDs] nanocomposite emulsions using the appropriate optical filter. The MR signals were discriminated solely on the basis PFC species (i.e., the resonance frequency) used in nanocomposite emulsions. Their results indicated that any specific spot point in the 12-spot array shown in Figure 2.27a could be readily designated by simultaneous tuning of the optical filter and the MR frequency. For example, the spot indicated by the white arrow in Figure 2.27a(i) could be easily selected using a green optical filter and the MR frequency of PFCE. To assess the correlation between ^{19}F-based MR signal and fluorescence intensity, a calibration curve was obtained from serial dilutions of PFD/ [CdSe/ZnS (596 nm) QDs] nanocomposites. The plot of ^{19}F-based MR signal intensity versus fluorescence intensity indicated a linear correlation with $r^2 = 0.99501$ (Figure 2.27b).

Based on *in vitro* experimental data, the labeled immune cells were subcutaneously injected into the different body parts of a mouse (Figure 2.28a). Using an optical filter (525WB20), green fluorescence signals were selectively detected at point A, where macrophage cells labeled with PFDOC/[CdSe/ZnS (525 nm) QDs] were injected (Figure 2.28b). After changing the optical filter with red filter (600WB20), red fluorescence signals were also detected at points B and C, where T cells labeled with PFDOC/[CdSe/ZnS (596 nm) QDs] and dendritic cells labeled with PFOB/ [CdSe/ZnS (596 nm) QDs] were injected, respectively (Figure 2.28c). When the magnetic excitation resonance frequency was matched with that of PFDOC, selective MR images were generated at points A and B where the macrophage cells labeled with PFDOC/[CdSe/ZnS (525 nm) QDs] and T cells labeled with PFDOC/[CdSe/ ZnS (596 nm) QDs] were injected, respectively (Figure 2.28e). Distinct MR image was also observed at point C where the dendritic cells labeled with PFOB/[CdSe/ZnS (596 nm) QDs] were injected (Figure 2.28f), with the matched resonance frequency of PFOB. While the ^{1}H-based MR image provides a whole body image, the ^{19}F-based MR image shows the only signals generated from the injected immune cells labeled with PFC/QD nanocomposite emulsions.

Kim et al. [94] described an easy but robust chemical strategy to synthesize high-performance MR/NIR multimodal imaging nanoprobes. A schematic representation for the facile synthesis of polyelectrolyte nanocomposites as high-performance MR/NIR dual-modality molecular imaging contrast agents is shown in Scheme 2.3. Negatively charged polyelectrolytes containing a carboxyl group could be used for the convenient phase transfer of magnetic nanoparticles ($MnFe_2O_4$) dispersed in organic solvents into aqueous solutions and could facilitate further ionic gelation with positively charged polyelectrolytes. During the ionic gelation process, $MnFe_2O_4$ nanoparticulate satellites could be encapsulated in the ionic gel nanocomplex, which could induce synergistic magnetism and result in huge T_2 relaxivity (r_2). The positively charged outer surface could be assembled with other negatively charged NIR-emitting fluorescent nanocrystals and could induce the highly efficient delivery of the magnetofluorescent polyelectrolyte nanocomposites (MagFL-PENs) into cancer cells [94].

Figure 2.29a and b shows the high-performance capability of the MagFL-PEN in HeLa cell labeling. Concerning MR performance, the cell-labeling efficiency of MagFL-PEN was compared with that of the commercialized MR contrast agent, Resovist. As shown in Figure 2.29a, the T_2-shortening effect in the MagFL-PEN-labeled cells (i and ii) was more dominant than that in Resovist-labeled cells (iii and iv). Note that the enhancement of negative contrast (i.e., darkening effect) of

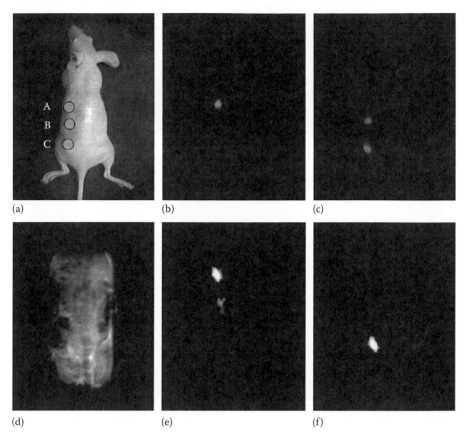

(a)   (b)   (c)

(d)   (e)   (f)

FIGURE 2.28 *In vivo* detection. (a) Black and white image of the mouse injected with three different types of immune cells (5×106 to 1×107 cells/mL) labeled with PFC/[CdSe/ZnS QDs] nanocomposite emulsions: (A) macrophage cells labeled with PFDOC/[CdSe/ZnS (525 nm) QDs]; (B) T cells labeled with PFDOC/[CdSe/ZnS (596 nm) QDs]; and (C) dendritic cells labeled with PFOB/[CdSe/ZnS (596 nm) QDs]; (b) image obtained by using a green filter (525WB20); (c) image obtained by using a red filter (600WB20); (d) ^{1}H MR image; (e) PFDOC-resonance selective MR image; and (f) PFOB-resonance selective MR image. (Reprinted with permission from Lim, Y.T., et al., 2009, 17145–54. Copyright 2009 American Chemical Society.)

MagFL-PEN at 2 µg/mL concentration was similar to that of Resovist at 20 µg/mL concentration. Considering that about 100 µg Fe/mL of Resovist is usually used for labeling cells in the clinical fields, the MagFL-PEN, even at a concentration of Fe (and Mn) content diluted by 50 times, can generate the similar MR contrast enhancement compared to Resovist. We also employed flow cytometry to quantify the labeling efficiency of HeLa cells by the MagFL-PEN or the QD800 (COOH) themselves. There was no distinct increase in QD800 (COOH) emissions over the background in cells treated with QD800 (COOH) alone [Figure 2.29b(i)], The enhancement of negative contrast of MagFL-PEN at 2 µg/mL concentration was similar to that of Resovist at 20 µg/mL concentration. The NIR fluorescence microscopy images

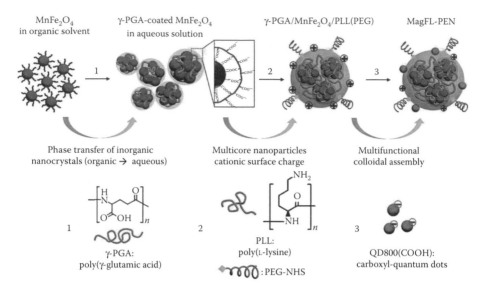

SCHEME 2.3   Schematic illustration of the facile fabrication of MR/NIR multimodal imaging nanoprobes based on MagFL-PENs via electrostatic assembly between polyelectrolytes and functional colloidal nanoparticles. (Reprinted with permission from Kim, H.M., et al., 2011, 8230–40. Copyright 2011 American Chemical Society.)

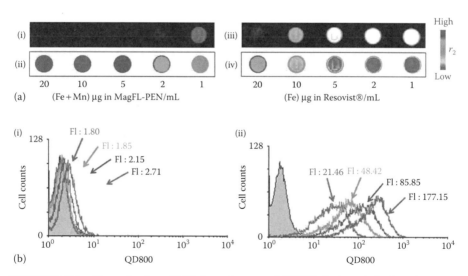

FIGURE 2.29   (See color insert.) High-performance MR/NIR dual-modality imaging properties of MagFL-PEN. (a) T_2-weighted MR images of HeLa cells treated with MagFL-PEN (i and ii) and Resovist (iii and iv); parts (i) and (iii) are in white and black and (ii) and (iv) in pseudo color. (b) Fluorescence-activated cell sorting (FACS) analysis of HeLa cells labeled with various concentrations of QD800 (COOH) and MagFL-PEN [i, QD800 (COOH); ii, MagFL-PEN] at 12.5 (red), 25 (green), 50 (blue), and 100 pM (purple). (Reprinted with permission from Kim, H.M., et al., 2011, 8230–40. Copyright 2011 American Chemical Society.)

of the MagFL-PEN-labeled cells even at 12.5 pM were able to be clearly observed. The labeling efficiency of MagFL-PEN was approximately 65-fold higher compared to that of the commercialized fluorescent nanocrystals, only after a 3-h incubation period, even at the test concentration (100 pM).

ACKNOWLEDGMENTS

This study was financially supported by research fund of Chungnam National University in 2011.

REFERENCES

1. Goldstein, A.N., Echer, C.M., and Alivisatos, A.P. (1992) Melting in semiconductor nanocrystals. *Science*, 256, 1425–7.
2. Alivisatos, A.P. (1996) Semiconductor clusters, nanocrystals, and quantum dots. *Science*, 271, 933–7.
3. Zhong, X., Han, M., Dong, Z., White, T.J., and Knoll, W. (2003) Composition-tunable $Zn_x Cd_{1-x}Se$ nanocrystals with high luminescence and stability. *Journal of the American Chemical Society*, 125, 8589–94.
4. Kim, S., Fisher, B., Eisler, H.-J., and Bawendi, M. (2003) Type II quantum dots: CdTe/CdSe(core/shell) and CdSe/ZnTe(core/shell) heterostructures. *Journal of the American Chemical Society*, 125, 11466–7.
5. Zhong, X., Feng, Y., Knoll, W., and Han, M. (2003) Alloyed $Zn_xCd_{1-x}S$ nanocrystals with highly narrow luminescence spectral width. *Journal of the American Chemical Society*, 125, 13559–63.
6. Pietryga, J.M., Schaller, R.D., Werder, D., Stewart, M.H., Klimov, V.I., and Hollingsworth, J.A. (2004) Pushing the band gap envelope: Mid-infrared emitting colloidal PbSe quantum dots. *Journal of the American Chemical Society*, 126, 11752–3.
7. Efros, A.L. and Rosen, M. (2000) The electronic structure of semiconductor nanocrystals. *Annual Review of Materials Science*, 30, 475–521.
8. Leatherdale, C.A., Woo, W.-K., Mikulec, F.V., and Bawendi, M.G. (2002) On the absorption cross section of CdSe nanocrystal quantum dots. *The Journal of Physical Chemistry B*, 106, 7619–22.
9. Gao, X., Yang, L., Petros, J.A., Marshall, F.F., Simons, J.W., and Nie, S. (2005) In vivo molecular and cellular imaging with quantum dots. *Current Opinion in Biotechnology*, 16, 63–72.
10. Dahan, M., Laurence, T., Pinaud, F., Chemla, D.S., Alivisatos, A.P., Sauer, M., and Weiss, S. (2001) Time-gated biological imaging by use of colloidal quantum dots. *Optics Letters*, 26, 825–7.
11. Gao, X., Cui, Y., Levenson, R.M., Chung, L.W., and Nie, S. (2004) In vivo cancer targeting and imaging with semiconductor quantum dots. *Nature Biotechnology*, 22, 969–76.
12. Maruvada, P., Wang, W., Wagner, P.D., and Srivastava, S. (2005) Biomarkers in molecular medicine: Cancer detection and diagnosis. *Biotechniques*, 38, S9–S15.
13. Kortan, A.R., Hull, R., Opila, R.L., Bawendi, M.G., Steigerwald, M.L., Carroll, P.J., and Brus, L.E. (1990) Nucleation and growth of CdSe on ZnS quantum crystallite seeds, and vice versa, in inverse micelle media. *Journal of the American Chemical Society*, 112, 1327–32.
14. Murray, C.B., Norris, D.J., and Bawendi, M.G. (1993) Synthesis and characterization of nearly monodisperse CdE (E = S, Se, Te) semiconductor nanocrystallites. *Journal of the American Chemical Society*, 115, 8706–15.

15. Talapin, D.V., Rogach, A.L., Komowski, A., Haase, M., and Weller, H. (2001) Highly luminescent monodisperse CdSe and CdSe/ZnS nanocrystals synthesized in a hexadecylamine–trioctylphosphine oxide–trioctylphospine mixture. *Nano Letters*, 1, 207–11.
16. Yang, H. and Holloway, P.H. (2004) Efficient and photostable ZnS-passivated CdS:Mn luminescent nanocrystals. *Advanced Functional Materials*, 14, 152–6.
17. Hines, M.A. and Guyot-Sionnest, P. (1996) Synthesis and characterization of strongly luminescing ZnS-capped CdSe nanocrystals. *The Journal of Physical Chemistry*, 100, 468–71.
18. Michalet, X., Pinaud, F.F., Bentolila, L.A., Tsay, J.M., Doose, S., Li, J.J., Sundaresan, G., Wu, A.M., Gambhir, S.S., and Weiss, S. (2005) Quantum dots for live cells, in vivo imaging, and diagnostics. *Science*, 307, 538–44.
19. Pellegrino, T., Manna, L., Kudera, S., Liedl, T., Koktysh, D., Rogach, A.L., Keller, S., Raldler, J., Natile, G., and Parak, W.J. (2004) Hydrophobic nanocrystals coated with an amphiphilic polymer shell: A general route to water soluble nanocrystals. *Nano Letters*, 4, 703–7.
20. Chan, W.C.W. and Nie, S. (1998) Quantum dot bioconjugates for ultrasensitive nonisotopic detection. *Science*, 281, 2016–18.
21. Pathak, S., Choi, S.-K., Arnheim, N., and Thompson, M.E. (2001) Hydroxylated quantum dots as luminescent probes for in situ hybridization. *Journal of the American Chemical Society*, 123, 4103–4.
22. Wu, X., Liu, H., Liu, J., Haley, K.N., Treadway, J.A., Larson, J.P., Ge, N., Peale, F., and Bruchez, M.P. (2003) Immunofluorescent labeling of cancer marker Her2 and other cellular targets with semiconductor quantum dots. *Nature Biotechnology*, 21, 41–6.
23. Dubertret, B., Skourides, P., Norris, D.J., Noireaux, V., Brivanlou, A.H., and Libchaber, A. (2002) In vivo imaging of quantum dots encapsulated in phospholipid micelles. *Science*, 298, 1759–62.
24. Hildebrandt, N. (2011) Biofunctional quantum dots: Controlled conjugation for multiplexed biosensors. *ACS Nano*, 5, 5286–90.
25. Algar, W.R., Prasuhn, D.E., Stewart, M.H., Jennings, T.L., Blanco-Canosa, J.B., Dawson, P.E., and Medintz, I.L. (2011) The controlled display of biomolecules on nanoparticles: A challenge suited to bioorthogonal chemistry. *Bioconjugate Chemistry*, 22, 825–58.
26. Lei, Y., Tang, H., Yao, L., Yu, R., Feng, M., and Zou, B. (2008) Applications of mesenchymal stem cells labeled with tat peptide conjugated quantum dots to cell tracking in mouse body. *Bioconjugate Chemistry*, 19, 421–7.
27. Yong, K.-T., Ding, H., Roy, I., Law, W.-C., Bergey, E.J., Maitra, A., and Prasad, P.N. (2009) Imaging pancreatic cancer using bioconjugated InP quantum dots. *ACS Nano*, 3, 502–10.
28. Nichols, L.S., Ashfaq, R., and Iacobuzio-Donahue, C.A. (2004) Claudin 4 protein expression in primary and metastatic pancreatic cancer: Support for use as a therapeutic target. *American Journal of Clinical Pathology*, 121, 226–30.
29. Argani, P., Rosty, C., Reiter, R.E., Wilentz, R.E., Murugesan, S.R., Leach, S.D., Ryu, B., et al. (2001) Discovery of new markers of cancer through serial analysis of gene expression: Prostate stem cell antigen is overexpressed in pancreatic adenocarcinoma. *Cancer Research*, 61, 4320–4.
30. Argani, P., Iacobuzio-Donahue, C., Ryu, B., Rosty, C., Goggins, M., Wilentz, R.E., Murugesan, S.R., et al. (2001) Mesothelin is overexpressed in the vast majority of ductal adenocarcinomas of the pancreas: Identification of a new pancreatic cancer marker by serial analysis of gene expression (SAGE). *Clinical Cancer Research*, 7, 3862–8.
31. Le Gac, S., Vermes, I., and van den Berg, A. (2006) Quantum dots based probes conjugated to Annexin V for photostable apoptosis detection and imaging. *Nano Letters*, 6, 1863–9.

32. Fadok, V.A., Voelker, D.R., Campbell, P.A., Cohen, J.J., Bratton, D.L., and Henson, P.M. (1992) Exposure of phosphatidylserine on the surface of apoptotic lymphocytes triggers specific recognition and removal by macrophages. *Journal of Immunology*, 148, 2207–16.

33. Bayles, A.R., Chahal, H.S., Chahal, D.S., Goldbeck, C.P., Cohen, B.E., and Helms, B.A. (2010) Rapid cytosolic delivery of luminescent nanocrystals in live cells with endosome-disrupting polymer colloids. *Nano Letters*, 10, 4086–92.

34. Kim, B.Y.S., Jiang, W., Oreopoulos, J., Yip, C.M., Rutka, J.T., and Chan, W.C.W. (2008) Biodegradable quantum dot nanocomposites enable live cell labeling and imaging of cytoplasmic targets. *Nano Letters*, 8, 3887–92.

35. Zhang, J., Campbell, R.E., Ting, A.Y., and Tsien, R.Y. (2003) Creating new fluorescent probes for cell biology. *Nature Reviews Molecular Cell Biology*, 3, 906–18.

36. Choi, Y., Kim, K., Hong, S., Kim, H., Kwon, Y.-J., and Song, R. (2011) Intracellular protein target detection by quantum dots optimized for live cell imaging. *Bioconjugate Chemistry*, 22, 1576–86.

37. Lee, J., Choi, Y., Kim, K., Hong, S., Park, H.-Y., Lee, T., Cheon, G.J., and Song, R. (2010) Characterization and cancer cell specific binding properties of anti-EGFR. *Bioconjugate Chemistry*, 21, 940–6.

38. Mendelsohn, J. (2002) Targeting the epidermal growth factor receptor for cancer therapy. *Journal of Clinical Oncology*, 20, 1–13.

39. Liu, A., Peng, S., Soo, J.C., Kuang, M., Chen, P., and Duan, H. (2011) Quantum dots with phenylboronic acid tags for specific labeling. *Analytical Chemistry*, 83, 1124–30.

40. Chen, X. and Varki, A. (2010) Advances in the biology and chemistry of sialic acids. *ACS Chemical Biology*, 5, 163–76.

41. Schauer, R. (2000) Achievements and challenges of sialic acid research. *Glycoconjugate Journal*, 17, 485–99.

42. Hahn, M.A., Tabb, J.S., and Krauss, T.D. (2005) Detection of single bacterial pathogens with semiconductor quantum dots. *Analytical Chemistry*, 77, 4861–9.

43. Delehanty, J.B., Bradburne, C.E., Susumu, K., Boeneman, K., Mei, B.C., Farrell, D., Blanco-Canosa, J.B., et al. (2011) Spatiotemporal multicolor labeling of individual cells using peptide-functionalized quantum dots and mixed delivery. *Journal of the American Chemical Society*, 133, 10482–9.

44. Giepmans, B.N., Adams, S.R., Ellisman, M.H., and Tsien, R.Y. (2006) The fluorescent toolbox for assessing protein location and function. *Science*, 312, 217–24.

45. Dieterich, D.C. (2010) Chemical reporters for the illumination of protein and cell dynamics. *Current Opinion in Neurobiology*, 21, 623–30.

46. Suzuki, T., Matsuzaki, T., Hagiwara, H., Aoki, T., and Takata, K. (2007) Recent advances in fluorescent labeling techniques for fluorescence microscopy. *Acta Histochemica et Cytochemica*, 40, 131–7.

47. Tsien, R.Y. and Miyawaki, A. (1998) Seeing the machinery of live cells. *Science*, 280, 1954–5.

48. Ghazani, A.A., Lee, J.A., Klostranec, J., Xiang, Q., Dacosta, R.S., Wilson, B.C., Tsao, M.S., and Chan, W.C.W. (2006) High throughput quantification of protein expression of cancer antigens in tissue microarray using quantum dot nanocrystals. *Nano Letters*, 6, 2881–6.

49. Klostranec, J.M., Xiang, Q., Farcas, G.A., Lee, J.A., Rhee, A., Lafferty, E.I., Perrault, S.D., Kain, K.C., and Chan, W.C.W. (2007) Convergence of quantum dot barcodes with microfluidics and signal processing for multiplexed high-throughput infectious disease diagnostics. *Nano Letters*, 7, 2812–18.

50. Fauci, A.S., Mavilio, D., and Kottilil, S. (2005) NK cells in HIV infection: Paradigm for protection or targets for ambush. *Nature Reviews Immunology*, 5, 835–43.

51. Lai, C.L., Ratziu, V., Yuen, M.F., and Poynard, T. (2003) Viral hepatitis B. *The Lancet*, 362, 2089–94.
52. Poynard, T., Yuen, M., Ratziu, V., and Lai, C. (2003) Viral hepatitis C. *The Lancet*, 362, 2095–100.
53. Erickson, D., Sinton, D., and Li, D. (2004) A miniaturized high-voltage integrated power supply for portable microfluidic applications. *Lab on a Chip*, 4, 87–90.
54. Giri, S., Sykes, E.A., Jennings, T.L., and Chan, W.C.W. (2011) Rapid screening of genetic biomarkers of infectious agents using quantum dot barcodes. *ACS Nano*, 5, 1580–7.
55. Hauck, T.S., Giri, S., Gao, Y., and Chan, W.C.W. (2010) Nanotechnology diagnostics for infectious diseases prevalent in developing countries. *Advanced Drug Delivery Reviews*, 62, 438–48.
56. Lopez, A.D., Mathers, C.D., Ezzati, M., Jamison, D.T., and Murray, C.J.L. (2006) Global and regional burden of disease and risk factors, 2001: Systematic analysis of population health data. *The Lancet*, 367, 1747–57.
57. Hufnagel, L., Brockmann, D., and Geisel, T. (2004) Forecast and control of epidemics in a globalized world. *Proceedings of the National Academy of Sciences of the United States of America*, 101, 15124–9.
58. Wei, H., Ratchford, D., Li, X., Xu, H., and Shih, C.-K. (2009) Propagating surface plasmon induced photon emission from quantum dots. *Nano Letters*, 9, 4168–71.
59. Fedutik, Y., Temnov, V.V., Schöps, O., and Woggon, U. (2007) Exciton-plasmon-photon conversion in plasmonic nanostructures. *Physical Review Letters*, 99, 136802–5.
60. Akimov, A.V., Mukherjee, A., Yu, C.L., Chang, D.E., Zibrov, A.S., Hemmer, P.R., Park, H., and Lukin, M.D. (2007) Generation of single optical plasmons in metallic nanowires coupled to quantum dots. *Nature*, 450, 402–6.
61. Barat, B., Sirk, S.J., McCabe, K.E., Li, J., Lepin, E.J., Remenyi, R., Koh, A.L., et al. (2009) Cys-diabody quantum dot conjugates (immunoQdots) for cancer marker. *Bioconjugate Chemistry*, 20, 1474–81.
62. Wu, A.M. and Senter, P.D. (2005) Arming antibodies: Prospects and challenges for immunoconjugates. *Nature Biotechnology*, 23, 1137–46.
63. Kenanova, V. and Wu, A.M. (2006) Tailoring antibodies for radionuclide delivery. *Expert Opinion on Drug Delivery*, 3, 53–70.
64. Yokota, T., Milenic, D.E., Whitlow, M., and Schlom, J. (1992) Rapid tumor penetration of a single-chain Fv and comparison with other immunoglobulin forms. *Cancer Research*, 52, 3402–8.
65. Holliger, P., Prospero, T., and Winter, G. (1993) "Diabodies": Small bivalent and bispecific antibody fragments. *Proceedings of the National Academy of Sciences of the United States of America*, 90, 6444–8.
66. Li, L., Olafsen, T., Anderson, A.L., Wu, A., Raubitschek, A.A., and Shively, J.E. (2002) Reduction of kidney uptake in radiometal labeled peptide linkers conjugated to recombinant antibody fragments. Site-specific conjugation of DOTA-peptides to a Cys-diabody. *Bioconjugate Chemistry*, 13, 985–95.
67. Olafsen, T., Cheung, C.W., Yazaki, P.J., Li, L., Sundaresan, G., Gambhir, S.S., Sherman, M.A., et al. (2004) Covalent disulfide-linked anti-CEA diabody allows site-specific conjugation and radiolabeling for tumor targeting applications. *Protein Engineering Design and Selection*, 17, 21–7.
68. Albrecht, H., Burke, P.A., Natarajan, A., Xiong, C.Y., Kalicinsky, M., DeNardo, G.L., and DeNardo, S.J. (2004) Production of soluble ScFvs with C-terminal-free thiol for site-specific conjugation or stable dimeric ScFvs on demand. *Bioconjugate Chemistry*, 15, 16–26.
69. Sirk, S.J., Olafsen, T., Barat, B., Bauer, K.B., and Wu, A.M. (2008) Site-specific, thiol-mediated conjugation of fluorescent probes to cysteine-modified diabodies targeting CD20 or HER2. *Bioconjugate Chemistry*, 19, 2527–34.

70. Gao, J., Chen, K., Luong, R., Bouley, D.M., Mao, H., Qiao, T., Gambhir, S.S., and Cheng, Z. (2012) A novel clinically translatable fluorescent nanoparticle for targeted molecular imaging of tumors in living subjects. *Nano Letters*, 12, 281–6.
71. Xie, R.G., Battaglia, D., and Peng, X.G. (2007) Colloidal InP nanocrystals as efficient emitters covering blue to near-infrared. *Journal of the American Chemical Society*, 129, 15432–3.
72. Zimmer, J.P., Kim, S.W., Ohnishi, S., Tanaka, E., Frangioni, J.V., and Bawendi, M.G. (2006) Size series of small indium arsenide-zinc selenide core-shell nanocrystals and their application to in vivo imaging. *Journal of the American Chemical Society*, 128, 2526–7.
73. He, X.X., Gao, J.H., Gambhir, S.S., and Cheng, Z. (2010) Near-infrared fluorescent nanoprobes for cancer molecular imaging: Status and challenges. *Trends in Molecular Medicine*, 12, 574–83.
74. Xiong, J.P., Stehle, T., Zhang, R.G., Joachimiak, A., Frech, M., Goodman, S.L., and Aranout, M.A. (2002) Crystal structure of the extracellular segment of integrin alpha Vbeta3 in complex with an Arg-Gly-Asp ligand. *Science*, 296, 151–5.
75. Weissleder, R., Kelly, K., Sun, E.Y., Shtatland, T., and Josephson, L. (2005) Cell-specific targeting of nanoparticles by multivalent attachment of small molecules. *Nature Biotechnology*, 23, 1418–23.
76. Kim, S.-W., Zimmer, J.P., Ohnishi, S., Tracy, J.B., Frangioni, J.V., and Bawendi, M.G. (2005) Engineering InAs$_x$P$_{1-x}$/InP/ZnSe III-V alloyed core/shell quantum dots for the near-infrared. *Journal of the American Chemical Society*, 127, 10526–32.
77. Kim, S., Lim, Y.T., Soltesz, E.G., De Grand, A.M., Lee, J., Nakayama, A., Parker, J.A., et al. (2004) Near-infrared fluorescent type II quantum dots for sentinel lymph node mapping. *Nature Biotechnology*, 22, 93–7.
78. Parungo, C.P., Ohnishi, S., Kim, S.-W., Kim, S., Laurence, R.G., Soltesz, E.G., Chen, F.Y., et al. (2005) Intraoperative identification of esophageal sentinel lymph nodes with near-infrared fluorescence imaging. *The Journal of Thoracic and Cardiovascular Surgery*, 129, 844–50.
79. Weng, K.C., Noble, C.O., Papahadjopoulos-Sternberg, B., Chen, F.F., Drummond, D.C., Kirpotin, D.B., Wang, D., Hom, Y.K., Hann, B., and Park, J.W. (2008) Targeted tumor cell internalization and imaging of multifunctional quantum dot-conjugated immunoliposomes in vitro and in vivo. *Nano Letters*, 8, 2851–7.
80. Park, J.W., Hong, K., Carter, P., Asgari, H., Guo, L.Y., Keller, G.A., Wirth, C., et al. (1995) Development of anti-p185[HER2] immunoliposomes for cancer therapy. *Proceedings of the National Academy of Sciences of the United States of America*, 92, 1327–31.
81. Park, J.W., Hong, K., Kirpotin, D.B., Colbern, G., Shalaby, R., Baselga, J., Shao, Y., et al. (2002) Anti-HER2 immunoliposomes: Enhanced efficacy attributable to targeted delivery. *Clinical Cancer Research*, 8, 1172–81.
82. Mamot, C., Drummond, D.C., Greiser, U., Hong, K., Kirpotin, D.B., Marks, J.D., and Park, J. W. (2003) Epidermal growth factor receptor (EGFR)-targeted immunoliposomes mediate specific and efficient drug delivery to EGFR- and EGFRvIII-overexpressing tumor cells. *Cancer Research*, 63, 3154–61.
83. Mamot, C., Drummond, D.C., Noble, C.O., Kallab, V., Guo, Z., Hong, K., Kirpotin, D.B., and Park, J.W. (2005) Epidermal growth factor receptor-targeted immunoliposomes significantly enhance the efficacy of multiple anticancer drugs in vivo. *Cancer Research*, 65, 11631–8.
84. Cho, H.-S., Dong, Z., Pauletti, G.M., Zhang, J., Xu, H., Gu, H., Wang, L., et al. (2010) Fluorescent, superparamagnetic nanospheres for drug storage, targeting, and imaging: A multifunctional nanocarrier system for cancer diagnosis and treatment. *ACS Nano*, 4, 5398–404.

85. Charron, G., Stuchinskaya, T., Edwards, D.R., Russell, D.A., and Nann, T. (2012) Insights into the mechanism of quantum dot-sensitized singlet oxygen production for photodynamic therapy. *The Journal of Physical Chemistry C*, 116, 9334–42.
86. Resch-Genger, U., Grabolle, M., Cavaliere-Jaricot, S., Nitschke, R., and Nann, T. (2008) Quantum dots versus organic dyes as fluorescent labels. *Nature Methods*, 5, 763–75.
87. Nann, T. (2011) Nanoparticles in photodynamic therapy. *Nano Biomedicine and Engineering*, 3, 137–42.
88. Dougherty, H., Gomer, C.J., Jori, G., Kessel, D., Korbelik, M., Moan, J., and Peng, Q.J. (1998) Photodynamic therapy. *National Cancer Institute*, 90, 889–905.
89. Sharman, W.M., Allen, C.M., and van Lier, J.E. (1999) Photodynamic therapeutics: Basic principles and clinical applications. *Drug Discovery Today*, 4, 507–17.
90. Brown, S.B., Brown, E.A., and Walker, I. (2004) The present and future role of photodynamic therapy in cancer treatment. *The Lancet Oncology*, 5, 497–508.
91. Samia, A.C.S., Chen, X., and Burda, C. (2003) Semiconductor quantum dots for photodynamic therapy. *Journal of the American Chemical Society*, 125, 15736–7.
92. Ma, J., Chen, J.-Y., Idowu, M., and Nyokong, T. (2008) Generation of singlet oxygen via the composites of water-soluble thiol-capped CdTe quantum dots-sulfonated aluminum phthalocyanines. *The Journal of Physical Chemistry B*, 112, 4465–9.
93. Lim, Y.T., Noh, Y.-W., Cho, J.-H., Han, J.H., Choi, B.S., Kwon, J., Hong, K.S., Gokarna, A., Cho, Y.-H., and Chung, B.H. (2009) Multiplexed imaging of therapeutic cells with multispectrally encoded magnetofluorescent nanocomposite emulsions. *Journal of the American Chemical Society*, 131, 17145–54.
94. Kim, H.M., Lee, H., Hong, K.S., Cho, M.Y., Sung, M.-H., Poo, H., and Lim, Y.T. (2011) Synthesis and high performance of magnetofluorescent polyelectrolyte nanocomposites as MR/near-infrared multimodal cellular imaging nanoprobes. *ACS Nano*, 5, 8230–40.

3 Biomedical Applications of Dendrimer Porphyrin or Phthalocyanine

Woo-Dong Jang and Won-Gun Koh
Yonsei University

CONTENTS

3.1 INTRODUCTION

Dendrimers are a class of regularly branched macromolecules having a unique topological aspect. Because dendrimers are synthesized by precisely controlled stepwise reactions, they do not have polydispersity.[1–3] In contrast to other linear, cross-linked, and branched polymers, dendrimers have a well-predictable three-dimensional (3D) shape, which often give plenty of unique properties and provide wide range of applications.[4–8] Dendrimers comprise three different topological parts, that is, focal core, layered building blocks, and multiple peripheral groups, which provide very fascinating chemical aspect.[9,10] The focal core in large dendrimer can be isolated from outer environment by extensive dendritic branching. The layered repeating units can preserve 3D structures of dendrimer. The multivalent surface can provide the integration of functionalities in small space and the congested surface functionalities only can interact with the external environment; therefore, the macroscopic properties of dendrimers can be tuned by the nature of peripheral functionalities.[11–13] During the past decade, a great number of dendrimer structures have been developed and investigated owing to their structural merit and fascinating aspect. Among them, ionic poly(benzyl ether) dendrimers, having a photofunctional porphyrin or phthalocyanine (Pc) core, have been developed and intensively investigated for their biomedical applications. In this chapter, the biomedical applications of dendrimer porphyrin (DP) and dendrimer Pc (DPc) are discussed.

3.2 DESIGN OF DENDRITIC MATERIALS

For the synthesis of dendritic materials, fully controlled stepwise reactions should be utilized. Two major synthetic strategies, that is, divergent and convergent approaches, are used to synthesize dendrimers. The divergent approach was first introduced by Tomalia et al.[14] and Newkome et al.[15] in the early 1980s. In the divergent strategy, reaction starts from the focal core to build up the molecule toward the periphery. A pair of basic operations, coupling reaction of building blocks and deprotection or modification reaction of end-functionalities onto the periphery to create new reactive functionalities, is repeated to build up dendritic structure. Because all the branching points should be reacted for the generation growth, the divergent approach often resulted in a number of defects. The convergent growth strategy, pioneered by Hawker and Fréchet,[16] developed as an alternative method to the divergent approach for producing precisely controlled dendritic architectures. The convergent growth strategy overcomes some of the problems associated with the divergent growth strategy. The reaction starts from the surface functional groups and proceeds to the core. In the convergent method, the simultaneous reactions in every step are relatively smaller than that of the divergent method. Therefore, the formation of defect can be remarkably reduced. Furthermore, the large mass difference between product and undesired by-product enables easy purification. However, the reactive site at the focal point can be buried by dendritic building blocks as the increase of generations. Therefore, the reaction times should be prolonged for the completion of the reaction.

For the synthesis of DP and DPc, convergent strategy was utilized. Schemes 3.1 and 3.2 show the synthetic procedures of water-soluble DP and DPc, respectively. DP was first synthesized by Aida et al. as a mimic of globular protein.[17] DPc was first synthesized by Ng et al. for the investigation of photophysical properties of isolated phtalocyanine.[18] Later, DP and DPc were utilized as photosensitizers (PSs) for photodynamic therapy (PDT) by Kataoka et al.

3.2.1 STRUCTURAL ASPECT OF DENDRIMERS

Unlike traditional polymeric materials, that is, linear, branched, and cross-linked polymers, dendrimers have unique chemical and physical properties, as described below.

1. Defect-free dendrimers do not have molecular weight distribution. Large dendrimers obtained by divergent synthesis eventually have some defects, but they also have very narrow molecular weight distribution.
2. The stepwise synthesis of dendrimers allows for site-selective functionalization.

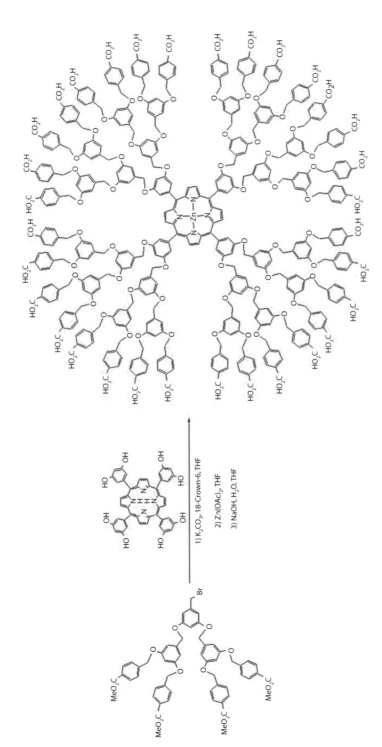

SCHEME 3.1 Synthesis of water-soluble DP.

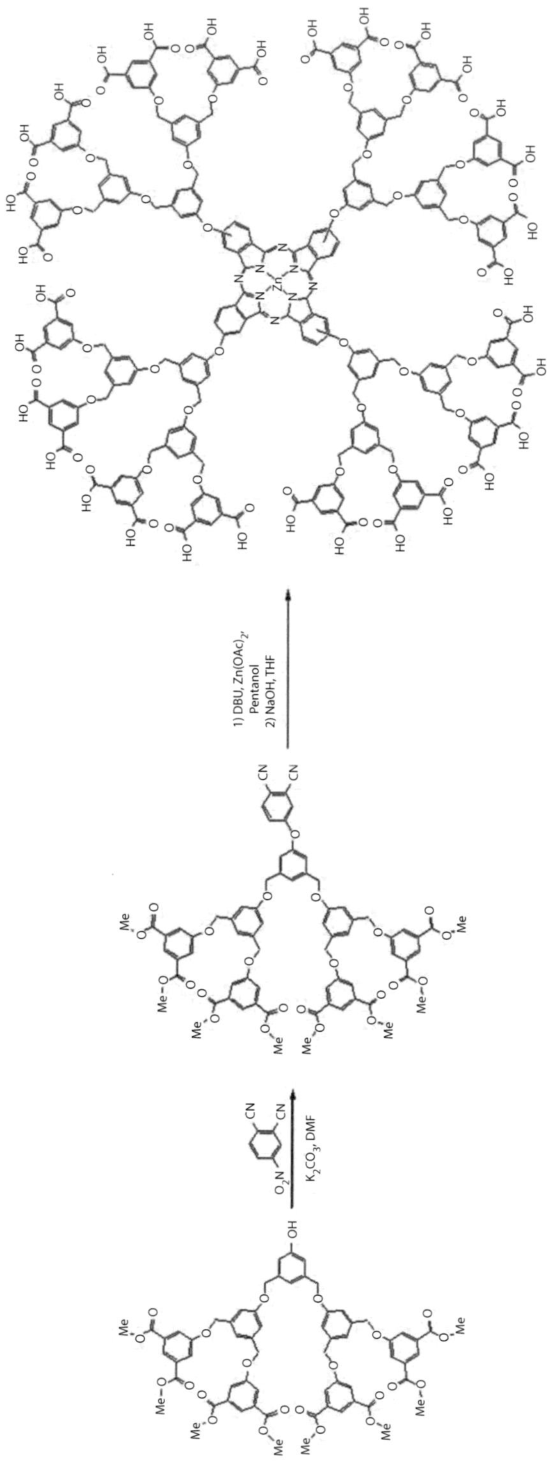

SCHEME 3.2 Synthesis of water-soluble DPc.

3. Because the number of branching systematically increases from the core to the periphery, the surface of a large dendrimer is highly congested, whereas a substantial free space can exist in the interior part. The free space often allows for various applications, such as site-specific pockets for selective reaction and guest molecule accommodation.
4. Unlike linear polymers, entanglement or interpenetration of dendrimers is generally unfavorable due to their densely packed surface. Thus, dendrimers tend to have smaller hydrodynamic volumes and lower solution viscosities compared to linear polymers having the same molecular weight.
5. Dendrimers have a predictable 3D architecture. Specifically, large dendrimers have a densely packed surface area, which provide site isolation effect of the focal core.
6. The solubility of dendrimers is predominately controlled by their peripheral functionalities.

The above unique chemical properties of dendrimers are well adapted to DP and DPc.

Although the benzyl ether building block has a hydrophobic nature, DP and DPc also have high solubility to aqueous medium owing to the large number of anionic functional groups of periphery. Also, large dendritic wedges can effectively prevent the formation of aggregates.

3.3 DENDRIMERS AS PSs FOR PDT

PDT is attracting attention as a promising technology for a less invasive cancer treatment.[19–21] PDT involves the systemic administration of a PS and successive laser light irradiation to the target tissue. According to the light irradiation, PSs are excited to the singlet state and are then transformed to a long-lived triplet state via intersystem crossing (Figure 3.1). The triplet state of PSs can transfer their excitation energy

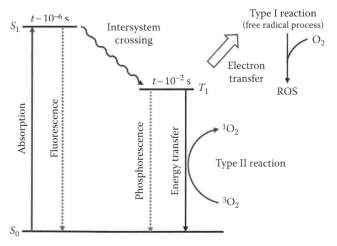

FIGURE 3.1   Photodynamic process.

or electron to oxygen molecules in the target tissue. Through the excitation energy or electron transfer, oxygen molecules transform to highly toxic reactive oxygen species (ROS), which eventually destroy the target tumor tissue. Unlike other malignant disease treatments, PDT has several distinguishable advantages. Most therapeutic agents influence on not only the therapeutic target but also normal tissue due to their poor selectivity. Therefore, chemotherapy eventually results in side effects or sequelae. Through the selective photoirradiation to the target tissue, it can be possible to minimize such adverse effects by PDT if PSs are nontoxic under light-free conditions. However, PDT also has several drawbacks in clinical applications.

For effective clinical applications, PSs need the following characteristics[22–25]:

1. Large absorption cross-section and high quantum yield for singlet oxygen generation
2. Long-wavelength absorption for the effective penetration of light into the target tissue
3. High solubility in aqueous media
4. Minimum toxicity under dark condition
5. Easiness of excretion after phototreatment
6. High chemical purity

For effective light absorption, PSs eventually need to have large π-conjugation domain. Most of the conventional PSs are composed of porphyrin derivatives due to their large absorption cross-section in visible light and effective generation of singlet oxygen. Therefore, PSs often have poor solubility in aqueous media due to π–π interaction and hydrophobic characteristics. PSs easily form aggregates at high local concentration in aqueous medium, which might result in decreased PDT efficacy due to a self-quenching of the excited state.[26–29] From the above viewpoint, dendrimers would be one of the promising materials because the substitution of large dendritic wedges can effectively prevent the formation of aggregates and provide high solubility in aqueous medium.[26,30] In fact, DP and DPc successfully exhibited high solubility in aqueous medium and effective cytotoxicity upon photoirradiation.[31,32] For example, Figure 3.2 shows cell viability curves of Lewis lung carcinoma (LLC) against the concentration of PSs after photoirradiation.[32] Compared to protoporphyrin IX (PIX), a conventional PS, DP exhibited 10–100 times higher photocytotoxicity. More recently, the ionic surfaces of DP and DPc have been utilized for the formation of polyion complex (PIC) micelles. The *in vitro* and *in vivo* experiments have been examined that PIC micelles are successful formulations for the PDT.

3.3.1 Properties of Dendritic PSs

As aforementioned, dendritic PSs have a unique photochemical property that the collisional quenching of focal PS unit is prevented by spatial isolation due to large dendritic wedges. Considering the short lifetime of singlet oxygen in aqueous medium, the maximum diffusion range of singlet oxygen is estimated to be less than 10 nm, indicating that the ROS generated by photoirradiation should be released from large dendritic wedges for effective PDT.[26,32] The singlet oxygen quantum

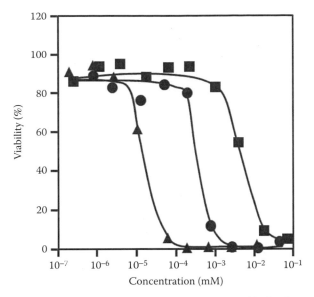

FIGURE 3.2 Viability of LLC cells treated with PIX (•), positively charged DP (▲), and negatively charged DP (■) after photoirradiation at incubation times of 8 h. (Reprinted with permission from Nishiyama, N., et al., 2003, 58–66. Copyright 2003 American Chemical Society.)

yield of DPs has been measured by direct observation of luminescence from singlet oxygen at 1270 nm in deutrated methanol (MeOD).[32] It has been demonstrated that ionic DPs showed successfully good singlet oxygen quantum yield compared to PIX in spite of the spatial isolation in dendritic wedges, indicating that the large dendritic wedges are not a barrier for singlet oxygen-induced photodynamic effect. This effect can possibly be explained by the prolonged lifetime of singlet oxygen in the hydrophobic environment of the dendrimer inside. Because the large dendritic wedges may prevent direct reaction of PS radicals with other molecules, singlet oxygen or other ROS should play essential roles for the PDT. The large hydrodynamic volume of DPs enables cellular uptake through endocytic pathways. The ionic DPs showed different cellular associations depending on the peripheral charges. For example, cationic DP rapidly associated with negatively charged plasma membrane through electrostatic attraction, followed by internalization by adsorptive endocytosis. Alternatively, anionic DP was slowly internalized by fluid-phase endocytosis due to electrostatic repulsion. Cationic DP exhibited 230 times higher photocytotoxicity than anionic DP because of the effective association of cationic DP to plasma membrane. Fluorescent microscopic observation revealed that DPs maintained the characteristic structure of cell membranes and intracellular organelles (the plasma membrane, mitochondrion, and lysosome) after photoirradiation. On the other hand, such organelles were severely disrupted by photoirradiation when conventional PSs were incubated with cells. Hypersensitivity of PS is one of the major problems in clinical PDT. For safe treatment, the patient should stay in a dark condition for a long time after PDT treatment. Ionic DPs showed extremely low dark toxicity even after prolonged incubation of 72 h. The extremely low dark toxicity of DPs may result from distinctive intracellular disposition characteristics due to their relatively large size.

For the effective penetration of light into target tissue, long-wavelength light absorption is also needed for PS.[33] However, DPs have relatively short excitation wavelengths (i.e., 430 and 560 nm), which might be a limitation for PDT except for the transparent tissues. Skin tissue has melanin dyes, which absorb short-wavelength light to prevent photochemical genetic disorder, and also heme proteins of red blood cells account for most of the light absorption in the visible region. Such light absorption by human bodies prevents the excitation of PSs for photochemical reactions. In this regard, several Pc-based PSs have been developed for practical PDT.[33] In this context, DPc has been synthesized and its photophysical properties evaluated. The DPc has absorption maximum at approximately 680 nm, where the light can penetrate tissues two times deeper than Photofrin, a conventional PS having absorption at 630 nm. DPc also showed almost negligible dark toxicity similar to DPs.

3.3.2 DEVELOPMENT OF DENDRITIC PS-LOADED MICELLES

Aggregate formation of PSs in aqueous medium severely decreases the quantum yield of ROS generation due to self-quenching of the excited state.[26–29] This property becomes one of the major problems for the design of delivery vehicles of PSs. The incorporation of PSs into nanocarriers, such as liposomes and polymeric micelles, eventually increases local concentration of the PSs. Therefore, the high local concentration of PSs induces aggregate formation, which results in their reduced PDT efficacy.[26] Also, hydrophobic compounds are generally difficult to incorporate into nanocarriers without compromising the nanocarrier's properties such as the size and surface properties, which are a critical issue for prolonged blood circulation. The dendritic PSs elicit effective ROS generation even at extremely high concentrations because the dendritic wedges effectively prevent aggregation of the focal photosensitizing units.[30,32] Also, ionic groups on the dendrimer periphery allow the formation of stable PIC micelle.[34] Several polymeric micelles containing antitumor agents have already progressed to clinical trials. The DP-loaded PIC micelles can be formed by electrostatic interaction of a pair of charged block copolymers of poly(ethylene glycol)-*block*-poly(L-lysine) (PEG-*b*-PLL) or PEG-*block*-poly(aspartic acid) (PEG-*b*-PAA) with oppositely charged DPs.[35] By simple mixing of charged block copolymers with oppositely charged DPs at a stoichiometric charge ratio, several tens of nanometers of size with core–shell architecture can be spontaneously formed. For example, the PIC micelles prepared from negatively charged DP and PEG-*b*-PLL had a diameter of approximately 60 nm with an extremely narrow size distribution in physiological saline solution (Figure 3.3).[35] The spherical shape of the DP-loaded PIC micelles was confirmed by observation with atomic force microscopy (AFM) and field emission-transmission electron microscopy (FE-TEM). The static light scattering (SLS) measurement revealed that each PIC micelle contains an average of 38 DP molecules. The resulting PIC micelles showed significantly high stability against remarkably high NaCl concentrations up to 1500 mM. The PIC micelles of DPs showed pH-dependent structural changes.[30] From the dynamic light scattering (DLS) and SLS measurements, the pH-dependent change of the

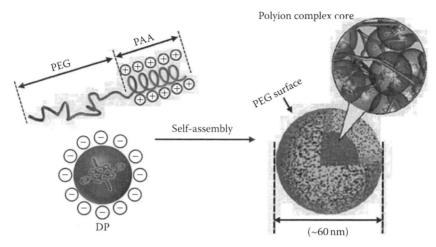

FIGURE 3.3   Formation of PIC micelle.

hydrodynamic diameter and the apparent molecular weight of PIC micelles have been observed. When the pH was below 6.4, the PIC micelles showed a gradual increase in the diameter and apparent molecular weight, and finally resulted in precipitation at pH 5.6, indicating the responsibility of the micelle to acidic environment. Such a pH-responsive behavior of the micelles allows their effective accumulation in solid tumors in response to a low pH condition in the tumor tissue[36] or an intracellular acidic endosomal compartment.

By the formation of PIC micelles, the anionic DP exhibited 5 nm of redshift with hypochromicity for the Soret absorption.[30] The diminished charge repulsion of the negatively charged DP surface may lead to shrinkage of the hydrophobic dendrimer frameworks, which may be related to the spectral shift.[37,38] Although the local concentration of DP is greatly high in the micellar core, the PIC micelles showed no fluorescent quenching.[30] It would be impossible to achieve the unique photochemical property of the DP-loaded PIC micelles by using other conventional PSs and PS formulations. To evaluate the efficiency of the photochemical reactions, oxygen consumption rate under light irradiation was investigated. The DP-loaded PIC micelle showed an almost comparable oxygen consumption rate to free DP in phosphate-buffered saline (PBS), containing fetal bovine serum (FBS) as a singlet oxygen acceptor, which suggests that the singlet oxygen molecules produced from DP can effectively escape from the micellar structure and react with proteins of FBS (Figure 3.4).[30]

Although the DP-loaded PIC micelle showed almost comparable oxygen consumption rate to free DP, DP-loaded PIC micelle exhibited significantly enhanced photocytotoxicity.

Although the cellular uptake amount of DP-loaded PIC micelle to LLC cells is only six to eight times greater than that of free anionic DP, the anionic DP-loaded PIC micelles exhibited approximately 280 times greater photocytotoxicity than free anionic DP. Such enhanced photocytotoxicity of DP-loaded PIC micelle can be explained by the high concentration of ROS generation in local site because

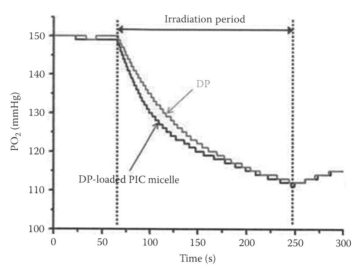

FIGURE 3.4 Oxygen depletion profiles by free DP and DP-loaded PIC micelle in PBS containing 10% FBS. The light irradiation and the oxygen partial pressure measurements were performed using an Hg lamp and a Clark-type oxygen microelectrode, respectively. (From Jang, W.-D., et al. Supramolecular nanocarrier of anionic dendrimer porphyrins with cationic block copolymers modified with polyethylene glycol to enhance intracellular photodynamic efficacy. *Angew. Chem. Int. Ed.*, 2005, 44, 419–423. Copyright Wiley-VCH Verlag GmbH & Co. KGaA. Reproduced with permission.)

large numbers of DPs are incorporated into the core of the micellar structure (Figure 3.5).

Recently, DPs with various generations [DP(Gn) = n-generation dendrimer, $n = 1$–3] have been explored for the formation of PIC micelles and their photochemical properties.[26] The DP-loaded PIC micelles were prepared by mixing of DP(Gn)s and PEG-PLL block copolymers at a stoichiometric charge ratio. DP(G3) formed 44-nm-sized particle with narrow distribution, which is consistent with the core–shell-type micellar structure. However, DP(G1) and DP(G2) exhibited the formation of relatively larger aggregates with diameters of 126 and 78 nm, respectively, indicating that the relatively open architectures and small dendritic wedges of DP(G1) and DP(G2) cannot perfectly prevent the aggregate formation of porphyrin cores. The fluorescence decay and oxygen consumption ability of DP(Gn)s and DP-loaded PIC micelles also showed clear generation dependency. The DP(G3)-loaded PIC micelle showed almost comparable fluorescence decay and oxygen consumption profiles to those of free DP(G3). However, the DP(G1)- and DP(G2)-loaded PIC micelles showed greatly shortened fluorescence lifetimes and decreased oxygen consumption rate compared with free DP(G1) and DP(G2), respectively.[26] Therefore, it can be concluded that the DP(G3) is the optimum size for the prevention of self-quenching of focal photosensitizing units in the micellar core. Similar to DP, the DPc-loaded PIC micelle, which has a size of approximately 50 nm, has also been prepared by electrostatic interaction between anionic DPc and PEG-*b*-PLL.[31] DPc-incorporated micelles were stable in a PBS containing 10%

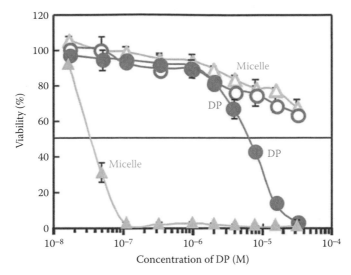

FIGURE 3.5   The cytotoxicity of LLC cells incubated with free DP (circle) and DP-loaded PIC micelles (triangle) compared with that of LLC cells under dark conditions (open symbol) and photoirradiation (closed symbol). Cells were photoirradiated for 10 min using broadband visible light from a xenon lamp (150 W) equipped with a filter passing light of 400–700 nm (fluence: 180 kJ/cm^2). (Reprinted with permission from Ideta, R., et al., 2005, 2426–2431. Copyright 2005 American Chemical Society.)

FBS, maintaining the size and polydispersity of the micelles. A shift of maximum absorption wavelength of DPc from 685 to 630 nm was accompanied by the formation of micellar structure, indicating that some interactions between the Pc units of DPc (i.e., aggregate formation) possibly happened in the micellar core. Considering the structure of DPc, the relatively small size of dendritic wedges in DPc may not be sufficient to prevent such interactions. Consequently, DPc-loaded PIC micelles showed reduced oxygen consumption rates compared with free DPc.[31] Nevertheless, DPc-incorporated micelles showed significant enhancement of the light-induced cytotoxicity, which greatly relied on the photoirradiation time. The DPc-loaded PIC micelles exhibited approximately 100 times higher photocytotoxicity than free DPc upon 60 min of photoirradiation.

3.3.3   *IN VITRO* PDT EFFECT OF DENDRITIC PS-LOADED MICELLES

To test the effectiveness of DPs in PDT, *in vitro* evaluations of DP(G*n*)s in a free or micellar form have been carried out against HeLa cells.[26] The DP(G1)-, DP(G2)-, and DP(G3)-loaded PIC micelles showed 7.5, 50, and 167 times higher photocytotoxicity, respectively, compared with the corresponding free DP(G*n*)s in the same condition (Figure 3.6). On the other hand, cellular uptake amounts of the DP(G1)-, DP(G2)-, and DP(G3)-loaded PIC micelles were 95, 53, and 15 times greater than those of the corresponding free DP(G*n*)s, respectively. The normalized PDT efficiencies based on the uptake amount of DP(G*n*)s were calculated to be 0.079, 0.94, and 11.1 for the DP(G1)-, DP(G2)-, and DP(G3)-loaded PIC micelles, respectively.

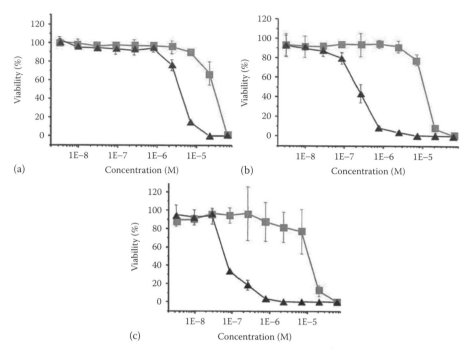

FIGURE 3.6   Cell viability of HeLa cells treated with DPs (■) of different generations—(a) DP(G1), (b) DP(G2), and (c) DP(G3)—and the corresponding DP(G*n*)-loaded micelles (▲) after photoirradiation. In this experiment, HeLa cells were incubated with DPs or DP-loaded micelles for 12 h, followed by photoirradiation for 30 min with broadband visible light using a halogen lamp equipped with a filter passing light of only 400–700 nm (fluence: 5.4 J/cm²). After 24 h, the cell viability was evaluated by 3-(4,5-dimethylthiazol-2-yl)-2,5-diphenyltetrazolium bromide (MTT) assay. (Reprinted with permission from Li, Y., et al., 2007, 5557–5562. Copyright 2007 American Chemical Society.)

The DP(G1)-loaded PIC micelle showed reduced PDT efficacy than that of free DP(G1), responsible for the shortened fluorescence lifetime and decreased oxygen consumption ability. However, the DP(G2)-loaded PIC micelle exhibited PDT efficiency comparable to that of free DP(G2) in spite of the shortened fluorescence lifetime and decreased oxygen consumption rate. Notably, the DP(G3)-loaded PIC micelle showed 11 times enhanced PDT efficiency, again indicating that the third-generation dendrimer of optimum size is required to obtain the best PDT efficacy due to the effective prevention of aggregate formation.

As aforementioned, DPc has been prepared for the prolonged wavelength absorption for effective light delivery.[12] By simple mixing of DPc and PEG-*b*-PLL, DPc also formed PIC micelle, which had a diameter of ~50 nm with narrow size distribution. The photocytotoxicity of the DPc-loaded PIC micelle was assessed against human lung adenocarcinoma A549 cells.[39] The DPc-loaded PIC micelle was 3.9 times more effective than Photofrin on a molar basis of photosensitizing units regardless of the quantum yields and cellular uptake amounts. Although the DPc-loaded PIC micelle showed only 7.6 times higher cellular uptake amounts than free

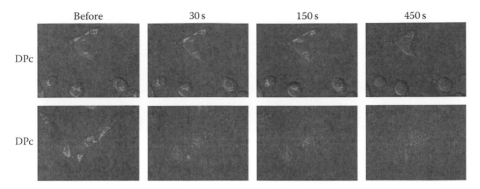

FIGURE 3.7   (See color insert.) Time-dependent morphological changes of A549 cells treated with free DPc or DPc-loaded PIC micelle during photoirradiation. A549 cells were incubated with free DPc or DPc-loaded PIC micelle for 24 h at a 99% growth inhibitory concentration (IC99). After the medium replacement, the morphological changes in the cells during photoirradiation by the light source of a time-lapse sectioning fluorescent microscope were continuously monitored using the microscope's differential interference contrast (DIC) mode. The fluorescent images from DPc (red) and Rhodamine 123 (Rh123) (green), a dye that specifically stains mitochondria, were monitored. (Reprinted from *J. Control. Release*, 133, Nishiyama, M., et al., Enhanced photodynamic cancer treatment by supramolecular nanocarriers charged with dendrimer phthalocyanine, 245–251, Copyright 2009, with permission from Elsevier.)

DPc, the DPc-loaded PIC micelle showed 78 times higher photocytotoxicity than free DPc under 10.8 J/cm^2 of light irradiation. Similar to the DP-loaded PIC micelle, the enhanced photocytotoxicity of the DPc-loaded PIC micelle cannot be explained by the intracellular concentration of DPc. Therefore, different mechanisms of light-induced cell death can be hypothesized between free DPc and DPc-loaded PIC micelle. In fact, there were significant differences in the light-induced morphological changes of cells when the cells were treated with IC99 of free DPc or DPc-loaded PIC micelle.[39] By the photoirradiation, DPc-loaded PIC micelle induced very rapid morphological changes of cells including swelling and membrane blebbing (Figure 3.7). On the other hand, free DPc-induced gradual shrinkage of the cells by photoirradiation. The rapid morphological changes of the cells induced by the DPc-loaded PIC micelle are similar to the characteristics of oncosis, which has been reported to be induced by several pathological conditions, such as hypoxia, inhibition of ATP production, and abnormal increase of plasma membrane permeability.[40] When the fluorescence of DPc and Rhodamine 123 (Rh123), a mitochondria-staining dye, was monitored by microscopy, the fluorescence of DPc became diffusive in cells treated by free DPc and DPc-loaded PIC micelle. Because the selective accumulation of DPc and the DPc-loaded PIC micelle in the endo/lysosomal compartments has already been confirmed, the fluorescence diffusion of DPc might indicate the translocation of both DPc and the DPc-loaded PIC micelle from the endo/lysosomal compartment to cytoplasm upon photoirradiation. This translocation was possibly explained by the photochemical disruption of the endo/lysosomal membranes.[41–43] Despite the similar intracellular behaviors of DPc and

DPc-loaded PIC micelle, only DPc-loaded PIC micelle caused rapid disappearance of the Rh123 fluorescence in the cell, suggesting that the DPc-loaded PIC micelle might affect mitochondrial functions during photoirradiation. Since the fluorescent intensity of Rh123 is correlated with the amount of ATP in the cells, PDT using the DPc-loaded PIC micelle may directly or indirectly influence the generation of ATP in the cell.[44] To determine whether the DPc-loaded PIC micelle induces direct photodamage to the mitochondria or not, ROS production in the mitochondria was monitored by using MitoSOX Red, which rapidly accumulates in the mitochondria and emits fluorescence when oxidized by ROS.[39] The cells treated by DPc-loaded PIC micelle displayed fluorescence from MitoSOX after 1 min of photoirradiation, whereas the free DPc-treated cells showed no fluorescence even after prolonged photoirradiation. Therefore, it can be concluded that DPc-loaded PIC micelle induces photodamage to the mitochondria. To summarize the cell death mechanism by DPc-loaded PIC micelle treatment, the following steps may be involved in the photoinduced cell death.[39] First, the DPc-loaded PIC micelle is internalized through the endocytic pathway and accumulated in the endo/lysosomes. Then, the translocation of DPc-loaded PIC micelle takes place from the endo/lysosomes to the cytoplasm through the photochemical disruption of the endo/lysosomal membranes upon photoirradiation. Finally, the DPc-loaded PIC micelle might induce photodamage to the mitochondria, which results in oncosis-like cell death through exhaustion of ATP in the cell. In addition to the unique intracellular localization and photochemical reactions, the high local concentration of DPc in micellar core may also contribute to the high PDT efficiency. The high local concentration of DPc might generate a high concentration of ROS at a local site, achieving a high photochemical oxidation level that exceeds the threshold of cell death.

3.3.4 *In Vivo* PDT Effect of Dendritic PS-Loaded Micelles

The DP- and DPc-loaded PIC micelles were treated to various disease models to evaluate their clinical availabilities. The exclusive age-related macular degeneration (AMD), a condition caused by choroidal neovascularization (CNV), is a major cause of visual loss in developed countries.[45] Recently, Visudyne, a liposomal formulation of verteporfin, has been approved for clinical use and demonstrated to prevent visual loss by means of PDT.[46] However, most patients of AMD require repeated treatments of PDT in every 3 months due to the intractableness, while still suffering from a reduced quality of life. Therefore, there is a strong need to develop more effective formulations of PSs for PDT treatment against AMD. For effective PDT against AMD, the selective accumulation of PS to the CNV lesions might be necessary.[46] In regard to the efficient delivery of PSs, low-density lipoproteins and antibodies have been used as a carrier molecule; however, PSs also distribute to normal tissues because normal tissues also express some extent of such biomarkers. Furthermore, the increased loading of PSs to the drug carriers often decreases the effect of PDT due to the formation of aggregates of PSs. Based on the above information, PDT using DP-loaded PIC micelle was carried out to the AMD model.[47] In this study, experimental CNV was delivered to the rats by laser photocoagulations to each eye. After 7 days of photocoagulation, 400 mL of DP-loaded

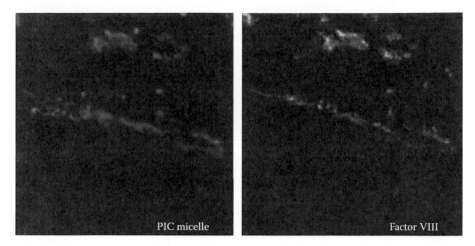

FIGURE 3.8   Selective accumulation of DP-loaded PIC micelle in experimental CNV lesion. Fluorescence is emitted from DP (left) and selective staining of endothelial cells by Factor VIII (right), respectively. (Reprinted with permission from Ideta, R., et al., 2005, 2426–2431. Copyright 2005 American Chemical Society.)

PIC micelle or PD, including 1.5 mg/mL of DP, was administered through tail vein injection into rats. The rats were sacrificed, and the eyes were immediately enucleated to observe the accumulation of DPs in the CNV lesions. As a result, an effective and selective accumulation of DP-loaded PIC micelle in the CNV lesions has been confirmed by fluorescence of DP, indicating that the CNV lesions may have characteristic features similar to solid tumor vasculatures, such as hyperpermeability and impaired lymphatic drainage (Figure 3.8).[48–51] The enhanced accumulation of DP-loaded PIC micelle into CNV lesions resulted in a significantly enhanced PDT effect, which was confirmed by fluorescein angiography.[47] When the PDT laser was applied 15 min after the DP-loaded PIC micelle injection, no fluorescein leakage has been found for 78% of the CNV lesions after 1 day of PDT. After 7 days of PDT, the hypofluorescence persisted, suggesting that the leakage from the CNV lesions was still reduced. More importantly, the photodamage of skin was not macroscopically observable when the rats were exposed to broadband visible light (Xenon lamp equipped with a filter passing light of 377–700 nm, incident light irradiance; approximately 30 mW/cm^2) at 4 h, after the DP-loaded PIC micelle injection. This is in sharp contrast to the results observed after the injection of Photofrin.

Alternatively, corneal neovascularization is another major cause of visual loss. The normal cornea is a vascular tissue, but under certain pathological conditions, capillaries from the limbal plexus invade the corneal tissue. A wide range of inflammatory, infectious, degenerative, and traumatic disorders may induce corneal neovascularization. Similar to the case of AMD, the DP-loaded PIC micelle was also selectively accumulated in the neovascular tissue in corneal tissue. PDT with 10 J/cm^2 of energy after the DP-loaded PIC micelle resulted in complete regression of all neovascular lesions at day 7. From these *in vivo* results, we can conclude that DP may have a great potential as a PS for the treatment of several ophthalmologic diseases.

Although the aforementioned results indicated that DP has a great potential to use as PSs for PDT in transparent ophthalmologic diseases, the absorption maxima of DP appear at 430 (Soret band) and 560 nm (Q-band), which might reduce the availability of DP in solid tumor due to the limitation of light delivery. As mentioned earlier, skin tissue has melanin dyes, which absorb short wavelength light to prevent photochemical genetic disorder, and also heme proteins that account for most of the absorption of light in the visible region. Therefore, the DPc-loaded PIC micelle has tested its availability to solid tumor model.[18,43,52,53] To the mice bearing subcutaneous A549 tumors, DPc-loaded PIC micelle (0.37 μmol/kg), free DPc, and Photofrin (2.7 μmol/kg) were administrated through intravenous (i.v.) injection; the relative tumor volumes were then monitored after the PDT treatment.[39] The DPc-loaded micelle showed significantly higher antitumor activity compared with DPc or Photofrin (Figure 3.9). Notably, the injected dose of the DPc-loaded micelle was 7.3 times lower than that of Photofrin on the basis of photosensitizing units. The enhanced PDT efficacy of the DPc-loaded PIC micelle might be attributed to the effective tumor accumulation based on the enhanced permeability and retention (EPR) effect as well as the enhanced photocytotoxicity. Similar to the DP-loaded PIC micelle, DPc-loaded PIC micelle also showed minimal skin toxicity upon broadband white light irradiation. This reduced skin phototoxicity of the DPc-loaded PIC micelle may be attributed to its lower accumulation in the skin and other normal organs.

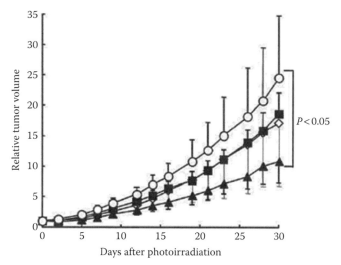

FIGURE 3.9 Growth curves of subcutaneous A549 tumors in control mice (o) and mice administered 0.37 μmol/kg DPc (■), 0.37 μmol/kg DPc-loaded PIC micelle (▲), and 2.7 μmol/kg Photofrin (◊) ($n = 6$). After 24 h administration, the tumors were photoirradiated using a diode laser (fluence: 100 J/cm²). (Reprinted from *J. Control. Release*, 133, Nishiyama, M., et al., Enhanced photodynamic cancer treatment by supramolecular nanocarriers charged with dendrimer phthalocyanine, 245–251, Copyright 2009, with permission from Elsevier.)

3.4　APPLICATION OF DPs OR PCs FOR DRUG DELIVERY

Light irradiation onto the PSs generates ROS, which disrupts tissues and organelles. When the PSs accumulated into the endo/lysosomal compartments, photoirradiation would selectively disrupt endo/lysosomal lipid bilayer membranes. Recently, such a concept has been applied to the drug delivery.[43] Endosomal escape of drugs would be one of the major obstacles in drug delivery, when the drug uptake relies on the endocytosis mechanism. Recently, several examples have been reported about light-induced endosomal escape of drugs by the combination of PSs. PS-loaded micelles can also be utilized for selective drug delivery using light irradiation. In this section, we are going to review the recent examples of DPc-loaded micelle or new formulations for photochemical drug delivery.

3.4.1　Photochemical Delivery Using Dendritic PS-Loaded Micelles

The DPc-loaded PIC micelles are taken up by the cells through the endocytic pathway, preferentially localizing in the endo/lysosome.[43] Upon photoirradiation, DPc-loaded PIC micelles may photochemically disrupt the endo/lysosomal membrane to translocate in the subcellular organelles susceptible to ROS-induced cell death. This process is available for the light-induced cytoplasmic delivery of macromolecular compounds such as plasmid DNA (pDNA), which are impermeable to cell membranes and easy to digest by enzymes in the endosome or lysosome.[41,42,54–57] This concept, photochemical internalization (PCI), has been proposed by Berg and Høgset et al. The light dose necessary for PCI is much lower than that for PDT, ensuring the low photocytotoxicity of PCI. Recently, PCI of pDNA by using the DPc-loaded PIC micelle has been carried out.[43] The PCI-mediated gene transfection was carried out using a combination of the DPc- and pDNA-loaded PIC micelles, and achieved 100 times enhancement of the transgene expression while maintaining 80% cell viability. By the optimization of chemical structures of PEG-*b*-polycations forming the pDNA-loaded PIC micelles, approximately 1000 times enhancement of gene transfection was achieved, where the PEG-*b*-polycations possessed repeated ethylenediamine units in the side chain. This result indicates that PCI may work synergistically with the so-called proton sponge effect to enhance the transfection efficiency.

Recently, a new type of polymeric micelle containing camptothecin (CPT), a hydrophobic anticancer agent, has been designed as a stimulus-responsive drug carrier.[58] The CPT is covalently conjugated to block copolymers via a disulfide bond that can be selectively cleaved by reductive condition in the cytosol due to 100–1000 times higher concentration of glutathione than that in the extracellular environment. The CPT-loaded micelle was prepared by the reaction of a thiolated CPT derivative (CPT-SH) with thiolated PEG-*b*-poly(glutamic acid) [PEG-*b*-P(Glu-SH)] block copolymers to form disulfide linkage. For the evaluation of *in vitro* cytotoxicity, the CPT-loaded micelle and the nontoxic concentration of the DPc-loaded PIC micelle were incubated with HeLa cells. When light was irradiated in this system, the cytotoxicity of the CPT-loaded micelle was significantly enhanced due to the effect of PCI by the DPc-loaded PIC micelle.[58] The light-selective activation

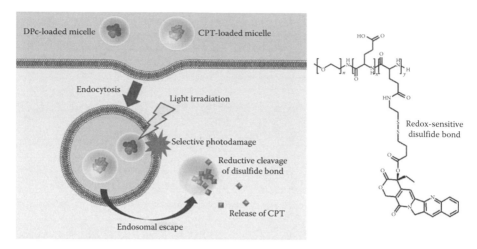

FIGURE 3.10   Photochemical delivery of CPT using DPc-loaded PIC and CPT-loaded micelles.

of chemotherapeutic agents by this system might be attributed to the selective photodamage to the endo/lysosomal membranes by the DPc-loaded PIC micelle and the selective release of CPT from CPT-loaded micelle by reductive cleavage of disulfide bonds after the endosomal escape by the PCI (Figure 3.10). Therefore, this system can minimize the drug leakage from the micelle during the circulation. This nanocarrier-based PCI system may have additional benefit in cancer treatment so that the drug released from the nanocarriers after the PCI can diffuse into deeper and hypoxic tumor tissues, which are known to be intractable by PDT alone due to limited light penetration and low oxygen concentration. As another benefit of the PCI-mediated chemotherapy, the strong potentials to overcome multidrug resistance mechanism have been proposed in many *in vivo* tumor models. Therefore, the above results indicate that utilization of DP- or DPc-loaded micelles has great potential in not only PDT but also PCI.

3.4.2   Design of Gene Carriers Using Dendritic PS

As previously mentioned, dendritic PSs have great potential for utilization in PDT and PCI. However, typically from the standpoint of *in vivo* application of the PCI-mediated transfection, the colocalization of therapeutic gene and PS unit would be of great importance. Therefore, a single-component system having a PS unit embedded in gene carriers would have great merit for light-activated gene expression. A ternary complex system composed of pDNA, quadruplicated cationic peptide (CP$_4$) containing nuclear localization signal (NLS) sequence, and anionic DPc has been designed based on this motivation.[59] The preparation of the ternary complex system was carried out by simple addition of anionic DPc to the cationic pDNA–CP$_4$ complex, which led to the spontaneous formation of the ternary complex having the pDNA–CP$_4$ core surrounded by the DPc envelope (Figure 3.11). The ternary complex thus obtained exhibited the diameter of 130 nm

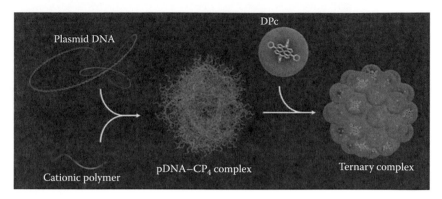

FIGURE 3.11 Formation of the pDNA–CP$_4$–DPc ternary complexes as light-responsive gene carriers for site-directed gene transfer.

with a narrow size distribution. In sharp contrast to the anionic DPc, such spherical nanoparticles (NPs) were not obtained when the PAA homopolymer that has 26 of polymerization degree was added to the pDNA–CP$_4$ complexes, which suggests that the 3D structure of DPc plays an essential role in the formation of the ternary complex. The ternary complex showed more than 100 times enhanced *in vitro* transgene expression effect by light irradiation without severe cellular toxicity. By contrast, when AlPcS$_{2a}$ (a conventional PS; aluminum Pc with two sulfonate groups on adjacent phthalate rings) was simply mixed with pDNA–CP$_4$ complex for PCI-mediated gene expression, severe cytotoxicity has been observed, which might be due to the nonselective adhesion of AlPcS$_{2a}$ to cells.[59] More importantly, the PCI-mediated transfection with the ternary complex was not accompanied by long-term toxicity, which was observed by transfection using polyethylenimine (PEI), a well-known transfecting agent. Thus, the ternary complexes might avoid the cytotoxicity induced by buffering polycations because the cytotoxic events might occur only during photoirradiation. The pDNA–CP$_4$–DPc ternary complex is assumed to activate the transgene expression in a light-inducible manner according to the following processes: (1) internalization into the cell of the ternary complex through endocytosis, (2) release of DPc from the ternary complex due to protonation of the peripheral carboxyl groups of DPc under acidic conditions in the endosome, (3) association of DPc into endosomal membrane due to the hydrophobic nature of the dendrimer framework, (4) light-induced disruption of endosomal membrane and escape of the pDNA–CP$_4$ complex to cytosol, and (5) nuclear transport of the pDNA–CP$_4$ complexes guided by the NLS sequence.[60] The ternary complex was subjected to subconjunctival injection in rats, followed by laser irradiation with a semiconductor laser (689 nm) at 2 h postinjection to demonstrate the potential of the ternary complex for *in vivo* gene transfection.[59] The PCI-mediated gene transfer with the ternary complexes resulted in appreciable gene expression of the fluorescent protein only at the laser-irradiated site in the conjunctiva, whereas the injection of pDNA–PEI complex did not show the evidence of gene expression.

3.4.3 NANODEVICES FOR COMBINATION CANCER THERAPY

Although PDT is a promising technology for noninvasive treatment of malignant tumors, we still need to improve the effectiveness of PDT to expand its application in a wide range of cancer modality. For this purpose, several nanodevices have been developed for combination cancer therapy. Recently, the combination of cisplatin [*cis*-dichlorodiammineplatinum(II); CDDP], a well-known anticancer drug, with radiotherapy or PDT has been proposed as a very effective cancer treatment.[61–63] For example, a combination of ionizing x-ray radiation with CDDP has been shown to lead to the enhancement of DNA damage.[64,65] As another example, the combination of CDDP with PSs, such as indocyanine green, and Photofrin led to significant increments in the cytotoxic and apoptotic deaths of cancer cells.[66–69] An important advance in combination cancer therapy was achieved with the fabrication of multifunctional nanomaterials, including polymeric micelles and NPs, which may be used to perform more than one therapy simultaneously.

For the effective combination of PDT and CDDP treatment, polymer–metal complex micelles (PMCMs) have been designed by coordination interaction of CDDP with DPc and PEG-*b*-PLA, where the formation of PMCMs was confirmed by TEM and laser light scattering (LLS) measurements.[70] The PMCMs are very stable in 10 mM PBS without NaCl and maintain their shape and size for over a month. However, they slowly released CDDP when they were incubated in physiological saline PBS at 37°C. To test the oxygen sensitizability of PMCM, the photoluminescence of singlet oxygen was observed under pulsed laser light irradiation with a wavelength of 615 nm. To effectively detect photoluminescence from singlet oxygen, the solution of PMCM was diluted with ethanol (PBS/ethanol: 5/95). Upon light irradiation condition, PMCM successfully generated singlet oxygen, which was observed by means of photoluminescence from singlet oxygen at a wavelength of 1270 nm. PMCMs have great potential as a biomedical nanodevice for combination cancer therapy as evidenced by the sustained release of CDDP from PMCMs under physiological saline conditions and the generation of singlet oxygen under light irradiation.

As a new type of biomedical nanodevice, hollow nanocapsule (NC) has been designed by alternative deposition of positive polyelectrolyte and negatively charged DP onto negatively charged polystyrene NP as the sacrificial template (Figure 3.12).[71] By alternative deposition of poly(allylamine hydrochloride) (PAH) and DP onto the polystyrene NP, stable layer-by-layer (LbL) structure was obtained. The sacrificial template was then removed by using tetrahydrofuran (THF) to obtain hollow NCs. Because the DP was successfully worked as a photosensitizing unit, the hollow NCs have strong potential for the utilization in PDT. Furthermore, the hollow NCs were filled with doxorubicin (DOX), a model anticancer drug, to implement chemotherapy. After the loading of DOX, the release rate of DOX from hollow NCs could be controlled by cross-linking of the NC surface using *N*-hydroxysuccinimide (NHS) and 1-ethyl-3-(3-dimethylaminopropyl)carbodiimide (EDC). To evaluate the feasibility of combination cancer therapy, HeLa cells were incubated with NCs or NCs with DOX under dark conditions and then irradiated light. These cell viability studies revealed that the combined treatment exerted higher toxicity than either chemotherapy or PDT alone. The viability of cell was decreased about 20% by the

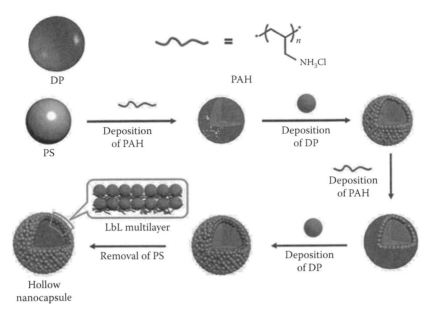

FIGURE 3.12   Procedure for the preparation of multilayer hollow NCs. PAH, poly(allylamine hydrochloride). (From Son, K. J., et al. Photosensitizing hollow nanocapsules for combination cancer therapy. *Angew. Chem. Int. Ed.*, 2011, 50, 11968–11971. Copyright Wiley-VCH Verlag GmbH & Co. KGaA. Reproduced with permission.)

effect of DOX. When photoirradiation was applied, both DOX-free NCs and NCs with DOX exhibited strong photocytotoxicity.

3.5   DIAGNOSTIC APPLICATIONS OF DP

Recently, dendrimers have been incorporated into various bioassay systems as a multifunctional linker to immobilize biomolecules.[72] The main motivation of using dendrimers in bioanalysis is that they have more binding capacity to immobilize biomolecules than conventional linear linkers due to their numerous functional groups, resulting in higher sensitivity and lower detection limits in biosensing applications.[73,74] Although most of the studies using dendrimers have been focused on DNA-based biosensors, many researches are moving forward to expand the use of dendrimer to protein-based biosensors with the thrust of scientific endeavor moving from genomics to proteomics. In this section, we first introduce the current state of art in the use of dendrimers for protein-based bioassay system and the use of DP-immobilized surfaces for biosensors.

3.5.1   IMMOBILIZATION OF DENDRIMER FOR HIGHLY SENSITIVE MICROARRAY

Protein microarrays were developed to address the realization that the investigation of genetic information alone cannot fully explain complex cellular networks and provide a powerful means of evaluating the activities of various proteins in a high-throughput manner.[75-77] The performance of protein microarray is dependent on various factors, including surface chemistry for protein immobilization, micro-fabrication technique for the array production, and detection techniques. Among these factors, surface chemistry is the most important because unlike DNA, structure and activity of proteins are very sensitive to the substrate materials and immobilization methods.[72] In most of protein microarrays, proteins were immobilized on the two-dimensional substrates through nonspecific adsorption or covalent binding to the tethered linear linkers on the surfaces.[78-81] However, in a fixed area on the planar substrate, the amount of protein that can be attached is limited, resulting in a relatively low sensitivity of assay, and immobilized proteins may dehydrate and denature due to rapid evaporation of the liquid environment and close contact with substrates, eventually losing their native structures and function. Dendrimer-coated surface is a potential candidate that can overcome problems associated with current protein microarray systems mentioned above because the 3D architecture of the dendrimer can provide numerous functional groups, which endows high density of protein immobilization.[71,74] Furthermore, the flexible nature of surface functional groups on dendrimers is suitable for minimizing protein denature. Beier and Hoheisel first reported on dendritic linker systems that were generated by direct chemical reaction on the substrates.[82] In spite of increased binding capacities, a major disadvantage of this system is that dendritic linker system must be generated *in situ* by time-consuming multiple chemical steps, precluding any quality control of the linkers during the process, and limiting a potential industrial development. Since Benters et al. reported that these problems could be resolved by employment of a presynthesized dendrimer, several researchers developed dendrimer-activated solid supports for protein microarray by covalent attachment of dendrimers to a substrate surface through self-assembled monolayers (SAMs) based on gold–sulfur or glass (silicon)–silane chemistry.[75,83-85] Among the various dendrimers, poly(amidoamine) (PAMAM) is most frequently studied due to a dense amine functional group that allows easy immobilization of dendrimers on the surface and protein to the dendrimer, but not many other dendrimers except PAMAM have been explored for protein immobilization. Furthermore, only limited examples were reported about creating dendrimer micropatterns and their subsequent use for protein microarrays.

3.5.2 DP-Immobilized Surface

Recently, DP has been utilized as a linker for immobilization of proteins on the solid substrates.[76] DP-coated silicon surfaces were prepared by electrostatic interaction. DP exhibits negative ζ potential (−31.0 mV) at pH 7 due to the 32 carboxylates on the periphery with a pK_a value of about 4.2. Therefore, when silicon surface was modified with positively charged amine groups using 3-aminopropyltriethoxysilane (APTES) by means of silanization reaction, negatively charged DP could be adsorbed to positively charged silicon surface via electrostatic interaction (Figure 3.13). Because of a focal porphyrin core that has strong fluorescence emission, the presence of DP on the substrates was easily confirmed with fluorescence microscopy and the relative amount of DP on the surface

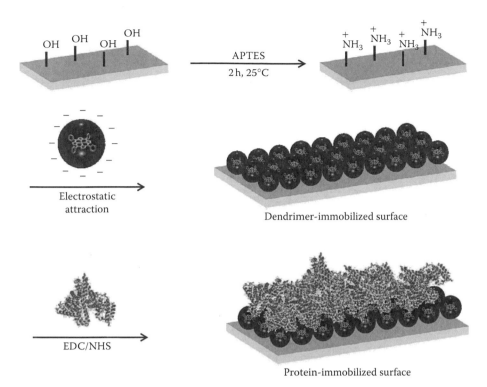

FIGURE 3.13 Schematic representation of protein immobilization on silicon/glass substrates coated with ionic DP.

could be easily monitored by fluorescence intensity. AFM study further revealed that the dendrimer was homogeneously coated onto the APTES-modified silicon surface as dome-shaped features that protruded 1.0–2.5 nm above the surface and had diameters that ranged from 50 to 100 nm, indicating that the collapsed dendrimer film reconfigures the planar silicon to create quasi-3D environments with nanomolecular dimensions. Compared with protein immobilization using linear linker systems, the DP-coating process increased the surface-binding capacity and activity of the surface-immobilized protein with lower nonspecific adsorption because the deposited DP can preserve the native conformation of immobilized proteins, perhaps by a "cushioning effect," and provide multiple carboxyl groups. Another attractive feature of DP is that it can also be used as a probe for environmental perturbations as well as multifunctional linkers because of fluorescent property of the porphyrin core. For example, glucose oxidase (GOx)-catalyzed reaction could be characterized using DP based on the fact that hydrogen peroxide generated from GOx-mediated glucose oxidation quenched fluorescence emission from the focal porphyrin core and there was a quantitative relationship between quenching and glucose concentration.

After confirming that DP could be effective linkers for protein immobilization with greater protein-binding capacity and higher protein activity than conventional linear linkers, and could play an additional role as a sensing element due

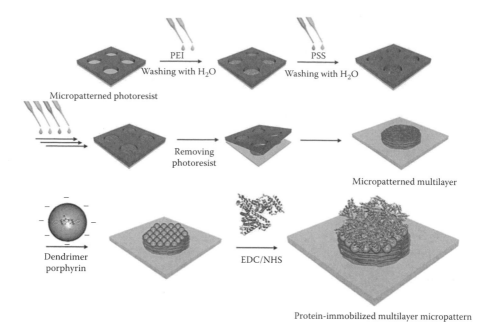

Micropatterned photoresist

PEI
Washing with H₂O

PSS
Washing with H₂O

Removing photoresist

Micropatterned multilayer

Dendrimer porphyrin

EDC/NHS

Protein-immobilized multilayer micropattern

FIGURE 3.14 Preparation of protein microarrays using patterned multilayer films with ionic DP coating.

to its fluorescence nature, protein microarrays with high sensitivity and stability have been fabricated by combining DP immobilization and microfabrication techniques. The DP-coated polyelectrolyte multilayer micropattern was prepared for protein microarrays through a combination of LbL self-assembly and liftoff methods (Figure 3.14).[86] A silicon substrate was micropatterned with a photoresist thin film using conventional photolithography, and then positively charged PEI and negatively charged poly(sodium 4-styrenesulfonate) (PSS) were alternatively deposited onto the substrate surface using spin-assisted self-assembly. A well-defined multilayer microarray was produced by subsequent removal of the photoresist template by a liftoff process. Negatively charged DP adsorbed more vigorously to positively terminated micropatterns (PEI/PSS)$_n$PEI, because of electrostatic attraction, resulting in the formation of multifunctional and quasi-3D micropatterns that could subsequently immobilize proteins. The amount of DP adsorbed on the multilayer micropatterns increased with the number of bilayers because increasing the number of bilayers allows more interaction with dendrimers due to the formation of more stable PEI layers on the micropattern, and eventually yields uniform and homogeneous PEI layers after multiple deposition. An immunoassay between immunoglobulin G (IgG) and anti-IgG demonstrated that the DP-coated microarrays showed better performance with better sensitivity and detection limit than the control microarrays coated with linear PAA polymer rather than DP, most likely due to the capability of DP to accommodate more proteins with higher activity.

REFERENCES

1. Gorman, C., 1998. Metallodendrimers: Structural diversity and functional behavior. *Adv. Mater.* 10: 295–309.
2. Zeng, F., et al., 1997. Dendrimers in supramolecular chemistry: From molecular recognition to self-assembly. *Chem. Rev.* 97: 1681–1712.
3. Fisher, M., et al., 1999. Dendrimers: From design to application—A progress report. *Angew. Chem. Int. Ed.* 38: 884–905.
4. Newkome, G. R., et al., 2001. *Dendrimers and Dendrons: Concepts, Syntheses, Applications.* Wiley-VCH, Weinheim.
5. Fréchet, J. M. J., et al., 2001. *Dendrimers and Other Dendritic Polymers.* Wiley-VCH, New York.
6. Bosman, A. W., et al., 1999. About dendrimers: Structure, physical properties, and applications. *Chem. Rev.* 99: 1665–1688.
7. Lee, I., et al., 2002. Structural molecular dynamics studies on polyamidoamine dendrimers for a therapeutic application: Effects of pH and generation. *Macromolecules* 35: 4510–4520.
8. Roy, R., et al., 1993. Solid-phase synthesis of dendritic sialoside inhibitors of influenza A virus haemagglutinin. *J. Chem. Soc., Chem. Commun.* 1869–1872.
9. Tekade, R. K., et al., 2009. Dendrimers in oncology: An expanding horizon. *Chem. Rev.* 109: 9–87.
10. Mintzer, M. A., et al., 2011. Biomedical applications of dendrimers: A tutorial. *Chem. Soc. Rev.* 40: 173–190.
11. Liu, M., et al., 2000. Water-soluble dendritic unimolecular micelles: Their potential as drug delivery agents. *J. Control. Release* 65: 121–131.
12. Stevelmans, S., et al., 1996. Synthesis, characterization, and guest–host properties of inverted unimolecular dendritic micelles. *J. Am. Chem. Soc.* 118: 7398–7399.
13. Gupta, U., et al., 2006. Dendrimers: Novel polymeric nanoarchitectures for solubility enhancement. *Biomacromolecules* 7: 649–658.
14. Tomalia, D. A., et al., 1985. A new class of polymers: Starburst-dendritic macromolecules. *Polym. J.* 17: 117–132.
15. Newkome, G. R., et al., 1985. Cascade molecules: A new approach to micelles. A [27]-Arborol. *J. Org. Chem.* 50: 2003–2004.
16. Hawker, C. J., et al., 1990. Preparation of polymers with controlled molecular architecture. A new convergent approach to dendritic macromolecules. *J. Am. Chem. Soc.* 112: 7638–7647.
17. Jin, R. H., et al., 1993. "Caged" porphyrin: The first dendritic molecule having a core photochemical functionality. *Chem. Commun.* 1260–1262.
18. Anthony, C. H., et al., 1999. Synthesis and photophysical properties of nonaggregated phthalocyanines bearing dendritic substituents. *Macromolecules* 32: 5292–5298.
19. Dolmans, D. E., et al., 2003. Photodynamic therapy for cancer. *Nat. Rev. Cancer* 3: 380–387.
20. Dougherty, T. J., et al., 1998. Photodynamic therapy. *J. Natl. Cancer Inst.* 90: 889–905.
21. Macdonald, I. J., et al., 2001. Basic principles of photodynamic therapy. *J. Porphyr. Phthalocyanines* 5: 105–129.
22. Bonnettt, R., 2000. *Chemical Aspects of Photodynamic Therapy.* Gordon and Breach Science Publishers, Amsterdam.
23. Pandey, R. K., et al., 2000. Porphyrins as photosensitizers in photodynamic therapy. In *The Porphyrin Handbook.* Kadishi, R. K., Smith, K. M., Guilard, R., Eds.; Academic Press, New York, vol. 6, pp. 157–230.
24. Derycke, A. S. L., et al., 2004. Liposomes for photodynamic therapy. *Adv. Drug Deliv. Rev.* 56: 17–30.

25. van Dongen, G. A. M. S., et al., 2004. Photosensitizer immunoconjugates for detection and therapy of cancer. *Adv. Drug Deliv. Rev.* 56: 31–52.
26. Li, Y., et al., 2007. Dendrimer generation effects on photodynamic efficacy of dendrimer porphyrins and dendrimer-loaded supramolecular nanocarriers. *Chem. Mater.* 19: 5557–5562.
27. Smith, G. J., 1985. The effects of aggregation on the fluorescence and triplet state yield of hematoporphyrin. *Photochem. Photobiol.* 41: 123–126.
28. Bennett, L. E., 1988. Singlet oxygen formation in monomeric and aggregated porphyrin c. *J. Photochem. Photobiol. B Biol.* 3: 81–89.
29. Cauchon, N., 2005. Structure-photodynamic activity relationships of substituted zinc trisulfophthalocyanines. *Bioconjug. Chem.* 16: 80–89.
30. Jang, W.-D., et al., 2005. Supramolecular nanocarrier of anionic dendrimer porphyrins with cationic block copolymers modified with polyethylene glycol to enhance intracellular photodynamic efficacy. *Angew. Chem. Int. Ed.* 44: 419–423.
31. Jang, W.-D., et al., 2006. Polyion complex micelle for photodynamic therapy: Incorporation of dendritic photosensitizer excitable at long wavelength relevant to improved tissue-penetrating property. *J. Control. Release* 113: 73–79.
32. Nishiyama, N., et al., 2003. Light-harvesting ionic dendrimer porphyrins as new photosensitizers for photodynamic therapy. *Bioconjug. Chem.* 14: 58–66.
33. O'Connor, A. E., et al., 2009. Porphyrin and nonporphyrin photosensitizers in oncology: Preclinical and clinical advances in photodynamic therapy. *Photochem. Photobiol.* 85: 1053–1074.
34. Zhang, G.-D., et al., 2003. Polyion complex micelles entrapping cationic dendrimer porphyrin: Effective photosensitizer for photodynamic therapy of cancer. *J. Control. Release* 93: 141–150.
35. Stapert, H. R., et al., 2000. Polyion complex micelles encapsulating light-harvesting ionic dendrimer zinc porphyrins. *Langmuir* 16: 8182–8188.
36. Tannock, I. F., et al., 1989. Acid pH in tumors and its potential for therapeutic exploitation. *Cancer Res.* 49: 4373–4384.
37. Maiti, N. C., et al., 1998. J- and H-aggregates of porphyrin–surfactant complexes: Time-resolved fluorescence and other spectroscopic studies. *J. Phys. Chem. B* 102: 1528–1538.
38. Kadish, K. M., et al., 1989. Micellar effects on the aggregation of tetraanionic porphyrins. Spectroscopic characterization of free-base meso-tetrakis(4-sulfonatophenyl) porphyrin, (TPPS)H2, and (TPPS)M (M = zinc(II), copper(II), and vanadyl) in aqueous micellar media. *Inorg. Chem.* 28: 2725–2731.
39. Nishiyama, M., et al., 2009. Enhanced photodynamic cancer treatment by supramolecular nanocarriers charged with dendrimer phthalocyanine. *J. Control. Release* 133: 245–251.
40. Majno, G., et al., 1995. Apoptosis, oncosis, and necrosis. An overview of cell death. *Am. J. Phathol.* 146: 3–15.
41. Berg, K., et al., 1999. Photochemical internalization: A novel technology for delivery of macromolecules into cytosol. *Cancer Res.* 59: 1180–1183.
42. Høgset, A., et al., 2004. Photochemical internalization in drug and gene delivery. *Adv. Drug Deliv. Rev.* 56: 95–115.
43. Nishiyama, N., et al., 2006. Photochemical enhancement of transgene expression by polymeric micelles incorporating plasmid DNA and dendrimer-based photosensitizer. *J. Drug Target.* 14: 413–424.
44. Downes, C. S., et al., 1985. Novobiocin inhibition of DNA excision repair may occur through effects on mitochondrial structure and ATP metabolism, not on repair topoisomerases. *Carcinogenesis* 6: 1343–1352.
45. Renno, R. Z., et al., 2001. Photosensitizer delivery for photodynamic therapy of choroidal neovascularization. *Adv. Drug Deliv. Rev.* 52: 63–78.

46. TAP and VIP Study Group, 2002. Guidelines for using verteporfin (visudyne(r)) in photodynamic therapy to treat choroidal neovascularization due to age-related macular degeneration and other causes. *Retina* 22: 6–18.
47. Ideta, R., et al., 2005. Nanotechnology-based photodynamic therapy for neovascular disease using a supramolecular nanocarrier loaded with a dendritic photosensitizer. *Nano Lett.* 5: 2426–2431.
48. Nishiyama, N., et al., 2003. Novel cisplatin-incorporated polymeric micelles can eradicate solid tumors in mice. *Cancer Res.* 63: 8977–8983.
49. Kwon, G., et al., 1994. Enhanced tumor accumulation and prolonged circulation times of micelle-forming poly(ethylene oxide-aspartate) block copolymer-adriamycin conjugates. *J. Control. Release* 29: 17–23.
50. Yokoyama, M., et al., 1999. Selective delivery of adiramycin to a solid tumor using a polymeric micelle carrier system. *J. Drug Target.* 7: 171–186.
51. Ideta, R., et al., 2004. Effective accumulation of polyion complex micelle to experimental choroidal neovascularization in rats. *FEBS Lett.* 557: 21–25.
52. Lo, P.-C., et al., 2004. New amphiphilic silicon(IV) phthalocyanines as efficient photosensitizers for photodynamic therapy: Synthesis, photophysical properties, and in vitro photodynamic activities. *Chem. Eur. J.* 10: 4831–4838.
53. Sheng, Z., et al., 2002. Transient absorption and fluorescence studies of disstacking phthalocyanine by poly(ethylene oxide). *Macromolecules* 35: 3681–3685.
54. Høgset, A., et al., 2000. Photochemical transfection: A new technology for light-induced, site-directed gene delivery. *Hum. Gene Ther.* 11: 869–880.
55. Prasmickaite, L., et al., 2001. Evaluation of different photosensitizers for use in photochemical gene transfection. *Photochem. Photobiol.* 73: 388–395.
56. Høgset, A., et al., 2002. Photochemical transfection: A technology for efficient light-directed gene delivery. *Somat. Cell Mol. Genet.* 27: 97–113.
57. Berg, K., et al., 2005. Site-specific drug delivery by photochemical internalization enhances the antitumor effect of bleomycin. *Clin. Cancer Res.* 11: 8476–8485.
58. Cabral, H., et al., 2009. A photo-activated targeting chemotherapy using glutathione sensitive camptothecin-loaded polymeric micelles. *Pharm. Res.* 26: 82–92.
59. Nishiyama, N., et al., 2005. Light-induced gene transfer from packaged DNA enveloped in a dendrimeric photosensitizer. *Nat. Mater.* 4: 934–941.
60. Rudolph, C., et al., 2003. Oligomers of the arginine-rich motif of the HIV-1 TAT protein are capable of transferring plasmid DNA into cells. *J. Biol. Chem.* 278: 11411–11418.
61. Prestayko, A. W., 1979. Cisplatin (cis-diamminedichloroplatinum II). *Cancer Treat. Rev.* 6: 17–39.
62. Kelland, L. R., 1993. New platinum antitumor complexes. *Crit. Rev. Oncol. Hematol.* 15: 191–219.
63. Rosenberg, B., 1985. Fundamental studies with cisplatin. *Cancer* 55: 2303–2316.
64. Kobayashi, K., et al., 2002. Enhancement of x-ray-induced breaks in DNA bound to molecules containing platinum: A possible application to hadrontherapy. *Radiat. Res.* 157: 32–37.
65. Lu, Q.-B., 2007. Molecular reaction mechanisms of combination treatments of low-dose cisplatin with radiotherapy and photodynamic therapy. *J. Med. Chem.* 50: 2601–2604.
66. Nonaka, M., et al., 2002. Effect of combined photodynamic and chemotherapeutic treatment on lymphoma cells in vitro. *Cancer Lett.* 184: 171–178.
67. Crescenzi, E., et al., 2004. Photodynamic therapy with indocyanine green complements and enhances low-dose cisplatin cytotoxicity in MCF-7 breast cancer cells. *Mol. Cancer Ther.* 3: 537–544.
68. Moorehead, R. A., et al., 1994. Cross-resistance to cisplatin in cells resistant to photofrin-mediated photodynamic therapy. *Cancer Res.* 54: 2556–2559.

69. Crescenzi, E., 2006. Low doses of cisplatin or gemcitabine plus Photofrin/photodynamic therapy: Disjointed cell cycle phase-related activity accounts for synergistic outcome in metastatic non-small cell lung cancer cells (H1299). *Mol. Cancer Ther.* 5: 776–785.

70. Kim, J., et al., 2009. Polymer–metal complex micelles for the combination of sustained drug releasing and photodynamic therapy. *J. Mater. Chem.* 19: 4627–4631.

71. Son, K. J., et al., 2011. Photosensitizing hollow nanocapsules for combination cancer therapy. *Angew. Chem. Int. Ed.* 50: 11968–11971.

72. Boas, U., et al., 2006. *Dendrimers in Medicine and Biotechnology: New Molecular Tools.* Springer, Berlin, pp. 130–151.

73. Satija, J., et al., 2011. Dendrimers in biosensors: Concept and applications. *J. Mater. Chem.* 21: 14367–14386.

74. Pathak, S., et al., 2004. Dendrimer-activated surfaces for high density and high activity protein chip applications. *Langmuir* 20: 6075–6079.

75. Benters, R., et al., 2001. Dendrimer-activated solid supports for nucleic acid and protein microarrays. *ChemBioChem* 2: 686–694.

76. Lee, Y., et al., 2009. Protein-conjugated, glucose-sensitive surface using fluorescent dendrimer porphyrin. *J. Mater. Chem.* 19: 5643–5647.

77. Angenendt, P., et al., 2003. Next generation of protein microarray support materials: Evaluation for protein and antibody microarray applications. *J. Chromatogr. A* 1009: 97–104.

78. Hoheisel, J. D., et al., 2006. Microarray technology: Beyond transcript profiling and genotype analysis. *Nat. Rev. Microbiol.* 7: 200–210.

79. Wilson, D. S., et al., 2003. Recent developments in protein microarray technology. *Angew. Chem. Int. Ed.* 42: 494–500.

80. Zhu, H., et al., 2001. Global analysis of protein activities using proteome chips. *Science* 293: 2101–2105.

81. Wolinsky, J. B., et al., 2008. Therapeutic and diagnostic applications of dendrimers for cancer treatment. *Adv. Drug Deliv. Rev.* 60: 1037–1055.

82. Beier, M., et al., 1999. Versatile derivatisation of solid support media for covalent bonding on DNA-microchips. *Nucleic Acids Res.* 27: 1970–1977.

83. Rozkiewicz, D. I., et al., 2007. Dendrimer-mediated transfer printing of DNA and RNA microarrays. *J. Am. Chem. Soc.* 129: 11593–11599.

84. Seok, H. J., et al., 2005. Mass spectrometric analysis of affinity-captured proteins on a dendrimer-based immunosensing surface: Investigation of on-chip proteolytic digestion. *Anal. Biochem.* 337: 294–307.

85. Yoon, H. C., 2002. Biocatalytic precipitation induced by an affinity reaction on dendrimer-activated surfaces for the electrochemical signaling from immunosensors. *Analyst* 127: 1082–1087.

86. Son, K. J., et al., 2010. Dendrimer porphyrin-terminated polyelectrolyte multilayer micropatterns for a protein microarray with enhanced sensitivity. *J. Mater. Chem.* 20: 6531–6538.

4 Polymeric Nanoparticles in Cancer Therapy

Heebeom Koo, Ji Young Yhee,
Ick Chan Kwon, and Kwangmeyung Kim
Korea Institute of Science and Technology

Ramesh Subbiah
University of Science and Technology
Korea Institute of Science and Technology

CONTENTS

4.1 INTRODUCTION

Chemotherapy is the clinical treatment of disease with chemical drugs, and has been researched and performed over several hundreds of years. Compared to surgery, it is regarded as noninvasive, relatively cheaper, easy for public assessment, and less dangerous. However, there are also some risks and side effects when drugs are not localized in the target disease site, but in another normal site, because most drugs can change the biological metabolism even in healthy tissues. Therefore, the efficient and accurate delivery of drugs to the target disease tissue and cells is highly important in chemotherapy. An ideal drug delivery system

(DDS) can provide expected clinical outcomes with a minimum amount of drugs so that its efficiency is valuable from the economic point of view. In addition, it can reduce the unintended side effect resulting from drug accumulation in normal healthy tissues. To realize this system, many biomedical researchers have made efforts for finding more efficient delivery methods or carriers and optimizing these systems (Xie et al. 2010).

Brilliant advances in nanoscience and biotechnology have revolutionized our view and approach to fight against disease and cure patients. In this century, nanoparticles (NPs) have been expected and researched as novel drug carriers to improve the pharmacokinetics of drugs (Petros and DeSimone 2010). Their large compartments such as large surface area or inner cores allow large amounts of drugs to be introduced into NPs through simple loading and chemical conjugation. These NPs can increase the circulation time of drugs in body and delay their excretion through the renal clearance by kidneys. Especially, there is fast angiogenesis in tumor tissue, and consequently, their vascular structures have a fenestrated structure different from normal vessels. High accumulation of NPs (below 500 nm) through these fenestrated vessels in tumor tissue has been proven, which is the so-called enhanced permeation and retention (EPR) effect (Figure 4.1) (Maeda et al. 2000). Furthermore, their accumulation in target tissue or uptake into target cells can be further enhanced using specific targeting moieties such as an antibody, an aptamer, or a particular sequence of peptides (Koo et al. 2011). For these advantages of NPs, many researchers have

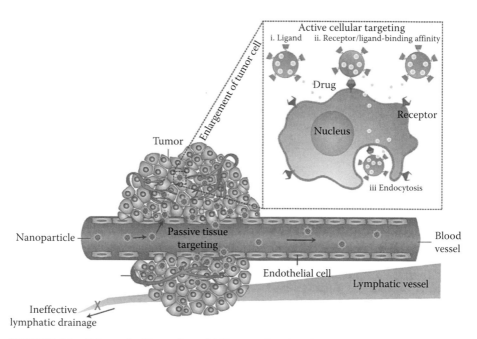

FIGURE 4.1 Schematic illustration of NPs targeting (passive tissue targeting and active cellular targeting). (Reprinted by permission from Macmillan Publishers Ltd. *Nature Nanotechnology*, Peer, D., et al. 2007, copyright 2007.)

paid much attention to NPs for more efficient and safe drug delivery and therapy (Lammers et al. 2011).

NPs have been developed for biomedical application using various organic or inorganic materials such as lipids, polymers, iron oxide, gold, silver, silica, or special carbon structures (Park et al. 2009). Among these base materials, polymers have been the most frequently used components for many years. The physicochemical properties of polymers depend on their molecular weight and chemical structures. These parameters can be easily controlled by researchers through simple chemistry, which means that the physicochemical properties of polymeric NPs such as surface size also can be controlled for their purpose. This variability of polymers has been used to fabricate various kinds of NP formulations.

Polymers are categorized into two types: natural polymers and synthetic polymers. Various NPs have been developed using both types of polymers, and they have distinct advantages for NP fabrication and application. In this chapter, we introduce the development of polymeric NPs based on these two types of natural and synthetic polymers and their biomedical application as drug carriers.

4.2 NATURAL POLYMER-BASED NPs FOR CANCER THERAPY

Many polymers are found in nature, and they are used as building blocks of living systems or sometimes perform more special functions such as carrying small molecules (Figure 4.2). Natural polymers are generally grouped into polysaccharides and proteins. For fabrication of NPs, the former are more advantageous due to easy handling compared to the latter with delicate three-dimensional folding. Here we introduce the five major natural polymers used for the development of NPs. We focus on the three polysaccharides, chitosan, hyaluronic acid, and dextran. In addition, albumin and gelatin (a protein and a protein/polypeptide mixture, respectively) will also be introduced as building blocks of NPs.

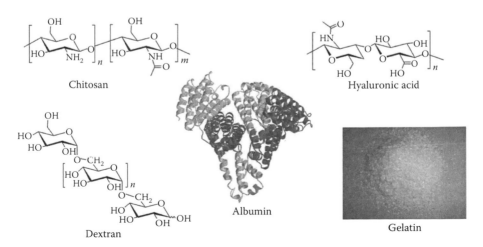

FIGURE 4.2 Natural polymers used in NP fabrication.

4.2.1 Chitosan NPs

Chitosan is β-(1,4)-2-amido-D-glucose linked via (1–4) glycosidic bonds, and it originates from chitin, the shell material found in crabs and shrimp. It is produced through a deacetylation procedure from chitin so that it has primary amine groups in its structure. This amine group can provide the possibility of conjugating various kinds of molecules to the chitosan backbone by amide bond linkage, enabling easy modification and wide application of chitosan (Park et al. 2010). Another useful property of chitosan for biomedical application is its biodegradability and biocompatibility. Chitosan is known to be degraded by various enzymes in the body and is excreted mainly by urine after several days.

The amine group in chitosan has pK_a value of about 6.5 so that it is soluble in acidic pH but not soluble in an aqueous condition with neutral pH. This low water-solubility of chitosan inhibits its application to various fields. Consequently, researchers have developed various chitosan derivatives such as carboxymethyl (CM) chitosan, trimethyl chitosan, PEGylated chitosan, or glycol chitosan (GC) by chemical modification. The kinds of chitosan derivatives and their application to biomedical fields such as drug delivery are well summarized by other researchers (Dash et al. 2011).

Among many chitosan derivatives, our group has focused on GC and developed GC NPs. These GC NPs showed biocompatibility and superior tumor-targeting ability after intravenous injection. Therefore, in this chapter, we introduce our GC NPs and their biomedical application for several years.

GC NPs were developed based on self-assembly of amphiphilic structure in aqueous condition. When hydrophobic moieties are conjugated to hydrophilic polymers such as GC, the resulting conjugates can self-assemble into NPs with hydrophobic multicores and hydrophilic polymer shells. Cho et al. (2007) synthesized amphiphilic NPs using GC, gelatin, and heparin as polymer backbones and compared their behavior during *in vivo* condition (Figure 4.3). FITC, doxorubicin, and lithocholic groups were used as hydrophobic substituents, and the size of these NPs was about 150–470 nm. They were intravenously injected into tumor-bearing mice models, and their biodistribution was evaluated using radio imaging with ^{131}I. Interestingly, GC NPs showed higher accumulation in tumor tissue compared to gelatin or heparin NPs. The amount of GC NPs in tumor tissue was gradually increased during 3 days, showing their long circulation and time-dependent accumulation in tumor tissue. Histological images showed their abundant localization in the perivascular region of the tumor, demonstrating their extravasation through fenestrated vascular structure in tumor tissue, the so-called EPR effect.

Park et al. (2007) synthesized GC NPs with different molecular weights and analyzed their tumor-targeting characteristics (Figure 4.4). Low molecular weight GC polymers were produced using an acidic degradation method, and three kinds of GC (20, 100, and 250 kDa) were used for NP fabrication. The resulting GC NPs showed a similar size from 231 to 310 nm, and the cationic zeta potential value was around 10 mV. To evaluate their biodistribution, we used optical imaging. Near-infrared (NIR) fluorescence dye, Cy5.5, was labeled to GC NPs for *in vivo* optical imaging, because NIR light can penetrate through deep tissue better than UV or visible light. After intravenous injection of these GC NPs into tumor-bearing mice models, their

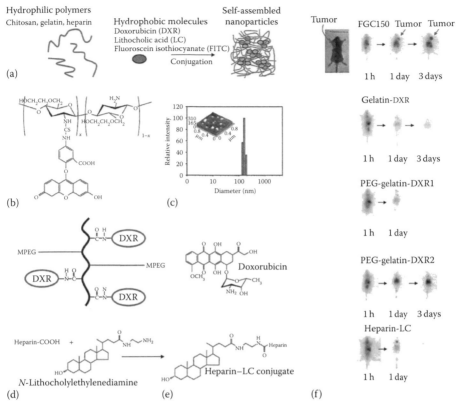

FIGURE 4.3 *In vivo* radionuclide imaging with self-assembled GC NPs. (a) Schematic illustration of amphiphilic NP synthesis and self-assembly. (b) Chemical structure of GC NPs. (c) Size and shape of GC NPs. (d) Chemical structure of gelatin NPs and doxorubicin (DXR). (e) Synthesis of heparin NPs. (f) Scintigraphic images of tumor-bearing mice models after intravenous injection of self-assembled NPs. (Reprinted from *Biomaterials*, 28, Cho, Y. W., S. A. Park, T. H. Han, D. H. Son, J. S. Park, S. J. Oh, D. H. Moon, et al., In vivo tumor targeting and radionuclide imaging with self-assembled nanoparticles: Mechanisms, key factors, and their implications, 1236–47, Copyright 2007, with permission from Elsevier.)

biodistribution and time-dependent accumulation in organs were analyzed by optical imaging. In both whole-body and excised organ images, GC NPs with higher molecular weight (250 kDa) showed longer circulation and higher accumulation in tumor tissue. These results demonstrated the importance of the physicochemical optimization of NPs and the usefulness of optical imaging for the development of tumor-targeting NPs.

The cellular uptake of GC NPs was studied by Nam et al. (2009) (Figure 4.5). For efficient drug delivery, drug-containing NPs should enter the target cells and release the drug inside. Consequently, the information about the cellular uptake of NPs and their mechanism is also meaningful. Interestingly, the amount of GC NPs inside human HeLa cells was higher compared to GC polymer or Cy5.5 dye after 1-h incubation. This result significantly demonstrated that the NP structure could facilitate

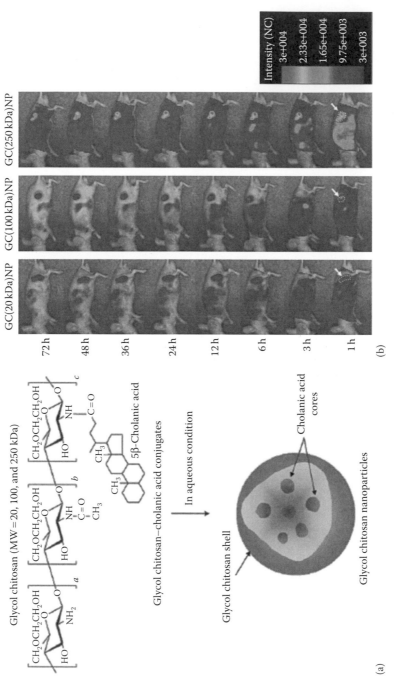

FIGURE 4.4 **(See color insert.)** Optimization of GC NPs for tumor targeting. (a) Chemical structure and schematic illustration of GC NPs. (b) *In vivo* optical images of tumor-bearing mice models after intravenous injection of GC NPs with different molecular weights. (Reprinted from *Journal of Controlled Release*, 122, Park, K., J.-H. Kim, Y. S. Nam, S. Lee, H. Y. Nam, K. Kim, J. H. Park, et al., Effect of polymer molecular weight on the tumor targeting characteristics of self-assembled glycol chitosan nanoparticles, 305–14, Copyright 2007, with permission from Elsevier.)

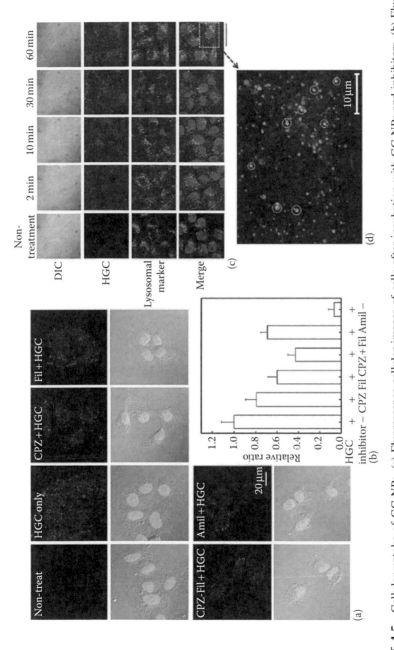

FIGURE 4.5 Cellular uptake of GC NPs. (a) Fluorescence cellular images of cells after incubation with GC NPs and inhibitors. (b) Fluorescence intensity of (a). (c) Cellular distribution of GC NPs with lysosome staining. (d) High-resolution image of (c). Amil, Amiloride; CPZ, chlorpromazine; Fil, filipin III; HGC, hydrophobically modified chitosan. (Reprinted from *Journal of Controlled Release*, 135, Nam, H. Y., S. M. Kwon, H. Chung, S.-Y. Lee, S.-H. Kwon, H. Jeon, Y. Kim, et al., Cellular uptake mechanism and intracellular fate of hydrophobically modified glycol chitosan nanoparticles, 259–67, Copyright 2009, with permission from Elsevier.)

the adhesion and uptake into cells. Then, the inhibitors related to the cellular uptake were tested with GC NPs for precise mechanism study. Chlorpromazine, filipin III, and amiloride were used as the inhibitors of clathrin-mediated endocytosis, caveolae, and macropinocytosis, respectively. The amount of GC NPs inside cells was reduced in all cases of inhibitor treatment, showing that GC NPs could internalize into cells by more than one mechanism. After cell staining with LysoTracker, some of GC NPs showed colocalization with lysosomes, but others did not. This result showed that the endosome–lysosome pathway is related to the uptake of GC NPs, but they could be dispersed in the cytoplasm.

Na et al. (2011) evaluated the tumor-targeting ability of GC NPs in various tumor models (Figure 4.6). In the flank tumor model, the movement of GC NPs through fenestrated vascular structure in tumor tissue was monitored by real-time video imaging. In the brain tumor model, GC NPs could not penetrate into brain tumor tissue due to the blood–brain barrier. However, they showed high accumulation in tumors after 3 weeks, demonstrating that the tumor-targeting ability of GC NPs

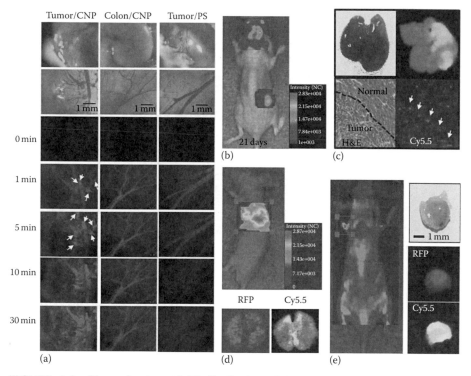

FIGURE 4.6 (See color insert.) Biodistribution of GC NPs in various tumor models. (a) Live imaging of vascular structures after NP injection. (b) GC NPs in brain tumor model. (c) Distribution of GC NPs in liver tumor. (d) GC NPs in lung metastasis model. (e) Unintended second metastasis tumor on forearm and the accumulation of GC NPs. CNP, chitosan nanoparticle; PS, polystyrene beads; RFP, red fluorescence protein. (Reprinted from *Biomaterials*, 32, Na, J. H., H. Koo, S. Lee, K. H. Min, K. Park, H. Yoo, S. H. Lee, et al., Real-time and non-invasive optical imaging of tumor-targeting glycol chitosan nanoparticles in various tumor models, 5252–61, Copyright 2011, with permission from Elsevier.)

is highly related with time-dependent angiogenesis in tumors. The liver is a major hurdle for tumor-targeting NPs due to the excretion metabolism of the reticuloendo-thelial system (RES). The superior tumor-targeting ability of GC NPs was success-fully reproduced in the liver tumor model. In addition, GC NPs were also highly accumulated in lung cancer and unintended second metastasis models, showing their possibility in clinical imaging. Furthermore, these overall results demonstrated that the stability, deformability, and rapid uptake into tumor cells resulted in the superior tumor-targeting ability of GC NPs.

Recently, Kim et al. (2010) showed optimized drug delivery using GC NPs (Figure 4.7). The biodistribution, tumor accumulation, and excretion of GC NPs were precisely monitored by noninvasive optical imaging system in tumor-bearing

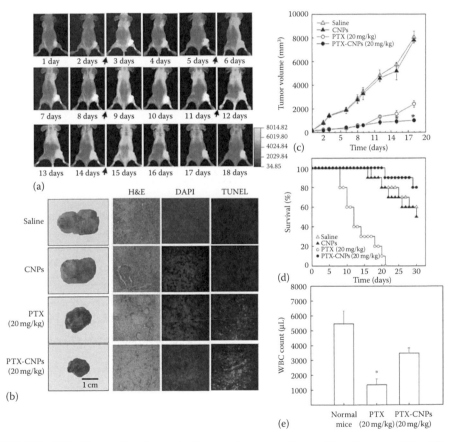

FIGURE 4.7 (See color insert.) Tumor therapy with paclitaxel-loaded GC NPs. (a) Determination of injection interval based on *in vivo* optical imaging data. (b) Analysis of excised tumors after therapy. (c) Tumor growth data. (d) Survival rates of mice models and (e) the concentration of WBCs after tumor therapy with paclitaxel-loaded GC NPs. CNP, chito-san nanoparticle; DAPI, 4′,6-diamidino-2-phenylindole. (Reprinted from *Journal of Controlled Release*, 146, Kim, K., J. H. Kim, H. Park, Y.-S. Kim, K. Park, H. Nam, S. Lee, et al., Tumor-homing multifunctional nanoparticles for cancer theragnosis: Simultaneous diagnosis, drug delivery, and therapeutic monitoring, 219–27, Copyright 2010, with permission from Elsevier.)

mice models. Thereafter, the injection interval of paclitaxel-loaded GC NPs was decided based on these imaging data. The overall results showed successful tumor suppression and increased survival rate in mice treated with these NPs. Hematoxylin and eosin (H&E) staining and terminal deoxynucleotidyl transferase dUTP nick end labeling (TUNEL) assay data significantly showed the increased apoptosis in tumor tissue based on the tumor-targeted delivery of paclitaxel by GC NPs. The acute toxicity of the different formulation of paclitaxel was evaluated by counting the number of white blood cells (WBCs) in blood 18 days postinjection. The number of WBCs in case of paclitaxel–GC NPs was higher than that of free paclitaxel in spite of improved tumor suppression. These studies demonstrated that GC NPs have superior tumor-targeting ability and great potential as drug carriers for tumor therapy.

4.2.2 Hyaluronic Acid NPs

Hyaluronic acid is a human body component abundant in the connective region and extracellular matrix. It is also called hyaluronan or hyaluronate, and is the only non-sulfated polysaccharide among the glycosaminoglycan family (Lapčik et al. 1998). Hyaluronic acid has two special advantages for biomedical application. First, it can bind to CD44 receptors on the cell surface, which are especially overexpressed in cancer cells. Consequently, hyaluronic acid-based NPs (HANPs) or micropar-ticles easily bind or internalize to cancer cells. Second, it can be easily degraded by hyaluronidase or reactive oxygen species in the human body (Stern and Jedrzejas 2006). This degradability is useful for NPs or hydrogels because they allow con-trolled release of inner cargo molecules such as drugs.

Choi et al. (2010) developed HANPs for tumor-targeted imaging or drug delivery (Figure 4.8). These particles were synthesized by the conjugation of hydrophobic 5β-cholanic acid groups similar to GC NPs. These amphiphilic polymer conjugates can self-assemble into stable NPs in aqueous condition. Their size could be reduced to about 240 nm, which is dependent on the ratio of conjugated 5β-cholanic acid groups. These HANPs showed superior tumor-targeting ability in cellular condi-tion and mice models. Their targeting strategy is based on both passive targeting due to their nano size and EPR effect and active targeting due to the binding between hyaluronic acid shell and CD44 receptors on the surface of cancer cells. In tumor-bearing mice models, the amount of accumulated NPs in tumor tissue was changed along with the ratio of 5β-cholanic acid groups, showing the importance of appropriate nano size. Furthermore, the preinjection of free hyaluronic acid inhib-ited tumor-targeting ability of HANPs, demonstrating the high accumulation of NPs partially originated from the interaction with CD44 receptors.

Choi et al. (2011a) optimized the tumor-targeting ability of HANPs by PEGylation (Figure 4.9). CD44 receptors that can bind to HANPs are abundant not only in cancer cells but also in liver tissue. They hypothesized that preventing liver uptake of NPs could increase their blood circulation time and tumor accumulation. PEGylation has been generally used to reduce the aggregation and unintended uptake into the liver or spleen, resulting in long circulation. As they expected, the amount of accumulated HANPs in tumor tissue is increased by the conjugation with the proper amount of polyethylene glycol (PEG). Intravital multicolor fluorescence images of NPs in tumor

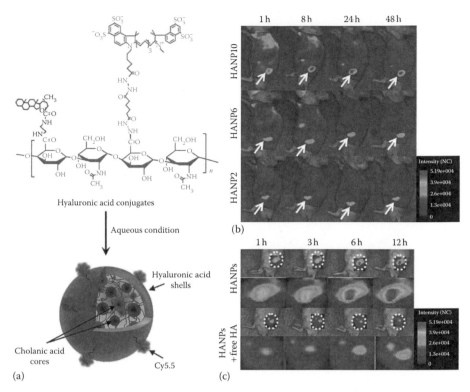

FIGURE 4.8 (See color insert.) Development of HANPs. (a) Chemical structure and schematic illustration of HANPs. (b) *In vivo* tumor accumulation of HANPs with different 5β-cholanic acid ratios. (c) *In vivo* tumor accumulation of HANPs after pretreatment of hyaluronic acids. (Reprinted from *Biomaterials*, 31, Choi, K. Y., H. Chung, K. H. Min, H. Y. Yoon, K. Kim, J. H. Park, I. C. Kwon, and S. Y. Jeong, Self-assembled hyaluronic acid nanoparticles for active tumor targeting, 106–14, Copyright 2010, with permission from Elsevier.)

vasculature significantly showed the penetration of HANPs through vessels and their accumulation around tumor tissue. These results demonstrated that PEGylation of NPs could improve their tumor-targeting ability and *in vivo* optical imaging techniques could be highly useful during these kinds of optimization.

In a recent paper, these HANPs were successfully used as tumor-targeted drug carriers (Figure 4.10) (Choi et al. 2011b). Camptothecin (CPT), a hydrophobic anticancer drug, was loaded into these NPs by simple dialysis. The loading contents and efficiency were about 34% and 85%, respectively. The release of CPT from HANPs highly increased in the presence of hyaluronidase under *in vitro* condition, showing the possibility of fast release in the cytosol of tumor cells. In a cell viability test, these CPT-loaded HANPs showed enhanced cytotoxicity in CD44 overexpressing cancer cells (MDA-MB-231) than in normal fibroblast cells (NIH3T3) due to their tumor cell-specific binding and uptake based on CD44 receptors. In MDA-MB-231 tumor-bearing mice models, they also showed superior tumor-targeting ability and successful therapeutic results. In addition, they resulted in higher cell death in tumor tissue and almost no damages compared to free CPT.

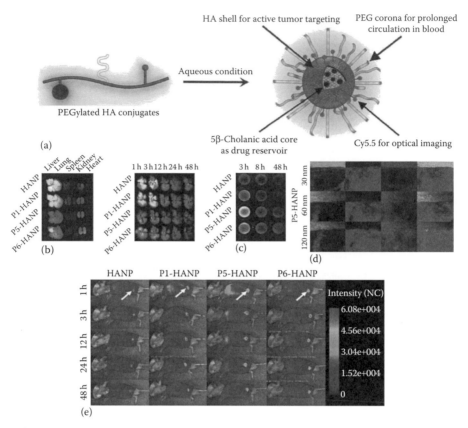

FIGURE 4.9 (See color insert.) PEGylation of HANPs. (a) Schematic illustration of PEGylated HANPs and their self-assembly in aqueous condition. (b) *Ex vivo* organ images. (c) Fluorescence intensity of blood samples. (d) Intravital live image. (e) Whole-body images of mice models treated with PEGylated HANPs. (Reprinted from *Biomaterials*, 32, Choi, K. Y., K. H. Min, H. Y. Yoon, K. Kim, J. H. Park, I. C. Kwon, K. Choi, and S. Y. Jeong, PEGylation of hyaluronic acid nanoparticles improves tumor targetability in vivo, 1880–89, Copyright 2011, with permission from Elsevier.)

Cho et al. (2011) developed another type of HANPs and tested its potential as a drug carrier with multidrug resistance (MDR) cell line (Figure 4.11). They conjugated hydrophobic ceramide group to hyaluronic acids, and NPs were prepared by the self-assembly of these conjugates and pluronic P85. Pluronic P85 was used to enhance the ability to overcome MDR and the stability of the micellar structure. The hydrophobic inner parts of these NPs can be used to carry hydrophobic molecules such as drugs. Coumarin 6 with green fluorescence was used as a model drug for cellular imaging. Using these NPs, a larger amount of coumarin 6 can be internalized in MCF-7/MDR cells compared to free coumarin 6. Relatively lower uptake of NPs in U87MG cells expressing a low level of CD44 and pretreatment of hyaluronic acid demonstrated the enhanced cellular uptake of NPs originated from the CD44 receptor-mediated endocytosis. In accordance with imaging data, docetaxel-loaded NPs could kill MCF-7/MDR cells more efficiently than free docetaxel. Also under *in vivo* conditions, the accumulation of these NPs in

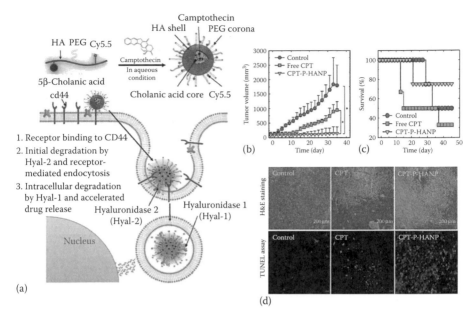

FIGURE 4.10 **(See color insert.)** Tumor-targeted drug delivery with HANPs. (a) Schematic illustration of drug loading into HANPs and their cellular uptake. (b) Tumor growth data. (c) Survival rates. (d) Histological analysis of tumor-bearing mice models after treatment with camptothecin-loaded HANPs. (Reprinted with permission from Choi, K. Y., et al., 2011, 8591–99. Copyright 2011 American Chemical Society.)

tumor tissue was reduced with pretreatment of hyaluronic acid. Taken together, we expect that HANPs will be consistently attractive drug carriers for tumor therapy.

4.2.3 DEXTRAN NPS

Dextran is produced in bacteria such as *Leuconostoc mesenteroides* or *Streptococcus mutans*, and its structure is mainly composed of linear α-(1,6)-D-glucose with some side chains linked by (1,3) positions. Dextran has a wide range of molecular weights and is highly soluble in water and many other solvents. Further modification of dextran is generally performed through its abundant hydroxyl groups, resulting in various dextran derivatives such as CM-dextran, diethylaminoethyl dextran (DEAE-dextran), or dextran sulfate. Basically, dextran is neutral in aqueous condition, but some of these derivatives have cationic or anionic charges depending upon their purpose. Dextran is easily biodegradable by natural enzymes such as dextran-(1,6)-glucosidase in the liver or spleen and dextranase in bacteria in the colon so that it is regarded as biocompatible even though it does not originate in the human body. It was also reported that dextran showed low cell binding and protein adsorption, which means it is safe after intravenous injection. These properties make dextran useful building blocks to fabricate NPs by many biomedical researchers.

Park et al. (2011) developed deoxycholic acid-conjugated dextran NPs and applied them to tumor therapy with doxorubicin. When hydrophobic deoxycholic acids were conjugated to a hydrophilic dextran backbone, they can self-assemble into an NP

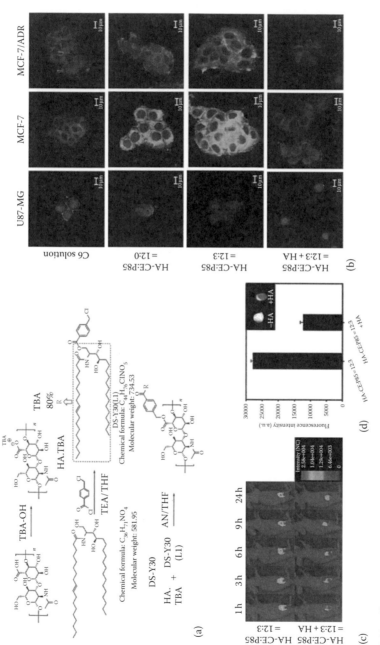

FIGURE 4.11 **(See color insert.)** HANPs for chemotherapy about MDR cell line. (a) Synthetic scheme of hyaluronic acid–ceramide conjugates. (b) Uptake of coumarin 6-loaded HANPs in MDR cells. (c) Whole-body images. (d) *Ex vivo* tumor images of MDR tumor-bearing mice models after intravenous injection of HANPs. AN, acetonitrile; TBA, tetra-*n*-butylammonium hydroxide; TEA, triethylamine; THF, tetrahydrofuran. (Reprinted from *Biomaterials*, 32, Cho, H.-J., H. Y. Yoon, H. Koo, S.-H. Ko, J.-S. Shim, J.-H. Lee, K. Kim, I. C. Kwon, and D.-D. Kim, Self-assembled nanoparticles based on hyaluronic acid–ceramide (HA-CE) and Pluronic® for tumor-targeted delivery of docetaxel, 7181–90, Copyright 2011, with permission from Elsevier.)

structure in an aqueous condition similar to chitosan-based nanoparticles (CNPs) or HANPs. Doxorubicin, a hydrophobic anticancer drug, could be successfully incorporated into these dextran NPs by dialysis. At optimal conditions, the loading efficiency and drug contents were 86.0% and 30.1% (w/w), respectively. The size of these NPs was about 150 nm, and the zeta potential value was about −10 mV. Incorporated doxorubicin could be slowly released in about 1 week, showing the stability of NPs. Their potential as drug carriers was evaluated in both cellular and animal studies. After incubation for 4 h, these dextran NPs showed fast cellular uptake into tumor cells, which was proved in fluorescence images based on the intrinsic red fluorescence of doxorubicin. Finally, they showed successful tumor suppression in CT26 tumor-bearing mice models through intravenous injection via the tail vein. The survival rate of mice treated with doxorubicin-incorporated dextran NPs was also improved compared to control groups with phosphate-buffered saline (PBS) or free doxorubicin. These data demonstrated that amphiphilic dextran NPs were good candidates for antitumor drug delivery.

Zhong group developed reversibly stabilized dextran NPs for efficient delivery of doxorubicin into the nuclei of cancer cells (Figure 4.12) (Li et al. 2009). The stability of NPs in blood flow is a critical problem for drug delivery, and an unintended burst release of drugs often results in unfavorable distribution of introduced drugs. To enhance stability, they used chemical cross-linking by degradable disulfide bonds. They conjugated lipoic acid to dextran as hydrophobic molecules for self-assembly as described in other papers. For cross-linking, these NPs were incubated with dithiothreitol (DTT), and the disulfide bond of lipoic acid was degraded into free thiol groups. Then, thiol groups interact with other thiol groups in the neighboring lipoic acid after removing DTT, resulting in cross-linking of lipoic acid molecules in hydrophobic cores of dextran NPs. After cross-linking, the stability of NPs was highly improved and they specifically degrade under a reductive condition such as cell cytosol. As expected, the release of doxorubicin from stabilized dextran NPs was extremely slower than that of non-cross-linked NPs, but it recovered in the presence of 10 mM DTT. The mechanism of doxorubicin is related to its interaction with DNA so that doxorubicin molecules are localized in the nuclei for their therapeutic effects. After a 2-h treatment, stabilized dextran NPs showed fast cellular uptake into HeLa cells, release of doxorubicin in cytosol, and their high accumulation in cell nuclei. Interestingly, the colocalization between doxorubicin and nuclei in the initial time was more enhanced in the case of NPs compared to free doxorubicin, demonstrating the enhanced stability of NPs and their fast release of doxorubicin.

Duan et al. developed another kind of dextran NP and showed its possible use of overcoming drug resistance in osteosarcoma cells (Figure 4.13) (Susa et al. 2009). Osteosarcoma is a common bone tumor that occurs in children and adolescents, and its 5-year survival rate has still remained at about 70%. Especially, the MDR tumor phenotype is frequently generated in this kind of tumor, which is the main obstacle to its therapy. Duan et al. showed the possibility of overcoming the MDR effect of osteosarcoma cells by sustained release of doxorubicin from their dextran NPs. They mixed doxorubicin, dextran–lipid conjugate, thiolated dextran, and thiolated PEG simultaneously. These molecules could be self-assembled into an NP structure based on hydrophobic interaction and further stabilized by disulfide bond formation with thiol groups. Quantitative analysis of internalized doxorubicin in cytosol showed that stable NP formulation could increase the amount of drug localized in

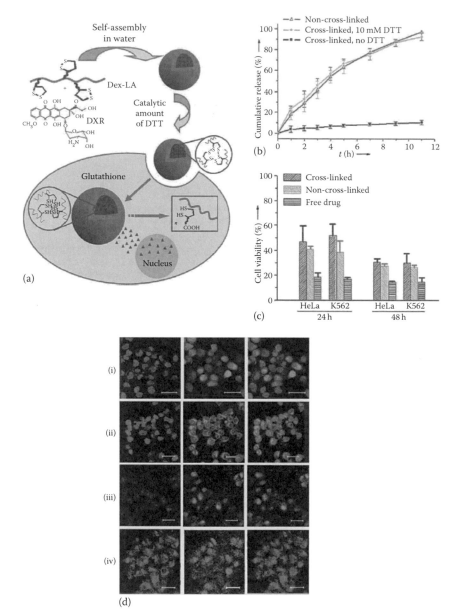

FIGURE 4.12 (See color insert.) Disulfide-stabilized dextran NPs for drug delivery. (a) Schematic illustration of disulfide-stabilized dextran NPs and triggered release in cell cytosol. (b) Triggered release of DXR from dextran NPs. (c) Cell viability. (d) Cellular uptake of DXR-loaded dextran NPs: (i) DXR-loaded dextran NPs (0.5-h incubation); (ii) DXR-loaded dextran NPs (2-h incubation); (iii) Free DXR (0.5-h incubation); (iv) Free DXR (2-h incubation). (From Li, Y.-L., Zhu, L., Liu, Z., Cheng, R., Meng, F., Cui, J.-H., Ji, S.-J., and Zhong, Z., Reversibly stabilized multifunctional dextran nanoparticles efficiently deliver doxorubicin into the nuclei of cancer cells. *Angew. Chem. Int. Ed.*, 2009, 48, 9914–18. Copyright Wiley-VCH Verlag GmbH & Co. KGaA. Reproduced with permission.)

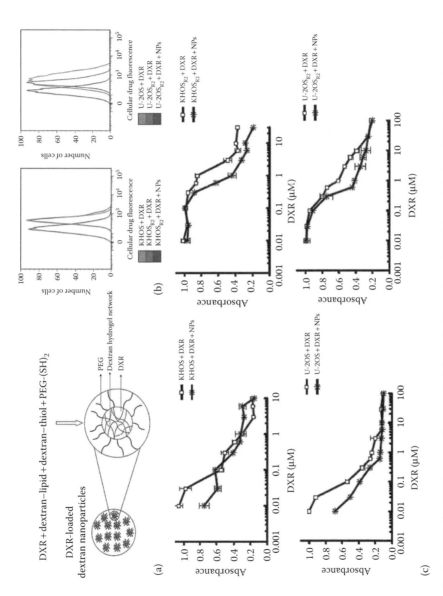

FIGURE 4.13 Dextran NPs for MDR tumor therapy. (a) Schematic illustration of DXR-loaded dextran NPs. (b) Cellular uptake and cell viability (MTT) data of DXR-loaded dextran NPs in MDR osteosarcoma cells. (Reprinted from Susa, M., et al., *BMC Cancer*, 9, 899, 2009. With permission.)

cell cytosol and overcome their strong efflux in MDR tumor cells. These data were in accordance with those of the Zhong group described earlier, which demonstrated an important potential of polymeric NPs as drug carriers against MDR tumor cells.

4.2.4 ALBUMIN NPs

Albumin is the most abundant human serum protein (about 35–50 g/L in human blood serum), and its half-life is approximately 20 days. The molecular weight of albumin is 66.5 kDa and it is 7.2 nm in diameter (He and Carter 1992). Albumin is originally bio-compatible and biodegradable because like hyaluronic acid, it is a component found in the human body. It has many amine groups in its structure and some of them are on the surface, which can be used for further chemical modification. Because of these charac-teristics, many researchers have paid much attention to albumin for biomedical applica-tions such as tissue engineering, drug delivery, and gene delivery (Hawkins et al. 2008).

The most famous albumin NP for drug delivery is albumin-bound paclitaxel (ABI-007), which is a commercialized formulation of paclitaxel for intravenous injection with the product name "Abraxane®" (Abraxis BioScience, Los Angeles, CA, USA) (Figure 4.14) (Kratz 2008). To prepare it, paclitaxel and human serum albumin are mixed in aque-ous condition and are passed through a jet under high pressure. This method is suitable for mass production in a factory compared to the dialysis method of other NPs. The size of the resulting NP, ABI-007, is about 100–200 nm, which enabled its free move-ment in blood vessels. ABI-007 showed increased circulation time, reduced toxicity, and enhanced tumor suppression in MX-1 breast cancer xenograft mice models compared to Taxol [paclitaxel solubilized in Cremophor EL (BASF Corp., Ludwigshafen, Germany)]. Moreover, intratumoral concentration of paclitaxel was also higher in the case of ABI-007 than in Taxol. In addition to these results, many preclinical and clinical studies have been performed with ABI-007, and it was finally approved in January 2005 for intra-venous injection in metastasis breast cancer patients. Now, it is commercially available and used clinically in many countries. Furthermore, it is being evaluated for the first-line treatment of nonsmall cell cancer, ovarian cancer, and pancreas cancer, and this type of albumin NP is under development with other drugs such as rapamycin or docetaxel.

Anhorn et al. (2008) developed trastuzumab-modified albumin NPs for enhanced drug delivery to human epidermal growth factor receptor 2 (HER2)-overexpressing breast cancer cells (Figure 4.15). They prepared doxorubicin-loaded albumin NPs by protein desolvation and cross-linking with glutaraldehyde. For chemical conjugation to trastuzumab, a monoclonical antibody targeting the HER2 receptor, the NP surface is modified with maleimide-functionalized PEG groups. After thiolation of trastuzumab, it was conjugated to prepared albumin NPs during 12 h of shaking. The amount of doxorubicin after uptake into SK-Br-3 tumor cells increased in the case of trastuzumab–albumin NPs compared to IgG–albumin NPs as controls. Even though the uptake of doxorubicin with trastuzumab–albumin NPs was not as high as free doxorubicin, the authors insisted that specific cellular uptake of doxorubicin into HER2-overexpressing tumor cells would be an important point of these NPs. In microscopic images, green spots of trastuzumab–albumin NPs were localized inside tumor cells, showing their efficient uptake. As expected, the cell viability test demonstrated that trastuzumab–albumin NPs showed more enhanced delivery of doxorubicin and cytotoxicity about

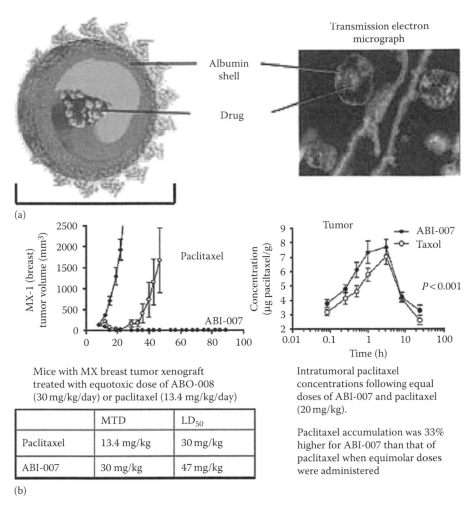

FIGURE 4.14 Commercialized albumin–paclitaxel NPs. (a) Schematic illustration and transmission electron microscopy (TEM) images of albumin–paclitaxel NPs. (b) *In vivo* therapeutic results in tumor-bearing mice models with albumin–paclitaxel NPs. LD_{50}, lethal dose 50; MTD, maximum tolerated dose; MX, mammary gland carcinoma. (Reprinted from *Journal of Controlled Release*, 132, Kratz, F., Albumin as a drug carrier: Design of prodrugs, drug conjugates and nanoparticles, 171–83, Copyright 2008, with permission from Elsevier.)

tumor cells compared to IgG–albumin NPs. Bare trastuzumab–albumin NPs showed negligible cytotoxicity, proving the biocompatibility of albumin again.

Recently, our group developed photosensitizer-conjugated albumin NPs for *in vivo* photodynamic therapy (PDT) (Jeong et al. 2011). We conjugated hydrophobic photosensitizer, chlorin e6 (Ce6), to human serum albumin for self-assembly and NP formation. The ratio between Ce6 and albumin molecules was determined based on grafting efficiency, and the optimized form has approximately 14 Ce6 molecules per one albumin. These Ce6-conjugated human serum albumin NPs (Ce6-HSA-NPs) were highly stable and showed no aggregation in aqueous condition in contrast with hydrophobic Ce6s.

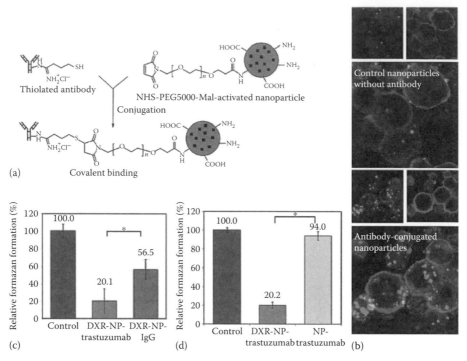

(a)   Covalent binding

(c)

(d)

(b)

FIGURE 4.15   **(See color insert.)** Antibody-conjugated albumin NPs. (a) Schematic illustration of antibody-conjugated albumin NPs. Cellular uptake (b) and cell viability assay (c and d) of antibody-conjugated albumin NPs. *The two samples are significantly different ($P < 0.01$; two-tailed Mann–Whitney U-test equivalent to the Wilcoxon rank-sum test). (Reprinted with permission from Anhorn, M. G., et al., 2008, 2321–31. Copyright 2008 American Chemical Society.)

The biodistribution of Ce6-HSA-NPs could be evaluated in tumor-bearing mice models based on intrinsic fluorescence of Ce6. Ce6-HSA-NPs significantly demonstrated higher tumor accumulation compared to free Ce6. Fluorescence analysis of excised organs also showed higher accumulation of Ce6-HSA-NPs in tumor tissue, but a large amount accumulated in the liver. This high accumulation of albumin NPs in the liver may be related to the metabolism of albumin in the liver, and this situation should be carefully considered and overcome for researchers to develop albumin NPs as tumor-targeted drug carriers. After laser irradiation, tumor tissue of mice treated with Ce6-HAS-NPs was effectively destroyed, and successful tumor suppression was proved. Free Ce6-treated group showed insufficient tumor therapy with the same amount of Ce6.

4.2.5   GELATIN NPs

Gelatin is a mixed compound of protein and polypeptide. It is generally produced by a hydrolysis procedure from collagen, which is the major component of animal skin or bone. During hydrolysis, large numbers of hydrogen or van der Walls bonds in collagen are broken so that gelatin shows more enhanced solubility than collagen in various solvents. However, it is viscous in water and easily undergoes gelation (as suggested by its name "gelatin"). This special gelation of gelatin is very useful in various applications such as food, cosmetics, drug capsules, or mechanical coating agents because of its biocompatibility and elastic property. Especially, gelatin can be obtained from the human body, and this is expected to have no immunogenicity after recombinant splicing (Olsen et al. 2003). This recombinant human gelatin is currently commercialized and used for biomedical researches.

Won et al. (2011) developed amphiphilic gelatin NPs based on hydrophilic recombinant human gelatin and hydrophobic alpha-tocopheryl succinate (α-TOS) (Figure 4.16), which was used as a drug carrier for tumor-targeted delivery of 17-AAG (17-allylamino-17-demethoxygeldanamycin), a small molecule anticancer drug to inhibit the function of heat shock protein 90. These gelatin NPs were about 235 nm in size and well dispersed in water without aggregation. Encapsulated 17-AAG in gelatin NPs showed sustained release for about 4 days, fast cellular uptake, and about 10% enhanced cytotoxicity to tumor cells compared to free 17-AAG. For their stable nanostructure, they showed high accumulation in the tumor site after systemic injection into tumor-bearing mice models. Their therapeutic efficacy was also evaluated in the same

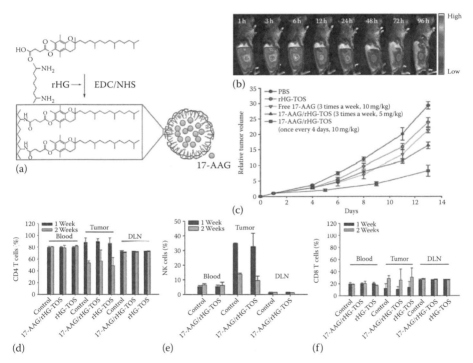

FIGURE 4.16   **(See color insert.)** α-Tocopherol-conjugated gelatin NPs for 17-AAG delivery. (a) Schematic illustration of α-tocopherol-conjugated gelatin NPs and 17-AAG loading. (b) *In vivo* whole-body distribution of gelatin NPs. (c) Tumor growth data and percentages of CD4 T (d), NK (e), and CD8 T (f) cells in tumor-bearing mice models after intravenous injection of 17-AAG-loaded gelatin NPs. DLN, draining lymph node; EDC, 1-ethyl-3-(3-dimethylaminopropyl)carbodiimide hydrochloride; NHS, *N*-hydroxysuccinimide; rHG, recombinant human gelatin. (Reprinted with permission from Won, Y.-W., et al., 2011, 3839–48. Copyright 2011 American Chemical Society.)

mice models. With half the amount of free 17-AAG, these gelatin NPs showed similar tumor suppression. In addition, they enabled reduced administration frequency of the same amount of 17-AAG and showed enhanced therapeutic results in this condition. The biological data surrounding the percentages of natural killer (NK) cells, CD8 T cells, and CD4 T cells also proved the negligible immunogenicity of these gelatin NPs.

Lin et al. developed biotinylated-EGF-modified gelatin NPs as carriers for anti-cancer drug cisplatin and applied these NPs to aerosol delivery for lung cancer therapy (Figure 4.17) (Tseng et al. 2009). The gelatin NPs were made through acetone desolvation and further cross-linked by glutaraldehyde. Cisplatin was incorporated into gelatin NPs via a ligand exchange reaction in distilled water. The surface of NPs was further modified by epidermal growth factor (EGF) using neutravidin/biotin

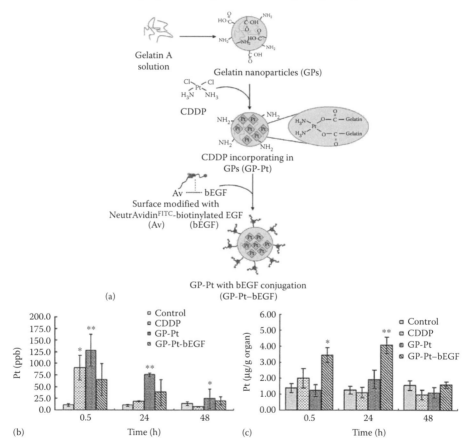

FIGURE 4.17 Cisplatin-incorporated gelatin NPs for pulmonary drug delivery. (a) Schematic illustration of cisplatin-incorporated gelatin NPs and epidermal growth factor (EGF) modification. (b) Time-dependent cisplatin accumulation in plasma (c) and lung (d) in mice models after inhalation of cisplatin-incorporated gelatin NPs. bEGF, biotinylated EGF. *$p < 0.05$, **$p < 0.01$ (one-way analysis of variance; significantly different). (Reprinted from *Biomaterials*, 30, Tseng, C.-L., W.-Y. Su, K.-C. Yen, K.-C. Yang, and F.-H. Lin, The use of biotinylated-EGF-modified gelatin nanoparticle carrier to enhance cisplatin accumulation in cancerous lungs via inhalation, 3476–85, Copyright 2009, with permission from Elsevier.)

binding. The EGF groups were expected to enhance the cellular uptake of gelatin NPs into tumor cells. The resulting NPs showed an efficient uptake and enhanced cytotoxicity in A549 human lung cancer cells. Their *in vivo* tumor suppression ability was proved in subcutaneous tumor-bearing mice models after subcutaneous injection. Finally, gelatin NPs were administrated into mice via inhalation and showed more enhanced accumulation in lung compared to free cisplatin. Especially, EGF-conjugated NPs showed highly increased accumulation, proving the effect of fast receptor-mediated endocytosis of NPs. These results successfully showed the potential of gelatin NPs as drug carriers for lung cancer treatment.

Shutava et al. (2009) developed gelatin NPs by a similar desolvation and cross-linking method, and used a layer-by-layer coating method for delivery of natural polyphenols (Figure 4.18). After the formation of gelatin NPs, their surface was positively charged (about +20 mV) at pH 6.0. This positive charge enabled the adsorption of negatively charged polymers and further adsorption of positively charged polymer again. Polyphenols such as curcumin, epigallocatechin gallate (EGCG), tannic acid (TA), and theaflavin (TF) could be adsorbed into inner gelatin NPs based on hydrogen bonding between hydrophobic amino acid in gelatin and phenol rings of polyphenols. The multilayer on gelatin NPs could provide sustained and pH-dependent release of adsorbed polyphenols. The loading amount of polyphenols could be controlled from 20 to 70 wt.%. In western blot analysis in MDA-MB-231 breast cancer cells, EGCG-containing gelatin NPs successfully blocked hepatocyte growth factor (HGF)-induced cell signaling, showing their potential for stable adsorption and sustained release of natural polyphenols.

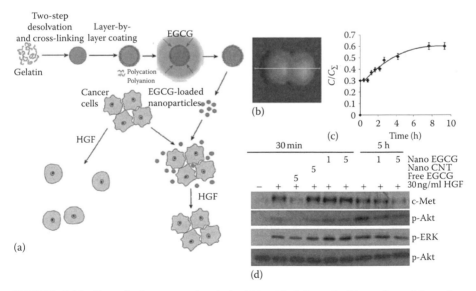

FIGURE 4.18 Layer-by-layer-coated gelatin NPs. (a) Schematic illustration of layer-by-layer-coated gelatin NPs and EGCG release. (b) Atomic force microscopy (AFM) image of layer-by-layer-coated gelatin NPs. (c) Time-dependent release of EGCG from gelatin NPs. (d) Inhibition of c-Met signaling in MDA-MB-231 cells treated with EGCG-loaded gelatin NPs. CNT, carbon nanotube; ERK, extracellular signal-regulated kinase. (Reprinted with permission from Shutava, T. G., et al., 2011, 1877–85. Copyright 2011 American Chemical Society.)

4.3 SYNTHETIC POLYMER-BASED NPs FOR CANCER THERAPY

Polymeric NPs have been formulated to augment drug concentrations in blood/ vascularized tissues to reduce the toxicity of the drug and improve its therapeutic effects for active anticancer therapy (Duncan 2003). Several types of NP functionalities have been explored with the goal of endocytosis in tumor cells (Subbiah et al. 2010). Polymeric NPs provide flexible chemistry for the attachment of cell-specific targeting agents that allow for both increased cell uptake and often cell specificity (Subbiah et al. 2010). Many membrane-bound receptors can be used for targeting via receptor-mediated endocytosis. Recent research has focused on developing NPs loaded with targeting, diagnostic and therapeutic agents. This novel construction will specifically recognize and bind to receptors in selected sites such as tumor cells along with the ability of *in vivo* tracking for biodistribution studies. Hence, the polymers used for NP formulation should have a pronounced structure along with pH-, thermo-, ultrasound-, or light-sensitive properties for controlled micelle dissociation and triggered drug release. Current cancer treatment strategy exhibits challenging barriers such as tumor size, location and presence of metastases in the case of surgical resection, motion of the tumor tissues in the case of external beam radiotherapy, and high tissue concentration associated with toxicity in the case of systemic chemotherapy (Osada et al. 2009). Developing chemotherapeutics with increased action and less toxicity can be achieved by either passively or actively targeting cancer cells utilizing NPs. Drug-loaded nanocarriers can overcome systemic toxicity due to their intrinsic physiochemical properties. The nanosized carriers show increased bioavailability, rapid elimination of entrapped low molecular weight drugs by kidneys or liver (Matsumura 2008), passive targeting by the EPR with increased concentration and minimized toxicity (Maeda et al. 2000), and administration of hydrophobic drugs without adjuvants that usually exhibit side effects. A nano-based targeting system reached clinical trials in the mid-1980s; then the first product based on polymeric liposome and polymer protein conjugates was marketed during the 1990s. More recent studies have focused on creating therapeutics based on the targeting strategy of NPs that have been approved for wider use. This can be achieved by conjugating nanocarriers to drugs and ligands that bind to overexpressed antigens or receptors on the target cells.

4.3.1 POLYMERIC NPs FOR ANTICANCER THERAPY

NP-based anticancer therapy and its formulations under clinical evaluation are listed in Table 4.1. Markedly, Genexol-PM was approved by FDA for breast cancer treatment. Figure 4.19 illustrates the targeting of tumor cells with functionalized NPs containing therapeutics and the numerous barriers that this technology encounters based on the principle of EPR (Osada et al. 2009). The most effective threshold size is <200 nm for NPs to exhibit effective extravasations into tumors (Hobbs et al. 1998; Torchilin 2005). Various polymeric NPs for cancer therapy are listed in Table 4.2, which provides information about the base material, size, loaded drug, and applicable tumors of the NPs.

TABLE 4.1
Representative Examples of PNP-Based Therapeutics for Cancer in Both Market and Clinical Development

Company	Drug
Ortho Biotech	Liposome-PEG DXR
Enzon	PEG-GCSF
Supratek Pharma	PEG-CPT
Callisto	PEG-L-asparginase
American Pharmaceutical Partners	Albumin-bound PTX
Samyang	Liposome-PEG DXR
Amgen	Methoxy-PEG-poly(D,L-lactide) taxol
Schering-Plough	Liposome-PEG DXR
Insert Therapeutics	Pluronic block copolymer DXR
NK105 micelles—P2 clinical stage	PEG-b-modified polyaspartate-PTX
NC-6004—P1/2	PEG-b-PGA
NK012—P2	PEG-b-PGA
Xyotax—P3	PLGA
CT-2106—P2	PLGA-glycine-CPT
SP1049C—P3	Pluronics-DXR
MCC465—P1	PEG-immunoliposome-DXR
CALAA-01—P1	Cyclodextrin-PEG-siRNA

CPT, camptothecin; DXR, doxorubicin; GCSF, granulocyte colony-stimulating factor; PEG, polyethylene glycol; PLGA, poly(D,L-lactide-co-glycolide); PTX, paclitaxel; siRNA, small interfering RNA.

Source: Matsumura et al. 2004; Uchino et al. 2005; Koizumi et al. 2006; Homsi et al. 2007; Davis 2009; Matsumura and Kataoka 2009; Kato et al. 2011; Valle et al. 2011.

4.3.2 POLYETHYLENE GLYCOL NPS

PEG exhibits a polymer structure similar to poly(ethylene oxide) (PEO), and is a widely accepted synthetic polymer because of its excellent properties that include water solubility, high hydration, efficient steric protection, biocompatibility, and low toxicity (van Vlerken et al. 2007). The structural formula of this linear polymer is $HO(-CH_2CH_2O-)_n-OH$. The repeating units determine the length and molecular weight of PEG, and unmodified PEG is generally nondegradable, which can be made degradable by copolymerizing with degradable polymers (Bourke and Kohn 2003). It can be synthesized from either the ring opening of ethylene oxide or condensation of ethylene glycol. Several forms of PEG can be synthesized via anionic, cationic, and UV irradiation polymerization. The backbone oxygen molecule makes the polymer water soluble, and it increases hydration volume and molecular mobility to minimize the binding interactions with proteins. Hence, it helps in increasing the bioavailability of bound drugs. PEG is nontoxic, bioinert, and nondegradable under physiological conditions, and its degraded soluble moieties are rapidly excreted by kidneys

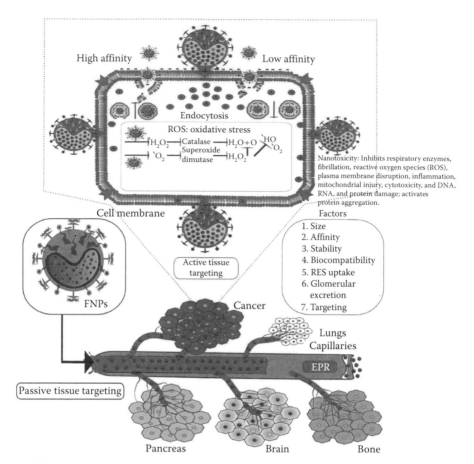

FIGURE 4.19 NP-based DDS for cancer targeting. (Reprinted from Subbiah, R., et al., *Current Medicinal Chemistry*, 17, 4559–77, 2010. Copyright 2010, with permission from Bentham Science Publishers.)

without any transformation. The terminal hydroxyl group can be activated for the attachment of various molecules and polymerizable groups for the synthesis of block copolymers. Therefore, it has been extensively used as an excipient in DDSs and other pharmaceutical formulations. The development of the NK911 system was reported (Figure 4.20), which demonstrates the attachment of PEG to conjugated doxorubicin–polyaspartic acid for hydrophobic anticancer DDSs (Nakanishi et al. 2001). Simple modification of PEG by cross-linking groups to form a micelle structure and creating degradable groups enhances its biomedical application. Several research groups have been working continuously on the synthesis of PEG copolymer using a variety of polymers. For instance, mixed micelles made of a PEG–phosphatidyl ethanolamine (PE) conjugate and D-α-tocopherylpolyetheylene glycol 1000 succinate (TPGS) were reported for the delivery of poorly soluble anticancer drugs such as CPT. The solubilization, stability, and cellular uptake of CPT by the mixed micelles (2:1 ratio of PEG–PE–TPGS) was more efficient and less toxic compared to the micelles made of PEG or PEG–PE alone (Mu et al. 2005). Smart polymeric micelles for site-specific gene/drug delivery and intracellular signals respond to PEG, and its copolymerized compounds have been extensively reviewed (Nishiyama et al. 2005). Doxorubicin-conjugated PEG–*b*-poly(aspartate) (PEG–PAsp) block copolymer micelles in aqueous media were reported in early 1987. These micelles

TABLE 4.2
Polymeric NPs for Cancer Therapy

Nanoparticles	Size (nm)	Drug	Indications
PCL	250–300	Tamoxifen	Breast cancer
PBCA	178	DXR	Dalton's lymphoma
PEG–PAsp	50	DXR	Leukemia
PLLA-*b*-PEG (folate targeted)	50–80	DXR	Solid tumors
PNIPA-*b*-PDLLA	60	PTX	Ovarian, lung, and breast cancers
PEG-PE/egg phosphatidylcholine (lipid conjugated)	100	PTX	Various cancers
MPEG-poly(β-amino ester)	62	DXR	Various cancers
MPEG-poly(β-amino ester)	122	Protoporphyrin	Photodynamic cancer therapy
PEG-PE	10–40	*m*-Porphyrin, tamoxifen, and PTX	Various cancers
Trimyristin-egg phosphatidylcholine-PEG-PE	217.4	PTX	Various cancers
PEG-phosphatidylethanolamine	10–100	CPT	Various cancers
PEG-lipid	10–40	Tamoxifen	Lung carcinoma
Poly(2-ethyl-2-oxazoline)-*b*-PCL	30–80	PTX	Various cancers
PCL-*b*-trimethylene carbonate-PEG (serum protein)	96	Ellipticin	Anticancer
PGA-*b*-PEG	40	DXR	Solid tumor
PDLLA *b*-methoxy PEG	30	PTX	Various cancers
Pluronics	10–100	Carboplatin	Colorectal cancer
PCL-*b*-methoxy-PEG	<200	PTX	Various cancers
PLGA-*b*-PEG	–	Docetaxel	Prostate cancer
PEG-PLGA	105	DXR	Various cancers
PEG-PCL	50–130	PTX	Various cancers
cGRD peptide in PEG-PCL	20–40	DXR	Various cancers
Galactose in poly(γ-benzyl L-glutamate)-PEG	104	PTX	Various cancers
Albumin-bound PEG NPs	–	DXR	Various cancers
poly(lysine) + poly(DEAP-Lys)-*b*-PEG-*b*-PLLA block copolymer	165	DXR	pH-sensitive tumor targeting
PLGA-*b*-PEG-COOH	70–250	PSMA based	Prostate cancer

(Continued)

TABLE 4.2 (continued)
Polymeric NPs for Cancer Therapy

Nanoparticles	Size (nm)	Drug	Indications
PLLA-PEG NPs	100–150	Biotin	Cancer cells—anticancer
PLA	250	Nucleic acid aptamer	Prostate epithelial cells—anticancer
PLGA	357	MP lipid A	Dentritic cells
MPEG/PLGA	50–300	Peptidomimetics	Brain cells

cGRD, cyclic Arg-Gly-Asp; CPT, camptothecin; DEAP, 3-diethylaminopropyl isothiocyanate; DXR, doxorubicin; MP, monophosphoryl; MPEG, methyl ether PEG; NP, nanoparticle; PAsp, poly(aspartic acid); PBCA, poly(butyl cyanoacrylate); PCL, poly(ε-caprolactone); PDLLA, poly(D,L-lactide); PGA, poly(glutamic acid); PE, phosphatidyl ethanolamine; PEG, polyethylene glycol; PLGA, poly(D,L-lactide-*co*-glycolide); PLLA, poly(L-lactic acid); PNIPA, poly(*N*-isopropylacrylamide); PSMA, prostate-specific membrane antigen; PTX, paclitaxel.

Source: Yokoyama et al. 1990; Nakanishi et al. 2001; Gao et al. 2002, 2003; Chawla and Amiji 2002; Fonseca et al. 2003; Lee et al. 2003, 2005, 2007; Wosikowski et al. 2003; Elamanchili et al. 2004; Farokhzad et al. 2004; Nasongkla et al. 2004; Reddy et al. 2004; Shuai et al. 2004; Yoo and Park 2004; Exner et al. 2005; Jeong et al. 2005; Liu et al. 2005; Mu et al. 2005; Olivier 2005; Park et al. 2005; Soga et al. 2005; Uchino et al. 2005; Wang et al. 2005; Emerich and Thanos 2006; Trimaille et al. 2006; Cheng et al. 2007; Ko et al. 2007; Zhang et al. 2008; Patil et al. 2009; Koo et al. 2010.

have shown less toxicity than the physically entrapped doxorubicin in the micelles (Yokoyama et al. 1987). Similarly, paclitaxel incorporated into the micelle proved to have higher efficacy with fewer side effects than free paclitaxel, and a phase II study is now under way in patients with advanced stomach cancer as NK105 (Kato et al. 2011). 7-Ethyl-10-hydroxycamptothecin (SN-38) is a biologically active metabolite of irinotecan hydrochloride (camptothecin) that is loaded into a polymeric micelle of PEG–poly(glutamate) (PEG–PGlu) by hydrophobic interaction (Koizumi et al. 2006). The SN-38-loaded micelle is currently being tested in a phase I clinical trial as NK012 in Japan and the United States. Yokoyama et al. (1996) reported the introduction of cisplatin into a micelle system by metal complexation between platinum and carboxyl groups of PEG–PAsp that yielded a very narrow size distribution. This cisplatin-loaded PEG–PAsp micelle exhibited a sixfold higher accumulation in tumor sites with the same anticancer activity compared to free cisplatin, and hence, further study was carried out using PEG–PGlu to enhance the activity by sustained release of drugs (Nishiyama et al. 2003). These micelles exhibited high plasma platinum level with enhanced accumulation at the tumor site, indicating tumor-selective targeting due to the EPR effect. The PEG–PGlu [*cis*-diamminedichloroplatinum(II) (CDDP)] micelle is currently undergoing a phase I clinical trial as NC-6004 in the United Kingdom (Uchino et al. 2005). Targeted anticancer micelles by conjugating folate to the distal end of PEG and doxorubicin into the PAsp in PEG–PAsp block copolymer were reported. The micelles showed increased cellular uptake with enhanced growth inhibitory activity of cancer cells, suggesting that this could be an effective approach

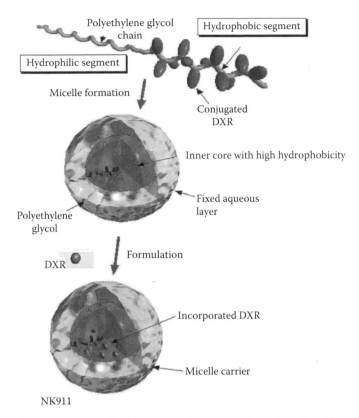

FIGURE 4.20 Development of NK911 system for drug delivery. (Reprinted from *Journal of Controlled Release*, 74, Nakanishi, T., S. Fukushima, K. Okamoto, M. Suzuki, Y. Matsumura, M. Yokoyama, T. Okano, Y. Sakurai, and K. Kataoka, Development of the polymer micelle carrier system for doxorubicin, 295–302, Copyright 2001, with permission from Elsevier.)

for ligand-mediated uptake for cancer treatment (Bae et al. 2005). Also, the micelles were tested to enhance the EPR effect by coadministration of tumor growth factor (TGF)-b type I receptor (TbR-I) inhibitor at low dose (Kano et al. 2007). The use of TbR-I inhibitor along with anticancer-loaded micelles might play a significant role in treating intractable cancers. Preparation of solid lipid NPs was reported to utilize egg phosphatidylcholine–PEG-PE (stabilizers) and trimyristin (solid lipid core) for the parenteral DDS of paclitaxel using a hot homogenization method (Lee et al. 2007). Moreover, pH-triggered drug release is another important strategy. Ko et al. reported the development of hydrophilic, biodegradable, and pH-responsive micelles composed of methyl ether PEG (MPEG)-poly(β-amino ester) block copolymer as a tumor-targeting DDS. A solvent evaporation method is used for loading 75.4% doxorubicin. The system showed a more rapid release of doxorubicin in a weak acidic environment than in a neutral pH condition (7.4). The doxorubicin release from the micelles could be controlled by pH-dependent micellization (slow release in physiologic pH 7.4) and demicellization (rapid release in weakly acidic pH 6.4) behavior of this unique copolymer that shows enriched doxorubicin concentration at the cancer

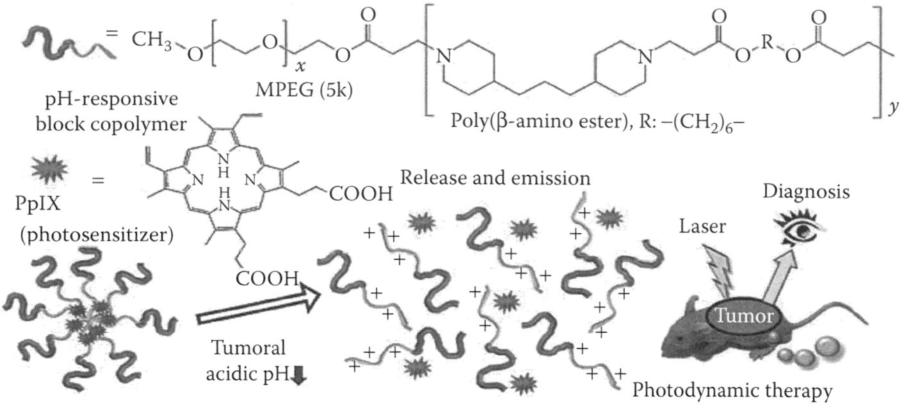

FIGURE 4.21 pH-responsive PEG-based block copolymer NPs as targeted theranostic agent. (Koo, H., H. Lee, S. Lee, K. H. Min, M. S. Kim, D. S. Lee, Y. Choi, I. C. Kwon, K. Kim, and S. Y. Jeong. In vivo tumor diagnosis and photodynamic therapy via tumoral pH-responsive polymeric micelles. *Chemical Communications*, 2010, 46: 5668–70. Reproduced by permission of The Royal Society of Chemistry.)

site of tumor-bearing mice (Ko et al. 2007). Recently, the same research group has developed a novel theranostic agent that consists of a photosensitizer such as protoporphyrin IX (PpIX)-encapsulated MPEG-poly(β-amino ester). Protoporphyrin in a nanocarrier system generates strong fluorescence and singlet oxygen on the targeted tumor site simultaneously on irradiation, and is therefore used in both diagnostics and PDT. Figure 4.21 demonstrates the merit and mechanism of micellization/demicellization transition of MPEG-poly(β-amino ester) block copolymer along with PpIX as a theranostic agent (Koo et al. 2010). The study revealed that nano-sized micelles could exhibit an EPR effect, demicellization associated with drug release at the acidic tumor site, photosensitized fluorescence imaging, and PDT. Simultaneously, pH-responsive 165-nm-sized flower-like micelles were developed to attain pH-triggered drug release using poly(N^ε-(3-diethylamino)propyl isothiocyanato-L-lysine)-*b*-PEG-*b*-poly(L-lactide). This self-assembled structure consisting of two hydrophobic blocks and a hydrophilic block is stable at physiological pH, but structural changes in the hydrophobic blocks are observed while the pH decreased to acidic levels (<pH 7.0) (Oh et al. 2009). Tumor-specific pH-sensitive core–shell block copolymer, which was made of poly(L-histidine) (polyHis)-*b*-PEG and poly(L-lactic acid) (PLLA)-*b*-PEG-*b*-polyHis-biotin for an anticancer DDS, was demonstrated (Lee et al. 2005).

4.3.3 Poly(d,l-Lactide-*co*-Glycolide) NPs

Polymer selection for formulating NPs is highly dependent on both the hydrophilic and hydrophobic characteristics of the copolymer. The hydrophilic nature provides steric stability and increased bioavailability by obviating the RES uptake in the body (Adams et al. 2003). Poly(d,l-lactide-*co*-glycolide) (PLGA) is the most extensively investigated polymer for drug delivery that is found to be the best biomaterial owing to its design (Shive and Anderson 1997). It is a copolymer synthesized using random ring-opening copolymerization of two different monomers, the cyclic dimers (1,4-dioxane-2,5-diones) of glycolic acid and lactic acid. The successive mono- mers are linked via ester formation to produce linear aliphatic polyester (PLGA) in the presence of catalysts including tin(II) 2-ethylhexanoate, tin(II) alkoxides, or aluminum isopropoxide. The beneficial characteristics of PLGA, such as bioabsorb- able, thermoplastic, biodegradability, good physiochemical properties, and porous structure, enhance its application in the biomedical arena, whereas the hydrophobic nature narrows it (Bennet and Kim 2011). PLGA is amorphous; hence, different forms and degradation rates of PLGA can be obtained by tuning the ratio of lactide to gly- colide used for the polymerization (PLGA 75:25 = 75% lactic acid and 25% glycolic acid). The homopolymers of lactic acid (PLA) and glycolic acid (PGA) show poor solubility, and the higher content of glycolide units reduces the degradation time. However, unlike PLA and PGA, PLGA can be dissolved by a wide range of common solvents including chlorinated solvents, tetrahydrofuran, and acetone or ethyl acetate (Jain 2000). PLGA polyester forms biologically compatible and metabolizable moi- eties on hydrolysis, and eventually gets removed from the body by the citric acid cycle without affecting normal cell function. Also, the drug that is loaded in PLGA is released at a controlled rate via diffusion, which slows the degradation rate of the polymer. The rate of drug release in PLGA can be modified by properly control- ling the porous structure of the polymers. After extensive animal toxicity and safety studies, PLGA is currently being applied to humans, and it has become a common choice in the biopharmaceuticals field including microparticles and NPs. Lupron Depot is the PLGA-based commercially available DDS marketed for the treatment of advanced prostate cancer (Panyam and Labhasetwar 2003). PLGA-based therapeu- tics and published anticancer DDSs are listed in Tables 4.1 and 4.2. Several PLGA NPs of various sizes have been successfully formulated using many strategies includ- ing the emulsification–evaporation method, the spontaneous emulsification–solvent diffusion method, the nanoprecipitation method, and the spray-drying method. A PLGA-based DDS for anticancer agents has been extensively reviewed elsewhere (Acharya and Sahoo 2011). The physical property and cellular uptake of PLGA NPs can be modulated by altering the factors and emulsifiers. The most commonly used emulsifier in PLGA NP synthesis is polyvinyl alcohol (PVA), which promotes homo- geneous nanosized particles and the ability of redispersion. PLGA NPs have reduced the plasma protein adsorption and hepatic filtration with enhanced cellular uptake. PLGA NPs less than 100 nm undergo less RES uptake, and the rapid RES uptake could be minimized by surface modification with PEG, resulting in prolonged NP circulation time (Gref et al. 1994). The endolysosomal escape mechanism of PLGA NPs is important for the cytoplasmic entry without serum effect. Most PLGA NPs were found in the endosomal or lysosomal compartment after internalization, which reduces the toxicity associated with cationic polymers (Clark and Hersh 1999).

Presently, so many drugs formulated in block copolymer micelles of PLGA and other polymers are in clinical trial development for the treatment of various cancers (Nakanishi et al. 2001). Nanosized block copolymer micelles comprise supramolecular assemblies of amphiphilic copolymers that consist of a hydrophobic core surrounded by a hydrophilic shell (Allen et al. 1999). The micelle core serves as a reservoir for the

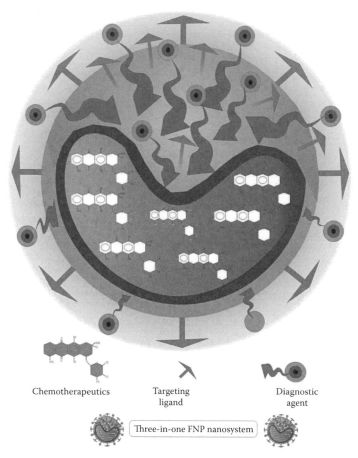

FIGURE 4.22 Schematic representation of the three-in-one NP construct and the structural composition of NPs for multimodality therapy. (Reprinted from Subbiah, R., et al., *Current Medicinal Chemistry*, 17, 4559–77, 2010. Copyright (2010), with permission from Bentham Science Publishers.)

incorporation of hydrophobic drugs, and the hydrophilic shell provides a protective interface between the core and the external medium. This copolymer has been generating attractive strategies in DDSs, for instance, the unique PLGA-PEG system was demonstrated for controlled and targeted delivery of docetaxel and cisplatin using the prostate-specific membrane antigen (PSMA) as a targeting agent. The result shows greater anticancer activity than that of free cisplatin (Dhar et al. 2011). A schematic illustration of the encapsulated anticancer agent, aptamer (targeting agent), and diagnostic agent is shown in Figure 4.22 (Subbiah et al. 2010).

4.3.4 POLY(CAPROLACTONE) NPS

Poly(caprolactone) (PCL) is the most widely studied polymer in the polyester class, which is basically designed as synthetic plastic for ecofriendly microbial degradation. PCL is a biodegradable, biocompatible, and semicrystalline polymer.

It is ideally suitable for a long-term controlled DDS in different forms, such as NPs, microspheres, and implants. The average molecular weight of PCL may vary from 10,000 to 42,500, and it could be classified according to its molecular weight. PCL is soluble in chloroform, dichloromethane, carbon tetrachloride, benzene, toluene cyclohexanone, and 2-nitropropane at room temperature. PCL has been synthesized from the anionic (low molecular weight polymer), cationic (high molecular weight of 15,000–50,000), and coordination (molecular weight of >50,000) polymerization of ε-caprolactone. Various initiators and polymerization conditions were utilized for each type of catalysts that include tertiary amines, alkali metal oxides, and carboxylates in nonpolar solvents for anionic reaction (Ito and Yamashita 1978) and $FeCl_3$, BF_3, Et_2O, and alkyl sulfonates in 1,2-dichloroethane for cationic reaction (Jenkins 1977). The di-*n*-butyl zinc, stannous octoate, and alkoxides and halides of Al, Mg, Ti, and Sn are also used for coordination polymerization (Hamitou et al. 1977). PCL is soluble in 2-nitropropane and aromatic and chlorinated hydrocarbons, but it is insoluble in aliphatic hydrocarbons, diethyl ether, and alcohols. The increased molecular weight of PCL decreases crystallinity. PCL and its copolymers undergo bulk hydrolysis *in vitro* and *in vivo*, and their biodegradation rate is influenced by the size and shape of the polymer.

The hydrophobic block of the copolymer system most often comprises PCL. Block copolymer micelles have been explored as delivery vehicles for a wide variety of anticancer agents including paclitaxel, ellipticine, doxorubicin, and aluminum phthalocyanine chloride. The influence of serum protein on the drug release kinetic from PCL micelles remains relatively unexplored. Yet many of the agents that have been formulated in micelles are hydrophobic and known to have a high affinity for plasma protein (Sparreboom et al. 1998). In this way, it is challenging for the micelles to function as true carriers rather than mere solubilizers, as the drug may have a tendency to quickly dissociate from the micelle following administration (Burt et al. 1999).

For anticancer therapy, tamoxifen-entrapped PCL NPs were prepared using solid displacement method to evince a targeted DDS toward breast cancer (Chawla and Amiji 2002). In order to make more efficient DDSs, a number of investigations were performed with the central objective of site specificity. This systematic localization showed minimized negative side effects (Torchilin 2000). Folic acid (FA)-bound PCL NPs are the attractive strategy for targeting cancer cell because it is an essential vitamin for the biosynthesis of nucleotide bases (Park et al. 2005). FA has high binding affinity, low immunogenicity, and stability during storage. Moreover, it is small in size, easy to modify for chemical reaction, and compatible with various organic and inorganic solvents. In particular, paclitaxel-loaded PCL micelles with the folate group showed similar cytotoxicity for both normal human fibroblasts and cancer cell lines, whereas folate conjugated with PCL showed more cytotoxicity on cancer cells than on normal cells (Leamon and Reddy 2004). PCL-Tween 80, a novel copolymeric NP, was also developed as potential DDS using modified solvent extraction/evaporation method (Ma et al. 2011). The relative amount of Tween 80 would be decreased after the incorporation of Tween 80 into a PCL-Tween 80 copolymer, and the advantages of PCL would be combined in this method.

Recently, small interfering RNA (siRNA)-based research is emerging in nanomedicine, particularly for cancer therapy, because of its high sensitivity, specificity, and low toxicity. However, it cannot be applied without a carrier system due to its rapid degradation in the environment with RNase. Moreover, siRNA shows poor cellular internalization for its negative surface charge, and it may induce type I interferon responses to stimulate the production of proinflammatory cytokines (Castanotto and Rossi 2009). The co-delivery of paclitaxel and siRNA for vascular endothelial growth factor (VEGF) has revealed improved therapeutic effect with anti-angiogenesis (Zhu et al. 2010). Cao et al. concluded that doxorubicin-loaded cationic nanomicelles were formed using polyethyleneimine (PEI)-PCL with intrinsic low toxicity, which is then conjugated with siRNA and FA-PEG-PGA to yield a hierarchical hybrid assembly. This simple approach is applied to introduce the targeting ligand with reduced vector toxicity and without affecting siRNA complexation. The hierarchical nano-assemblies were capable of simultaneously transporting siRNA and doxorubicin into Bel-7402 cells, and FA-directed internalization significantly increased the delivery efficiency. Systemic biological experiments revealed that B-cell lymphoma 2 (BCL-2) expression in Bel-7402 cells was significantly suppressed by the co-delivery of BCL-2 siRNA. Consequently, cell apoptosis was enhanced and the potency of doxorubicin in inducing cell death was greatly potentiated through the synergistic effect of the two therapeutic agents (Cao et al. 2011).

4.3.5 PLURONIC NPs

Block copolymers based on PEG-poly(propylene glycol)-PEG are generically known as poloxamer. A pluronic is a triblock copolymer consisting of hydrophilic PEO and hydrophobic poly(propylene oxide) (PPO) blocks arranged in an A–B–A triblock structure (PEO–PPO–PEO), and is available in various lengths and compositions. These polymers can be tuned as thermally reversible gels to be formed at body temperature. Pluronic NPs have been extensively used as vehicles in a variety of pharmaceutical formulations for both diagnostic and therapeutic agents including anticancer drugs, low molecular weight drugs, and polypeptides. Pluronics can implement several inert carrier functions by being biological response modifiers that cause various functional alterations in the cell. The hydrophilic segments form the corona that surrounds the hydrophobic core, and the chemical cross-linking of pluronic micelle cores or shells has been used to increase the stability of the micelles. This property enables the internalization of NPs by cancer cells more efficiently, and thus, higher anticancer activity would be expected (Xu et al. 2006). Pluronics show promising application in the treatment of drug-resistant tumors by interacting with MDR cancer tumors. This definite property of pluronics results in drastic sensitization of MDR tumors with respect to various anticancer agents with enhanced drug transport across physiological barriers. It causes transcriptional activation of gene expression both *in vitro* and *in vivo* (Kabanov et al. 2002). Pluronics affect drug resistance mechanisms, such as abolishing drug sequestration in acidic vesicles, inhibition of drug efflux transporters, and glutathione/glutathione *S*-transferase detoxification system. They also affect several cellular functions

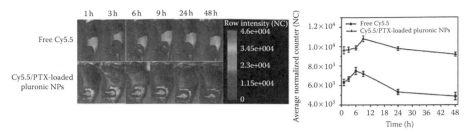

FIGURE 4.23 *In vivo* non-invasive NIR images and quantification analysis of Cy5.5/PTX NPs. (Reprinted from *Journal of Controlled Release*, 148, Oh, K. S., J. Y. Song, S. H. Cho, B. S. Lee, S. Y. Kim, K. Kim, H. Jeon, I. C. Kwon, and S. H. Yuk, Paclitaxel-loaded Pluronic nanoparticles formed by a temperature-induced phase transition for cancer therapy, 344–50, Copyright 2010, with permission from Elsevier.)

including ATP synthesis, mitochondrial respiration, apoptotic signal transduction, and gene expression. Solubility, stability, pharmacokinetics, and biodistribution of drugs can be achieved by incorporating low molecular weight drugs into pluronics (Kabanov et al. 2003). Several studies were reported for tumor-specific delivery of antineoplastic agents using PCL NPs (Kabanov and Alakhov 2002).

Doxorubicin in the mixed micelles (SP1049C) of pluronics L61 and F127 accounts for the first clinically evaluated anticancer micellar formulation (Valle et al. 2004). Drug resistance time is increased with sustained doxorubicin release in SP1049C system, which indicates that pluronics enhance anticancer activity. Pluronics exhibit chemosensitizing activity, enhanced release profile by sustained micelle disintegration, and facilitated cellular uptake (Oh et al. 2010). Tumor-targeting pluronic (F68 and PEG-paclitaxel)-based NPs were prepared by temperature-induced phase transition solvent-free process. This system demonstrated the real-time quantification of tumor-localized NPs using NIR fluorescence imaging technology in tumor-bearing mice (Figure 4.23). Folate-conjugated pluronic F127 improves the targeting capability with enhanced tumor specificity and reduced side effects of paclitaxel (Li et al. 2010). Collectively, pluronics can be a promising DDS to overcome MDR in several cancers and suggest a broad spectrum of biological response-modifying activities, resulting in a remarkable impact on cancer treatment.

4.4 CONCLUSION

In summary, we have introduced the recent progress in the development and biomedical application of NPs. They have attracted much attention as targeted drug carriers for efficient and safe delivery. To fabricate these NPs, researchers have used various materials such as lipids, polymers, carbon nanotubes, graphenes, iron oxide, gold, silver, and silica. Among them, we focused on polymers because they have a very long history and are the most frequently used materials for easy handling and modification. We introduced the NPs based on natural and synthetic polymers, and both groups have shown promising potential for drug delivery. Various brilliant researchers have made improvement in this technology, and knowledge about targeted delivery of NPs has also been accumulated. Therefore, we expect that more advanced NPs will provide better clinical results in the near future, and polymers are still one of their main components.

ACKNOWLEDGMENTS

This work was supported by Global Research Laboratory (GRL) project of the Ministry of Education, Science, and Technology (MEST).

REFERENCES

Acharya, S., and S. K. Sahoo. PLGA nanoparticles containing various anticancer agents and tumour delivery by EPR effect. *Advanced Drug Delivery Reviews* 63, no. 3 (2011): 170–83.

Adams, M. L., A. Lavasanifar, and G. S. Kwon. Amphiphilic block copolymers for drug delivery. *Journal of Pharmaceutical Sciences* 92, no. 7 (2003): 1343–55.

Allen, C., D. Maysinger, and A. Eisenberg. Nano-engineering block copolymer aggregates for drug delivery. *Colloids and Surfaces B: Biointerfaces* 16, no. 1–4 (1999): 3–27.

Anhorn, M. G., S. Wagner, J. Kreuter, K. Langer, and H. von Briesen. Specific targeting of HER2 overexpressing breast cancer cells with doxorubicin-loaded trastuzumab-modified human serum albumin nanoparticles. *Bioconjugate Chemistry* 19, no. 12 (2008): 2321–31.

Bae, Y., W. D. Jang, N. Nishiyama, S. Fukushima, and K. Kataoka. Multifunctional polymeric micelles with folate-mediated cancer cell targeting and pH-triggered drug releasing properties for active intracellular drug delivery. *Molecular BioSystems* 1, no. 3 (2005): 242–50.

Bennet, D., and S. Kim. Implantable microdevice for peripheral nerve regeneration: Materials and fabrications. *Journal of Materials Science* 46, no. 14 (2011): 4723–40.

Bourke, S. L., and J. Kohn. Polymers derived from the amino acid L-tyrosine: Polycarbonates, polyarylates and copolymers with poly(ethylene glycol). *Advanced Drug Delivery Reviews* 55, no. 4 (2003): 447–66.

Burt, H. M., X. C. Zhang, P. Toleikis, L. Embree, and W. L. Hunter. Development of copolymers of poly(D,L-lactide) and methoxypolyethylene glycol as micellar carriers of paclitaxel. *Colloids and Surfaces B: Biointerfaces* 16, no. 1–4 (1999): 161–71.

Cao, N., D. Cheng, S. Y. Zou, H. Ai, J. M. Gao, and X. T. Shuai. The synergistic effect of hierarchical assemblies of sirna and chemotherapeutic drugs co-delivered into hepatic cancer cells. *Biomaterials* 32, no. 8 (2011): 2222–32.

Castanotto, D., and J. J. Rossi. The promises and pitfalls of RNA-interference-based therapeutics. *Nature* 457, no. 7228 (2009): 426–33.

Chawla, J. S., and M. M. Amiji. Biodegradable poly(epsilon-caprolactone) nanoparticles for tumor-targeted delivery of tamoxifen. *International Journal of Pharmaceutics* 249, no. 1–2 (2002): 127–38.

Cheng, J., B. A. Teply, I. Sherifi, J. Sung, G. Luther, F. X. Gu, E. Levy-Nissenbaum, A. F. Radovic-Moreno, R. Langer, and O. C. Farokhzad. Formulation of functionalized PLGA-PAG nanoparticles for in vivo targeted drug delivery. *Biomaterials* 28, no. 5 (2007): 869–76.

Cho, H.-J., H. Y. Yoon, H. Koo, S.-H. Ko, J.-S. Shim, J.-H. Lee, K. Kim, I. C. Kwon, and D.-D. Kim. Self-assembled nanoparticles based on hyaluronic acid-ceramide (HA-CE) and Pluronic® for tumor-targeted delivery of docetaxel. *Biomaterials* 32, no. 29 (2011): 7181–90.

Cho, Y. W., S. A. Park, T. H. Han, D. H. Son, J. S. Park, S. J. Oh, D. H. Moon, et al. In vivo tumor targeting and radionuclide imaging with self-assembled nanoparticles: Mechanisms, key factors, and their implications. *Biomaterials* 28, no. 6 (2007): 1236–47.

Choi, K. Y., H. Chung, K. H. Min, H. Y. Yoon, K. Kim, J. H. Park, I. C. Kwon, and S. Y. Jeong. Self-assembled hyaluronic acid nanoparticles for active tumor targeting. *Biomaterials* 31, no. 1 (2010): 106–14.

Choi, K. Y., K. H. Min, H. Y. Yoon, K. Kim, J. H. Park, I. C. Kwon, K. Choi, and S. Y. Jeong. Pegylation of hyaluronic acid nanoparticles improves tumor targetability in vivo. *Biomaterials* 32, no. 7 (2011a): 1880–89.

Choi, K. Y., H. Y. Yoon, J.-H. Kim, S. M. Bae, R.-W. Park, Y. M. Kang, I.-S. Kim, et al. Smart nanocarrier based on pegylated hyaluronic acid for cancer therapy. *ACS Nano* 5, no. 11 (2011b): 8591–99.

Clark, P. R., and E. M. Hersh. Cationic lipid-mediated gene transfer: Current concepts. *Current Opinion in Molecular Therapeutics* 1, no. 2 (1999): 158–76.

Dash, M., F. Chiellini, R. M. Ottenbrite, and E. Chiellini. Chitosan—A versatile semi-synthetic polymer in biomedical applications. *Progress in Polymer Science* 36, no. 8 (2011): 981–1014.

Davis, M. E. The first targeted delivery of sirna in humans via a self-assembling, cyclodextrin polymer-based nanoparticle: From concept to clinic. *Molecular Pharmacology* 6, no. 3 (2009): 659–68.

Dhar, S., N. Kolishetti, S. J. Lippard, and O. C. Farokhzad. Targeted delivery of a cisplatin prodrug for safer and more effective prostate cancer therapy in vivo. *Proceedings of the National Academy of Sciences of the United States of America* 108, no. 5 (2011): 1850–55.

Duncan, R. The dawning era of polymer therapeutics. *Nature Reviews Drug Discovery* 2, no. 5 (2003): 347–60.

Elamanchili, P., M. Diwan, M. Cao, and J. Samuel. Characterization of poly(D,L-lactic-co-glycolic acid) based nanoparticulate system for enhanced delivery of antigens to dendritic cells. *Vaccine* 22, no. 19 (2004): 2406–12.

Emerich, D. F., and C. G. Thanos. The pinpoint promise of nanoparticle-based drug delivery and molecular diagnosis. *Biomolecular Engineering* 23, no. 4 (2006): 171–84.

Exner, A. A., T. M. Krupka, K. Scherrer, and J. M. Teets. Enhancement of carboplatin toxicity by pluronic block copolymers. *Journal of Controlled Release* 106, no. 1–2 (2005): 188–97.

Farokhzad, O. C., S. Jon, A. Khademhosseini, T. N. Tran, D. A. Lavan, and R. Langer. Nanoparticle-aptamer bioconjugates: A new approach for targeting prostate cancer cells. *Cancer Research* 64, no. 21 (2004): 7668–72.

Fonseca, M. J., J. C. Jagtenberg, H. J. Haisma, and G. Storm. Liposome-mediated targeting of enzymes to cancer cells for site-specific activation of prodrugs: Comparison with the corresponding antibody-enzyme conjugate. *Pharmaceutical Research* 20, no. 3 (2003): 423–28.

Gao, Z. G., A. N. Lukyanov, A. Singhal, and V. P. Torchilin. Diacyllipid-polymer micelles as nanocarriers for poorly soluble anticancer drugs. *Nano Letters* 2, no. 9 (2002): 979–82.

Gao, Z., A. N. Lukyanov, A. R. Chakilam, and V. P. Torchilin. PEG-PE/phosphatidylcholine mixed immunomicelles specifically deliver encapsulated taxol to tumor cells of different origin and promote their efficient killing. *Journal of Drug Targeting* 11, no. 2 (2003): 87–92.

Gref, R., Y. Minamitake, M. T. Peracchia, V. Trubetskoy, V. Torchilin, and R. Langer. Biodegradable long-circulating polymeric nanospheres. *Science* 263, no. 5153 (1994): 1600–03.

Hamitou, A., T. Ouhadi, R. Jerome, and P. Teyssie. Soluble bimetallic μ-oxoalkoxides.7. Characteristics and mechanism of ring-opening polymerization of lactones. *Journal of Polymer Science Part A: Polymer Chemistry* 15, no. 4 (1977): 865–73.

Hawkins, M. J., P. Soon-Shiong, and N. Desai. Protein nanoparticles as drug carriers in clinical medicine. *Advanced Drug Delivery Reviews* 60, no. 8 (2008): 876–85.

He, X. M., and D. C. Carter. Atomic structure and chemistry of human serum albumin. *Nature* 358, no. 6383 (1992): 209–15.

Hobbs, S. K., W. L. Monsky, F. Yuan, W. G. Roberts, L. Griffith, V. P. Torchilin, and R. K. Jain. Regulation of transport pathways in tumor vessels: Role of tumor type and microenvironment. *Proceedings of the National Academy of Sciences of the United States of America* 95, no. 8 (1998): 4607–12.

Homsi, J., G. R. Simon, C. R. Garrett, G. Springett, R. De Conti, A. A. Chiappori, P. N. Munster, et al. Phase I trial of poly-L-glutamate camptothecin (Ct-2106) administered weekly in patients with advanced solid malignancies. *Clinical Cancer Research* 13, no. 19 (2007): 5855–61.

Ito, K., and Y. Yamashita. Propagation and depropagation rates in anionic-polymerization of epsilon-caprolactone cyclic oligomers. *Macromolecules* 11, no. 1 (1978): 68–72.

Jain, R. A. The manufacturing techniques of various drug loaded biodegradable poly(lactide-co-glycolide) (PLGA) devices. *Biomaterials* 21, no. 23 (2000): 2475–90.

Jenkins, V. F. Caprolactone and its polymers. *Polymers Paint Colour Journal* 167 (1977): 622–27.

Jeong, H., M. Huh, S. J. Lee, H. Koo, I. C. Kwon, S. Y. Jeong, and K. Kim. Photosensitizer-conjugated human serum albumin nanoparticles for effective photodynamic therapy. *Theranostics* 1 (2011): 230–39.

Jeong, Y. I., S. J. Seo, I. K. Park, H. C. Lee, I. C. Kang, T. Akaike, and C. S. Cho. Cellular recognition of paclitaxel-loaded polymeric nanoparticles composed of poly(gamma-benzyl L-glutamate) and poly(ethylene glycol) diblock copolymer endcapped with galactose moiety. *International Journal of Pharmaceutics* 296, no. 1–2 (2005): 151–61.

Kabanov, A. V., and V. Y. Alakhov. Pluronic block copolymers in drug delivery: From micellar nanocontainers to biological response modifiers. *Critical Reviews in Therapeutic Drug Carrier Systems* 19, no. 1 (2002): 1–72.

Kabanov, A. V., E. V. Batrakova, and V. Y. Alakhov. Pluronic block copolymers for overcoming drug resistance in cancer. *Advanced Drug Delivery Reviews* 54, no. 5 (2002): 759–79.

Kabanov, A. V., E. V. Batrakova, and D. W. Miller. Pluronic(R) block copolymers as modulators of drug efflux transporter activity in the blood-brain barrier. *Advanced Drug Delivery Reviews* 55, no. 1 (2003): 151–64.

Kano, M. R., Y. Bae, C. Iwata, Y. Morishita, M. Yashiro, M. Oka, T. Fujii, et al. Improvement of cancer-targeting therapy, using nanocarriers for intractable solid tumors by inhibition of TGF-beta signaling. *Proceedings of the National Academy of Sciences of the United States of America* 104, no. 9 (2007): 3460–65.

Kato, K., K. Chin, T. Yoshikawa, K. Yamaguchi, Y. Tsuji, T. Esaki, K. Sakai, et al. Phase II study of NK105, a paclitaxel-incorporating micellar nanoparticle, for previously treated advanced or recurrent gastric cancer. *Investigational New Drugs* 30, no. 4 (2011): 1621–7.

Kim, K., J. H. Kim, H. Park, Y.-S. Kim, K. Park, H. Nam, S. Lee, et al. Tumor-homing multifunctional nanoparticles for cancer theragnosis: Simultaneous diagnosis, drug delivery, and therapeutic monitoring. *Journal of Controlled Release* 146, no. 2 (2010): 219–27.

Ko, J., K. Park, Y. S. Kim, M. S. Kim, J. K. Han, K. Kim, R. W. Park, et al. Tumoral acidic extracellular pH targeting of pH-responsive MPEG-poly(beta-amino ester) block copolymer micelles for cancer therapy. *Journal of Controlled Release* 123, no. 2 (2007): 109–15.

Koizumi, F., M. Kitagawa, T. Negishi, T. Onda, S. Matsumoto, T. Hamaguchi, and Y. Matsumura. Novel SN-38-incorporating polymeric micelles, NK012, eradicate vascular endothelial growth factor-secreting bulky tumors. *Cancer Research* 66, no. 20 (2006): 10048–56.

Koo, H., H. Lee, S. Lee, K. H. Min, M. S. Kim, D. S. Lee, Y. Choi, I. C. Kwon, K. Kim, and S. Y. Jeong. In vivo tumor diagnosis and photodynamic therapy via tumoral pH-responsive polymeric micelles. *Chemical Communications* 46, no. 31 (2010): 5668–70.

Koo, H., M. S. Huh, I.-C. Sun, S. H. Yuk, K. Choi, K. Kim, and I. C. Kwon. In vivo targeted delivery of nanoparticles for theranosis. *Accounts of Chemical Research* 44, no. 10 (2011): 1018–28.

Kratz, F. Albumin as a drug carrier: Design of prodrugs, drug conjugates and nanoparticles. *Journal of Controlled Release* 132, no. 3 (2008): 171–83.

Lammers, T., S. Aime, W. E. Hennink, G. Storm, and F. Kiessling. Theranostic nanomedicine. *Accounts of Chemical Research* 44, no. 10 (2011): 1029–38.

Lapčik, L., S. De Smedt, J. Demeester, and P. Chabreček. Hyaluronan: Preparation, structure, properties, and applications. *Chemical Reviews* 98, no. 8 (1998): 2663–84.

Leamon, C. P., and J. A. Reddy. Folate-targeted chemotherapy. *Advanced Drug Delivery Reviews* 56, no. 8 (2004): 1127–41.

Lee, E. S., K. Na, and Y. H. Bae. Polymeric micelle for tumor pH and folate-mediated targeting. *Journal of Controlled Release* 91, no. 1–2 (2003): 103–13.

Lee, E. S., K. Na, and Y. H. Bae. Super pH-sensitive multifunctional polymeric micelle. *Nano Letters* 5, no. 2 (2005): 325–9.

Lee, M. K., S. J. Lim, and C. K. Kim. Preparation, characterization and in vitro cytotoxicity of paclitaxel-loaded sterically stabilized solid lipid nanoparticles. *Biomaterials* 28, no. 12 (2007): 2137–46.

Li, N., X. Yang, G. Zhai, and L. Li. Multifunctional pluronic/poly(ethylenimine) nanoparticles for anticancer drug. *Journal of Colloid and Interface Science* 350, no. 1 (2010): 117–25.

Li, Y.-L., L. Zhu, Z. Liu, R. Cheng, F. Meng, J.-H. Cui, S.-J. Ji, and Z. Zhong. Reversibly stabilized multifunctional dextran nanoparticles efficiently deliver doxorubicin into the nuclei of cancer cells. *Angewandte Chemie International Edition* 48, no. 52 (2009): 9914–18.

Liu, J., F. Zeng, and C. Allen. Influence of serum protein on polycarbonate-based copolymer micelles as a delivery system for a hydrophobic anti-cancer agent. *Journal of Controlled Release* 103, no. 2 (2005): 481–97.

Ma, Y., Y. Zheng, X. Zeng, L. Jiang, H. Chen, R. Liu, L. Huang, and L. Mei. Novel docetaxel-loaded nanoparticles based on PCL-Tween 80 copolymer for cancer treatment. *International Journal of Nanomedicine* 6 (2011): 2679–88.

Maeda, H., J. Wu, T. Sawa, Y. Matsumura, and K. Hori. Tumor vascular permeability and the EPR effect in macromolecular therapeutics: A review. *Journal of Controlled Release* 65, no. 1–2 (2000): 271–84.

Matsumura, Y. Poly (amino acid) micelle nanocarriers in preclinical and clinical studies. *Advanced Drug Delivery Reviews* 60, no. 8 (2008): 899–914.

Matsumura, Y., M. Gotoh, K. Muro, Y. Yamada, K. Shirao, Y. Shimada, M. Okuwa, et al. Phase I and pharmacokinetic study of MCC-465, a doxorubicin (DXR) encapsulated in PEG immunoliposome, in patients with metastatic stomach cancer. *Annals of Oncology* 15, no. 3 (2004): 517–25.

Matsumura, Y., and K. Kataoka. Preclinical and clinical studies of anticancer agent-incorporating polymer micelles. *Cancer Science* 100, no. 4 (2009): 572–79.

Mu, L., T. A. Elbayoumi, and V. P. Torchilin. Mixed micelles made of poly(ethylene glycol)-phosphatidylethanolamine conjugate and D-alpha-tocopheryl polyethylene glycol 1000 succinate as pharmaceutical nanocarriers for camptothecin. *International Journal of Pharmaceutics* 306, no. 1–2 (2005): 142–49.

Na, J. H., H. Koo, S. Lee, K. H. Min, K. Park, H. Yoo, S. H. Lee, et al. Real-time and non-invasive optical imaging of tumor-targeting glycol chitosan nanoparticles in various tumor models. *Biomaterials* 32, no. 22 (2011): 5252–61.

Nakanishi, T., S. Fukushima, K. Okamoto, M. Suzuki, Y. Matsumura, M. Yokoyama, T. Okano, Y. Sakurai, and K. Kataoka. Development of the polymer micelle carrier system for doxorubicin. *Journal of Controlled Release* 74, no. 1–3 (2001): 295–302.

Nam, H. Y., S. M. Kwon, H. Chung, S.-Y. Lee, S.-H. Kwon, H. Jeon, Y. Kim, et al. Cellular uptake mechanism and intracellular fate of hydrophobically modified glycol chitosan nanoparticles. *Journal of Controlled Release* 135, no. 3 (2009): 259–67.

Nasongkla, N., X. Shuai, H. Ai, B. D. Weinberg, J. Pink, D. A. Boothman, and J. Gao. Crgd-functionalized polymer micelles for targeted doxorubicin delivery. *Angewandte Chemie International Edition* 43, no. 46 (2004): 6323–27.

Nishiyama, N., Y. Bae, K. Miyata, S. Fukushima, and K. Kataoka. Smart polymeric micelles for gene and drug delivery. *Drug Discovery Today: Technologies* 2, no. 1 (2005): 21–26.

Nishiyama, N., S. Okazaki, H. Cabral, M. Miyamoto, Y. Kato, Y. Sugiyama, K. Nishio, Y. Matsumura, and K. Kataoka. Novel cisplatin-incorporated polymeric micelles can eradicate solid tumors in mice. *Cancer Research* 63, no. 24 (2003): 8977–83.

Oh, K. S., J. Y. Song, S. H. Cho, B. S. Lee, S. Y. Kim, K. Kim, H. Jeon, I. C. Kwon, and S. H. Yuk. Paclitaxel-loaded pluronic nanoparticles formed by a temperature-induced phase transition for cancer therapy. *Journal of Controlled Release* 148, no. 3 (2010): 344–50.

Oh, K. T., Y. T. Oh, N. M. Oh, K. Kim, D. H. Lee, and E. S. Lee. A smart flower-like polymeric micelle for pH-triggered anticancer drug release. *International Journal of Pharmaceutics* 375, no. 1–2 (2009): 163–69.

Olivier, J. C. Drug transport to brain with targeted nanoparticles. *NeuroRx* 2, no. 1 (2005): 108–19.

Olsen, D., C. Yang, M. Bodo, R. Chang, S. Leigh, J. Baez, D. Carmichael, et al. Recombinant collagen and gelatin for drug delivery. *Advanced Drug Delivery Reviews* 55, no. 12 (2003): 1547–67.

Osada, K., R. J. Christie, and K. Kataoka. Polymeric micelles from poly(ethylene glycol)-poly(amino acid) block copolymer for drug and gene delivery. *Journal of the Royal Society Interface* 6, no. Suppl 3 (2009): S325–39.

Panyam, J., and V. Labhasetwar. Biodegradable nanoparticles for drug and gene delivery to cells and tissue. *Advanced Drug Delivery Reviews* 55, no. 3 (2003): 329–47.

Park, E. K., S. Y. Kim, S. B. Lee, and Y. M. Lee. Folate-conjugated methoxy poly(ethylene glycol)/poly(epsilon-caprolactone) amphiphilic block copolymeric micelles for tumor-targeted drug delivery. *Journal of Controlled Release* 109, no. 1–3 (2005): 158–68.

Park, J. H., G. Saravanakumar, K. Kim, and I. C. Kwon. Targeted delivery of low molecular drugs using chitosan and its derivatives. *Advanced Drug Delivery Reviews* 62, no. 1 (2010): 28–41.

Park, K. B., Y.-I. Jeong, K. C. Choi, S. G. Kim, and H. K. Kim. Adriamycin-incorporated nanoparticles of deoxycholic acid-conjugated dextran: Antitumor activity against Ct26 colon carcinoma. *Journal of Nanoscience and Nanotechnology* 11, no. 5 (2011): 4240–49.

Park, K., J.-H. Kim, Y. S. Nam, S. Lee, H. Y. Nam, K. Kim, J. H. Park, et al. Effect of polymer molecular weight on the tumor targeting characteristics of self-assembled glycol chitosan nanoparticles. *Journal of Controlled Release* 122, no. 3 (2007): 305–14.

Park, K., S. Lee, E. Kang, K. Kim, K. Choi, and I. C. Kwon. New generation of multifunctional nanoparticles for cancer imaging and therapy. *Advanced Functional Materials* 19, no. 10 (2009): 1553–66.

Patil, Y. B., U. S. Toti, A. Khdair, L. Ma, and J. Panyam. Single-step surface functionalization of polymeric nanoparticles for targeted drug delivery. *Biomaterials* 30, no. 5 (2009): 859–66.

Peer, D., J. M. Karp, S. Hong, O. C. Farokhzad, R. Margalit, and R. Langer. Nanocarriers as an emerging platform for cancer therapy. *Nature Nanotechnology* 2 (2007): 751–60.

Petros, R. A., and J. M. DeSimone. Strategies in the design of nanoparticles for therapeutic applications. *Nature Reviews Drug Discovery* 9, no. 8 (2010): 615–27.

Reddy, L. H., R. K. Sharma, and R. S. Murthy. Enhanced tumour uptake of doxorubicin loaded poly(butyl cyanoacrylate) nanoparticles in mice bearing Dalton's lymphoma tumour. *Journal of Drug Targeting* 12, no. 7 (2004): 443–51.

Shive, M. S., and J. M. Anderson. Biodegradation and biocompatibility of PLA and PLGA microspheres. *Advanced Drug Delivery Reviews* 28, no. 1 (1997): 5–24.

Shuai, X. T., T. Merdan, A. K. Schaper, F. Xi, and T. Kissel. Core-cross-linked polymeric micelles as paclitaxel carriers. *Bioconjugate Chemistry* 15, no. 3 (2004): 441–48.

Shutava, T. G., S. S. Balkundi, P. Vangala, J. J. Steffan, R. L. Bigelow, J. A. Cardelli, D. P. O'Neal, and Y. M. Lvov. Layer-by-layer-coated gelatin nanoparticles as a vehicle for delivery of natural polyphenols. *ACS Nano* 3, no. 7 (2009): 1877–85.

Soga, O., C. F. van Nostrum, M. Fens, C. J. Rijcken, R. M. Schiffelers, G. Storm, and W. E. Hennink. Thermosensitive and biodegradable polymeric micelles for paclitaxel delivery. *Journal of Controlled Release* 103, no. 2 (2005): 341–53.

Sparreboom, A., O. van Tellingen, W. J. Nooijen, and J. H. Beijnen. Preclinical pharmacokinetics of paclitaxel and docetaxel. *Anti-Cancer Drugs* 9, no. 1 (1998): 1–17.

Stern, R., and M. J. Jedrzejas. Hyaluronidases: Their genomics, structures, and mechanisms of action. *Chemical Reviews* 106, no. 3 (2006): 818–39.

Subbiah, R., M. Veerapandian, and K. S. Yun. Nanoparticles: Functionalization and multi-functional applications in biomedical sciences. *Current Medicinal Chemistry* 17, no. 36 (2010): 4559–77.

Susa, M., A. Iyer, K. Ryu, F. Hornicek, H. Mankin, M. Amiji, and Z. Duan. Doxorubicin loaded polymeric nanoparticulate delivery system to overcome drug resistance in osteosarcoma. *BMC Cancer* 9, no. 1 (2009): 399.

Torchilin, V. P. Drug targeting. *European Journal of Pharmaceutical Sciences* 11, no. Suppl 2 (2000): S81–91.

Torchilin, V. P. Recent advances with liposomes as pharmaceutical carriers. *Nature Reviews Drug Discovery* 4, no. 2 (2005): 145–60.

Trimaille, T., K. Mondon, R. Gurny, and M. Moller. Novel polymeric micelles for hydrophobic drug delivery based on biodegradable poly(hexyl-substituted lactides). *International Journal of Pharmaceutics* 319, no. 1–2 (2006): 147–54.

Tseng, C.-L., W.-Y. Su, K.-C. Yen, K.-C. Yang, and F.-H. Lin. The use of biotinylated-EGF-modified gelatin nanoparticle carrier to enhance cisplatin accumulation in cancerous lungs via inhalation. *Biomaterials* 30, no. 20 (2009): 3476–85.

Uchino, H., Y. Matsumura, T. Negishi, F. Koizumi, T. Hayashi, T. Honda, N. Nishiyama, K. Kataoka, S. Naito, and T. Kakizoe. Cisplatin-incorporating polymeric micelles (NC-6004) can reduce nephrotoxicity and neurotoxicity of cisplatin in rats. *British Journal of Cancer* 93, no. 6 (2005): 678–87.

Valle, J. W., A. Armstrong, C. Newman, V. Alakhov, G. Pietrzynski, J. Brewer, S. Campbell, P. Corrie, E. K. Rowinsky, and M. Ranson. A phase 2 study of SP1049C, doxorubicin in P-glycoprotein-targeting pluronics, in patients with advanced adenocarcinoma of the esophagus and gastroesophageal junction. *Investigational New Drugs* 29, no. 5 (2011): 1029–37.

Valle, J. W., J. Lawrance, J. Brewer, A. Clayton, P. Corrie, V. Alakhov, and M. Ranson. A phase II, window study of SP1049C as first-line therapy in inoperable metastatic adenocarcinoma of the oesophagus. *Journal of Clinical Oncology* 22, no. 14S (2004): 4195.

van Vlerken, L. E., T. K. Vyas, and M. M. Amiji. Poly(ethylene glycol)-modified nanocarriers for tumor-targeted and intracellular delivery. *Pharmaceutical Research* 24, no. 8 (2007): 1405–14.

Wang, J., D. Mongayt, and V. P. Torchilin. Polymeric micelles for delivery of poorly soluble drugs: Preparation and anticancer activity in vitro of paclitaxel incorporated into mixed micelles based on poly(ethylene glycol)-lipid conjugate and positively charged lipids. *Journal of Drug Targeting* 13, no. 1 (2005): 73–80.

Won, Y.-W., S.-M. Yoon, C. H. Sonn, K.-M. Lee, and Y.-H. Kim. Nano self-assembly of recombinant human gelatin conjugated with α-tocopheryl succinate for Hsp90 inhibitor, 17-AAG, delivery. *ACS Nano* 5, no. 5 (2011): 3839–48.

Wosikowski, K., E. Biedermann, B. Rattel, N. Breiter, P. Jank, R. Loser, G. Jansen, and G. J. Peters. In vitro and in vivo antitumor activity of methotrexate conjugated to human serum albumin in human cancer cells. *Clinical Cancer Research* 9, no. 5 (2003): 1917–26.

Xie, J., S. Lee, and X. Chen. Nanoparticle-based theranostic agents. *Advanced Drug Delivery Reviews* 62, no. 11 (2010): 1064–79.

Xu, P. S., E. A. Van Kirk, S. Y. Li, W. J. Murdoch, J. Ren, M. D. Hussain, M. Radosz, and Y. Q. Shen. Highly stable core-surface-crosslinked nanoparticles as cisplatin carriers for cancer chemotherapy. *Colloids and Surfaces B: Biointerfaces* 48, no. 1 (2006): 50–57.

Yokoyama, M., S. Inoue, K. Kataoka, N. Yui, and Y. Sakurai. Preparation of adriamycin-conjugated poly(ethylene glycol)-poly(aspartic acid) block copolymer—A new type of polymeric anticancer agent. *Die Makromolekulare Chemie-Rapid Communications* 8, no. 9 (1987): 431–35.

Yokoyama, M., M. Miyauchi, N. Yamada, T. Okano, Y. Sakurai, K. Kataoka, and S. Inoue. Polymer micelles as novel drug carrier—Adriamycin-conjugated poly(ethylene glycol) poly(aspartic acid) block copolymer. *Journal of Controlled Release* 11, no. 1–3 (1990): 269–78.

Yokoyama, M., T. Okano, Y. Sakurai, S. Suwa, and K. Kataoka. Introduction of cisplatin into polymeric micelle. *Journal of Controlled Release* 39, no. 2–3 (1996): 351–56.

Yoo, H. S., and T. G. Park. Folate receptor targeted biodegradable polymeric doxorubicin micelles. *Journal of Controlled Release* 96, no. 2 (2004): 273–83.

Zhang, L., F. X. Gu, J. M. Chan, A. Z. Wang, R. S. Langer, and O. C. Farokhzad. Nanoparticles in medicine: Therapeutic applications and developments. *Clinical Pharmacology & Therapeutics* 83, no. 5 (2008): 761–69.

Zhu, C. H., S. Jung, S. B. Luo, F. H. Meng, X. L. Zhu, T. G. Park, and Z. Y. Zhong. Co-delivery of sirna and paclitaxel into cancer cells by biodegradable cationic micelles based on PDMAEMA-PCL-PDMAEMA triblock copolymers. *Biomaterials* 31, no. 8 (2010): 2408–16.

5 Carbon Nanotube Bioconjugates

Monica Samal and Dong Kee Yi
Kyungwon University

Shashadhar Samal
S.B.R. Government (Autonomous) Women's College

CONTENTS

5.1 INTRODUCTION

The carbon nanotubes (CNTs) categorized as multiwalled CNTs (MWNTs)[1-3] and single-walled CNTs (SWNTs)[4,5] exhibit unique mechanical, structural, and electrical properties. They have a high aspect ratio, lengths from several hundred nanometers to several micrometers, and diameters of 0.4–2 nm for SWNTs and 2–100 nm for coaxial MWNTs. These one-dimensional carbon allotropes are the ultimate carbon fibers. They are ultra lightweight, have the highest mechanical strength of all known materials, highest thermal conductivity, outstanding field emission properties, and can function as the active semiconductors in nanoscale devices. Metallic CNTs conduct electricity without dissipating heat. The nanotubes can absorb gas molecules as nano capillaries, be dissolved in surfactants, and undergo chemical derivatization for a myriad of additional functions. The last two decades have witnessed tremendous academic interest in CNTs, due largely to their attractive properties and potential applications in diverse fields, resulting in an avalanche of literature, summarized in several state-of-the-art reviews,[6-11] books, and monographs.[12-27] Initial interest in application of CNTs stemmed from their exceptionally high tensile strength and stiffness, leading to CNT-based advanced composite materials,[28] while in recent times their unique geometry offers promising applications in biology and medicine.[29-36] In this chapter, syntheses of some CNT bioconjugates and their biological and biomedical applications are discussed with a brief introduction on the structure and reactivity of the nanotubes.

5.2 STRUCTURE

CNTs are seamlessly folded-up graphene sheets. Graphene is a one-atom-thick planar sheet of sp^2-bonded carbon atoms. Graphite consists of many graphene sheets stacked up through van der Waal interactions with an interplanar spacing

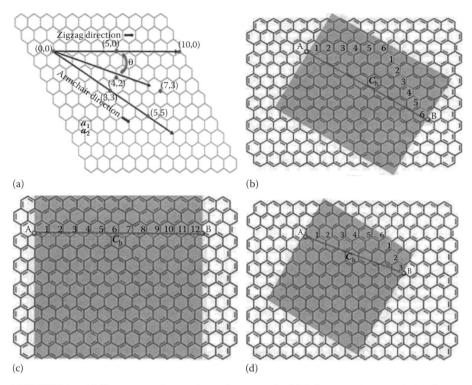

FIGURE 5.1 (a) Three ways the graphene sheets can be folded, generating armchair, zigzag, and chiral SWNTs. The unit vectors a_1 and a_2 are also shown. (b–d) Schematically drawn graphene sheets with two lattice points A and B. Folding up of the graphene sheet is done in a manner that point A comes over point B leading to, for example, armchair (6,6) (b), zigzag (12,0) (c), and chiral (6,3) (d) SWNTs of circumference C_h.

of 0.335 nm. There are three ways of folding graphene sheets (Figure 5.1a), which generate three distinctly different tubes that are named armchair, zigzag, and chiral SWNTs. The names armchair and zigzag simply reflect the shape of the open edges of the CNTs. Figure 5.1b–d shows schematically drawn graphene sheets with two crystallographically equivalent lattice points A and B. Folding up of the graphene sheet is done in a manner that point A comes over point B, that is, both points coincide. This leads to SWNTs being characterized by circumference C_h, the chirality vector, described for an SWNT as chiral indices (n,m) by the expression: $C_h = na_1 + ma_2$, where a_1 and a_2 are the unit vectors, as defined in Figure 5.1a.

To realize the (n,m) tube, point B is defined from point A, the origin $(0,0)$, as moving n times a_1 and m times a_2 to get to the lattice point B and rolling up the sheet so that A and B coincide. If both n and m are positive integers and equal $(n = m \neq 0)$, it results in an armchair nanotube. For a (6,6) armchair nanotube, the chirality vector and the lattice points A and B are shown in Figure 5.1b. The zigzag tubes are defined by the chirality vector $C_h = na_1 + ma_2$, where n is a positive integer and m is zero or vice versa $(n \neq 0, m = 0, \text{ or } n = 0, m \neq 0)$. Thus, for example, a

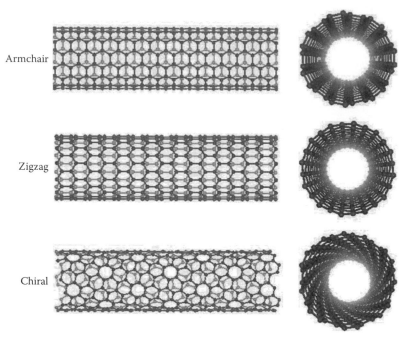

Armchair

Zigzag

Chiral

FIGURE 5.2   Three types of SWNTs with their prospective views.

(12,0) zigzag SWNT results from folding up of the graphene sheet moving 12 times a_1 and 0 time a_2 (Figure 5.1c). When both n and m are positive integers and not equal ($n \neq m \neq 0$), the resulting nanotube is termed as chiral because these tubes lack symmetry. The armchair and zigzag nanotubes are achiral due to their symmetrical structures. The three types of SWNTs with their prospective views are shown in Figure 5.2.

The chiral angle θ, defined as the angle between vectors a_1 (zigzag direction) and $na_1 + ma_2$ (chiral direction), is 30° for armchair and 0° for zigzag, and varies in the range 0°–30° for chiral nanotubes. The armchair nanotubes are (n,n) with a chiral angle of 30°, the zigzag nanotubes correspond to $(n,0)$ or $(0,m)$ and have a chiral angle of 0°, while chiral nanotubes have general (n,m) values and a chiral angle between 0° and 30°. The diameter and the chiral angle of a (n,m) nanotube can be calculated from the following relations:

$$d_t = C_h / \pi = \frac{\sqrt{3}a_{C-C}\left(n^2 + nm + m^2\right)^{1/2}}{\pi}$$

$$\theta = \tan^{-1}\left[\sqrt{3m}\left(2n + m\right)\right]$$

where a_{C-C} is the nearest-neighbor C–C distance (1.421Å in graphite) and C_h is the length of the chiral vector.

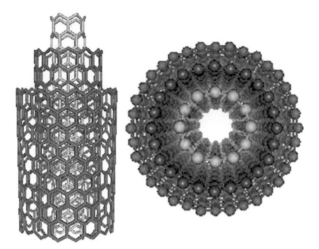

FIGURE 5.3 Views of MWNTs made up of three concentric SWNTs. The spacing between the tubes is ~3.4Å.

MWNTs are multiple rolled layers of graphene forming concentric tubes with an interlayer spacing of ~3.4Å, close to the distance between graphene layers in graphite (Figure 5.3). The concentric tubes are SWNTs, which can be metallic or semiconducting. The number of concentric tubes can be significantly high, and hence, MWNTs are graphite-like and usually zero-gap metals. When there are just two concentric tubes, it results in a double-walled CNT (DWNT). DWNTs form a special class of nanotubes because their properties are similar to those of SWNTs, but unlike the SWNTs, their resistance to chemicals is significantly improved.

5.2.1 END CAPS

The ends of the as-produced CNTs are closed by hemispheres of C_n (Figure 5.4). If C_{60} is bisected normal to a fivefold axis, and the two halves are filled up by adding a cylinder of graphene, an armchair tube is formed. If C_{60} is bisected normal to a threefold axis, and the two halves are filled up by adding a cylinder of graphene, a zigzag tube is formed. The size of the end-cap fullerene hemispheres varies with the tube size. For example, the diameter of a (10,10) nanotube requires that the ends be capped by hemispheres of C_{240}.

The end caps of the raw MWNTs can be seen in high-resolution transmission electron microscopy (TEM) images. The purified nanotubes, particularly the SWNTs, are open-ended tubes because during purification the end caps get destroyed. The tubes are not perfect as they seem to be from the simple pictures presented above. CNTs are not made up of hexagons exclusively. Rings other than hexagons, such as pentagons and heptagons, may be present. There may be defect sites with missing carbon atoms either present in the formation stage or introduced during the purification process.

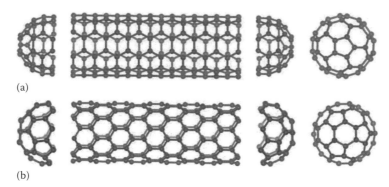

(a)

(b)

FIGURE 5.4   SWNT end caps: (a) armchair SWNT with C_{60} hemisphere caps having five-fold axis of symmetry; (b) zigzag SWNT with C_{60} hemisphere caps having threefold axis of symmetry.

5.2.2   DEFECTS

A pentagon defect site bends the tube. An SWNT with a 7–5 defect, where the two rings are located at the opposite walls of the nanotube, results in bending of the tube (Figure 5.5). If the 7–5 defect is such that the seven- and six-membered rings share a common bond, the tube diameter changes at the defect site. These defect sites are highly vulnerable to chemical attack. Simple sonication can degrade the tubes breaking bonds at the defects. Fortunately, defects are desirable as reactive functionalities can be easily introduced at these sites.

5.2.3   OXIDATION

When the raw CNT soot is refluxed or sonicated in the presence of strong oxidizing agents such as HNO_3 or H_2SO_4 or a mixture of the two, the end caps of the nanotubes as well as the defect sites in the sidewalls are oxidized to carboxylic acids or other weak acidic functionalities such as quinones.[37–43] Nitric acid treatment purifies the raw nanotubes by removal of the metal catalysts and amorphous carbon.

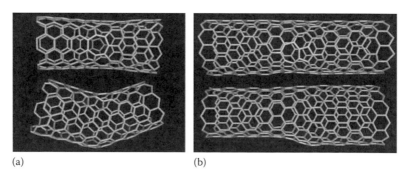

(a)   (b)

FIGURE 5.5   7–5 Defects: (a) Two rings are located at the opposite sides of the nanotube. This results in a bend. (b) The two rings may share a common bond. Note the change in tube diameter upon introduction of the defect.

Once oxidized, the SWNTs can be dispersed ultrasonically in various amide-type organic solvents. Oxidation introduces new defects on the nanotube surface[44] and produces impurity states at the Fermi level,[45] with consequent effects in the electronic properties of the nanotubes.[46,47] The process shortens the CNTs,[48-51] and prolonged treatment can eventually destroy it. However, sonication in organic solvents alone does least damage to the pristine structure of the nanotube and produces dangling bonds that undergo further chemical reactions.[52] Purification of raw soot to remove the metal catalysts and amorphous carbon is thus associated with the removal of the end caps and the oxidation of defect sites in the sidewalls. This disrupts the aromatic ring system of the SWNTs. All the nanotubes are not similarly affected by the oxidizing agents, the size and nature of the tube being an important factor. The largest diameter tubes require the strong oxidative conditions, whereas the smaller diameter HiPco tubes get extensively damaged by such harsh treatment.[53,54]

5.2.4 Semiconducting and Metallic CNTs

In SWNTs, the possible bond alternation patterns are illustrated in Figure 5.6. If all the bonds in the nanotubes are isodistant (uniform delocalization of π-electrons), then all three types of SWNTs will have zero bandgap. If the bonds are not isodistant (Alt 1, Alt 2, Kekulé), only for the armchair (n,n) SWNTs with Alt 1 bond pattern, the bandgap is zero; that is, armchair nanotubes with the typical π-bond arrangement pattern are metallic. Thus, the armchair (n,n) SWNTs with the Alt 1 bond pattern will be metallic, and the zigzag $(n,0)$ tubes with the Alt 1 bond alternation pattern are metallic when $n/3$ is a positive integer. If the bond alternation pattern is Alt 2, the nanotubes are quasimetallic (narrow bandgap). The chiral (n,m) SWNTs are metallic or narrow gap semiconductors when $(2n + m)/3$ is a positive integer. The nanotubes not conforming to the above conditions are wide-gap semiconductors.

The density of states (DOS) of metallic and semiconducting SWNTs are shown in Figure 5.7 for armchair (5,5) and zigzag (7,0) SWNTs as illustrative examples.[55]

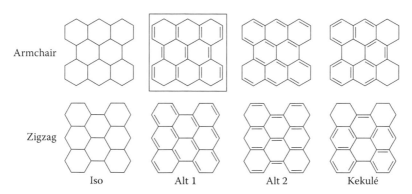

FIGURE 5.6 Bond alternation patterns of SWNTs: isodistant (Iso), bond alternant 1 (Alt 1), bond alternant 2 (Alt 2), and Kekulé patterns.

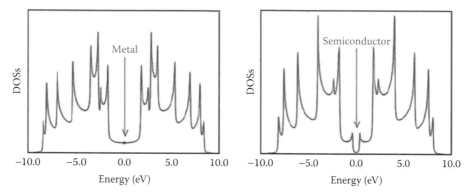

FIGURE 5.7 The DOS exhibiting the valence band (negative values), the conduction band (positive values), and the Fermi energy (centered at 0 eV) of metallic and semiconducting carbon nanotubes. The armchair (5,5) nanotube exhibits metallic behavior and the zigzag (7,0) nanotube is a small gap semiconductor. Sharp spikes in the DOS are van Hove singularities, the energy states determining optical excitation and emission transitions. (Reprinted with permission from Charlier, J.-C., 2002, 1063–1069. Copyright 2002 American Chemical Society.)

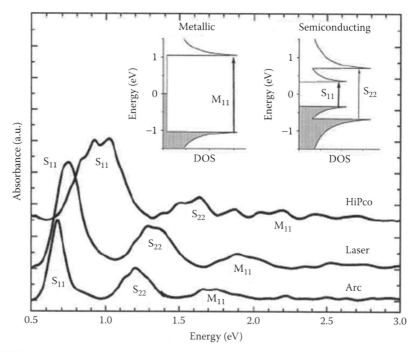

FIGURE 5.8 Electronic transitions between the energy bands of SWNTs, observed by transmission spectroscopy of films, together with a schematic of the nomenclature (S_{11}, S_{22}, M_{11}) used to designate the interband transitions. (Reprinted with permission from Hamon, M. A., et al., 2001, 11292–11293. Copyright 2001 American Chemical Society.)

The armchair (5,5) nanotube exhibits a metallic behavior with finite value of charge carriers in the DOS at the Fermi energy located at zero. The zigzag (7,0) nanotube is a small-gap semiconductor with no charge carriers in the DOS at the Fermi energy. The sharp spikes in the DOS are van Hove singularities that determine the gap between the valence bands and the conduction bands. Electronic transitions between the energy bands of SWNTs, observed by TEM of films, together with a schematic of the nomenclature S_{11}, S_{22}, and M_{11} used to designate the interband transitions, are shown in Figure 5.8 for SWNTs from three different sources of preparation.[56] Fermi level electronic structure of common forms of SWNTs with characteristic low-energy (~0.01 eV) features arises from a combination of transitions that are intrinsic to the metallic SWNTs, transitions due to the curvature-induced gap in the chiral metallic SWNTs, and transitions due to purification-induced acid doping of the semiconducting SWNTs.[45]

5.3 REACTIVITY

The reactivity of a perfect SWNT without any structural defects and with fullerene hemisphere end caps is not the same for the three types of nanotubes. Further, the reactivity of the same nanotube will be different at the sidewalls and the end caps. The reactivity of the end caps is primarily driven by strain arising out of the spherical geometry. Since all the carbon atoms in graphene are sp^2 hybridized and hence of planar geometry, the rolling of the graphene sheet into an SWNT induces strain, and the extent of strain will be related to the extent of deviation from planarity. To explain it further, let us consider two neighboring carbon atoms of a graphene sheet. The angle between the π-orbital and the σ-molecular plane ($\theta_{\sigma\pi}$) is 90° (Figure 5.9a). For such planar sp^2-hybridized carbon atoms, the pyramidization angle θ_P, defined as $\theta_P = \theta_{\sigma\pi} - 90°$, is 0°. The angle between the π-orbital of a carbon atom in C_{60} and the σ-skeleton forming the curved surface of the molecule is 101.6° (Figure 5.9b), and hence the θ_P, which is a measure of deviation from the planarity for the C_{60} carbon atoms, is 11.6°. For a tetrahedral sp^3-hybridized carbon atom, the pyramidization angle is 19.5° ($\theta_P = 109.5° - 90°$). Because the θ_P of 11.6° for the C_{60} carbon

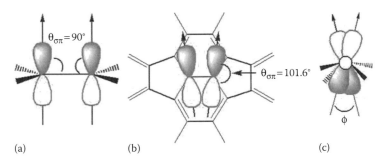

(a)   (b)   (c)

FIGURE 5.9 (a) Angle between the π-orbital and the π-molecular plane ($\theta_{\sigma\pi}$) is 90° for two neighboring carbon atoms of a graphene sheet; (b) $\theta_{\sigma\pi}$ for the π-orbitals and the σ-molecular surface of C_{60} is 101.6°; and (c) misalignment angle ϕ for π-bonds running at an angle to the nanotube circumference.

atoms is close to the tetrahedral geometry, any structural modification arising out of a chemical reaction that changes the hybridization of carbon atoms of the SWNT caps from sp^2 to sp^3 is strongly preferred. This not only relieves strain at the specific carbon atom, the remaining carbon atoms also feel the relieving strain.[57,58]

The carbon atoms of SWNT walls are sp^2 hybridized. Being curved, the wall π-bonds are also strained; the extent of strain is inversely related to the degree of curvature. Thus, the diameters of the nanotube are inversely related to the pyramidization angles. In addition, the π-bonds on the walls of SWNTs experience another kind of strain arising out of misalignment of the π-orbitals (Figure 5.9c). Hence, the extent of pyramidization on the caps and walls and the π-orbital misalignment on the walls[59–63] define the strain of an SWNT. To realize

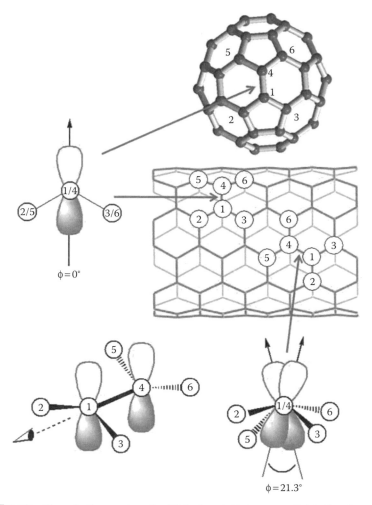

FIGURE 5.10 The misalignment angles (φ) for bonds that run parallel to the circumference (or perpendicular to the nanotube axis) (φ = 0°) to the nanotube axis and those at an angle (φ = 21.3°) to the circumference for a (5,5) SWNT.

which of the above two sources of strain determines the reactivity of an SWNT, a comparison of the tube diameter and the cap size is relevant. For example, in the (5,5) SWNT, the end caps are hemispheres of C_{60}, for which θ_p is 11.6°. That for a (10,10) SWNT is a hemisphere of C_{240}, for which θ_p is 9.7°. For any fullerene, θ_p cannot be lower than 9.7°, which means that the end caps will always be quite reactive irrespective of the diameter of the nanotube. There is very little π-orbital misalignment in the fullerenes,[64,65] for which the pyramidalization angle alone governs their reactivity.

In CNTs, there are two types of bonds: those that run parallel to the circumference (or perpendicular to the nanotube axis) and those at an angle to the circumference (Figure 5.10).[66] For all SWNTs, the π-orbital misalignment angles for bonds that run parallel to the circumference are 0°. However, for bonds at an angle to the circumference the extent of orbital misalignment depends on the tube diameter. For the (5,5) and (10,10) SWNTs, these are 21.3° and 10.4°, respectively.

The θ_p values of carbon atoms of CNT walls vary in the range 2.59°–5.97°, but ϕ varies in the range 9.1°–21.3°. Since the pyramidization angles are small compared to those for fullerenes (Figure 5.11), the π-orbital misalignment is likely to be the main source of strain in CNTs. The π-orbital misalignment angles of SWNTs vary inversely with the diameter of the tubes, and hence, CNTs of different diameters will exhibit reactivity in that order.

While molecules are nanoscopic in all dimensions, SWNTs are nanoscopic in two dimensions, being thousands of times longer in the third dimension. Depending on how the graphene sheets are wrapped up, SWNTs can be either small- or medium-gap semiconductors, or truly metallic conductors. Again, for the

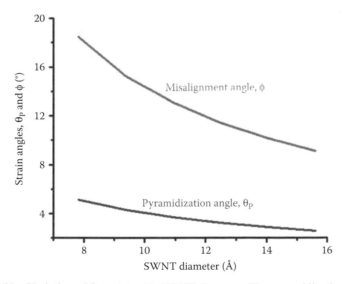

FIGURE 5.11 Variation of θ_p and ϕ with SWNT diameter. The pyramidization angles are small compared to that for fullerenes (11.6° for C_{60} and cannot be less than 9.7°). The misalignment angle ϕ for π-bonds making an angle with the tube circumference is much larger than θ_p.

semiconducting tubes the conductivity varies with the diameter. The basic structure visualized as an ideal defect-free hexagonal array of graphene wrapped into a seamless tube is indeed laden with defects. These have direct bearing on the reactivity of the π-bonds. Thus, a sample of raw SWNT is a mixture of tubes varying in their diameter, length, electrical conductivity, and so on. Therefore, working on such a material is a challenging task since no two tubes are identical in all respects. Nevertheless, simple laboratory techniques for purification of the CNTs, such as nitric acid oxidation or sonication in the presence of a suitable solvent or a combination of both, lead to CNTs that can be easily dissolved in water after suitable functionalization, paving the way for numerous applications in diverse fields.

5.4 FUNCTIONALIZATION

To functionalize SWNTs by covalent or noncovalent strategies for any targeted application, the crude nanotube is first purified by oxidation to remove metal particles or amorphous carbon. Under oxidative conditions, in addition to removal of impurities, the SWNTs themselves break up into very short tubes of 100–300 nm length and about 1.5 nm diameter.[38] The purified SWNTs are still bundles of tubes held together by strong hydrophobic interactions. The nanotubes can be dispersed in various nonpolar and polar solvents including water. During functionalization, the functional species that binds SWNTs noncovalently or covalently outweigh the attractive forces existing among the tubes, resulting in debundling of the tubes. Functionalization of the purified nanotubes carried out under sonication may further break the tubes into still smaller ones.

A large variety of SWNTs with biological molecules covalently linked to the nanotubes have been synthesized. In the covalent functionalization strategy, after chemical reactions, the nanotube structure gets extensively disrupted. Hence, the intrinsic physical properties of CNTs such as photoluminescence and Raman scattering are often destroyed. The intensities of Raman scattering and photoluminescence of SWNTs are drastically decreased, reducing the potential of their applications based on these optical methods. Thus, a careful control over the extent of functionalization is essential, particularly when the optical characteristics of the nanotube become determinant in the biological application.

Unless the tubes are degraded to very small pieces, in the noncovalent functionalization approach, the chemical structure of the π-network of CNTs is not disrupted significantly; hence, the physical properties of CNTs are essentially preserved. Thus, a number of bioactive molecules including DNA have been used to noncovalently functionalize the purified SWNTs. Nevertheless, there is a limitation to this approach. Once an SWNT loaded with a bioactive molecule is introduced into a target site such as the cell, tissue, or organ, and the loaded molecule is delivered, the SWNTs aggregate once again forming insoluble bundles that may be toxic to the target site.[67,68] It is reported that DNA molecules coated on SWNTs can be cleaved by nucleases in the serum, suggesting that DNA functionalization of SWNTs might not be stable in such biological environments.[69] In spite of the above limitations, many soluble CNTs have been developed through noncovalent interactions, which are quite stable in biological environments.

5.4.1 Covalent Functionalization: Reaction at the COOH Groups

Nitric acid oxidation of SWNT introduces carboxylic acid groups at the tube ends and defect sites in the sidewalls, which are anchors for further functionalization. The COOH groups of the SWNTs (1) can be easily converted to amides or esters (2) via acid chloride or carbodiimide-activated coupling (Figure 5.12).[70] The solubility of SWNTs in organic solvents is significantly influenced by the nature of the hydrocarbon chain introduced on amidation or esterification. The SWNT amides and esters with long alkyl chains are soluble in tetrahydrofuran (THF), CS_2, and aromatic solvents. The long-chain hydrocarbons appended to the ends and sidewalls disrupt the strong hydrophobic attractions, resulting in debundling of the nanotubes. Direct reaction of acid-purified shortened SWNTs with long-chain amines leads to soluble materials by the formation of zwitterions (3) with the COOH groups.[71] Such ionic functionalization has several advantages. Unlike the covalent amide bond, the cation in the ionic bond is readily exchanged by other organic and inorganic cations. This feature has been explored to study electrostatic interactions between SWNTs and biological molecules. In the functionalization of the SWNTs through amidation, esterification, and ionic interaction with the carboxylic acid group, the nanotube electronic structure is generally retained. On the other hand, sidewall functionalization by addition onto the π-bonds alters conjugated nanotube surface electronic structure.[8]

5.4.1.1 Attaching Biopolymers to COOH Groups

Modifying the terminal and defect site COOH groups to amides and esters is further extended, appending the purified and activated nanotubes with polymers and dendrimers having amino or hydroxy group functions (Figure 5.13).[72–75] A number of such amphiphilic polymers are used to functionalize the SWNTs through acylation–amidation or carbodiimide-activated amidation of the COOH groups so as to make the nanotubes soluble in water and other polar solvents. One of the first water- and chloroform-soluble CNT samples is obtained by covalent attachment of an amphiphilic aminopolymer, poly(propionylethyleneimine-*co*-ethyleneimine) (PPEI-EI).[76] The PPEI-EI-functionalized CNTs are strongly luminescent. Functionalization with

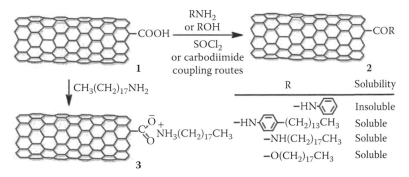

FIGURE 5.12 Functionalization of the SWNTs through amidation, esterification, and ionic interaction of the carboxylic acid groups.

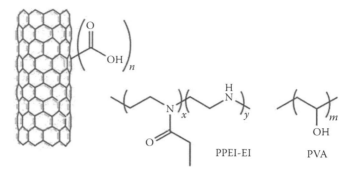

PPEI-EI   PVA

FIGURE 5.13 Modifying the terminal and defect site COOH groups to amides and esters by reacting the purified and activated nanotubes with polymers having amino or hydroxy group functions.

aminopolymer through ionic interaction is affected by directly heating nanotubes and aminopolymers. These samples are also soluble in water. Sonication during the reaction significantly improves the nanotube solubilization, though the nanotubes are shortened if sonication is prolonged.[77]

The aminopolymer attached to the tube ends and the sidewalls interacts very strongly with the SWNT surface. High-resolution TEM analysis of the PPEI-EI-functionalized SWNTs shows that the polymer chains cover the nanotube surface significantly.[78] The SWNT bundles are exfoliated into thinner ones and individual tubes and get completely wrapped up by the polymer. As a consequence, the tubes get passivated and become soluble in water and other polar solvents. The soluble sample from the carbodiimide activation scheme contains more bundled SWNTs.[79] Like PEG, poly(vinyl alcohol) (PVA) has properties useful to biomedical applications. PVA is a water-soluble vinyl polymer that undergoes biodegradation under suitable conditions. Thus, SWNTs are functionalized with PVA[80] and poly(vinyl acetate-*co*-vinyl alcohol),[72] which are highly water soluble.

Attaching poly(ethylene glycol) (PEG) chains to SWNTs is of particular interest because PEG possesses many properties useful to biomedical and biotechnical applications. Functionalization of SWNTs with diamine-terminated oligomeric PEG (**4**) (Figure 5.14)[81] shows that the functionalization and solubilization of smaller SWNTs are favored. The insoluble component gets enriched with the nanotubes of larger diameters.[82] For MWNTs, no preferential functionalization and solubilization are observed as in case of SWNTs.[83] A number of studies have been carried out focusing on functionalization of CNTs with oligomeric and polymeric species-containing PEG chains.[84,85] These include amine-terminated PEG-functionalized SWNTs soluble in water and organic solvents, microwave heating to obtain amine-terminated PEG-functionalized SWNTs, and synthesis of derivatized SWNTs via reaction with 2-aminomethyl-18-crown-6 ether soluble in various solvents, including water. The water solubility of the PEG-functionalized SWNT samples also allows further chemical manipulations and bioconjugations in an aqueous medium.

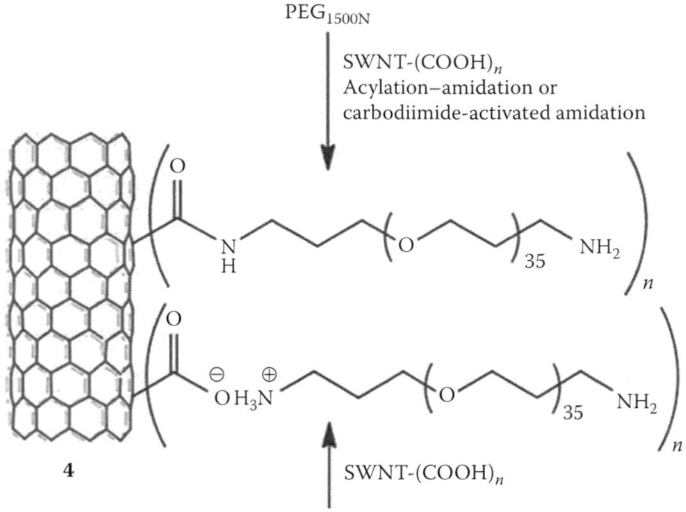

FIGURE 5.14 Functionalization of COOH groups with diamine-terminated oligomeric PEG via acylation–amidation or carbodiimide-activated amidation as well as zwitterion formation.

5.4.2 COVALENT SIDEWALL FUNCTIONALIZATION

The C=C π-bonds on the sidewalls and defect sites in SWNTs are initially considered inert to chemical reactions. Subsequently, it is found that these bonds readily undergo a number of reactions. The reactivity of the π-bonds depends on the curvature of the nanotube. An increase in curvature leads to more pronounced pyramidization of the sp^2-hybridized carbon atoms and an increased tendency to undergo addition reactions. One of the first reactions attempted on SWNTs is fluorination. Purified SWNTs in the form of bucky paper (SWNT over a polytetrafluoroethylene membrane) are electrochemically reacted with elemental fluorine between 150°C and 600°C.[86,87] Fluorinated SWNTs are appreciably soluble in alcoholic solvents and the nanotube bundles exfoliate into individual tubes. Fluorination drastically changes the electronic properties of the CNTs; the samples synthesized at 250°C are insulators. The C–F bonds in SWNTs are vulnerable to nucleophilic substitution reactions. Strong nucleophiles such as Grignard and alkyl lithium reagents and metal alkoxides displace the fluorine substituents. The reactions apparently proceed via a concerted, allylic displacement mechanism, as S_N2 attack is not possible, and the stability of a carbocation for S_N1 pathway is questionable, considering that the SWNT surface is highly curved.

Fluorinated SWNTs react with amino acids, $NH_2(CH_2)_nCOOH$, where $n = 1$ (glycine), 5 (6-aminohexanoic acid), and 10 (11-aminoundecanoic acid), and the resulting carboxylic acid-functionalized SWNTs are characterized by magic angle spinning (MAS) ^{13}C NMR spectroscopy.[88] In the amino acid-functionalized SWNTs, the resolution of the aliphatic CH_2 carbon signal depends on the length of the aliphatic chain of the amino acid. When substituent chains are short, NMR data collection becomes difficult. To alleviate this problem, the amino acid-functionalized SWNTs are esterified with an appropriate alcohol to ensure parity of the overall substituent length. It is concluded that increasing the length of SWNT sidewall functional groups enhances the ability to observe the sidewall sp^3 carbon.

Covalent functionalizations with radicals and anions have also been demonstrated. The reactivity of SWNTs with aryl diazonium compounds presumably proceeds via the aryl radical generated on one-electron reduction of the diazonium salt.[89,90] The degree of functionalization is sufficient to cause a complete loss of electronic structure in SWNTs. Functionalization of SWNTs utilizing radical sources other than aryl diazoniums has also been reported, including perfluoroalkyl iodides.[91] In the functionalization of SWNTs with a nucleophilic carbene generated by deprotonation of the stable imidizolinium cation, no cyclopropanation occurs. Each added group is bound through just one covalent bond to the tube. The added group is positively charged and one negative charge per added groups is transferred to the nanotube framework. Due to mutual electrostatic repulsion of these charges, the nanotubes get debundled, rendering these adducts highly soluble.

The reactions of SWNTs with succinic or glutaric acid acyl peroxides in o-dichlorobenzene at 80–90°C result in the addition of 2-carboxyethyl or 3-carboxypropyl groups, respectively, to the sidewalls of the SWNT.[92] These acid-functionalized SWNTs are converted to amides with terminal diamines such as ethylenediamine, 4,4′-methylenebis(cyclohexylamine), and diethyltoluenediamine. The acid-functionalized SWNTs show an improved solubility in alcohol and water, which enables their processing for a variety of biomedical applications.

Cycloaddition turns out to be a very attractive route for functionalization of SWNTs. Carbene-generating compounds can conduct [2+1] cycloadditions via the Bingel reaction,[93,94] or by photochemical reaction of CNTs with azides, leading to the corresponding products **6** (bridging carbon) and **8** (bridging nitrogen), respectively (Figure 5.15).[95,96] A 1,3-dipolar cycloaddition reaction on CNTs developed by Prato et al. is a very versatile reaction.[97,98] In this reaction, azomethine ylides generated by condensation of an α-amino acid and an aldehyde are added to the SWNT surface, forming a pyrrolidine ring (**9**). These reactions have paved ways to introduce additional functionalities to CNTs for a variety of applications including those in bio-related fields.[99,100]

5.4.2.1   Carbon Bridging

SWNTs undergo cyclopropanation reactions with dichlorocarbene generated from $CHCl_3$ and KOH and from phenyl(bromodichloromethyl)mercury furnishing **7**.[101,102] However, the degree of functionalization in these cases is low. On the other hand, the Bingel reaction affords SWNT-malonates readily. Unambiguous characterization of SWNT-malonate synthesized in the Bingel reaction conditions by conventional spectroscopy and electron microscopy is difficult mainly due to low solubility, electron beam sensitivity and resolution, and metallic behavior of the nanotubes. This problem of imaging has been elucidated by attaching chemical markers to SWNTs. By this technique, surface sites that have undergone cyclopropanation reaction can be visualized by atomic force microscopy (AFM) and other spectroscopic techniques.[93] Transesterification of SWNT-malonates (**10**) (Figure 5.16) is carried

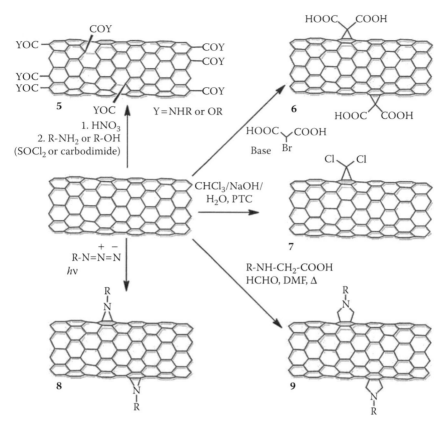

FIGURE 5.15 Various routes to covalent functionalization of SWNTs.

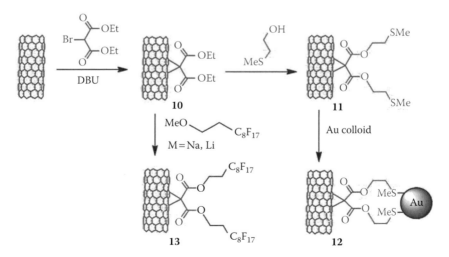

FIGURE 5.16 Cyclopropanation of SWNTs and introduction of chemical markers. (Reprinted with permission from Coleman, K. S., et al., 2003, 8722–8723. Copyright 2003 American Chemical Society.)

out with 2-(methylthio)ethanol, followed by introduction of preformed ~5-nm gold colloids (**12**). Transesterification is also carried out with the sodium or lithium salt of 1*H*,1*H*,2*H*,2*H*-perfluorodecan-1-ol leading to the corresponding SWNT-bearing perfluorodecan moiety (**13**). The chemically tagged products are suitable for identifying the presence of reacted surface sites using AFM, and ¹⁹F NMR and x-ray photoelectron spectroscopies.

The characteristic electronic properties of the acid-purified nanotubes have a direct bearing on the number of π-bonds retained on the sidewalls. It is demonstrated that covalent functionalization of the sidewalls of SWNTs with one functional group per 10–100 carbon atoms on the sidewall leads to loss of the characteristic electronic properties of the nanotubes.[71,104] When the number of functional groups is reduced to one per 75–300 carbon atoms, the electronic properties of SWNTs are largely retained. Sidewalls of acid-treated, shortened SWNTs with long alkyl chains at the open ends and defect sites (**14**) facilitate functionalization by microwave-assisted Bingel reaction due to enhanced solubility imparted by the long alkyl chain (Figure 5.17).[94] The degree of sidewall functionalization is controllable by changing the output power of the microwave. AFM and TEM showed the progressive exfoliation of SWNT bundles. Resonant Raman and UV–Vis–near-infrared

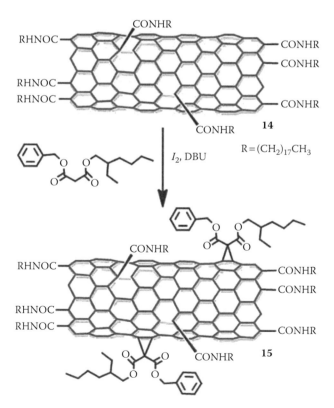

FIGURE 5.17 Synthetic strategy for repeat functionalization of the SWNTs with benzyl 2-ethylhexyl malonate.

(NIR) absorption spectroscopies of **15** reveal that the electronic properties of SWNT are largely retained.

5.4.2.2 Nitrogen Bridging

Sidewall functionalization of SWNTs by nitrenes generated by thermolysis of alkyl azidoformates is a facile route to introduction of a variety of groups onto the nanotube. The azidoformates under thermal conditions generate oxycarbonyl nitrenes *in situ* by N_2 extrusion. Addition of (R-)-oxycarbonyl nitrenes, where R is the desired functionality, allows covalent binding of a variety of different groups such as alkyl chains, aromatic groups, dendrimers, crown ethers, and oligoethylene glycol units (**16**) (Figure 5.18).[104] Such additions lead to a considerable increase in solubility in organic solvents. The highest solubilities of 1.2 mg/mL are found for SWNT adducts with nitrenes containing crown ether of oligoethylene glycol moieties. The chelating donor groups of oligoethylene glycol and crown ether allow complexation of Cu^{2+} and Cd^{2+}. Raman and UV–Vis–NIR studies show that the electronic properties of SWNTs are mostly retained after functionalization, indicating a low degree of addition.

A facile route of growing DNA oligonucleotide of a desired base sequence on the sidewalls of MWNTs, which renders the MWNTs water soluble, involves first reacting MWNTs photochemically with azidothymidine (AZT).[96] The aligned MWNTs on the solid support are coated with a solution of AZT and are UV irradiated to produce photoadducts, each with a hydroxyl group. The hydroxyl group

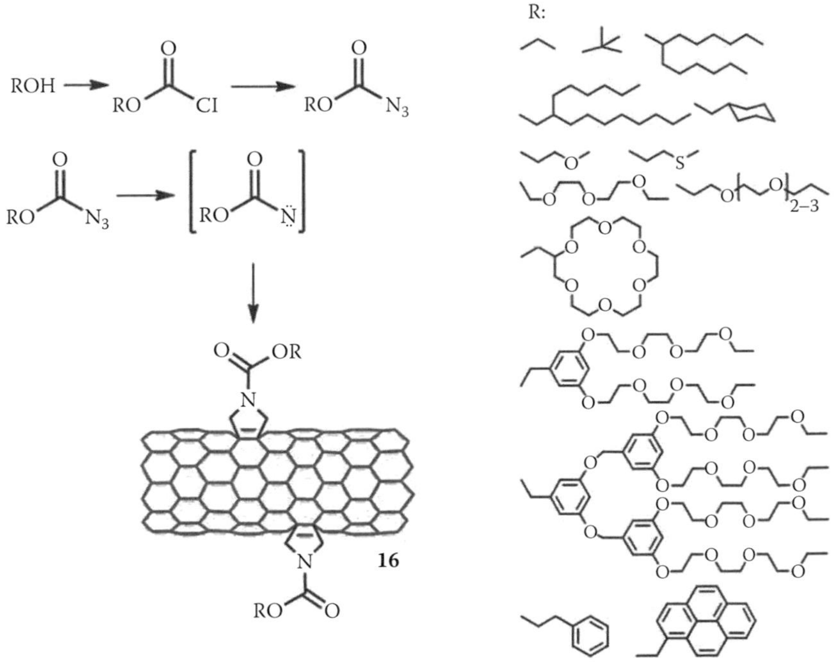

FIGURE 5.18 Sidewall functionalization of SWCNTs with nitrenes generated by thermolysis of alkyl azidoformates.

of the photoadduct is reacted with a phosphoramidite mononucleotide, and thus, a nucleotide base is introduced. The protected hydroxyl group is deprotected for reaction with the next nucleotide, and the cycle is repeated until MWNT with the desired base sequence is made. Finally, the supported nanotubes are heated in ammonia solution to remove blocking groups from the nucleotides to produce DNA-coated nanotubes. These water-soluble DNA-coated nanotubes are further hybridized with gold nanoparticles modified with complementary single-stranded DNA. The DNA-coated vertically aligned nanotubes offer the architecture for a highly loaded three-dimensional DNA chip.

5.4.2.3 Addition of Azomethine Ylides

Azomethine ylides are reactive intermediates generated *in situ* by thermal condensation of aldehydes and α-amino acids. These transient species efficiently react with the π-system of both MWNTs and SWNTs. Treatment of CNTs suspended in dimethylformamide (DMF) with an aldehyde and an N-substituted glycine derivative at 130°C results in substituted pyrrolidine moieties on the nanotube surface (**17**) (Figure 5.19). In this facile 1,3-dipolar cycloaddition reaction, a large number of pyrrolidine rings are fused to the carbon–carbon π-bonds of CNTs. Depending on R_1 and R_2, a variety of products can be synthesized. Based on this scheme, Prato et al. devised protocols for synthesis of a vast library of functional nanotubes for diverse applications leading to highly soluble functional CNT materials (**18–23**) (Figure 5.20).[97,98,105] Solubility as high as 50 mg/mL is achieved by suitably choosing the substitutent on pyrrolidone nitrogen. Solubilizing chains such as oligoethylene glycol moieties as substituents on nitrogen leads to highly water-soluble CNTs.[106]

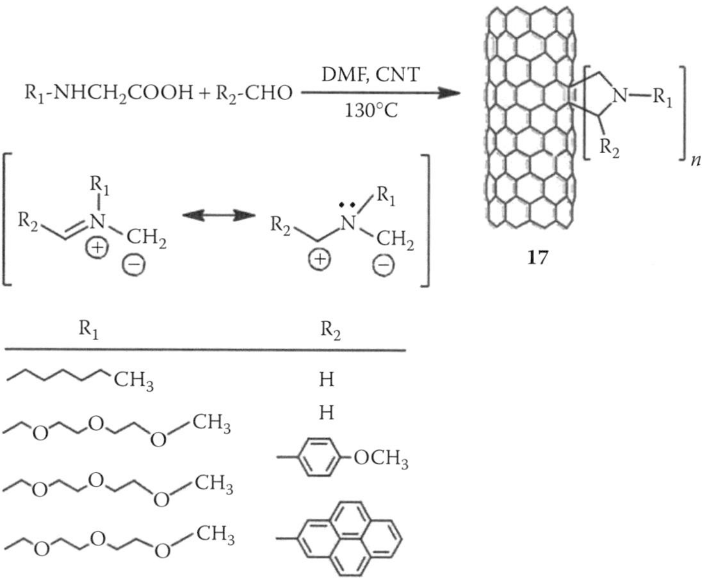

FIGURE 5.19 1,3-Dipolar cycloaddition of azomethine ylides on the CNTs affording a variety of products by varying R_1 and R_2.

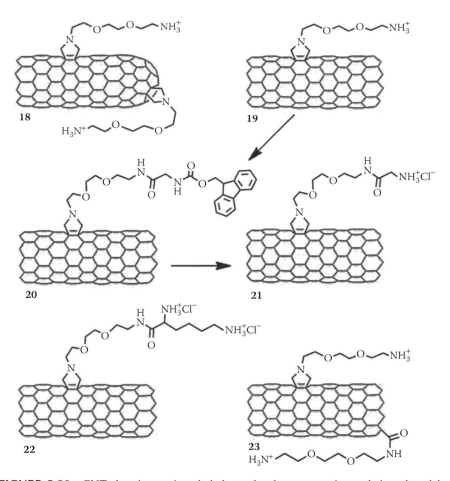

FIGURE 5.20 CNTs bearing aminotriethylene glycol as ammonium salt introduced by Prato reaction as well as reaction with the COOH groups leading to highly water-soluble precursors for synthesis of a variety of biologically relevant macromolecules.

To generate new amine functionality, initially N-functionalized glycine, bearing *tert*-butyloxycarbonyl (Boc)-protected amino end group, is used. After acid treatment, this leads to the removal of the protecting group forming the related ammonium salt **21**, which is also highly soluble in water. Similarly, for CNT derivative with N-functionalized lysine bearing Boc-protected amino group, acid treatment leads to **22**. The COOH groups of **19** are also functionalized with aminotriethylene glycol ammonium group affording **23**. Once these protocols are perfected, a number of functional moieties are appended to MWNTs and SWNTs, furnishing an exciting array of nanoconstructs that have expanded the prospects of these highly water-soluble and noncytotoxic materials as biomedicines. The ammonium moiety allows the formation of supramolecular complexes with biologically relevant macromolecules and substrates based on electrostatic interactions. Neutralized terminal amino groups give access to a wide variety of functional CNT-based nanohybrid materials utilizing the versatile chemistry of the aliphatic amine groups. In fact, a series of amino acids, fluorescent probes, and bioactive peptides and drugs have been covalently linked to the $-NH_2$ group.

5.4.3 NONCOVALENT FUNCTIONALIZATION

The surface of CNTs is polyaromatic network of hexagons, and hence can noncovalently bind other molecules through hydrophobic and π–π interactions.[107,108] Taking advantage of these interactions, pristine CNTs have been solubilized by a variety of molecules. A number of commercially available surfactants such as sodium dodecylsulfate (SDS), sodium dodecylsulfonate (SDSA), sodium dodecylbenzenesulfonate (SDBS), dodecyltrimethyl ammonium bromide (DTAB), and cetyltrimethylammonium bromide (CTAB) have been used for preparing CNT suspensions in water. PEG-based surfactants (Figure 5.21) such as Pluronic and Tween-20 are also very effective in forming stable suspensions. The surfactants having long hydrocarbon tails interact with the CNTs, whereas the hydrophilic head groups extend into water. Mixture of the nanotube with the surfactant in water is sonicated for several hours, during which the intertube hydrophobic interactions are outweighed by the CNT–surfactant interactions, resulting in debundling of the tubes. These suspensions have been used for biological experiments. In a biological environment, however, the surfactant coating is not sufficiently stable. Thus, once SWNT–Pluronic conjugates are injected intravenously, the surfactant masking the nanotube is replaced by serum proteins. This problem is particularly worse for surfactants of high critical micelle concentration (CMC). In such cases, the CNTs require an excess of surfactant molecules to form a stable suspension. If applied in biological systems, large amounts of surfactants can denature proteins and damage the cell membranes. Upon removal of the excess coating molecules, the suspension is not stable as the nanotubes again get bundled. Thus, such suspensions are not suitable in biological environments.

Polymers such as poly(vinylpyrrolidone) and poly(styrenesulfonate),[109] poly(m-phenylenevinylene),[110] and polysaccharides[111,112] interact strongly with CNTs. The polymers supramolecularly encapsulate the nanotubes (Figure 5.22)

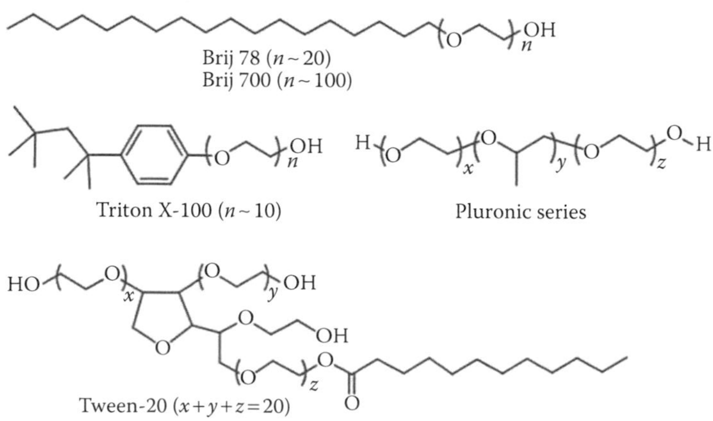

FIGURE 5.21 Some commercial surfactants used to prepare CNT suspensions in water.

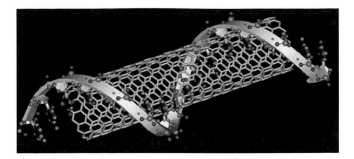

FIGURE 5.22 Schematic model of polymers wrapping up an SWNT.

so as to maximize interaction. Like polymers, many macromolecules also strongly interact with CNTs. Solubility has been achieved in varying degrees using macromolecules such as peptides,[113,114] oligonucleotides,[115,116] lipid derivatives,[117] surfactants,[118,119] and cyclodextrins.[120,121] Due to supramolecular masking, CNTs get debundled and become soluble in polar solvents.

Molecules bearing aromatic rings such as pyrene interact strongly with SWNTs. Derivatives of pyrene-bonded proteins[107] and glycodendrimers are immobilized on SWNTs.[122] Aromatic molecules such as porphyrin derivatives[123] solubilize SWNTs with the aromatic domain π–π stacked on the nanotube surface. Like pyrene, bases of DNA, being aromatic, strongly interact with the nanotube surface.[115] Single-stranded DNA molecules are demonstrated to efficiently solubilize SWNTs. However, the DNA molecules coated on SWNTs are cleaved by nucleases in the serum, suggesting that DNA functionalization of SWNTs is not stable in biological environments.[69]

Thus, an ideal noncovalently functionalized coating on CNTs for biological applications should require the coating molecule to be biocompatible, nontoxic, and sufficiently stable, and resist detachment from the nanotube surface in biological solutions, especially in serum with a high salt and protein content. The amphiphilic coating molecule should have very low CMC values. Furthermore, the coating molecule should have functional groups available for bioconjugation to create various functional CNT conjugates.

To meet the above requirements, Dai and coworkers developed a number of PEGylated phospholipids (PL-PEGs), which are used to noncovalently functionalize SWNTs (**24**) (Figure 5.23).[36] Phospholipids generally consist of hydrophobic tails and a hydrophilic head, and are a major component of cell membranes. The two hydrocarbon chains of the phospholipid strongly anchor onto the nanotube surface through hydrophobic interactions. The SWNTs with the PL-PEG are rendered water soluble as the PEG chain extends into the aqueous phase. The PEGylated SWNTs prepared by this method are highly stable in various biological solutions including serum, and even under harsh conditions without requiring the presence of excess PL-PEG, that is, they are stable without coating detachment upon heating in phosphate-buffered saline at 70°C for weeks. PL-PEGs with different PEG lengths and structures have been used to obtain specific PEGylated SWNTs for desired applications.

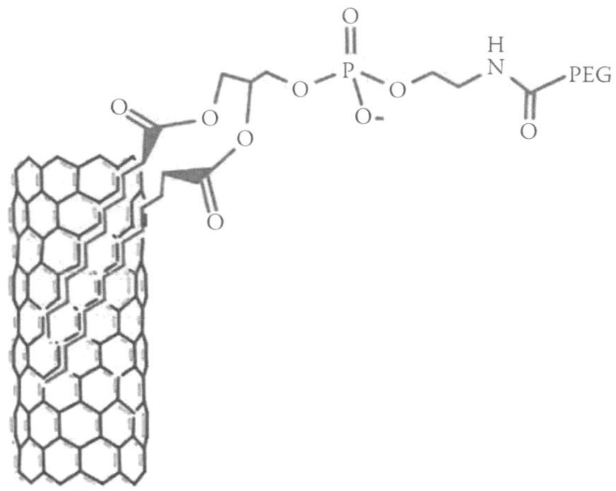

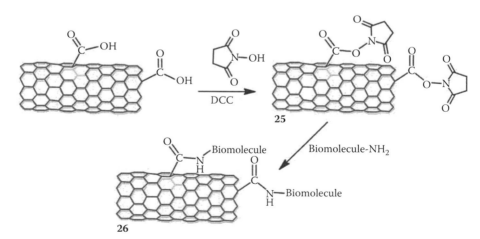

FIGURE 5.23 SWNTs noncovalently functionalized by PEGylated phospholipids.

5.4.4 N-HYDROXY SUCCINIMIDE- AND MALEIMIDE-MEDICATED FUNCTIONALIZATION

A facile approach to appending biomolecules to the carboxylic acid groups at the tube ends and defect sites of the purified CNTs is first activating the COOH groups with maleimide by treating the CNT with *N*-hydroxy succinimide (NHS) in the presence of *N,N'*-dicyclohexylcarbodiimide (DCC) as the coupling agent. The NHS-activated carboxylic acid (**25**) (Figure 5.24) is then treated with a biomolecule bearing a free and accessible −NH₂ (e.g., lysine) or thiol (e.g., cysteine) group leading to the corresponding CNT bioconjugate (**26**).

Covalent binding of biomolecules bearing the thiol group (e.g., cysteine or 5′-thiol-modified single-stranded DNA) on the sidewalls of SWNTs has been

FIGURE 5.24 Covalent binding of biomolecules bearing amine (e.g., lysine or protein having lysine) or thiol (e.g., cysteine or thiol-terminated ssDNA) with NHS-activated carboxylic acid groups of SWNTs in the tube ends or defect sites.

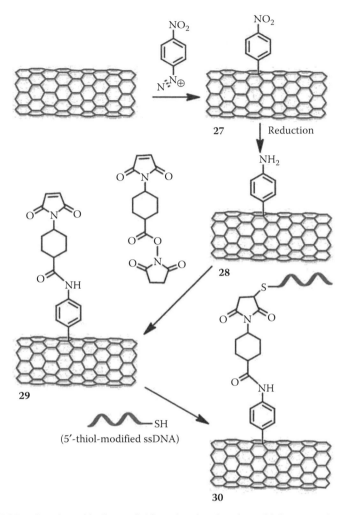

FIGURE 5.25 Covalent binding of biomolecules bearing thiol group (e.g., cysteine, peptide-SH, or 5′-thiol-modified ssDNA) on the sidewalls of SWNTs. Nitrobenzene diazonium salt reacts with SWNT sidewalls that is then reduced and reacted with a heterofunctional spacer to introduce a maleimide group that reacts with the free peptide-SH or the ssDNA-spacer-SH.

carried out on SWNTs bearing an amino group. Nitrobenzene diazonium salt reacts with the sidewalls of SWNT, reduces to an amino group (**28**), and then reacts with a heterofunctional spacer to introduce a maleimide group (**29**) (Figure 5.25). The π-bond in the maleimide group reacts readily with the thiol group of single-stranded DNA leading to the CNT–DNA conjugate (**30**).

Yet another approach is to use a pristine, purified nanotube, and attach NHS-functionalized pyrene to its walls (**31**) (Figure 5.26). The pyrene moiety is adsorbed onto the CNT wall very securely through strong π–π interaction. The NHS-activated carboxylic acid on the pyrene derivative can then be functionalized with the biomolecule such as the lysine residue of a protein leading to the CNT–protein bioconjugate (**33**).

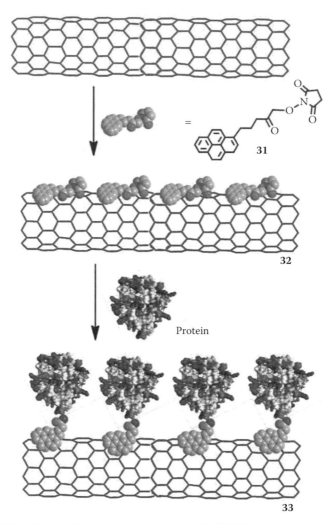

FIGURE 5.26 Noncovalent functionalization of SWNT: *N*-Hydroxy succinimide-functionalized pyrene is adsorbed onto the SWNT followed by reaction with the lysine residue of a protein.

In this approach, the electronic property of the CNT is retained. Hence, methods based on this property for detection and quantitative assessment of the nanotubes introduced into the cells *in vitro* and *in vivo* become an accurate estimate of the CNT concentration.

5.5 TOXICITY

For CNTs to be used in biomedical fields, the materials must be carefully screened by conducting toxicity tests *in vitro* and *in vivo*. CNTs have a very high surface area that enables loading large quantities of active materials for delivery into the biological environment. The CNT bioconjugate must penetrate the cell wall and enter the cytoplasm, and possibly the nucleus, to deliver the cargo load of bioactive material, which would not have been possible without the carrier CNT. There remains a genuine concern that the raw CNTs may be quite toxic, and hence probably their handling right from the production stage to the laboratory use necessitates stringent precautions. In fact, unfunctionalized raw CNTs are very light, become airborne easily, and can potentially reach the lungs. Raw CNTs are toxic to mice after inhalation into the lung. To evaluate the acute lung toxicity of intratracheally instilled SWNTs in rats, the lungs of rats were instilled with either 1 or 5 mg/kg of SWNTs.[124] Instillation in a high dose (5 mg/kg) produced mortality in ~15% of the rats within 24 h. Fortunately, it was found that the mortality results from the mechanical blockage of the airways by the SWNTs and was not due to inherent pulmonary toxicity of the instilled SWNTs. Pulmonary exposures to SWNTs produce a non-dose-dependent series of multifocal granulomas, which are evident from a foreign tissue body reaction and are nonuniform in distribution and not progressive beyond 1 month postexposure.

To evaluate occupational health hazards in chronic inhalation exposures, a study on a raw HiPco SWNT sample on mice was conducted and the results compared with carbon black and quartz.[125] The lungs of some animals 7 days after a single exposure revealed peribronchial inflammation and necrosis that persisted even after 90 days (Figure 5.27). The lungs of mice treated with carbon black were normal, whereas those treated with high-dose quartz revealed mild to moderate inflammation. On an equal-weight basis, and under identical exposure conditions, if CNTs reach the lungs, they are much more toxic than carbon black and quartz. Hence, raw CNT is considered a serious occupational health hazard in chronic inhalation exposures and should be handled with due caution.

The acid-purified SWNTs without any functionality are also quite toxic. Pharyngeal aspiration of acid-purified HiPco SWNTs elicits unusual pulmonary effects on mice.[126] Acute inflammation with early-onset yet progressive fibrosis and granulomas is observed. A dose-dependent increase in the protein, lactate dehydrogenase (LDH), and γ-glutamyl transferase activities in bronchoalveolar lavage are

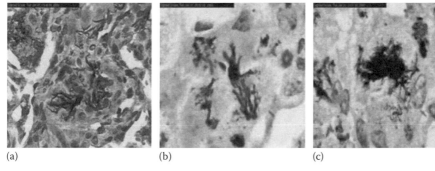

(a)   (b)   (c)

FIGURE 5.27 Lung tissues from mice instilled with 0.5 mg of SWNT per mouse showing presence of SWNT fibers 90 days after the single treatment. (a) Raw SWNT—SWNT fibers in a granuloma. (b) Purified SWNT—SWNT fibers in a granuloma. (c) Purified SWNT—clumps of SWNT fibers in a granuloma. (Reprinted with permission from Lam, C. W., et al., *Toxicol. Sci.* 77, 126–134, 2004. Copyright 2004 Society of Toxicology.)

found along with accumulation of 4-hydroxynonenal and depletion of glutathione in lungs. *In vitro* experiments to study the effects of SWNTs on cells include cytokine production, stimulation of reactive oxidant species, and particle uptake.

Purified MWNTs and ground CNTs were administered intratracheally to rats. Lung persistence, inflammation, and fibrosis were estimated biochemically and histologically.[127] The CNTs were still present in the lungs after 60 days and both induced inflammatory and fibrotic reactions. At 2 months, pulmonary lesions induced by CNTs were characterized by the formation of collagen-rich granulomas protruding in the bronchial lumen, in association with alveolitis in the surrounding tissues. Furthermore, unfunctionalized, long MWNTs may pose a carcinogenic risk in mice.[128] A comparison of the toxicity of pristine and oxidized MWNTs on human T cells[129] reveals that the latter are more toxic and induce massive loss of cell viability through programmed cell death. It should, however, be noted that no toxic effect is observed for shorter and smaller MWNTs (length: 1–20 μm, diameter: 10–14 nm), indicating that the toxicology profiles may significantly differ among CNTs of various sizes. So, properly functionalized CNTs having short dimensions (length: 50–300 nm, diameter: 1–2 nm) should be used for further evaluation of toxicity.

The initial studies on the cytotoxicity of the CNTs used pristine, nonfunctionalized CNTs, usually dispersed in an aqueous buffer with the aid of a surfactant. SWNTs suspended in various surfactants, SDS and SDBS, are toxic to 1321N1 human astrocytoma cells.[130] The toxicity is not due to SWNTs, rather due to the surfactant on the nanotube surfaces. When cells are exposed to SDS or SDBS solution having a concentration as low as 0.05 mg/mL for 30 min, this toxicity is observed. The proliferation and viability of the cells are not affected by SWNTs. The cells proliferate similarly to untreated cells when surrounded by SWNTs as they grow, which indicates that the nanotubes do not affect cells adversely.

The metal catalyst content in CNTs can also be responsible for the toxicity of CNTs,[131] and hence, the samples must be thoroughly purified. In toxicity tests, interference of CNTs with the assay reagents may lead to erroneous conclusions. Cytotoxicity of HiPco SWNTs is evaluated in the A549 human alveolar carcinoma cell line. The degree of interaction between SWNTs and the dyes used in cytotoxicity studies is assessed in order to estimate their applicability for measuring cell viability following cell exposure to the SWNT.[132] The indicator dyes used in the study are Coomassie Blue (Coomassie), Alamar Blue™ (AB), Neutral Red (NR), 3-(4,5-dimethylthiazol-2-yl)-2,5-diphenyltetrazolium bromide (MTT), and 2-(4-iodophenyl)-3-(4-nitrophenyl)-5-(2,4-disulfophenyl)-2*H*-tetrazolium (WST-1). Exposure of the cells reveals the nanotubes to have low acute toxicity; however, considerable variation is found depending on the cell viability with the dyes employed. In yet another study, A549 cells incubated with CNTs show strong cytotoxic effect, whereas the same treatment with SWNTs, but detection with WST-1, reveals no cytotoxicity.[133] The results comprehensively confirm that the dyes used in this study (Coomassie, AB, NR, MTT, and WST-1) are not appropriate for the quantitative toxicity assessment of CNTs.

The above studies suggest that CNTs indeed can be very toxic at sufficiently high concentrations and that careful toxicity studies need to be undertaken particularly when nanomedical applications of CNTs are desired. Since raw or purified unfunctionalized CNTs are potentially toxic to humans, strict industrial hygiene measures should be taken to limit exposure during their manipulation. However, properly functionalized CNTs afford stable aqueous solutions, and such samples are not cytotoxic as seen from a number of elegant studies discussed below.

5.5.1 Noncytotoxic CNT Bioconjugates

Pristine SWNTs are modified via the 1,3-dipolar cycloaddition reaction, or via the oxidation–amidation route, obtaining ammonium-functionalized CNTs (f-CNTs) (Figure 5.28).[134] The first type of nanotube (19) (see Figure 5.20) is highly soluble under physiological conditions. Oxidized nanotubes, derivatized with PEG_{1500} chains at the carboxylic functions (35), form homogeneous suspensions. Both f-CNTs 19 and 35 are further modified with fluorescein isothiocyanate (FITC) to generate fluorescent nanotubes 34 and 36, respectively, which are used for the immune cell uptake study.

The water-soluble f-CNTs, functionalized according to the 1,3-dipolar cyclo-addition, are not cytotoxic. The f-CNTs (19) cause neither cell death nor activation of lymphocytes and macrophages, and do not disturb normal cell functions. In contrast, PEG-functionalized CNT (35) suspensions activate the primary immune cells, especially on macrophages, and modify their subsequent capacity to respond to a physiological stimulus. Thus, stable aqueous solutions of f-CNTs do not exert toxic effects on immortalized cell lines from different origins, whereas SWNT suspensions are cytotoxic. The degree of functionalization density has a direct bearing on the solubility. A study demonstrates that with increasing functionalization density, the cytotoxicity of SWNTs toward human dermal fibroblasts decreases.[135] This clearly means that the SWNT surface must be completely passivated such that the integrity of the structure is retained in the biological medium.

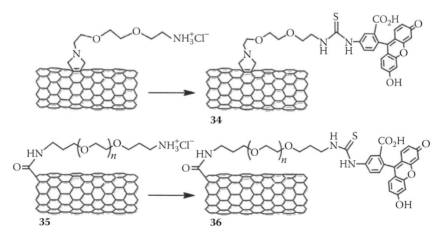

FIGURE 5.28 Ammonium-functionalized SWNTs and their respective FITC derivatives used for cell imaging and cytotoxicity study.

The highly water-soluble *f*-CNTs have been used in a number of imaging studies that reveal their noncytotoxic nature. The capacity of *f*-CNTs to penetrate transformed cell lines from different origins including 3T3 (mouse fibroblasts),[99] HeLa (human cervical carcinoma cells),[136] MCF7 (human breast cancer cells),[137] and Jurkat cells (human T-cell leukemia)[100,138] has been nicely demonstrated through imaging studies. The *f*-CNTs are also efficient in imaging the primary immune cells isolated from mouse lymphoid organs. These cells are involved in the mechanisms that allow the protection of the body against pathogens and foreign particles. Figure 5.29 shows confocal microscopy images of the localization of *f*-CNTs **34** and **36** inside the B and T lymphocytes as well as macrophages. The bundles of *f*-CNTs **36** that are located outside lymphocytes but inside the cytoplasm of macrophages affect the functioning of the immune cells and microphages. On the other hand, **34** forms a stable aqueous solution for which it does not exert toxic effects on the cell lines.

Since SWNTs functionalized with PEG attached through an amide linkage to the carboxylic acid groups at the tube ends and defect sites (SWNT-CONH-PEG) form

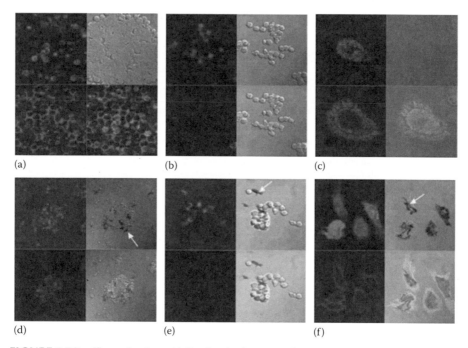

(a)   (b)   (c)

(d)   (e)   (f)

FIGURE 5.29 **(See color insert.)** Confocal microscopy images. *f*-CNTs **34** and **36** localize inside B and T lymphocytes as well as macrophages. Three major immune cell populations, that is, B lymphocytes (a and d), T lymphocytes (b and e), and macrophages (c and f), were isolated from the spleen, lymph nodes, and peritoneal cavity of mice, respectively. They were then incubated with either *f*-CNT **34** (a–c) or **36** (d–f) (green fluorescence). The white arrows indicate the bundles of *f*-CNT **36** that are located outside lymphocytes (d and e) but inside the cytoplasm of macrophages (f). (Reprinted with permission from Dumortier, H., et al., 2006, 1522–1528. Copyright 2006 American Chemical Society.)

suspension in water, and such suspension is cytotoxic as it activates the primary immune cells, a dose-dependent experiment taking the solubility limit of the SWNTs and the maximum volume that can be injected into mice without causing potential cardiovascular effects has been carried out with SWNT-PEG.[139] The results are compared with noncovalently PEGylated SWNTs mediated by phospholipid (SWNT-PL-PEG) developed by Dai and coworkers. The results reveal that both SWNT-PEG and SWNT-PL-PEG are not cytotoxic, showing near-identical behavior. Histology (Figure 5.30) and Raman microscopic mapping demonstrate that the functionalized SWNTs persist within liver and spleen macrophages for 4 months without apparent toxicity.

There are a number of CNT bioconjugates that are now proven to be noncytotoxic. In all such cases, it has been inadvertently established that the nanotubes upon functionalization are extensively debundled and become highly water soluble. Further, in the biological environment, the solubilizing moiety keeps the nanotube passivated, which, in particular, is an important issue for water-soluble bioconjugates synthesized via noncovalent interactions. For example, the glycodendrimers can function as homogeneous bioactive coatings for SWNTs through noncovalent interaction of the CNT walls with the pyrene

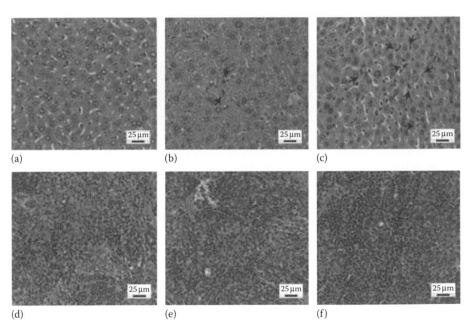

(a)   (b)   (c)

(d)   (e)   (f)

FIGURE 5.30 Liver and spleen histology. (a–f) Hematoxylin and eosin stains of liver (a–c) and spleen (d–f) tissues of mice injected with PBS (a and d), SWNT-PL-PEG (b and e), or SWNT-CONH-PEG (c and f). Finely granular pigments are seen in sinusoidal liver cells of SWNT-PL-PEG (b, arrows) and SWNT-CONH-PEG (c, arrows), as well as in spleen macrophages of SWNT-PL-PEG and SWNT-CONH-PEG (e and f) without signs of cellular or tissue damage. (Reprinted by permission from Macmillan Publishers Ltd. [*Nature Nanotechnology*] Schipper, M. L., et al., *Nat. Nanotechnol.* 3, 216–221, 2008, copyright 2008.)

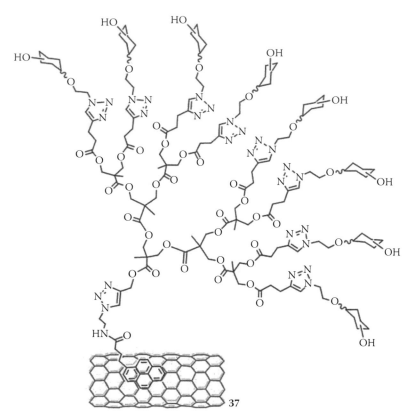

FIGURE 5.31 Glycodendrimers generation 3 (G-3) used for functionalization of SWNTs via noncovalent interaction with pyrene moiety.

moiety (**37**) (Figure 5.31).[122] The glycodendrimer-coated SWNTs are co-cultured with HEK293 cells for 4 days. In control experiments, the cells are incubated with unmodified SWNTs or with media alone. Cells cultured with glycodendrimer-coated SWNTs proliferate at the same rate as cells grown in the absence of SWNTs. By contrast, unmodified SWNTs greatly hamper the growth of HEK293 cells.

Purified CNTs without proper functionalization have a highly hydrophobic surface and tend to remain as aggregate in the cell culture. The free hydrophobic surface facilitates the interaction with cells by binding to various biomolecules, including proteins, and induces cell toxicity. Other factors that make SWNTs cytotoxic are the presence of metal catalysts as impurities even after following standard purification protocols and the toxicity induced by the solubilizing component, particularly when it is attached to the nanotube surface through noncovalent interaction. Thus, surfactants used as solubilizing agents when present in large excess in the suspension can be cytotoxic. Toxicity evaluation is also dose dependent, and hence, the concentration of the CNTs *in vitro* and *in vivo* is to be carefully determined before any conclusion is drawn on the toxicity of the material. Furthermore, SWNT constructs may prove to be noncytotoxic within the time duration set for the study, but may show acute toxicity in the long term. In toxicity tests, proper assay reagents must be employed to avoid interference with the CNTs. In many studies, intensity of fluorescence emission is a method of choice for evaluation of CNT toxicity. In the fluorescence method, dyes such as Coomassie, AB, NR, MTT, and WST-1 are used as a reporter of cell viability. It is shown that these dyes can bind to CNTs, quenching their fluorescence, thereby introducing uncertainty in assessment of toxicity.[133] There are many careful studies undertaken in exploring these aspects and there are roughly as many publications reporting no apparent cytotoxicity, as there are reports of varying degrees of significant cytotoxicity. Early reports raising the alarm of toxicity in model cell culture systems have not been adequately verified. However, recently a number of highly water-soluble CNTs have been successfully tried for cell imaging and targeted drug delivery, and as anticancer agents; careful pharmacokinetic studies indicate that these sophisticated nanoconstructs are not toxic at least for the duration of their monitoring *in vitro* and *in vivo*. Nevertheless, the question of whether CNTs have long-term toxicity in biomedical applications requires further research.

5.6 CELL IMAGING

Cell imaging studies provide critical insight into the nature of cellular and tissue function. They are an analytical tool in diverse biomedical research disciplines such as cell biology, developmental biology, neurobiology, pharmacology, and other related fields. Rapid advances in live cell imaging currently being witnessed using fluorescent protein and synthetic fluorophore techniques are further expanded using CNT derivatives.

5.6.1 Cell Imaging Using Intrinsic NIR Fluorescence of CNTs

SWNTs covalently linked to visible-wavelength fluorophores, such as functional nanoparticles, have been used in cell imaging studies.[99,138] In this approach, however, the chemical linkage of the fluorophore must resist enzymatic cleavage in the biological fluid. Emission from the visible-wavelength fluorophore must be detected above the background fluorescence. Besides, chemical processing of nanoparticles may dramatically change their biological fate. To circumvent this limitation, a method for observing pristine, hydrophobic SWNTs in biological media relies on their intrinsic NIR fluorescence.[140,141] The debundled SWNTs show fluorescence emission in the range 1125–1600 nm upon excitation at 660 nm. Peritoneal macrophage-like cells of cultured mouse are incubated for varying periods in a growth medium containing various concentrations of SWNTs in Pluronic surfactant. The cells actively ingest SWNTs without showing toxic effects. Cell cultures with added surfactant or added surfactant plus SWNTs show equivalent population growth and normal adhesion, morphology, and confluence. The ingested nanotubes remain fluorescent, showing emission in the range 1125–1400 nm (Figure 5.32). The cells also can be imaged through NIR fluorescence microscopy at wavelengths beyond 1100 nm. High-contrast imaging is aided by very low levels of endogenous

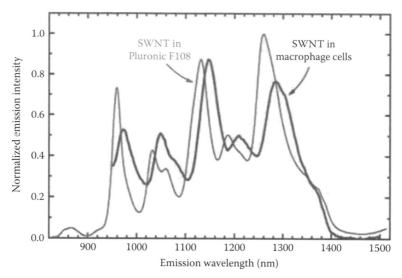

FIGURE 5.32 NIR emission spectra of SWNT in an aqueous Pluronic F108 suspension, and in macrophage cells incubated in SWNT suspension and then washed. Samples are excited at 660 nm. The emission beyond 1350 nm is strongly attenuated by H_2O absorption. (Reprinted with permission from Cherukuri, P., et al., 2004, 15638–15639. Copyright 2004 American Chemical Society.)

fluorescence. Imaging selective SWNT–antibody binding to cells is achieved by detecting the intrinsic NIR photoluminescence of HiPco SWNTs functionalized with PL-PEG-NH$_2$. Cell imaging by using this biologically inert SWNT-PL-PEG conjugated with antibodies such as Rituxan selectively recognizes the CD20 cell surface receptor on B cells.[142]

5.6.2 Cell Imaging by FITC Fluorescent Probe on CNTs

FITC has been traditionally known as a fluorescent probe in cell imaging studies. The aminotriethylene glycol chains of *f*-CNTs are modified with FITC for both MWNTs and SWNTs (Figure 5.33), which are found to be excellent candidates for the cell imaging studies.[134] FITC is also attached to the COOH groups (**39**) in which some of the amino groups of aminotriethylene glycol are left unlabeled to improve aqueous solubility. It is observed that the FITC-functionalized CNTs are more toxic than those with free amino groups. The *f*-CNTs bearing FITC (**38**) penetrate the cell membrane and are mainly distributed into the cytoplasm but slowly move toward the nucleus. In order that the SWNT derivative rapidly gets introduced to the cell nucleus, it is attached to FITC via a peptide linker (**40**). This peptide belongs to the α-subunit of G$_s$ protein corresponding to the sequence 384–394. Cellular uptake of the G$_s$ protein is extremely poor. The C-terminus of this protein is modified with cysteine for conjugation to the nanotubes, and lysine in the N-terminus binds FITC. The peptide mimics the G$_s$ protein; when incubated with HeLa cells, it is rapidly translocated into the cell nucleus.

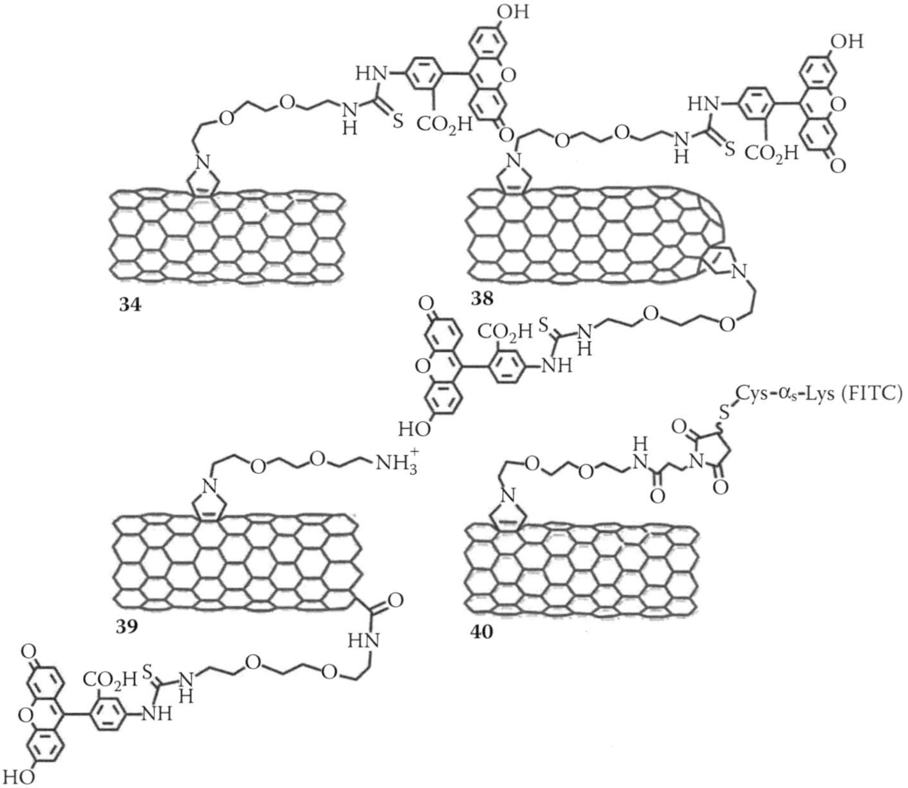

FIGURE 5.33 The aminotriethylene glycol chains of f-CNTs modified with fluorescent probes with FITC. In **40**, α_s represents α-subunit of G_s protein corresponding to the sequence 384–394 modified with cysteine at the C-terminus and lysine at the N-terminus.

5.6.3 Cell Imaging by Cyanine Dye as Probe on CNTs

SWNT suspension obtained by noncovalent interaction with cyanine dye–single-stranded DNA (SWNT–Cy3–ssDNA) conjugate incubated with HeLa cells in a fetal bovine serum (FBS) medium shows high fluorescence intensity from the cells, indicative of the high-level inclusion of SWNT–Cy3–ssDNA. However, the fluorescence intensity is remarkably reduced if SWNT–Cy3–ssDNA is incubated with cells in the FBS-free medium. Systematic control experiments reveal that Cy3 dye molecules are released from SWNT–Cy3–ssDNA conjugates by nuclease, and the free Cy3 dyes penetrate into HeLa cells with high efficiency.[143] The actual amounts of SWNTs internalized in the cells are almost identical for both cells incubated in the FBS-present and FBS-absent media according to the Raman studies. However, the degree of SWNT internalization based on the fluorescence intensities, especially when the coloring dye molecules are linked to oligonucleotides in nuclease-containing media, should be determined with caution. It is possible that the fluorescence intensity from cells does not necessarily reflect the actual amount of SWNTs internalized in the cells. Instead, it is more likely to indicate the amount of free Cy3 dye that is released from SWNT–Cy3–ssDNA.

Hence, an appropriate selection of the cell culture and incubation environment is necessary for systematic studies of the inclusion of nanomaterials including SWNTs in cells, especially when they are passivated with oligonucleotides.

5.6.4 PHOTOACOUSTIC IMAGING

Photoacoustic imaging is a biomedical imaging technique based on the photoacoustic effect, in which biological tissues are exposed to nonionizing radiofrequency laser pulses. The portion of the energy absorbed is converted into heat leading to emission of ultrasonic waves, which is detected by ultrasonic transducers to form 2D or 3D images. Compared with most optical imaging techniques, photoacoustic imaging of living subjects offers higher spatial resolution and allows deeper tissues to be imaged.[144–147] Many diseases do not exhibit a natural photoacoustic contrast, especially in their early stages. It is necessary to administer a photoacoustic contrast agent for cell imaging. A number of contrast agents for photoacoustic imaging are known,[148–150] but most are not shown to target a disease site in living subjects. The noncovalently functionalized SWNTs via phospholipids and PEG_{5000}, $SWNT-PL-PEG_{5000}$ (plain SWNT), are conjugated with cyclic Arg-Gly-Asp (RGD) peptides and the $SWNT-PL-PEG_{5000}-RGD$ (SWNT-RGD) is used as a contrast agent for photoacoustic imaging of tumors (Figure 5.34).[151] RGD allows SWNTs to bind to tumor cells. Intravenous administration of these targeted nanotubes to mice bearing tumors shows eight times greater photoacoustic signal in the tumor than mice injected with nontargeted nanotubes. The signal produced by SWNT-RGD is observed to be linearly dependent on its concentration. The spectral overlap between plain SWNT and SWNT-RGD suggests that the RGD conjugation does not perturb the photoacoustic signal. The photoacoustic image (green) is overlaid on the corresponding slice in the ultrasound image (gray). The skin is visible in the ultrasound images, and the photoacoustic images show the SWNTs.

5.6.5 MECHANISM OF CNT INTERNALIZATION

Before proceeding further, it is important to understand the mechanistic pathway the CNT bioconjugates follow for cell internalization so that ideal conditions can be set for it. The purified and oxidized nanotubes contain negatively charged carboxylates along the sidewalls and tube ends. Covalent or noncovalent functionalization of the purified CNTs still leaves unoxidized areas in the nanotubes, which are regions of appreciable hydrophobicity. When the nanotube bioconjugates are incubated with the cells, there can be nonspecific interaction with the hydrophobic regions of the cell surface. For internalization of the CNT bioconjugates, the mechanism of uptake is suggested to be via insertion and diffusion through the lipid bilayer of cell membrane.[137,152] The CNTs function as nanoneedles that inject the biomaterial through the cell membranes.[35,136,153] MWNTs functionalized by 1,3-dipolar cycloaddition reaction (**38**) (see Figure 5.33) show the CNTs crossing the cell membranes as nanoneedles (Figure 5.35).

In several other works discussed below, an endocytosis mechanism is proposed.[141,154–156] In studies on delivery of protein and DNA,[157,158] it is observed that

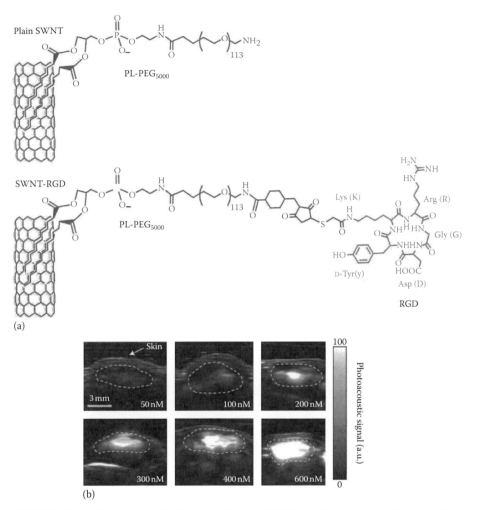

FIGURE 5.34 Noncovalently functionalized SWNTs and characterization of their photoacoustic properties. (a) Structures of plain SWNTs and SWNT–RGD. (b) The photoacoustic image is overlaid on the corresponding slice in the ultrasound image. (Reprinted by permission from Macmillan Publishers Ltd. Zerda, A., et al., *Nat. Nanotechnol.* 3, 557–562, 2008, copyright 2008.)

fluorescently labeled CNTs readily enter cells after incubation for 1 h at 37°C, but only very weak green fluorescence is detected after incubation for 1 h at 4°C, confirming that the uptake mechanism is energy-dependent endocytosis.

5.7 PHARMACOKINETICS

The long-term fate of CNTs *in vivo* when intravenously injected into animals is an issue critical to potential clinical applications of these materials. CNTs can readily redistribute from their site of deposition, enter the respiratory tract,

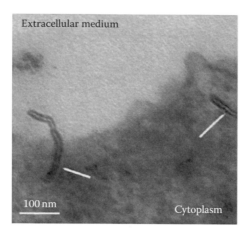

FIGURE 5.35 Ultrathin transverse section of a HeLa cell treated with ammonium-functionalized CNT **38** (see Figure 5.33). Carbon nanotubes are crossing the cell membrane or visible in the cytoplasm (white arrows). (Reprinted with permission from Prato, M., et al., 2008, 60–68. Copyright 2008 American Chemical Society.)

deposit in the lung tissue, escape from the normal phagocytic defenses, modify the structure of proteins, and activate inflammatory and immunological responses, affecting normal organ function. Hence, the pharmacological profiles of administered CNTs must be determined *in vivo* and the safety of their formulation unequivocally ensured. Pristine SWNTs are highly hydrophobic and are thus retained in biological systems indefinitely. Studies on biodistribution of intravenously injected pristine ^{13}C-enriched SWNTs in mice show that nanotubes are retained in the lung as well as the reticuloendothelial system (RES) in high concentrations for a long time (Figure 5.36).[159] It is highly desirable that the CNTs are effectively debundled to individual tubes and the hydrophobicity of SWNTs is reduced significantly or eliminated entirely by suitable functionalization for use *in vivo*.

Pluronic F108, a nonionic poloxamer surfactant physisorbed on raw HiPco SWNTs, leads to the debundling of the nanotubes furnishing individual tubes. The SWNT–Pluronic F108 is intravenously administered to rabbits and the nanotube concentration is monitored through their characteristic NIR fluorescence.[160] *In vitro* experiments show that blood proteins displace the nanotube coating of synthetic surfactant molecules within seconds. The nanotube concentration in the blood serum decreases exponentially with a half-life of 1.0 ± 0.1 h (Figure 5.37). At 24 h after intravenous administration, significant concentrations of nanotubes are found only in the liver.

Functionalization of biomolecules relying on noncovalent interaction should be such that the structural features of the SWNT bioconjugate are retained in the systemic circulation. Chemical functionalization of SWNTs with biocompatible PEG coatings makes the biologically inert SWNTs hydrophilic. Circulation and long-term fate of highly water-soluble SWNTs obtained by

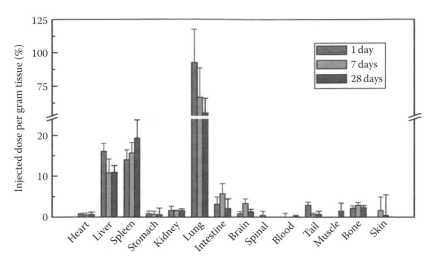

FIGURE 5.36 The biodistribution of pristine SWNTs (^{13}C-SWNTs) in mice at different time points postexposure. (Reprinted with permission from Yang, S. T., et al., 2007, 17761–17764. Copyright 2007 American Chemical Society.)

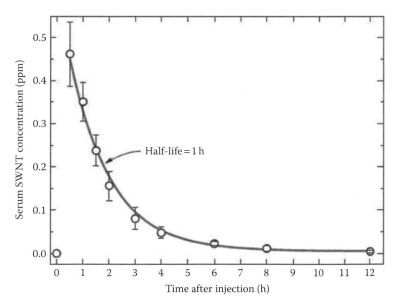

FIGURE 5.37 Time dependence of blood serum SWNT concentration after injection monitored through their characteristic NIR fluorescence, as measured for rabbits showing a half-life of 1 h. (Reprinted with permission from Cherukuri, P., et al., 2006. Mammalian pharmacokinetics of carbon nanotubes using intrinsic near-infrared fluorescence. *Proc. Natl. Acad. Sci. USA* 103:18882–18886. Copyright 2006 National Academy of Sciences, U.S.A.)

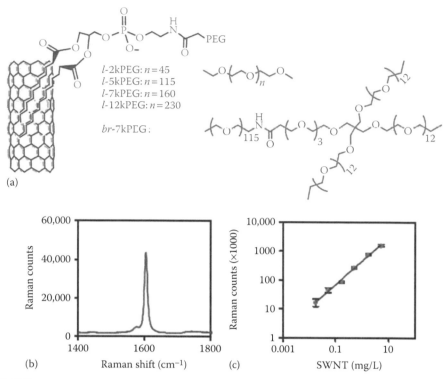

FIGURE 5.38 Noncovalently functionalized SWNTs by various PEGylated phospholipids. (a, left) Scheme of functionalization by various PL-PEGs with linear or branched PEG chains. (Right) A photo of the SWNT-*br*-7kPEG saline solution used for injection. (b) Raman spectrum of a solution of SWNT-*l*-2kPEG. The G band peak at 1590 cm⁻¹ is used for SWNT detection. (c) Raman intensity vs. SWNT concentration calibration curve. (Reprinted with permission from Liu, Z., et al., 2008. Circulation and long-term fate of functionalized, biocompatible single-walled carbon nanotubes in mice probed by Raman spectroscopy. *Proc. Natl. Acad. Sci. USA* 105:1410–1415. Copyright 2008 National Academy of Sciences, U.S.A.)

noncovalent interaction with various PL-PEG in mice are probed by Raman spectroscopy (Figure 5.38).[161]

The G-band peak at 1590 cm⁻¹ is used for SWNT detection and concentration calibration. When administered *in vivo*, these SWNT-PEGs show long blood circulation, low RES uptake, and relatively fast clearance from organs and excretion from the body. SWNTs with both linear (SWNT-*l*-2kPEG, SWNT-*l*-5kPEG, SWNT-*l*-7kPEG, SWNT-*l*-12kPEG) and branched (SWNT-*br*-7kPEG) PEGs are administered *in vivo* and the results show that SWNT-*br*-7kPEG with the branched chain PEG is most effective. SWNT-*l*-5kPEG, SWNT-*l*-7kPEG, and SWNT-*l*-12kPEG show similar blood circulation time, significantly longer than that of SWNT-*l*-2kPEG. The longest blood circulation of ~24 h is observed for SWNT-*br*-7kPEG. SWNTs are detected in various organs and tissues of mice *ex vivo* over a period of 3 months. The SWNT-PEG conjugates are retained in the blood circulation up to 1 day, shown by the relatively low uptake in the RES and near-complete clearance from the main organs in ~2 months. Raman spectroscopy is used to detect SWNTs in the intestine, feces, kidney, and bladder of mice. The results suggest excretion and clearance of SWNTs from mice via the biliary and renal pathways. No toxic side effects of SWNTs in mice are observed in necropsy, histology, and blood chemistry measurements. SWNT-PL-PEGs obtained via noncovalent interaction are known to escape the capture of RES for a blood circulation half-life of up to 2 h.[162] Covalent function-alization of ^{13}C-enriched SWNTs with the diamine-terminated PEG oligomers (PEG$_{1500N}$)[81,163,164] furnishes individual tubes.[134] The SWNT-PL-PEG$_{1500N}$ has a pro-longed blood circulation time and low hepatic uptake[165] compared to SWNTs func-tionalized by other PEGylation techniques making them ideal stealth nanotubes.

Covalently functionalized SWNTs through 1,3-dipolar cycloaddition reaction and bearing radiotracers are intravenously administered and their tissue biodistribution and blood clearance rates are studied (Figure 5.39).[166] These highly water-soluble SWNTs are functionalized with the chelating molecule diethylenetriaminepenta-acetic (DTPA) dianhydride leading to **41** that is labeled with radioactive indium (^{111}In) furnishing **42** (and **43**) for monitoring the concentration of the CNT conju-gate in various organs. Intravenous administration of these functionalized SWNTs (*f*-SWNTs) followed by radioactivity tracing indicates that *f*-CNTs are not retained

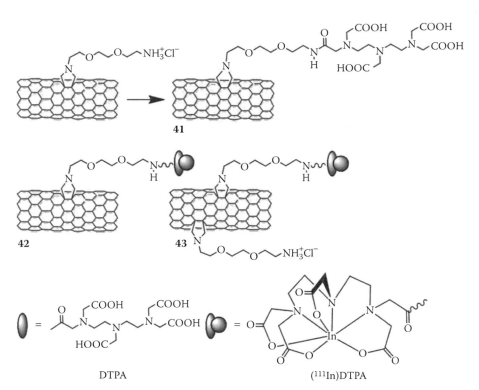

FIGURE 5.39 Synthesis of ^{111}In-labeled SWNT through chelating DTPA using ^{111}InCl$_3$. Compound **42** is completely saturated with DTPA. Compound **43** presents only 60% of DTPA functionalization and 40% of free amine groups.

in any of the RES organs (liver or spleen) and are rapidly cleared from systemic blood circulation (half-life 3 h) through the renal excretion route. The observed rapid blood clearance of *f*-SWNTs has major implications for all potential clinical uses of CNT. Moreover, urine excretion studies using both *f*-SWNTs and functionalized MWNTs followed by electron microscopy analysis of urine samples reveal that both types of nanotubes are excreted as intact nanotubes. Intravenously administered MWNTs functionalized with DTPA (DTPA-MWNTs) and radio-labeled with ^{111}In are dynamically tracked *in vivo* using a micro-single photon emission tomography (microSPECT) scanner.[167] Imaging showed that nanotubes enter the systemic blood circulation and within 5 min begin to permeate through the renal glomerular filtration system into the bladder. Urinary excretion of DTPA-MWNTs is confirmed at 24 h postadministration.

The functionalized MWNTs are labeled with ^{125}I and the biodistribution study *in vivo* shows that radio iodine is very effective in tracing the nanotubes. 2-Aminoethanesulfonic acid (taurine), a biological molecule, is used to covalently functionalize MWNTs (tau-MWNTs). MWNTs are also noncovalently wrapped by Tween-80 (Tween-MWNTs). These are labeled with ^{125}I, and their distributions in mice are then determined.[168] As expected, Tween-80 reduces the RES uptake of MWNTs remarkably. In contrast to tau-MWNTs, Tween-MWNTs distribute not only into the liver, spleen, and lung, but also into other organs such as the stomach, kidney, large intestine, and small intestine. After 30 min postdosing, the lung uptake of Tween-MWNTs declines remarkably.

Pharmacokinetic and biodistribution studies involve *in vivo* monitoring of the SWNTs by NIR measurement or by radiochemical assay. NIR measurement is noninvasive and measures the concentration of SWNTs. However, measurement of SWNT concentration using the characteristic NIR requires that the nanotubes should be debundled and individualized. PEGylation via nonconvalent interaction of phospholipids with SWNTs appears to afford individual tubes completely wrapped up by PEG. Also PEGs appended covalently to SWNTs act as a very effective sheath for which they are retained in the biological fluid for a long duration. Individual, highly water-soluble nanotubes, synthesized by 1,3-dipolar cycloaddition, are also very safe as they are almost entirely devoid of any toxicity. PEGylated SWNTs obtained through the covalent functionalization route have long blood circulation time several orders higher than noncovalently functionalized nanotubes. While long blood circulation time facilitates better chance of the nanotubes getting retained in the tumor cells, shorter blood circulation time means lower long-term toxicity. The use of radioisotopes in tracing studies also has benefits as well as limitations. While the Raman measurement requires that the nanotubes must remain individualized during their lifetime in systemic circulation, the radio tracing method is not affected by this issue. However, the isotopes, such as ^{111}In, require special chelating agents, and ^{111}In, ^{125}I, ^{59}Cu, ^{14}C, and ^{13}C vary in their respective half-lives, leading to issues relating to their long-term effect *in vivo* and their safe environment disposal. ^{13}C-enriched SWNTs in many ways appear to be promising as their detection by mass spectrometry is less cumbersome and equally reliable. Besides, the original nature of SWNTs remains intact, which makes them suitable for long-term tracing owing to their high stability *in vivo*.

5.8 PROTEIN AND ANTIGEN TRANSFECTION

Peptide and protein transfection is a growing area of research as it relates to current and emerging routes for delivery of therapeutics. A number of different macromolecules, fluorescently labeled antibodies, and enzymes, as well as other low and high molecular weight species, are delivered by this technique. The CNT–protein conjugates are remarkably effective for delivering a number of these bioactive materials into the cytoplasm of the cell.

5.8.1 DELIVERY OF PROTEINS NONSPECIFICALLY BOUND TO CNTS

The purified and oxidized nanotubes have unoxidized areas that are regions of appreciable hydrophobicity. A general phenomenon of protein nonspecifically binding to as-grown and acid-oxidized SWNTs is attributed to interactions between the proteins and the hydrophobic regions of the nanotubes,[169–172] a finding exploited for the application of SWNTs in protein sensing. A number of proteins exhibit nonspecific binding (NSB) interacting noncovalently with the nanotube sidewalls.[173] The proteins investigated include streptavidin (SA), protein A (SpA), bovine serum albumin (BSA), and cytochrome c (cyt-c) as well as adherent and nonadherent mammalian cell lines, including HeLa, NIH-3T3 fibroblast, HL60, and Jurkat cells. Simple mixing of oxidized SWNTs with protein solutions leads to NSB of proteins to the nanotubes (Figure 5.40).

The loading appears to be the highest for cyt-c. Cyt-c has an isoelectric point p$I \approx 9.2$ that facilitates attractive electrostatic interactions with the oxidized SWNTs. Proteins with p$I < 7$ such as SA and BSA also exhibit affinity for

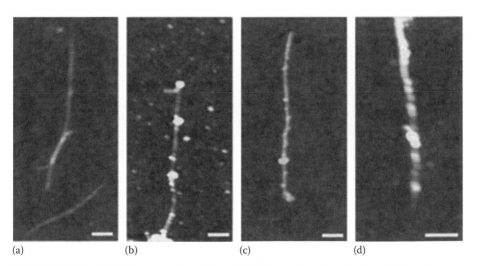

(a)   (b)   (c)   (d)

FIGURE 5.40 AFM images of various SWNT samples deposited on SiO_2 substrate. (a) Oxidized SWNT prior to conjugation with proteins and after conjugation to BSA (b), spA (c), and cyt-c (d). The loading appears to be the highest for cyt-c. Scale bar = 100 nm. (Reprinted with permission from Kam, N. W. S.; Dai, H., 2005, 6021–6026. Copyright 2005 American Chemical Society.)

oxidized SWNT sidewalls. This is attributed to the binding to either electrostatic forces between carboxylate groups on SWNTs and positively charged domains on proteins or hydrophobic interactions. To investigate the fate of the protein–SWNT conjugates *in vitro*, proteins fluorescently labeled by FITC are conjugated to SWNTs and treated with the cells. It is observed that while proteins in solutions are unable to traverse across cell membranes by themselves, SWNTs are effective in transporting protein cargos inside cells. Once released from the endosomes, the internalized protein–nanotube conjugates enter the cytoplasm of cells and perform biological functions, evidenced by apoptosis induction by transported cyt-*c*. The observed internalization of the noncovalently bound proteins via oxidized SWNT transporters is the endocytosis pathway, which is a well-known mechanism for a wide range of species traversing cell membranes, including large liposomes and nanoparticles, and is an energy-dependent internalization mechanism hindered at low temperatures.[154–156] Indeed, by incubating cells in protein–SWNT conjugates at 4°C, little uptake of the conjugates is observed (Figure 5.41), suggesting the endocytosis mechanism for the cellular uptake of protein–nanotube conjugates.

5.8.2   INTERNALIZATION BASED ON SA–BIOTIN RECOGNITION

Cell internalization of SWNTs functionalized with biotin is facilitated when conjugated with SA. Biotin is composed of a tetrahydroimidizalone ring fused with a tetrahydrothiophene ring. A valeric acid substituent is attached to one of the carbon atoms of the tetrahydrothiophene ring. SA, a protein (MW ~ 60 kDa), in the form of a tetramer has an extraordinarily high affinity for biotin. The attachment of biotin to various chemical sites, biotinylation, is used as an important laboratory technique

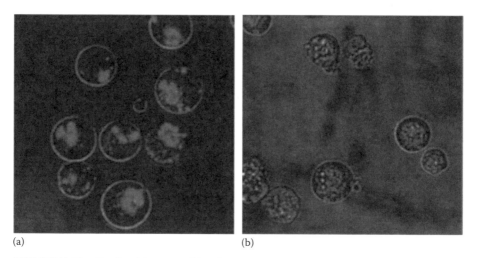

(a)   (b)

FIGURE 5.41   Confocal images of HL60 cells after incubation in cyt-*c*-SWNTs for 2 h at 37°C (a) and 4°C (b). (Reprinted with permission from Kam, N. W. S.; Dai, H., 2005, 6021–6026. Copyright 2005 American Chemical Society.)

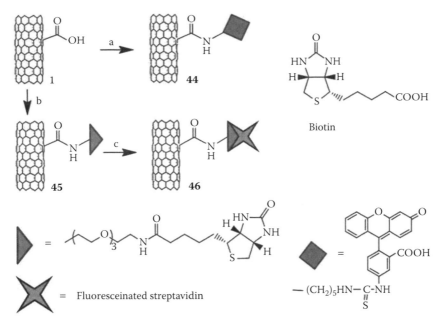

FIGURE 5.42 Synthesis and schematic of various SWNT conjugates. (a) EDC, 5-(5-amino-pentyl)thioureidyl fluorescein, phosphate buffer saline; (b) EDC, biotin-LC-PEO-amine, phosphate buffer; (c) fluoresceinated streptavidin.

to study various processes, including protein localization, protein interactions, DNA transcription, and replication. The reaction of an aqueous suspension of purified, shortened nanotubes (**1** in Figure 5.12) with 1-ethyl-3-(3-dimethylamino-propyl)carbodiimide) (EDC) and 5-(5-aminopentyl)thioureidyl fluorescein affords fluorescein-functionalized SWNTs, **44** (Figure 5.42).[174] When human promyelocytic leukemia (HL60) cells are incubated with **44**, appreciable fluorescence on the surface and in the cell interior (Figure 5.2a) confirms that the fluorescently labeled SWNTs can enter the cells. Treatment of **1** with EDC and biotinyl-3,6,9-trioxaun-decanediamine (biotin-LC-PEO-amine) furnishes biotin-functionalized SWNTs **45**. This is reacted with fluoresceinated SA to afford SWNT–biotin–SA conjugate **46**. Incubation of HL60 cells with **46** shows intense fluorescence inside the cells. The mechanism of internalization is proved to be endocytosis as incubation carried out at 4°C showed little cell fluorescence compared to incubation at 37°C.

The functionalized SWNTs **1**, **44**, and **45** show no appreciable toxicity toward HL60 cells. On the other hand, the SWNT–biotin–SA conjugate **46** causes extensive cell death ~12 h after the incubation of HL60 cells. When the amount of SA on the SWNT is reduced from 2.5 to <1.25 µM, the observed toxicity is nearly nonexistent. Fluoresceinated SA by itself cannot enter cells. Hence, no toxicity is observed after cells are incubated even in highly concentrated solutions of SA. It readily enters cells when complexed to an SWNT–biotin transporter and its cytotoxicity is dose dependent.

5.8.3 DELIVERY OF ANTIGENS

As CNTs are very effective in delivering proteins to cells synthetic peptides are linked to CNTs to study their antigenic and immunogenic properties. As a model antigen, a B-cell epitope from foot-and-mouth disease (FMDV) is chosen. This peptide corresponds to the sequence 141–159 of the VP1 protein of the FMDV virus. The peptide is linked to *f*-CNTs either as a monoconjugate (**47**) or a bisconjugate (**48**) (Figure 5.43).[175]

In the first case, *f*-CNT with the amino function is derivatized with a maleimido group using *N*-succinimidyl-3-maleimidopropionate. The FMDV peptide is linked to the product by reaction of cysteine with the maleimide moiety. The bisconjugate is obtained by first derivatizing it with lysine, which is subsequently modified with maleimido groups. The FMDV peptide is then linked to the maleimide moieties via reaction with cysteine of the peptide. The CNT–FMDV peptide conjugates thus mimic as though they are FMDV virus. Once interacted into the cell, the

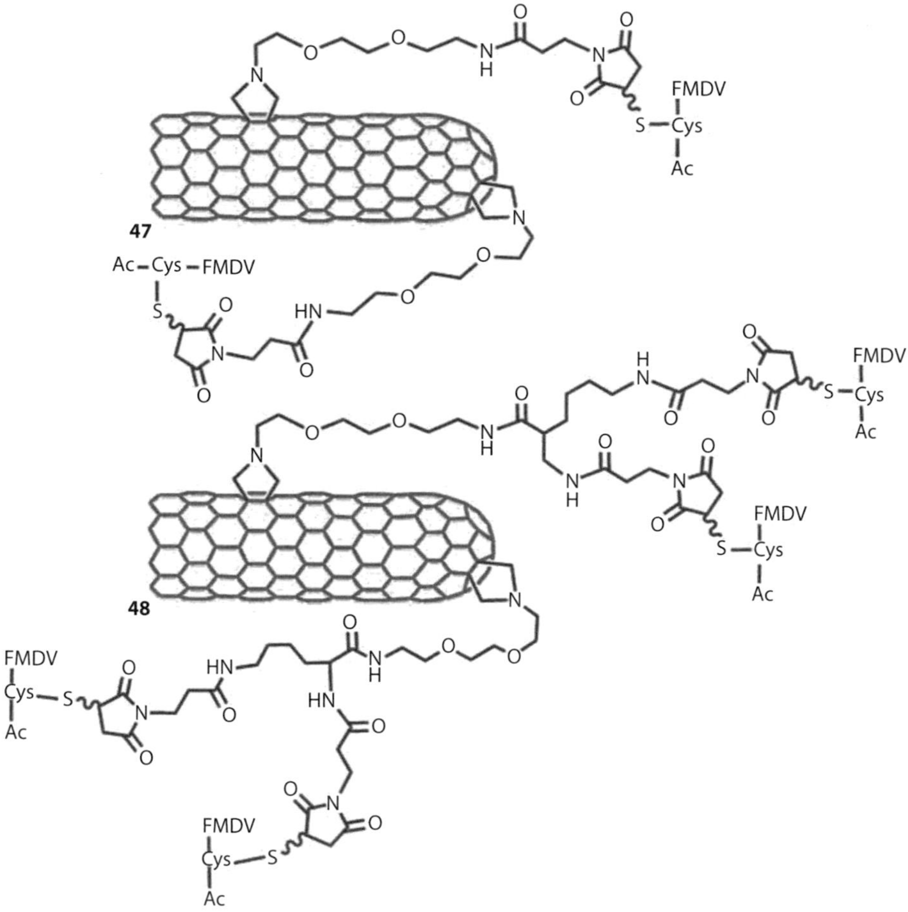

FIGURE 5.43   MWNT-FMDV peptide conjugates for antigenic and immunogenic properties.

latter should show immunogenic response. When cells come in contact with foreign bodies such as viruses, bacteria, and fungi, the B cells produce immunoglobulin, a Y-shaped protein, which is called the antibody. It recognizes a unique part of the invading foreign body mimicking the lock-and-key principle, and this part of the foreign target is called the antigen. Each tip of the antibody is the lock, called paratope, which is specific for one particular key, called epitope, on the antigen. Here, the CNT–FMDV peptide conjugate is the antigen and its antigenicity, the capacity to be recognized by an antibody, is evaluated using the enzyme-linked immunosorbent assay (ELISA) test with specific monoclonal and polyclonal antibodies. The CNT–FMDV peptide conjugates are recognized by the antibodies, whereas in control experiments, the f-CNTs without the FMDV peptide are recognized. The immunogenicity of the CNT–FMDV peptide conjugates is also evaluated. The anti-FMDV peptide antibody response is clearly enhanced in mice immunized with the CNT–FMDV peptide conjugates.

5.9   DELIVERY OF NUCLEIC ACIDS

Introduction of a DNA molecule into a host cell nucleus is an advanced field of genetic engineering. Of specific importance is the introduction of a plasmid into a nucleus. A plasmid is a DNA molecule separated from the chromosomal DNA. It has the unique capability of replicating autonomously within a suitable host. When integrated into a host gene, it can make many copies of that particular gene, a process called gene expression. A number of applications are possible through plasmid vectors. For example, it is possible to genetically engineer embryonic stem cells. Therapeutic genes can be inserted at the appropriate chromosomal target sites, a process well known as gene therapy.

Transfection is the process of deliberately introducing nucleic acids into cells. Genetic material, such as supercoiled plasmid DNA or small interfering RNA (siRNA), may be transfected. The siRNA (also known as short interfering RNA or silencing RNA) is a double-stranded RNA 20–25 nucleotides in length. If introduced into a host cell, it interferes with the expression of specific genes having a complementary nucleotide sequence. This is called the RNA interference (RNAi) pathway that leads to gene knockdown by which the expression of one or more genes of an organism is reduced. Gene knockdown by RNAi by introduction of siRNAs has generated a great deal of interest in view of potential applications.[176] For example, suppressing a particular gene expression may initiate a therapeutic benefit *in vivo*.

In one of the earliest approaches for DNA transfection, buffered saline solution containing phosphate ions is combined with a $CaCl_2$ solution containing the DNA.[177,178] The suspension of the precipitate is then added to the cells to be transfected when the cells take up some of the precipitate, and with it, the DNA, by a process not entirely understood. Several chemical methods of transfection have been developed since then using cyclodextrins,[179] polymers,[180,181] dendrimers,[182] nanoparticles,[183,184] and nanogels[185] as biocompatible transporters. This field has evoked much interest in recent years because of the attractive outcome of such exercises, and hence, new improved methods for efficient transfection to a broad range of cell types remain a high priority. SWNTs are attractive materials for gene transfection in view of their strong attraction for biomolecules such as DNA, RNA, and protein. CNTs have been found to enhance DNA amplification,[186] affect the growth pattern of neurons,[29] and deliver genes into cells,[136] with no apparent toxic effects.

There are two broad approaches to immobilize DNA onto the surface of CNTs, through noncovalent interactions[187–190] or covalent bonds,[191–195] with each method having advantages and limitations. Covalent bond approaches might compromise and even spoil the functions of DNA owing to chemical reactions, and releasing DNA may prove to be difficult. Noncovalent approaches also have limitations as immobilization of DNA onto the surface of CNTs may not form a stable sheath strong enough to sustain the biochemical environment. Here are some illustrative examples.

5.9.1 Delivery of Nucleic Acids Bound Noncovalently to CNTs

Both SWNTs and MWNTs are covalently modified by using the method based on the 1,3-dipolar cycloaddition of azomethine ylides. These f-CNTs carrying positively charged ammonium functions associate with the negatively charged phosphate groups of plasmid DNA through electrostatic interactions. When a solution of f-SWNTs in water is mixed with plasmid DNA in a 6:1 charge ratio, globular and supercoiled structures are observed in different regions of the nanotube surface.[136] These f-CNTs penetrate the mammalian cell membranes and f-CNT-associated plasmid DNA is delivered to cells efficiently. Gene expression becomes 10 times higher than that achieved with DNA alone.

The interactions of three types of f-CNTs, ammonium-functionalized SWNTs and MWNTs (SWNT-NH$_3^+$, MWNT-NH$_3^+$), and lysine-functionalized SWNTs (SWNTLys-NH$_3^+$), with plasmid DNA have been explored.[187] All three types of cationic CNTs are able to condense DNA to varying degrees, indicating that both nanotube surface area and charge density are critical parameters that determine the interaction and electrostatic complex formation between f-CNTs with DNA. All three different f-CNT types exhibited upregulation of marker gene expression over naked DNA using a mammalian (human) cell line. The study indicates that both f-CNT surface area, due to differences in both length and width of nanotubes, and charge density are critical parameters for determining the interaction and electrostatic complex formation between f-CNTs with DNA.

5.9.1.1 Enhancing Transfection Efficiency of DNA

Attempts have been made to enhance transfection efficiency of DNA into different type of cells.[157] MWNT-NH$_2$ (in short for MWNT-COCH$_2$CH$_2$NH$_2$) is obtained by treating MWNT-COCl with ethylenediamine. Polyethylenimine (PEI, -[-(CH$_2$-CH$_2$-NH-]$_n$-) has a high density of secondary amines. PEI is grafted onto the surface of MWNTs by performing a cationic polymerization of aziridine (cyclopropane with NH replacing a CH$_2$) in the presence of MWNT-NH$_2$. The PEI-grafted MWNTs (PEI-g-MWNTs) are easily dispersed in water, and the resulting suspension is stable even after 6 months. Interaction of PEI-g-MWNTs with DNA leads the DNA to immobilize onto the surface of MWNTs through strong multiple electrostatic interactions as demonstrated by the total inhibition of the migration of DNA in gel electrophoresis. PEI-g-MWNTs show transfection efficiency for delivery of DNA that is similar to or even several times higher than that of PEI and several orders of magnitude higher than that of naked DNA. The optimal weight ratio for PEI-g-MWNTs to DNA is about 45:1. Under these conditions, the transfection efficiency of PEI-g-MWNTs toward human embryonic kidney 293 cells (HEK 293 or 293 cells) is more than 3 times higher than that of PEI (25 K), and 4 orders of magnitude higher than that of naked DNA. PEI-g-MWNTs show good transfection efficiency of DNA in other cells as well. The transfection efficiencies of PEI-g-MWNTs in COS7 (derived from monkey kidney tissue) and HepG2 cells (derived from human liver tissue with differentiated hepatocellular carcinoma) are around twice and half, respectively, of those of PEI (25 K) and much higher than those of naked DNA. The high transfection efficiency of PEI-g-MWNTs is attributed to (1) the secure immobilization of DNA onto the surface of MWNTs, which leads to the formation of stable complexes that protect DNA from degradation, and (2) proton sponge effect of the grafted PEI that allows the PEI-g-MWNTs/DNA complexes to escape easily from endosomes or other vesicles in cells.[196]

That the positive charge on the nanotube surface is critical for gene delivery is proved from comparison of DNA interaction with MWNTs bearing OH, COOH, NH_2, and $CH_2CH_2CH_3$ functions. Only the amino-functionalized MWNTs are able to interact with plasmid DNA and deliver the green fluorescent protein (GFP) gene into cultured human cells.[197] Little or no cytotoxicity is observed with MWNT-NH_2-mediated gene transfer.

5.9.2 Delivery of Nucleic Acids Covalently Attached to CNTs

Various biological molecules are attached to phospholipid-functionalized SWNTs via cleavable disulfide linkage. Stable aqueous suspensions of short SWNTs prepared by noncovalent adsorption of phospholipid with PEG chains and terminal amine or maleimide groups (PL-PEG-NH_2 or PL-PEG-maleimide) are used to conjugate with a wide range of biological molecules. For incorporation of a disulfide bond, a heterobifunctional cross-linker is employed for any thiol-containing biomolecule (X), such as DNA and siRNA with a thiol functional group and a six-carbon long spacer at the 5′ end (49) (Figure 5.44).[198,199] Specifically, SWNT-PL-PEG-SS-X is prepared, where X is a 15-mer DNA with fluorescence label Cy3 (cyanine dye, yellow-green fluorescence, ~550 nm excitation, ~570 nm emission), or siRNA. For comparison, SWNT-PL-PEG-X (X = DNA, siRNA) conjugates (50) as control with no disulfide linkage are prepared by conjugating X to SWNT-PL-PEG-maleimide. Transportation, release, and nuclear translocation of DNA oligonucleotides in mammalian cells with SWNT transporters are demonstrated via the cleavage of the disulfide linkage (Figure 5.45). Highly efficient delivery of siRNA by SWNTs, more than lipofectamine, a widely used transfection agent, is shown.

5.10 TUMOR TARGETING AND CANCER THERAPY

In cancer treatment, conventional chemotherapy or radiotherapy damages both cancerous and noncancerous cells, with significant side effects. Over a period of time, tumor cells develop resistance to many chemotherapeutic agents. Besides, most chemotherapeutic drugs kill dividing cancer cells and not the dormant ones.

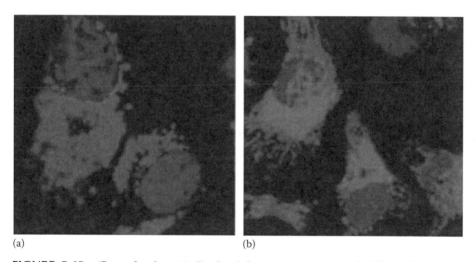

FIGURE 5.44 Two schemes of SWNT functionalization by thiolated biological molecule X with and without disulfide bond.

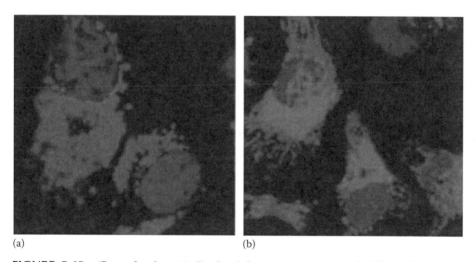

(a)   (b)

FIGURE 5.45 (**See color insert.**) Confocal fluorescence images of HeLa cells (nucleus stained with blue by Draq 5) after incubation in **49** (a) and **50** (b). Red color surrounding the nucleus corresponds to Cy3-labeled DNA molecules transported inside cells by SWNT carriers. (Reprinted with permission from Kam, N. W. S., et al., 2005, 12492–12493. Copyright 2005 American Chemical Society.)

Targeted therapies are being developed to decrease nonspecific toxic effects and to kill nondividing cancer cells. Targeted drug delivery, that is, delivery of high doses of drug molecules to tumor sites for maximum treatment efficacy while minimizing the side effects to normal organs, has remained a challenge.[200,201] There are two approaches of targeted delivery of anticancer drugs into the tumor tissue. One is passive targeting and the other is active targeting. In passive targeting, the drug is directly administered *in vivo* into the tumor tissue. In the process of active targeting, the anticancer drugs are administered *in vivo* into the systemic blood circulation. The drug is guided by tumor-targeting ligands such that they get preferentially retained in the tumor tissue before being drained out. The retention of the drug in the tumor tissue relies on a phenomenon referred to as the "enhanced permeability and retention (EPR) effect".[202–205] The cancer cells are known to multiply quickly. For their nutritional and oxygen supply, they stimulate the production of blood vessels. The newly formed blood vessels are indeed tumor vessels and are usually abnormal in form and architecture. Furthermore, the tumor tissues usually lack effective lymphatic drainage. These factors lead to abnormal molecular transport of the administered macromolecular drugs. These drugs are preferentially retained in the cancerous tissues as compared to normal tissues, which is called the EPR effect.

5.10.1 Thermal Ablation of Tumor Cells by NIR

SWNTs absorb NIR radiation in the range 700–1100 nm. Biological systems are highly transparent to NIR radiation in this spectral range. Experiments conducted *in vitro* show that SWNTs can be used for optical stimulation of nanotubes inside living cells. Continuous NIR radiation can cause cells to heat up (Figure 5.46), and eventually lead to death because of excessive local heating.[206] The ability of CNTs to convert NIR light into heat provides an opportunity to create a new generation of drugs for cancer phototherapy with high performance and efficacy.

In the above study, as-grown HiPco SWNTs are noncovalently functionalized by phospholipids with a PEG-bearing FITC fluorescent label for cell imaging. For selective internalization, SWNT-PL-PEG is endowed with folic acid terminal group (Figure 5.47). These highly sophisticated functional SWNTs selectively enter cells

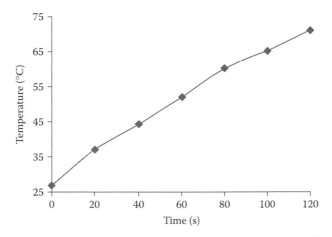

FIGURE 5.46 Heating of DNA-SWNT solution caused by absorption of 808-nm NIR laser light by SWNTs in the solution. (Reprinted with permission from Kam, N. W. S., et al., 2005. Carbon nanotubes as multifunctional biological transporters and near-infrared agents for selective cancer cell destruction. *Proc. Natl. Acad. Sci. USA* 102:11600–11605. Copyright 2005 National Academy of Sciences, U.S.A.)

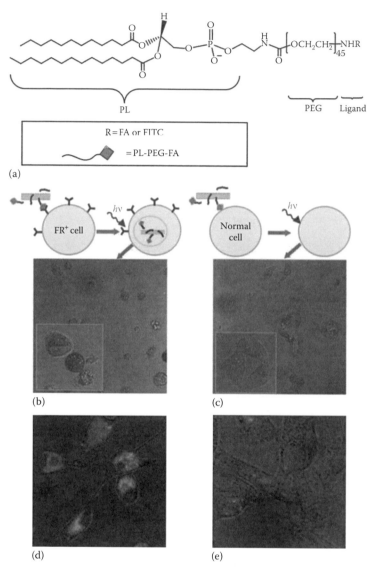

FIGURE 5.47 Selective targeting and killing of cancer cells. (a) Chemical structure of PL-PEG-FA and PL-PEG-FITC. (b and c) Schematic of selective internalization of SWNT-PL-PEG-FA into folate-overexpressing (FR+) cells and normal cells without available FRs. The lower images show death of FR+ cells after NIR 808-nm laser radiation. The FR+ cells show rounded morphology, whereas the shapes of cells without FRs are not affected. (d) Confocal image of FR+ cells after incubation in SWNT-PL-PEG-FA and SWNT-PL-PEG-FITC. The strong FITC fluorescence inside cells confirms the SWNT uptake with FA and FITC cargos. (e) Image for normal cells without abundant FRs on cell surfaces. There is little fluorescence inside cells, confirming little uptake of SWNTs with FA and FITC cargos. (Reprinted with permission from Kam, N. W. S., et al., 2005. Carbon nanotubes as multifunctional biological transporters and near-infrared agents for selective cancer cell destruction. *Proc. Natl. Acad. Sci. USA* 102:11600–11605. Copyright 2005 National Academy of Sciences, U.S.A.)

labeled with the folate receptor (FR⁺) tumor markers, which have a high affinity for folic acid and several of its reduced derivatives. The oligonucleotide transported inside living cells by the SWNTs translocates into cell nucleus upon rupture triggered by NIR laser pulses. NIR-triggered cancer cell death is carried out very efficiently without harming normal cells.

In another study, monoclonal antibodies (mAbs) are used with SWNTs for selectively targeting cancer cells.[207] The mAbs are monospecific as these are the same because they are made using identical immune cells that are all clones of a unique parent cell. These antibodies have monovalent affinity, in that they bind to the same part of an antigen. Specific binding of antibody-coupled CNTs to tumor cells *in vitro*, followed by their highly specific ablation with NIR light, is demonstrated. Water-soluble CNTs functionalized with biotinylated polar lipids are stable, biocompatible, noncytotoxic CNT dispersions that are then attached to avidin-derivatized mAbs directed against either human or Daudi cells. Only the specifically targeted cells are killed after exposure to NIR light.

5.10.2 Tumor Targeting by CNT Conjugates Bearing Radionuclides

Targeting tumor cells by RGD peptides is a promising strategy for delivering cytotoxic drugs for cancer therapy.[208] SWNTs with two different PEG coatings PEG_{5000} and PEG_{2000} conjugated with both peptide (RGD) and ^{64}Cu radiolabels complex in the ligand 1,4,7,10-tetraazacyclododecane-1,4,7,10-tetraacetic acid (DOTA) are intravenously injected into tumor-bearing mice, which are monitored by micro-positron emission tomography (micro-PET) over a period of time (Figure 5.48).[209] SWNTs conjugated to RGD with a long PEG chain (SWNT-PEG_{5400}-RGD) show a high tumor uptake ~13% injected dose per gram (ID/g) (second column). By contrast, SWNT-PEG_{2000}-RGD shows a lower tumor uptake (first column). The third column is a control experiment showing blocking of SWNT-PEG_{5400}-RGD tumor uptake by co-injection of free cyclic peptide c(RGDyK). The fourth column is a control experiment showing low uptake of SWNT-PEG_{5400}-RGD in HT-29 tumor. It is important to note here that efficient tumor targeting is realized when SWNTs are coated with long PEG (SWNT-PEG_{5400}-RGD) but not with short PEG (SWNT-PEG_{2000}-RGD). The latter had short blood circulation time, and thus lower probability of being trapped in tumors or of binding the tumor receptors.

Immunoglobulin G (IgG) is an antibody, a protein complex composed of four peptide chains. It is the main antibody found in blood and extracellular fluid and controls infection of body tissues. It binds viruses, bacteria, and fungi, and protects the body against them. SWNTs conjugated with specific IgG antibody can efficiently target tumor tissue. Tumor-targeting multifunctional CNT constructs are synthesized from sidewall-functionalized, water-soluble SWNTs (Figure 5.49) by covalently attaching tumor-specific IgG (**51**), radio metal-ion chelate (^{111}In) (**52**), and fluorescent probes.[210] These nanoconstructs with the specific appended antibodies are reactive with the human cancer cells *in vivo* and *in vitro*. The antibodies drive the nanoconstructs to the specific tumor target, the radio metal ion is delivered on site, and the fluorescent probes report the location of the cancer cells.

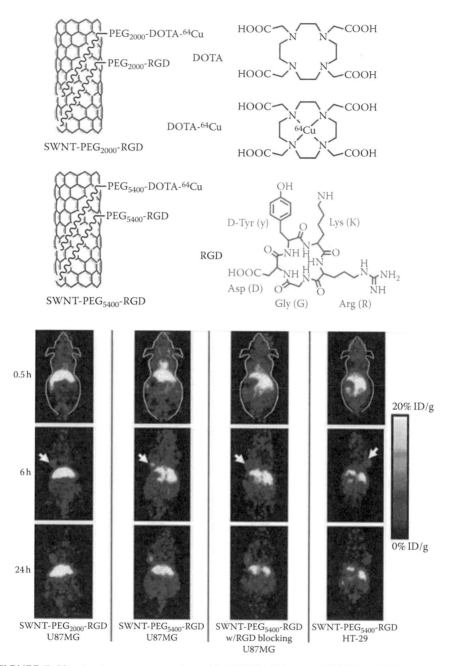

FIGURE 5.48 *In vivo* tumor targeting with SWNTs. Scheme of PEGylated SWNTs with RGD conjugation and radio labeling and micro-PET images of mice. The arrows point to the tumors. (Reprinted by permission from Macmillan Publishers Ltd. Liu, Z., et al., *Nat. Nanotechnol.*, 2, 47–52, 2007, copyright 2007.)

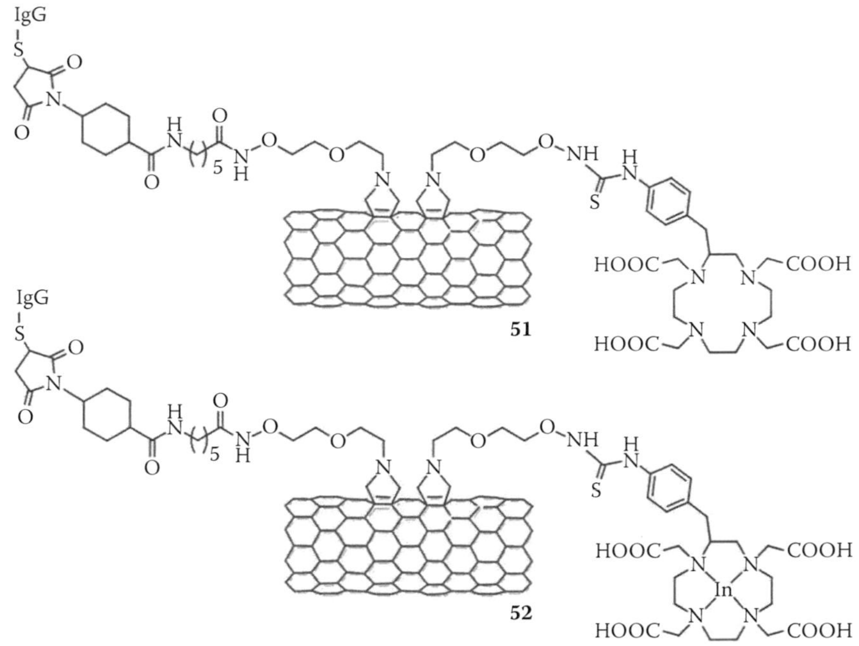

FIGURE 5.49 Synthetic CNT constructs.

5.10.3 *In Vitro* Cancer Treatment

Telomerase is a ribonucleoprotein, the key enzyme for the stabilization of chromosomes by adding TTAGGG repeats to the telomere ends.[211,212] Telomerase activation is detected in the majority of malignant tumors but not in most normal somatic cells. Therefore, inhibition of telomerase activity and knockdown of telomerase expression are attractive approaches for targeted cancer therapy. SWNTs-CONH-$(CH_2)_6$-$NH_3^+Cl^-$ carrying complexed siRNA efficiently enters into tumor cells and releases the siRNA to silence the targeted gene.[213] The functionality -CONH-$(CH_2)_6$-$NH_3^+Cl^-$ mediates the conjugation of telomerase reverse transcriptase (TERT) siRNA to SWNTs to form the mouse TERT (mTERT) siRNA:SWNT+ complexes. The ability of TERT siRNA delivered via SWNT complexes to silence the expression of TERT is assessed by their effects on the proliferation and growth of tumor cells both *in vitro* and in mouse models (Figure 5.50). It is observed that mTERT siRNA:SWNT+ complexes rapidly enter the cultured murine tumor cell lines, suppress mTERT expression, and produce growth arrest. Injection of mTERT siRNA:SWNT+ complexes into lung tumors reduces tumor growth. Furthermore, human TERT siRNA:SWNT+ complexes also suppress the growth of human HeLa cells both *in vitro* and when injected into tumors in nude mice. In this study, siRNA:SWNT+ complexes are directly injected into tumors.

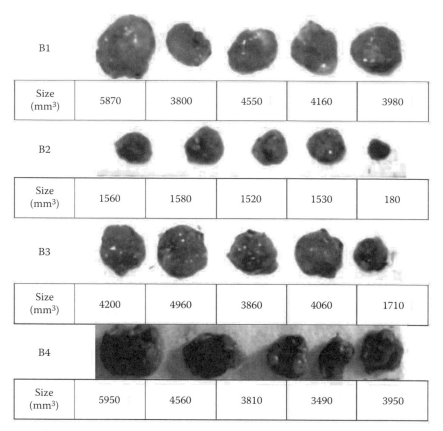

B1					
Size (mm³)	5870	3800	4550	4160	3980
B2					
Size (mm³)	1560	1580	1520	1530	180
B3					
Size (mm³)	4200	4960	3860	4060	1710
B4					
Size (mm³)	5950	4560	3810	3490	3950

FIGURE 5.50 Injection of mTERT siRNA:SWNT+ complexes suppresses tumor growth *in vivo*. Tumor size at day 7 after injection. B1, control; B2, mTERT siRNA:SWNT+ complexes; B3, mTERT siRNA alone; B4, mock siRNA:SWNT+ complexes. (Reprinted with permission from Zhang, Z. H., et al., 12, 4933–4939, 2006. Copyright 2006 American Association for Cancer Research.)

5.10.4 *In Vivo* Cancer Treatment

Active SWNT drug delivery *in vivo* for tumor suppression in mice has been demonstrated with paclitaxel (PTX), the widely used cancer chemotherapy drug (Figure 5.51).[214] PTX is conjugated to branched polyethylene glycol chains on SWNTs via a cleavable ester bond. First the PTX molecules are reacted with succinic anhydride to form cleavable ester bonds followed by carbodiimide coupling of the carboxylic acid end to the termini of branched PEG-NH$_2$. PTX is released from nanotubes by ester cleavage *in vivo*. The water-soluble SWNT–PTX conjugate affords higher efficacy in suppressing tumor growth than clinical Taxol® in a murine 4T1 breast cancer model. This is due to prolonged blood circulation and 10-fold higher tumor PTX uptake by SWNT delivery likely through the EPR effect. Drug molecules carried into the system are released from SWNTs and excreted without causing toxic effects to normal organs. This is the first successful report that CNTs are used as drug delivery vehicles to achieve *in vivo* tumor treatment efficacy with mice.

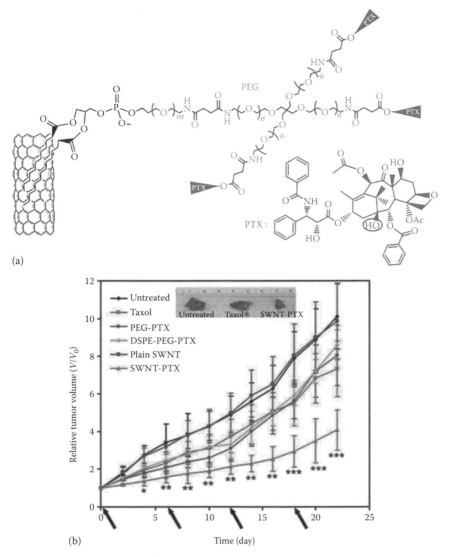

(a)

(b)

FIGURE 5.51 *In vivo* drug delivery with CNTs for cancer treatment. (a) Schematic illustration of PTX conjugation (at the circled OH site) to SWNT functionalized by phospholipids with branched-PEG chains. (b) Tumor growth curves of 4T1 tumor-bearing mice receiving the different treatments indicated. DSPE, 1,2-distearoyl-*sn*-glycero-3-phosphoethanolamine. Inset: A photo of representative tumors taken out of an untreated mouse, a Taxol-treated mouse and an SWNT-PTX-treated mouse at the end of the treatments. (Reprinted with permission from Liu, Z., et al., 68, 6652–6660. Copyright 2008 American Association for Cancer Research.)

In a novel SWNT-based tumor-targeted drug delivery system (DDS), a functionalized SWNT is linked to tumor-targeting biotin as well as an anticancer agent taxoid with a cleavable linker as prodrug (**53**) (Figure 5.52).[215] Taxoids are derivatives of PTX, which are anticancer drugs that inhibit cell division. The prodrug module activates to its cytotoxic form inside the tumor cells (L1210FR leukemia cell line) upon

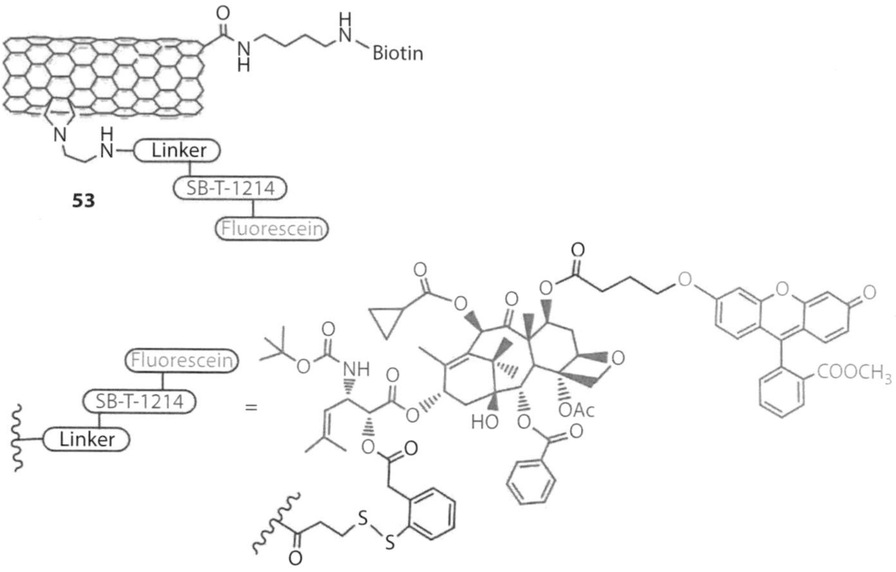

FIGURE 5.52   Structure of biotin–SWNT–linker–(taxoid-fluorescein) conjugate.

internalization and releases *in situ*. The tumor-targeting DDS shows high potency toward specific cancer cell lines. Internalization of the whole conjugate takes place via receptor-mediated endocytosis and the drug releases through cleavage of the disulfide linker moiety by intracellular thiol binding of the free taxoid molecules to tubulins/microtubules, forming stabilized microtubules that block cell mitosis and trigger apoptosis. Since each taxoid molecule is fluorescently labeled with fluorescein, the internalized biotin–SWNT–linker–taxoid conjugate in the cytoplasm and the taxoid-bound microtubules are fluorescent.

5.10.4.1   *In Vivo* Cancer Treatment Using CNT–Pt(IV) Complex

Cisplatin is an anticancer drug that reacts *in vivo*, binding to and causing cross-linking of DNA, ultimately triggering programmed cell death. The release of cisplatin *in vivo* is demonstrated using the cell-sensitizing estradiol units attached to Pt(IV) compounds, which, upon entry into the cell, are reduced to release the cytotoxic Pt(II) compound *cis*-[Pt(NH$_3$)$_2$Cl$_2$].[216] Following this principle, an SWNT–Pt(IV) conjugate is shown to effectively deliver a lethal dose of cisplatin upon reduction inside the cell. The Pt(IV) complex *cis,cis,trans*-[Pt(NH$_3$)$_2$Cl$_2$(OEt) (OOCCH$_2$CH$_2$COOH)] is tethered through the carboxylic acid group on one of its axial ligands to an amine-functionalized SWNT.[217] This complex, which is nearly nontoxic to testicular cancer cells, displays a significantly enhanced cytotoxicity profile when attached to the surface of amine-functionalized soluble SWNTs. The soluble SWNT–Pt(IV) conjugate internalizes through endocytosis. Once confined within the endosomes, the lower pH environment facilitates the release of cisplatin by reduction and concomitant loss of the axial ligands by which it is tethered to the SWNT surface.

The above Pt(IV) complex is further modified with FR for targeted delivery. The Pt(IV) complex of the formula *cis,cis,trans*-[Pt(NH$_3$)$_2$Cl$_2$(OOCCH$_2$CH$_2$COOH)

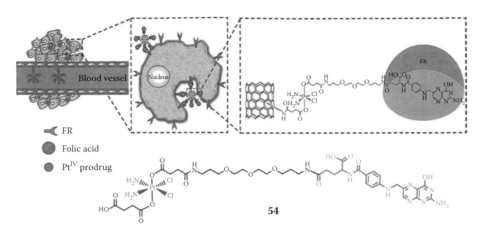

FIGURE 5.53 FR-mediated targeting and SWNT-mediated delivery of **1** by endocytosis and structure of **54**. (Reprinted with permission from Dhar, S., et al., 2008, 11467–11476. Copyright 2008 American Chemical Society.)

(OOCCH₂CH₂CONH-PEG-FA)] (54), containing a folate derivative (FA) at an axial position, is conjugated with SWNT and used as a prodrug for targeted delivery.[218] Compound **54** is attached to an amine-functionalized SWNT (SWNT-PL-PEG-NH₂) through amide linkages (Figure 5.53). The SWNT–Pt(IV) bioconjugate targets the tumor cells since folic acid offers a means of targeting human cells that highly over-express the FR. The prodrug releases cisplatin upon intracellular reduction of Pt(IV) to Pt(II). The SWNT-tethered **54** selectively destroys cells with FR, leaving cells unaffected without FR. That the SWNTs deliver the folate-bearing Pt(IV) cargos into FR⁺ cancer cells by endocytosis is demonstrated by the localization of fluoro-phore-labeled SWNTs using fluorescence microscopy. Once inside the cell, cisplatin, formed upon reductive release, enters the nucleus and reacts with its target nuclear DNA leading to death of tumor cells.

SWNTs have been proven to selectively target head and neck squamous cell carcinomas (HNSCCs), head and neck cancers originating from the mucosal lining of these regions. Treating HNSCCs is a long-standing problem, since the drugs used lack specificity and cause severe side effects.[219,220] Targeted *in vivo* killing of HNSCCs has been demonstrated using SWNT-cisplatin-epidermal growth factor (EGF) and SWNT-quantum dot-EGF (SWNT-Qdot-EGF) bioconjugates (Figure 5.54).[221]

EGF attached to SWNT-cisplatin or SWNT-Qdot specifically targets squamous cancer. Imaging studies *in vitro* with HNSCC overexpressing EGF receptors (EGFRs) using Qdot luminescence and confocal microscopy show that SWNT-Qdot-EGF bio-conjugates internalize rapidly into the cancer cells. Limited uptake occurs for control cells without EGF. Imaging *in vivo* shows that SWNT-Qdot-EGF injected into live mice is selectively taken up by HNSCC tumors, but SWNT-Qdot controls with no EGF are cleared from the tumor region in less than 20 min. HNSCC cells treated with SWNT-cisplatin-EGF are also killed selectively, while control systems do not influence cell proliferation. Regression of tumor growth is rapid in mice treated with targeted SWNT-cisplatin-EGF relative to SWNT-cisplatin without EGF.

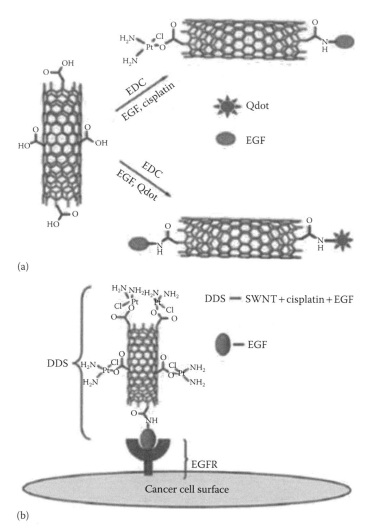

(a)

(b)

FIGURE 5.54 SWNT-based delivery system. (a) Illustration of chemical reactions used to attach EGF, cisplatin, and Qdots onto carboxylated SWNTs using EDC as the coupling agent. (b) Schematic showing SWNT bundles bioconjugated with EGF and cisplatin targeting the cell surface receptor EGFR on a single HNSCC cell. (Reprinted with permission from Bhirde A. A., et al., 2009, 307–316. Copyright 2009 American Chemical Society.)

5.11 TARGETED DELIVERY OF POTENT DRUGS

The CNTs can be ideal candidates for targeted delivery of potent drug molecules, such as amphotericin B (AmB). This drug is considered to be the most effective antibiotic in the treatment of chronic fungal infections.[222,223] However, the drug is highly toxic to mammalian cells, likely cause being formation of aggregates as a result of the lower solubility of AmB in water. Conjugation of this drug to water-soluble functional SWNTs increases the solubility of the molecule, decreases

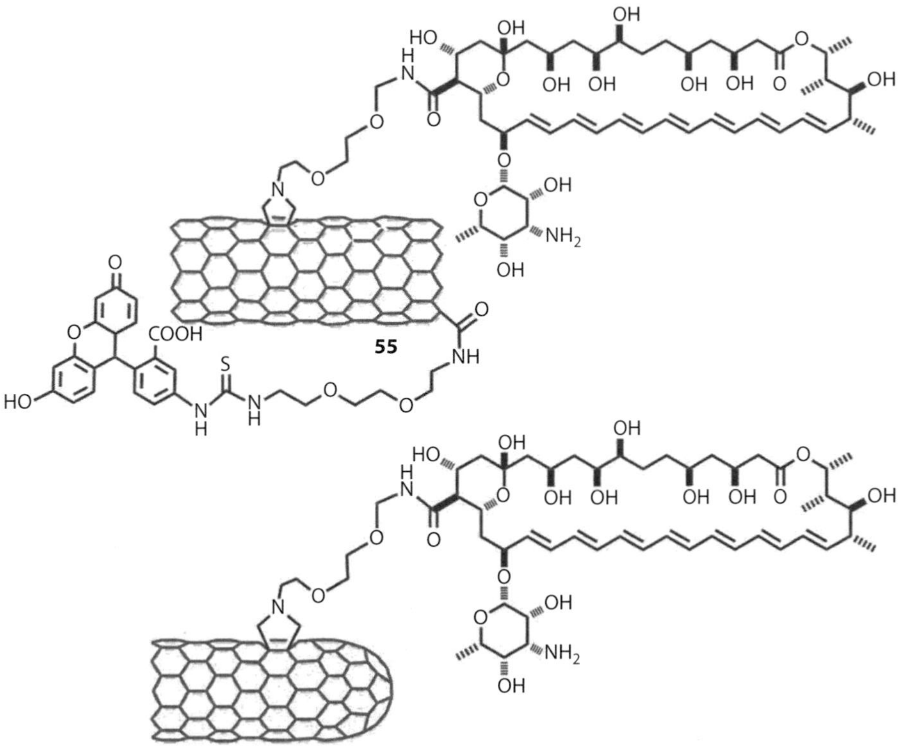

FIGURE 5.55 Attaching AmB, a potent commercially available antifungal agent, to the CNTs. SWNT double functionalized with AmB and fluorescein (**55**) for evaluation of antifungal activity toward mammalian cells. Attaching AmB to MWNT (**56**).

the aggregation phenomena, and improves the efficacy owing to the internalization capacity of the CNTs. The activity of CNTs double functionalized with AmB and fluorescein (**55** and **56**) toward different types of cells (mammalian, bacterial, and fungal) is evaluated (Figure 5.55).[224] This finding paves the way for the development of CNTs as nanovectors to carry therapeutic agents with recognition capacity to a target site for treatment of different types of ailments.

5.12 CONCLUDING REMARKS

CNTs, initially envisioned for applications based on their optical and electronic properties in the early years of investigation, have become highly attractive candidates for applications in biology and medicine in recent times. The high surface area of nanotubes with controllable density of functionality translates into the materials being highly unique as very efficient drug delivery vehicles. Being made up of carbon, the nanotubes are resistant to biochemical degradation, and hence, there are genuine concerns for their safety. However, recent results show that if the nanotubes are pure, are of a desirable size, and are effectively sheathed to furnish highly water-soluble bioconjugates that are stable in biological fluid, they are retained in the systemic circulation without registering any toxicity. This evokes further research to find new CNT materials that can be loaded with drugs and can have additional functions of recognition. Fortunately, there is now a library of such CNT-based materials tested for targeted drug delivery for treating life-threatening diseases. These nanoconstructs are capable of delivering a cargo load of drugs at the target site and drain out of the systemic circulation in over a period of time without causing harm to healthy vital organs. In spite of these promising results, the use of CNTs for drug delivery of small molecules, such as anticancer, antibacterial, or antiviral agents, remains still unexplored. In years to come, for large-scale use of CNT nanoconstructs for addressing human ailments, it becomes crucial that their long-term safety be thoroughly evaluated. This write-up is an introduction to CNT bioconjugates presented at a rudimentary level. For exhaustive accounts on each aspect, opinions of the experts in the field[30–36] are more defining and should be pursued. Applications based on electronic properties of CNTs, such as sensing of biomolecules, not covered in this chapter, are highly attractive. Development of CNT biosensors is a very interesting and highly rewarding research arena due to its academic as well as commercial implications.

ACKNOWLEDGMENTS

This chapter was prepared with the support of the Ministry of Education Science and Technology (MEST) and the Korean Federation of Science and Technology Societies (KOFST) 121S-4-3-0409. Help rendered by the members of our research groups, past and present, is gratefully acknowledged. Our thanks are to Miss Sudipta Mallick for her contribution during the preparation of the manuscript.

REFERENCES

1. Bacon, R. J. 1960. Growth, structure, and properties of graphite whiskers. *J. Appl. Phys.* 31:283–291.
2. Iijima, S. 1991. Helical microtubules of graphitic carbon. *Nature* 354:56–58.
3. Zhao, X.; Ohkohchi, M.; Wang, M.; Iijima, S.; Ichihashi, T.; Ando, Y. 1997. Preparation of high-grade carbon nanotubes by hydrogen arc discharge. *Carbon* 35:775–781.
4. Iijima, S.; Ichihashi, T. 1993. Single-shell carbon nanotubes of 1-nm diameter. *Nature* 363:603–605.
5. Bethune, D. S.; Ohkohchi, M.; Wang, M.; Iijima, S.; Ichihashi, T.; Ando, Y.; Kiang, C. H.; et al. 1993. Cobalt-catalysed growth of carbon nanotubes with single-atomic-layer walls. *Nature* 363:605–607.
6. Haddon, R. C. (Ed.). 2002. Special issue on carbon nanotubes. *Acc. Chem. Res.* 35:997–1113.
7. Ajayan, P. M. 1999. Nanotubes from carbon. *Chem. Rev.* 99:1787–1800.
8. Bahr, J. L.; Tour, J. M. 2002. Covalent chemistry of single-wall carbon nanotubes. *J. Mater. Chem.* 12:1952–1958.
9. Hirsch, A. 2002. Functionalization of single-walled carbon nanotubes. *Angew. Chem. Int. Ed.* 41:1853–1859.
10. Baughman, R. H.; Zakhidov, A. A.; de Heer, W. A. 2002. Carbon nanotubes—The route toward applications. *Science* 297:787–792.
11. Joselevich, E. 2004. Electronic structure and chemical reactivity of carbon nanotubes: A chemist's view. *ChemPhysChem* 5:619–624.
12. Dresselhaus, M. S.; Dresselhaus, G.; Eklund, P. C. 1996. *Science of Fullerenes and Carbon Nanotubes: Their Properties and Applications.* Academic Press: San Diego, CA.

13. Ebbesen, T. W. 1997. *Carbon Nanotubes: Preparation and Properties*. CRC Press: Boca Raton, FL.
14. Saito, R.; Dresselhaus, G.; Dresselhaus, M. S. 1998. *Physical Properties of Carbon Nanotubes*. Imperial College Press: London.
15. Tanaka, K.; Yamabe, T.; Fukui, K. (Eds.). 1999. *The Science and Technology of Carbon Nanotubes*. Elsevier: Amsterdam, The Netherlands.
16. Tománek, D.; Enbody, R. J. 2000. *Science and Application of Nanotubes*. Kluwer Academic/Plenum Publishers: New York.
17. Harris, P. J. F. 2001. *Carbon Nanotubes and Related Structures: New Materials for the Twenty-First Century*. Cambridge University Press: Cambridge, UK.
18. Dresselhaus, M. S.; Dresselhaus, G.; Avouris, P. 2001. *Carbon Nanotubes: Synthesis, Structure, Properties, and Applications*. Springer: New York.
19. Reich, S.; Thomsen, C.; Maultzsch, J. 2004. *Carbon Nanotubes: Basic Concepts and Physical Properties*. John Wiley & Sons: Weinheim, Germany.
20. Meyyappan, M. 2005. *Carbon Nanotubes: Science and Applications*. CRC Press: Westborough, MA.
21. Popov, V. N.; Lambin, P. 2006. *Carbon Nanotubes: From Basic Research to Nanotechnology*. Springer: Dordrechet, The Netherlands.
22. O'Connel, M. J. (Ed.). 2006. *Carbon Nanotubes: Properties and Applications*. CRC Press (Taylor & Francis): Boca Raton, FL.
23. Loiseau, A. 2006. *Understanding Carbon Nanotubes: From Basics to Applications*. Springer: New York.
24. Saitō, S. 2008. *Carbon Nanotubes: Quantum Cylinders of Graphene*. Elsevier: Amsterdam, The Netherlands.
25. Hierold, C. 2008. *Carbon Nanotube Devices: Properties, Modeling, Integration and Applications*. Wiley-VCH: Weinheim, Germany.
26. Rafii-Tabar, H. 2008. *Computational Physics of Carbon Nanotubes*. Cambridge University Press: New York.
27. Colbert, D. T.; Smalley, R. E. 2002. Past, present and future of fullerene nanotubes: Buckytubules. In Osawa, E. (Ed.), *Prospective of Fullerene Nanotechnology*. Kluwer Academic Publishers: Dordrechet, The Netherlands, pp. 3–10.
28. Wong, E. W.; Zakhidov, A. A.; de Heer, W. A.; Sheehan, P. E.; Lieber, C. M. 1997. Nanobeam mechanics: Elasticity, strength, and toughness of nanorods and nanotubes. *Science* 277:1971–1975.
29. Mattson, M. P.; Zakhidov, A. A.; de Heer, W. A.; Haddon, R. C.; Rao, A. M. 2000. Molecular functionalization of carbon nanotubes and use as substrates for neuronal growth. *J. Mol. Neurosci.* 14:175–182.
30. Bianco, A.; Prato, M. 2003. Can carbon nanotubes be considered useful tools for biological applications? *Adv. Mater.* 15:1765–1768.
31. Bianco, A. 2004. Carbon nanotubes for the delivery of therapeutic molecules. *Expert Opin. Drug Deliv.* 1:57–65.
32. Bianco, A.; Zakhidov, A. A.; de Heer, W. A.; Kostarelos, K.; Pratidos, C. D.; Prato, M. 2005. Biomedical applications of functionalised carbon nanotubes. *Chem. Commun.* 571–577.
33. Lin, Y.; Zakhidov, A. A.; de Heer, W. A.; Taylor, S.; Li, H.; Fernando, K. A. S.; Qu, L.; et al. 2004. Advances toward bioapplications of carbon nanotubes. *J. Mater. Chem.* 14:527–541.
34. Lacerda, L.; Zakhidov, A. A.; de Heer, W. A.; Bianco, A.; Prato, M.; Kostarelos, K. 2008. Carbon nanotube cell translocation and delivery of nucleic acids *in vitro* and *in vivo*. *J. Mater. Chem.* 18:17–22.
35. Prato, M.; Zakhidov, A. A.; de Heer, W. A.; Kostarelos, K.; Bianco, A. 2008. Functionalized carbon nanotubes in drug design and discovery. *Acc. Chem. Res.* 41:60–68.
36. Liu, Z.; Tabakman, S.; Welsher, K.; Dai, H. 2009. Carbon nanotubes in biology and medicine: *In vitro* and *in vivo* detection, imaging and drug delivery. *Nano Res.* 2:85–120.

37. Ebbesen, T. W. 1998. Cones and tubes: Geometry in the chemistry of carbon. *Acc. Chem. Res.* 31:558–566.
38. Liu, J.; Zakhidov, A. A.; de Heer, W. A.; Rinzler, A. G.; Dai, H.; Hafner, J. H.; Bradley, R. K.; et al. 1998. Fullerene pipes. *Science* 280:1253–1255.
39. Mawhinney, D. B.; Zakhidov, A. A.; de Heer, W. A.; Naumenko, V.; Kuznetsova, A.; Yates, J. T. J.; Liu, J.; Smalley, R. E. 2000. Surface defect site density on single walled carbon nanotubes by titration. *Chem. Phys. Lett.* 324:213.v–216.v.
40. Hu, H.; Bhowmik, P.; Zhao, B.; Hamon, M. A.; Itkis, M. E.; Haddon, R. C. 2001. Determination of the acidic sites of purified single-walled carbon nanotubes by acid-base titration. *Chem. Phys. Lett.* 345:25–28.
41. Hiura, H.; Zakhidov, A. A.; de Heer, W. A.; Ebbesen, T. W.; Tanigaki, K. 1995. Opening and purification of carbon nanotubes in high yields. *Adv. Mater.* 7:275–276.
42. Ebbesen, T. W.; Hiura, H.; Bisher, M. E.; Treacy, M. M. J.; Shreeve-Keyer, J. L.; Haushalter, R. C. 1996. Decoration of carbon nanotubes. *Adv. Mater.* 8:155–157.
43. Kuznetsova, A.; Zakhidov, A. A.; de Heer, W. A.; Popova, I.; Yates, J. T.; Bronikowski, M. J.; Huffman, C. B.; et al. 2001. Oxygen-containing functional groups on single-walled carbon nanotubes: NEXAFS and vibrational spectroscopic studies. *J. Am. Chem. Soc.* 123:10699–10704.
44. Monthioux, M.; Smith, B. W.; Burteaux, B.; Claye, A.; Fischer, J. E.; Luzzi, D. E.; Zakhidov, A. A.; de Heer, W. A. 2001. Sensitivity of single-wall carbon nanotubes to chemical processing: An electron microscopy investigation. *Carbon* 39:1251–1272.
45. Itkis, M. E.; Niyogi, S.; Meng, M.; Hamon, M.; Hu, H.; Haddon, R. C.; Zakhidov, A. A.; de Heer, W. A. 2002. Spectroscopic study of the Fermi level electronic structure of single-walled carbon nanotubes. *Nano Lett.* 2:155–159.
46. Ausman, K. D.; Piner, R.; Lourie, O.; Ruoff, R. S.; Korobov, M.; Zakhidov, A. A.; de Heer, W. A. 2000. Organic solvent dispersions of single-walled carbon nanotubes: Toward solutions of pristine nanotubes. *J. Phys. Chem. B* 104:8911–8915.
47. Bower, C.; Kleinhammes, A.; Wu, Y.; Zhou, O.; Zakhidov, A. A.; de Heer, W. A. 1998. Intercalation and partial exfoliation of single-walled carbon nanotubes by nitric acid. *Chem. Phys. Lett.* 288:481–486.
48. Tohji, K.; Zakhidov, A. A.; de Heer, W. A.; Takahashi, H.; Shinoda, Y.; Shimizu, N.; Jeyadevan, B.; et al. 1997. Purification procedure for single-walled nanotubes. *J. Phys. Chem. B* 101:1974–1978.
49. Bandow, S.; Asaka, S.; Zhao, X.; Ando, Y.; Zakhidov, A. A.; de Heer, W. A. 1998. Purification and magnetic properties of carbon nanotubes. *Appl. Phys. A* 67:23–27.
50. Dujardin, E.; Zakhidov, A. A.; de Heer, W. A.; Ebbesen, T. W.; Krishnan, A.; Treacy, M. M. J. 1998. Purification of single-shell nanotubes. *Adv. Mater.* 10:611–613.
51. Dillon, A. C.; Gennet, T.; Jones, K. M.; Alleman, J. L.; Parilla, P. A.; Heben, M. J.; Zakhidov, A. A.; de Heer, W. A. 1999. A simple and complete purification of single-walled carbon nanotube materials. *Adv. Mater.* 11:1354–1358.
52. Koshio, A.; Yudasaka, M.; Zhang, M.; Iijima, S.; Zakhidov, A. A.; de Heer, W. A. 2001. A simple way to chemically react single-wall carbon nanotubes with organic materials using ultrasonication. *Nano Lett.* 1:361–363.
53. Chiang, I. W.; Zakhidov, A. A.; de Heer, W. A.; Brinson, B. E.; Huang, A. Y.; Willis, P. A.; Bronikowski, M. J.; Margrave, J. L.; Smalley, R. E.; Hauge, R. H. 2001. Purification and characterization of single-wall carbon nanotubes (SWNTs) obtained from the gas-phase decomposition of CO (HiPco process). *J. Phys. Chem. B* 105:8297–8301.
54. Zhou, W.; Zakhidov, A. A.; de Heer, W. A.; Ooi, Y. H.; Russo, R.; Papanek, P.; Luzzi, D. E.; Fischer, J. E.; Bronikowski, M. J.; Willis, P. A.; Smalley, R. E. 2001. Structural characterization and diameter-dependent oxidative stability of single wall carbon nanotubes synthesized by the catalytic decomposition of CO. *Chem. Phys. Lett.* 350:6–14.
55. Charlier, J.-C. 2002. Defects in carbon nanotubes. *Acc. Chem. Res.* 35:1063–1069.

56. Bachilo, S. M.; Zakhidov, A. A.; de Heer, W. A.; Strano, M. S.; Kittrell, C.; Hauge, R. H.; Smalley, R. E.; Weisman, R. B. 2002. Structure-assigned optical spectra of single-walled carbon nanotubes. *Science* 298:2361–2366.

57. Haddon, R. C. 1993. Chemistry of the fullerenes: The manifestation of strain in a class of continuous aromatic molecules. *Science* 261:1545–1550.

58. Taylor, R.; Walton, D. M. R. 1993. The chemistry of the fullerenes. *Nature* 363:685–693.

59. Hamon, M. A.; Zakhidov, A. A.; de Heer, W. A.; Itkis, M. E.; Niyogi, S.; Alvaraez, T.; Kuper, C.; Menon, M.; Haddon, R. C. 2001. Effect of rehybridization on the electronic structure of single-walled carbon nanotubes. *J. Am. Chem. Soc.* 123:11292–11293.

60. Haddon, R. C. 1990. Measure of nonplanarity in conjugated organic molecules: Which structurally characterized molecule displays the highest degree of pyramidalization? *J. Am. Chem. Soc.* 112:3385–3389.

61. Rabideau, P. W.; Sygula, A. 1996. Buckybowls: Polynuclear aromatic hydrocarbons related to the buckminsterfullerene surface. *Acc. Chem. Res.* 29:235–242.

62. Srivastava, D.; Zakhidov, A. A.; de Heer, W. A.; Brenner, D. W.; Schall, J. D.; Ausman, K. D.; Yu, M.; Ruoff, R. S. 1999. Predictions of enhanced chemical reactivity to regions of local conformational strain on carbon nanotubes: Kinky chemistry. *J. Phys. Chem. B* 103: 4330–4337.

63. Haddon, R. C. 1988. pi-Electrons in three-dimensions. *Acc. Chem. Res.* 21:243–249.

64. Haddon, R. C. 1986. Hybridization and the orientation and alignment of pi-orbitals in nonplanar conjugated organic molecules: Pi-orbital axis vector analysis (POAV2). *J. Am. Chem. Soc.* 108:2837–2842.

65. Kroto, H. W. 1987. The stability of the fullerenes C_n. *Nature* 329:529–531.

66. Niyogi, S.; Hamon, M. A.; Hu, H.; Zhao, B.; Bhowmik, P.; Sen, R.; Itkis, M. E.; et al. 2002. Chemistry of single-walled carbon nanotubes. *Acc. Chem. Res.* 35:1105–1113.

67. Colvin, V. J. 2003. The potential environmental impact of engineered nanomaterials. *Nat. Biotech.* 21:1166–1170.

68. Shvedova, A. A.; Castranova, V.; Kisin, E. R. 2003. Exposure to carbon nanotube cytotoxicity using human keratinocyte cells. *Toxicol. Environ. Health Part A* 66:1909–1926.

69. Moon, H. K.; Zakhidov, A. A.; de Heer, W. A.; Brenner, D. W.; Schall, J. D.; Ausman, K. D.; Yu, M.; et al. 2008. Effect of nucleases on the cellular internalization of fluorescent labelled DNA-functionalized single-walled carbon nanotubes. *Nano Res.* 1:351–360.

70. Hamon, M. A.; Zakhidov, A. A.; de Heer, W. A.; Brenner, D. W.; Schall, J. D.; Ausman, K. D.; Yu, M.; et al. 2009. Dissolution of single-walled carbon nanotubes. *Adv. Mater.* 11:834–840.

71. Niyogi, S.; Zakhidov, A. A.; de Heer, W. A.; Brenner, D. W.; Schall, J. D.; Ausman, K. D.; Yu, M.; et al. 2002. Chemistry of single-walled carbon nanotubes. *Acc. Chem. Res.* 35:1105–1113.

72. Riggs, J. E.; Zakhidov, A. A.; de Heer, W. A.; Brenner, D. W.; Schall, J. D.; Ausman, K. D.; Yu, M.; et al. 2000. Strong luminescence of solubilized carbon nanotubes. *J. Am. Chem. Soc.* 122:5879–5880.

73. Sun, Y.-P.; Zakhidov, A. A.; de Heer, W. A.; Brenner, D. W.; Schall, J. D.; Ausman, K. D.; Yu, M.; et al. 2001. Soluble dendron-functionalized carbon nanotubes: Preparation, characterization, and properties. *Chem. Mater.* 13:2864–2869.

74. Fu, K.; Huang, W.; Lin, Y.; Riddle, L. A.; Carroll, D. L.; Sun, Y.-P.; Zakhidov, A. A.; et al. 2001. Defunctionalization of functionalized carbon nanotubes. *Nano Lett.* 1:439–441.

75. Sano, M.; Zakhidov, A. A.; de Heer, W. A.; Brenner, D. W.; Schall, J. D.; Ausman, K. D.; Yu, M.; et al. 2001. Self-organization of PEO-*graft*-single-walled carbon nanotubes in solutions and Langmuir–Blodgett films. *Langmuir* 17:5125–5128.

76. Riggs, J. E.; Zakhidov, A. A.; de Heer, W. A.; Brenner, D. W.; Schall, J. D.; Ausman, K. D.; Yu, M.; et al. 2000. Optical limiting properties of suspended and solubilized carbon nanotubes, *J. Phys. Chem. B* 104:7071–7076.

77. Huang, W.; Zakhidov, A. A.; de Heer, W. A.; Brenner, D. W.; Schall, J. D.; Ausman, K. D.; Yu, M.; et al. 2002. Sonication-assisted functionalization and solubilization of carbon nanotubes. *Nano Lett.* 2:231–234.
78. Lin, Y.; Zakhidov, A. A.; de Heer, W. A.; Brenner, D. W.; Schall, J. D.; Ausman, K. D.; Yu, M.; et al. 2003. Characterization of functionalized single-walled carbon nanotubes at individual nanotube-thin bundle level. *J. Phys. Chem. B* 107:10453–10457.
79. Shim, M. A.; Zakhidov, A. A.; de Heer, W. A.; Brenner, D. W.; Schall, J. D.; Ausman, K. D.; Yu, M.; et al. 2001. Polymer functionalization for air-stable *n*-type carbon nanotube field-effect transistors. *J. Am. Chem. Soc.* 123:11512–11513.
80. Lin, Y.; Zakhidov, A. A.; de Heer, W. A.; Brenner, D. W.; Schall, J. D.; Ausman, K. D.; Yu, M.; et al. 2003. Polymeric carbon nanocomposites from carbon nanotubes functionalized with matrix polymer. *Macromolecules* 36:7199–7204.
81. Huang, W.; Zakhidov, A. A.; de Heer, W. A.; Brenner, D. W.; Schall, J. D.; Ausman, K. D.; Yu, M.; et al. 2003. Solubilization of single-walled carbon nanotubes with diamine-terminated oligomeric poly(ethylene glycol) in different functionalization reactions. *Nano Lett.* 3:565–568.
82. Huang, W.; Zakhidov, A. A.; de Heer, W. A.; Brenner, D. W.; Schall, J. D.; Ausman, K. D.; Yu, M.; et al. 2003. Preferential solubilization of smaller single-walled carbon nanotubes in sequential functionalization reactions. *Langmuir* 19:7084–7088.
83. Lin, Y.; Zakhidov, A. A.; de Heer, W. A.; Brenner, D. W.; Schall, J. D.; Ausman, K. D.; Yu, M.; et al. 2003. Characterization of fractions from repeated functionalization reactions of carbon nanotubes. *J. Phys. Chem. B* 107:914–919.
84. Jin, Z.; Zakhidov, A. A.; de Heer, W. A.; Brenner, D. W.; Schall, J. D.; Ausman, K. D.; Yu, M.; et al. 2000. Nonlinear optical properties of some polymer/multi-walled carbon nanotube composites. *Chem. Phys. Lett.* 318:505–510.
85. Negra, D.; Zakhidov, A. A.; de Heer, W. A.; Brenner, D. W.; Schall, J. D.; Ausman, K. D.; Yu, M.; et al. 2003. Microwave-assisted synthesis of a soluble single wall carbon nanotube derivative. *Fullerenes Nanotubes Carbon Nanostruct.* 11:25–34.
86. Boul, P. J.; Liu, J.; Mickelson, E. T.; Huffman, C. B. Ericson, L. M.; Chiang, I. W.; Smith, K. A.; et al. 1999. Reversible sidewall functionalization of buckytubes. *Chem. Phys. Lett.* 310:367–372.
87. Mickelson, E. T.; Chiang, I. W.; Zimmerman, J. L.; Boul, P. J.; Lozano, J.; Liu, J.; Smalley, R. E.; Hauge, R. H.; Margrave, J. L. 1999. Solvation of fluorinated single-wall carbon nanotubes in alcohol solvents. *J. Phys. Chem. B* 103:4318–4322.
88. Zeng, L.; Alemany, L. B.; Edwards, C. L.; Barron, A. R. 2008. Demonstration of covalent sidewall functionalization of single wall carbon nanotubes by NMR spectroscopy: Side chain length dependence on the observation of the sidewall sp^3 carbons. *Nano Res.* 1:72–88.
89. Bahr, J. L.; Yang, J.; Kosynkin, D. V.; Bronikowski, M. J.; Smalley, R. E.; Tour, J. M. 2001. Functionalization of carbon nanotubes by electrochemical reduction of aryl diazonium salts: A bucky paper electrode. *J. Am. Chem. Soc.* 123:6536–6542.
90. Bahr, J. L.; Tour, J. M. 2001. Highly functionalized carbon nanotubes using *in situ* generated diazonium compounds. *Chem. Mater.* 13:3823–3824.
91. Holzinger, M.; Vostrowsky, O.; Hirsch, A.; Hennrich, F.; Kappes, M.; Weiss, R.; Jellen, F. 2001. Sidewall functionalization of carbon nanotubes. *Angew. Chem. Int. Ed.* 40:4002–4005.
92. Peng, H.; Alemany L. B.; Margrave, J. L.; Khabashesku, V. N. 2003. Sidewall carboxylic acid functionalization of single-walled carbon nanotubes. *J. Am. Chem. Soc.* 125:15174–15182.
93. Coleman, K. S.; Bailey, S. R.; Fogden, S.; Green, M. L. H. 2003. Functionalization of single-walled carbon nanotubes via the Bingel reaction. *J. Am. Chem. Soc.* 125:8722–8723.

94. Umeyama, T.; Tezuka, N.; Fujita, M.; Matano, Y.; Takeda, N.; Murakoshi, K.; Yoshida, K.; Isoda, S.; Imahori, H. 2007. Retention of intrinsic electronic properties of soluble single-walled carbon nanotubes after a significant degree of sidewall functionalization by the Bingel reaction. *J. Phys. Chem. C* 111:9734–9741.

95. Lee, K. M.; Li, L. C.; Dai, L. M. 2005. Asymmetric end-functionalization of multi-walled carbon nanotubes. *J. Am. Chem. Soc.* 127:4122–4123.

96. Moghaddam, M. J.; Taylor, S.; Gao, M.; Huang, S. M.; Dai, L. M.; McCall, M. J. 2004. Highly efficient binding of DNA on the sidewalls and tips of carbon nanotubes using photochemistry. *Nano Lett.* 4:89–93.

97. Georgakilas, V.; Kordatos, K.; Prato, M.; Guldi, D. M.; Holzinger, M.; Hirsch, A. 2002. Organic functionalization of carbon nanotubes. *J. Am. Chem. Soc.* 124:760–761.

98. Tagmatarchis, N.; Prato, M. 2004. Functionalization of carbon nanotubes via 1,3-dipolar cycloadditions. *J. Mater. Chem.* 14:437–439.

99. Pantarotto, D.; Briand, J. P.; Prato, M.; Bianco, A. 2004. Translocation of bioactive peptides across cell membranes by carbon nanotubes. *Chem. Commun.* 2004:16–17.

100. Pastorin, G.; Wu, W.; Wieckowski, S.; Briand, J. P.; Kostarelos, K.; Prato, M.; Bianco, A. 2006. Double functionalisation of carbon nanotubes for multimodal drug delivery. *Chem. Commun.* 2006:1182–1184.

101. Chen, Y.; Haddon, R. C.; Fang, S.; Rao, A. M.; Eklund, P. C.; Lee, W. H.; Dickey, E. C.; et al. 1998. Chemical attachment of organic functional groups to single-walled carbon nanotube. *Mater. J. Mater. Res.* 13:2423–2431.

102. Chen, J.; Hamon, M. A.; Hu, H.; Chen, Y.; Rao, A. M.; Eklund, P. C.; Haddon, R. C. 1998. Solution properties of single-walled carbon nanotubes. *Science* 282:95–98.

103. Sun, Y.-P.; Fu, K.; Lin, Y.; Huang, W. 2002. Functionalized carbon nanotubes: Properties and applications. *Acc. Chem. Res.* 35:1096–1104.

104. Holzinger, M.; Abraham, J.; Whelan, P.; Graupner, R.; Ley, L.; Hennrich, F.; Kappes, M.; Hirsch, A. 2003. Functionalization of single-walled carbon nanotubes with (R-)oxycarbonyl nitrenes. *J. Am. Chem. Soc.* 125:8566–8580.

105. Georgakilas, V.; Voulgaris, D.; Vazquez, E.; Prato, M.; Guldi, D. M.; Kukovecz, A.; Kuzmany, H. 2002. Purification of HiPco carbon nanotubes via organic functionalization. *J. Am. Chem. Soc.* 124:14318–14319.

106. Guldi, D. M.; Marcaccio, M.; Paolucci, D.; Paolucci, F.; Tagmatarchis, N.; Tasis, D.; Vázquez, E.; Prato, M. 2003. Single-wall carbon nanotube-ferrocene nanohybrids: Observing intramolecular electron transfer in functionalized SWNTs. *Angew. Chem. Int. Ed.* 42:4206–4209.

107. Chen, R. J.; Zhang, Y. G.; Wang, D. W.; Dai, H. J. 2001. Noncovalent sidewall functionalization of single-walled carbon nanotubes for protein immobilization. *J. Am. Chem. Soc.* 123:3838–3839.

108. Chen, J.; Liu, H. Y.; Weimer, W. A.; Halls, M. D.; Waldeck, D. H.; Walker, G. C. 2002. Noncovalent engineering of carbon nanotube surfaces by rigid, functional conjugated polymers. *J. Am. Chem. Soc.* 124:9034–9035.

109. O'Connell, M. J. 2001. Reversible water-solubilization of single-walled carbon nanotubes by polymer wrapping. *Chem. Phys. Lett.* 342:265–271.

110. Star, A.; Stoddart, J. F.; Steuerman, D.; Diehl, M.; Boukai, A.; Wong, E. W.; Yang, X.; Chung, S. W.; Choi, H.; Heath, J. R. 2001. Preparation and properties of polymer-wrapped single-walled carbon nanotubes. *Angew. Chem. Int. Ed.* 40:1721–1725.

111. Kim, O. K.; Je, J.; Baldwin, J. W.; Kooi, S.; Pehrsson, P. E.; Buckley, L. J. 2003. Solubilization of single-walled carbon nanotubes by supermolecular encapsulation of helical amylose. *J. Am. Chem. Soc.* 125:1426–1427.

112. Star, A.; Steuerman, D. W.; Heath, J. R.; Stoddard, J. F. 2002. Starched carbon nanotubes. *Angew. Chem. Int. Ed.* 41:2508–2512.

113. Dieckmann, G. R.; Dalton, A. B.; Jonson, P. A.; Razal, J.; Chen, J.; Giordano, G. M.; Muñoz, E.; Musselman, I. H.; Baughman, R. H.; Draper, R. K. 2003. Controlled assembly of carbon nanotubes by designed amphiphilic peptide helices. *J. Am. Chem. Soc.* 125:1770–1777.

114. Wang, S.; Humphreys, E. S.; Chung, S. Y. 2003. Peptides with selective affinity for carbon nanotubes. *Nat. Mater.* 2:196–200.

115. Zheng, M.; Jagota, A.; Semke, E. D. 2003. DNA-assisted dispersion and separation of carbon nanotubes. *Nat. Mater.* 2:338–342.

116. Zheng, M.; Jagota, A.; Strano, M. S.; Santos, A. P.; Barone, P.; Chou, S. G.; Diner, B. A.; et al. 2003. Structure-based nanotube sorting by sequence-dependent DNA assembly. *Science* 302:1545–1548.

117. Richard, C.; Balavoine, F.; Schultz, P.; Ebbesen, T. W.; Mioskowski, C.; 2003. Supramolecular self-assembly of lipid derivatives on carbon nanotubes. *Science* 300:775–778.

118. Kang, Y.; Taton, T. A. 2003. Micelle encapsulated carbon nanotubes: A route to nanotube composites. *J. Am. Chem. Soc.* 125:5650–5651.

119. Wang, H.; Zhou, W.; Ho, D. L.; Winey, K. I.; Fischer, J. E.; Glinka, C. J.; Hobbie, E. K. 2004. Dispersing single-walled carbon nanotubes with surfactants: A small angle neutron scattering study. *Nano Lett.* 4:1789–1793.

120. Chambers, G.; Carroll, C.; Farrell, G. F. 2003. Characterization of the interaction of gamma cyclodextrin with single-walled carbon nanotubes. *Nano Lett.* 3:843–846.

121. Dodziuk, H.; Ejchart, A.; Anczewski, W. 2003. Water solubilization, determination of the number of different types of single-wall carbon nanotubes and their partial separation with respect to diameters by complexation with η-cyclodextrin. *Chem. Commun.* 2003:986–987.

122. Wu, P.; Chen, X.; Hu, N.; Tam, U. C.; Blixt, O.; Zettl, A.; Bertozzi, C. R. 2008. Biocompatible carbon nanotubes generated by functionalization with glycodendrimers. *Angew. Chem. Int. Ed.* 47:5022–5025.

123. Guldi, D. M.; Taieb, H.; Rahman, G. M. A.; Tagmatarchis, N.; Prato, M. 2005. Novel photoactive single-walled carbon nanotube-porphyrin polymer wraps: Efficient and long-lived intracomplex charge separation. *Adv. Mater.* 17:871–875.

124. Warheit, D. B.; Laurence, B. R.; Reed, K. L.; Roach, D. H.; Reynolds, G. A. M.; Webb, T. R. 2004. Comparative pulmonary toxicity assessment of single-wall carbon nanotubes in rats. *Toxicol. Sci.* 77:117–125.

125. Lam, C. W.; James, J. T.; McCluskey, R.; Hunter, R. L. 2004. Pulmonary toxicity of single-wall carbon nanotubes in mice 7 and 90 days after intratracheal instillation. *Toxicol. Sci.* 77:126–134.

126. Shvedova, A. A.; Kisin, E. R.; Mercer, R.; Murray, A. R.; Johnson, V. J.; Potapovich, A. I.; Tyurina, Y. Y.; et al. 2005. Unusual inflammatory and fibrogenic pulmonary responses to single-walled carbon nanotubes in mice. *Am. J. Phys. Lung Cell. Mol. Physiol.* 289:L698–L708.

127. Muller, J.; Huaux, F.; Moreau, N.; Misson, P.; Heilier, J. F.; Delos, M.; Arras, M.; et al. 2005. Respiratory toxicity of multi-wall carbon nanotubes. *Toxicol. Appl. Pharmacol.* 207:221–231.

128. Poland, C. A.; Duffin, R.; Kinloch, I.; Maynard, A.; Wallace, W. A. H.; Seaton, A.; Stone, V.; Brown, S.; MacNee, W.; Donaldson, K. 2008. Carbon nanotubes introduced into the abdominal cavity of mice show asbestos-like pathogenicity in a pilot study. *Nat. Nanotechnol.* 3:423–428.

129. Bottini, M.; Bruckner, S.; Nika, K.; Bottini, N.; Bellucci, S.; Magrini, A.; Bergamaschi, A.; Mustelin, T. 2006. Multi-walled carbon nanotubes induce T lymphocyte apoptosis. *Toxicol. Lett.* 160:121–126.

130. Dong, L.; Joseph, K. L.; Witkowski, C. M.; Craig, M. M. 2008. Cytotoxicity of single-walled carbon nanotubes suspended in various surfactants. *Nanotechnology* 19:255702.

131. Plata, D. L.; Gschwend, P. M.; Reddy, C. M. 2008. Industrially synthesized single-walled carbon nanotubes: Compositional data for users, environmental risk assessments, and source apportionment. *Nanotechnology* 19:185706.
132. Casey, A.; Herzog, E.; Davoren, M.; Lyng, F. M.; Byrne, H. J.; Chambers, G. 2007. Spectroscopic analysis confirms the interactions between single walled carbon nanotubes and various dyes commonly used to assess cytotoxicity. *Carbon* 45:1425–1432.
133. Worle-Knirsch, J. M.; Pulskamp, K.; Krug, H. F. 2006. Oops they did it again! Carbon nanotubes hoax scientists in viability assays. *Nano Lett.* 6:1261–1268.
134. Dumortier, H.; Lacotte, S.; Pastorin, G.; Marega, R.; Wu, W.; Bonifazi, D.; Briand, J. P.; Prato, M.; Muller, S.; Bianco, A. 2006. Functionalized carbon nanotubes are noncytotoxic and preserve the functionality of primary immune cells. *Nano Lett.* 6:1522–1528.
135. Sayes, C. M.; Liang, F.; Hudson, J. L.; Mendez, J.; Guo, W.; Beach, J. M.; Moore, V. C.; et al. 2006. Functionalization density dependence of single-walled carbon nanotubes cytotoxicity in vitro. *Toxicol. Lett.* 161:135–142.
136. Pantarotto, D.; Singh, R.; McCarthy, D.; Erhardt, M.; Briand, J. P.; Prato, M.; Kostarelos, K.; Bianco, A. 2004. Functionalized carbon nanotubes for plasmid DNA gene delivery. *Angew. Chem. Int. Ed.* 43:5242–5246.
137. Lu, Q.; Moore, J. M.; Huang, G.; Mount, A. S.; Rao, A. M.; Larcom, L. L.; Kc, P. C. 2004. RNA polymer translocation with single-walled carbon nanotubes. *Nano Lett.* 4:2473–2477.
138. Kam, N. W. S.; Jessop, T. C.; Wender, P. A.; Dai, H. J. 2004. Nanotube molecular transporters: Internalization of carbon nanotube-protein conjugates into mammalian cells. *J. Am. Chem. Soc.* 126:6850–6851.
139. Schipper, M. L.; Nakayama-Ratchford, N.; Davis, C. R.; Kam, N. W. S.; Chu, P.; Liu, Z.; Sun, X.; Dai, H.; Gambhir, S. S. 2008. A pilot toxicology study of single-walled carbon nanotubes in a small sample of mice. *Nat. Nanotechnol.* 3:216–221.
140. O'Connell, M.; Bachilo, S. M.; Huffman, C. B.; Moore, V.; Strano, M. S.; Haroz, E.; Rialon, K.; et al. 2002. Band gap fluorescence from individual single-walled carbon nanotubes. *Science* 297:593–596.
141. Cherukuri, P.; Bachilo, S. M.; Litovsky, S. H; Weisman, R. B. 2004. Near-infrared fluorescence microscopy of single-walled carbon nanotubes in phagocytic cells. *J. Am. Chem. Soc.* 126:15638–15639.
142. Welsher, K.; Liu, Z.; Daranciang, D.; Dai, H. 2008. Selective probing and imaging of cells with single walled carbon nanotubes as near-infrared fluorescent molecules. *Nano Lett.* 8:586–590.
143. Moon, H. K.; Chang, C. I.; Lee, D.-K.; Choi, H. C. 2008. Effect of nucleases on the cellular internalization of fluorescent labelled DNA-functionalized single-walled carbon nanotubes. *Nano Res.* 1:351–360.
144. Xu, M. H.; Wang, L. H. V. 2006. Photoacoustic imaging in biomedicine. *Rev. Sci. Instrum.* 77:41–101.
145. Zhang, H. F.; Maslov, K.; Stoica, G.; Wang, L. V. 2006. Imaging acute thermal burns by photoacoustic microscopy. *J. Biomed. Opt.* 11:054033.
146. Wang, X.; Xie, X.; Ku, G.; Wang, L. V.; Stoica, G. 2006. Noninvasive imaging of haemoglobin concentration and oxygenation in the rat brain using high-resolution photoacoustic tomography. *J. Biomed. Opt.* 11:024015.
147. Zhang, H. F.; Maslov, K.; Stoica, G.; Wang, L. V. 2006. Functional photoacoustic microscopy for high-resolution and noninvasive in vivo imaging. *Nat. Biotechnol.* 24:848–851.
148. Eghtedari, M. 2007. High sensitivity of in vivo detection of gold nanorods using a laser optoacoustic imaging system. *Nano Lett.* 7:1914–1918.
149. Yang, X.; Skrabalak, S. E.; Li, Z. Y.; Xia, Y.; Wang, L. V. 2007. Photoacoustic tomography of a rat cerebral cortex in vivo with Au nanocages as an optical contrast agent. *Nano Lett.* 7:3798–3802.

150. Zharov, V. P. 2007. Photoacoustic flow cytometry: Principle and application for real-time detection of circulating single nanoparticles, pathogens and contrast dyes in vivo. *J. Biomed. Opt.* 12:051503.

151. Zerda, A.; Zavaleta, C.; Keren, S.; Vaithilingam, S.; Bodapati, S.; Liu, Z.; Levi, J.; Ma, T.-J.; Oralkan, O.; Cheng, Z. 2008. Photoacoustic molecular imaging in living mice utilizing targeted carbon nanotubes. *Nat. Nanotechnol.* 3:557–562.

152. Bianco, A.; Hoebeke, J.; Godefroy, S.; Chaloin, O.; Pantarotto, D.; Briand, J.-P.; Muller, S.; Prato, M.; Partidos, C. D. 2005. Cationic carbon nanotubes bind to CpG oligodeoxynucleotides and enhance their immunostimulatory properties. *J. Am. Chem. Soc.* 127:58–59.

153. Singh, R.; Pantarotto, D.; McCarthy, D.; Chaloin, O.; Hoebeke, J.; Partidos, C. D.; Briand, J. P.; Prato, M.; Bianco, A.; Kostarelos, K. 2005. Binding and condensation of plasmid DNA onto functionalized carbon nanotubes: Toward the construction of nanotube-based gene delivery vectors. *J. Am. Chem. Soc.* 127:4388–4396.

154. Silverstein, S. C.; Steinman, R. M.; Cohn, Z. A. 1977. Endocytosis. *Annu. Rev. Biochem.* 46:669–722.

155. Vida, T. A.; Emr, S. D. 1995. A new vital stain for visualizing vacuolar membrane dynamics and endocytosis in yeast. *J. Cell Biol.* 128:779–792.

156. Mukherjee, S.; Ghosh, R. N.; Maxfield, F. R. 1997. Endocytosis. *Physiol. Rev.* 77:759–803.

157. Liu, Y.; Wu, D. C.; Zhang, W. D.; Jiang, X.; He, C. B.; Chung, T. S.; Goh, S. H.; Leong, K. W. 2005. Polyethylenimine-grafted multiwalled carbon nanotubes for secure noncovalent immobilization and efficient delivery of DNA. *Angew. Chem. Int. Ed.* 44:4782–4785.

158. Kam, N. W. S.; Liu, Z. A.; Dai, H. J. 2006. Carbon nanotubes as intracellular transporters for proteins and DNA: An investigation of the uptake mechanism and pathway. *Angew. Chem. Int. Ed.* 45:577–581.

159. Yang, S. T.; Guo, W.; Lin, Y.; Deng, X. Y.; Wang, H. F.; Sun, H. F.; Liu, Y. F.; et al. 2007. Biodistribution of pristine single-walled carbon nanotubes *in vivo*. *J. Phys. Chem. C* 111:17761–17764.

160. Cherukuri, P.; Gannon, C. J.; Leeuw, T. K.; Schmidt, H. K.; Smalley, R. E.; Curley, S. A.; Weisman, R. B. 2006. Mammalian pharmacokinetics of carbon nanotubes using intrinsic near-infrared fluorescence. *Proc. Natl. Acad. Sci. USA* 103:18882–18886.

161. Liu, Z.; Davis, C.; Cai, W.; He, L.; Chen, X.; Dai, H. 2008. Circulation and long-term fate of functionalized, biocompatible single-walled carbon nanotubes in mice probed by Raman spectroscopy. *Proc. Natl. Acad. Sci. USA* 105:1410–1415.

162. Liu, Z.; Cai, W. B.; He, L. N.; Nakayama, N.; Chen, K.; Sun, X. M.; Chen, X. Y.; Dai, H. J. 2007. *In vivo* biodistribution and highly efficient tumor targeting of carbon nanotubes in mice. *Nat. Nanotechnol.* 2:47–52.

163. Fernando, K. A. S.; Lin, Y.; Sun, Y. P. 2004. High aqueous solubility of functionalized single-walled carbon nanotubes. *Langmuir* 20:4777–4778.

164. Fernando, K. A. S.; Lin, Y.; Wang, W.; Cao, L.; Meziani, M. J.; Wang, X.; Veca, M. L.; et al. 2007. Diameter-selective fractionation of HiPco single-walled carbon nanotubes in repeated functionalization reactions. *J. Phys. Chem. C* 111:10254–10259.

165. Yang, S. T.; Fernando, K. A.; Liu, J. H.; Wang, J.; Sun, H. F.; Liu, Y.; Chen, M.; et al. 2008. Covalently PEGylated carbon nanotubes with stealth character *in vivo*. *Small* 4:940–944.

166. Singh, R.; Pantarotto, D.; Lacerda, L.; Pastorin, G.; Klumpp, C.; Prato, M.; Bianco, A.; Kostarelos, K. 2006. Tissue biodistribution and blood clearance rates of intravenously administered carbon nanotube radiotracers. *Proc. Nat. Acad. Sci. USA* 103:3357–3362.

167. Lacerda, L.; Soundararajan, A.; Singh, R.; Pastorin, G.; Al-Jamal, K. T.; Turton, J.; Frederik, P.; et al. 2008. Dynamic imaging of functionalized multi-walled carbon nanotube systemic circulation and urinary excretion. *Adv. Mater.* 20:225–230.

168. Deng, X. Y.; Yang, S. T.; Nie, H. Y.; Wang, H. F.; Liu, Y. F. 2008. A generally adoptable radiotracing method for tracking carbon nanotubes in animals. *Nanotechnology* 19:075101.

169. Balvavoine, F.; Schultz, P.; Richard, C.; Mallouh, V.; Ebbeson, T. W.; Mioskowski, C. 1999. Helical crystallization of proteins on carbon nanotubes: A first step towards the development of new biosensors. *Angew. Chem. Int. Ed.* 38:1912–1915.
170. Shim, M.; Kam, N. W. S.; Chen, R.; Li, Y.; Dai, H. 2002. Functionalization of carbon nanotubes for biocompatibility and biomolecular recognition. *Nano Lett.* 2:285–288.
171. Azamian, B. R.; Davis, J. J.; Coleman, K. S.; Bagshaw, C. B.; Green, M. L. H. 2002. Bioelectrochemical single-walled carbon nanotubes. *J. Am. Chem. Soc.* 124:12664–12665.
172. Chen, R. J.; Bangsaruntip, S.; Drouvalakis, K. A.; Kam, N. W. S.; Shim, M.; Li, Y. M.; Kim, W.; Utz, P. J.; Dai, H. J. 2003. Noncovalent functionalization of carbon nanotubes for highly specific electronic biosensors. *Proc. Natl. Acad. Sci. USA* 100:4984–4989.
173. Kam, N. W. S.; Dai, H. 2005. Carbon nanotubes as intracellular protein transporters: Generality and biological functionality. *J. Am. Chem. Soc.* 127:6021–6026.
174. Hussey, S. L.; Peterson, B. R. 2002. Efficient delivery of streptavidin to mammalian cells: Clathrin-mediated endocytosis regulated by a synthetic ligand. *J. Am. Chem. Soc.* 124:6265–6273.
175. Pantarotto, D.; Hoebeke, J.; Graff, R.; Partidos, C. D.; Briand, J.-P.; Prato, M.; Bianco, A. 2003. Synthesis, structural characterization, and immunological properties of carbon nanotubes functionalized with peptides. *J. Am. Chem. Soc.* 125:6160–6164.
176. Alekseev, O. M.; Richardson, R. T.; Alekseev, O.; O'Rand, M. G. 2009. Analysis of gene expression profiles in HeLa cells in response to overexpression or siRNA-mediated depletion of NASP. *Reprod. Biol. Endocrinol.* 7:45.
177. Graham, F. L.; van der Eb, A. J. 1973. A new technique for the assay of infectivity of human adenovirus 5 DNA. *Virology* 52:456–467.
178. Bacchetti, S.; Graham, F. 1977. Transfer of the gene for thymidine kinase to thymidine kinase-deficient human cells by purified herpes simplex viral DNA. *Proc. Natl. Acad. Sci. USA* 74:1590–1594.
179. Menuel, S.; Fontanay, S.; Clarot, I.; Duval, R. E.; Diez, L.; Marsura, A. 2008. Synthesis and complexation ability of a novel bis-(guanidinium)-tetrakis-(β-cyclodextrin) dendrimeric tetrapod as a potential gene delivery (DNA and siRNA) system. Study of cellular siRNA transfection. *Bioconjug. Chem.* 19:2357–2362.
180. Fischer, D.; von Harpe, A.; Kunath, K.; Petersen, H.; Li, Y. X.; Kissel, T. 2002. Copolymers of ethylene imine and N-(2-hydroxyethyl)-ethylene imine as tools to study effects of polymer structure on physicochemical and biological properties of DNA complexes. *Bioconjug. Chem.* 13:1124–1133.
181. Funhoff, A. M.; van Nostrum, C. F.; Lok, C. M.; Fretz, M. M.; Crommelin, D. J. A.; Hennink, W. E. 2004. Poly(3-guanidinopropyl methacrylate): A novel cationic polymer for gene delivery. *Bioconjug. Chem.* 15:1212–1220.
182. Zhang, X. Q.; Wang, X. L.; Huang, S. W.; Zhuo, R. X.; Liu, Z. L.; Mao, H. Q.; Leong, K. W. 2005. *In vitro* gene delivery using polyamidoamine dendrimers with a trimesyl core. *Biomacromolecules* 6:341–350.
183. Jen, C. P.; Chen, Y. H.; Fan, C. S.; Yeh, C. S.; Lin, Y. C.; Shieh, D. B.; Wu, C. L.; Chen, D. H.; Chou, C. H. 2004. A nonviral transfection approach in vitro: The design of Au nanoparticle vector joint with MEMS. *Langmuir* 20:1369–1374.
184. Kumar, M. N. R.; Sameti, M.; Mohapatra, S. S.; Kong, X.; Lockey, R. F.; Bakowsky, U.; Lindenblatt, G.; Schmidt, H.; Lehr, C. M. 2004. Cationic silica nanoparticles as gene carriers: Synthesis, characterization and transfection efficiency *in vitro* and *in vivo*. *J. Nanosci. Nanotechnol.* 4:876–881.
185. Vinogradov, S. V.; Batrakova, E. V.; Kabanov, A. V. 2004. Nanogels for oligonucleotide delivery to the brain. *Bioconjug. Chem.* 15:50–60.
186. Cui, D.; Tian, F.; Kong, Y.; Titushikin, I.; Gao, H. 2004. Effects of single-walled carbon nanotubes on the polymerase chain reaction. *Nanotechnology* 15:154–157.

187. Tsang, S. C.; Guo, Z.; Chen, Y. K.; Green, M. L. H.; Hill, H. A. O.; Hambley, T. W.; Sadler, P. J. 1997. Immobilization of platinated and iodinated oligonucleotides on carbon nanotubes. *Angew. Chem. Int. Ed.* 36:2198–2200.

188. Guo, Z.; Sadler, P. J.; Tsang, S. C. 1998. Immobilization and visualization of DNA and proteins on carbon nanotubes. *Adv. Mater.* 10:701–703.

189. Taft, B. J.; Lazareck, A. D.; Withey, G. D.; Yin, A.; Xu, J. M.; Kelley, S. O. 2004. Site-specific assembly of DNA and appended cargo on arrayed carbon nanotubes. *J. Am. Chem. Soc.* 126:12750–12751.

190. McKnight, T. E.; Melechko, A. V.; Griffin, G. D.; Guillorn, M. A.; Merkulov, V. I.; Serna, F.; Hensley, D. K.; et al. 2003. Intracellular integration of synthetic nanostructures with viable cells for controlled biochemical manipulation. *Nanotechnology* 14:551–556.

191. Nguyen, C. V.; Delzeit, L.; Cassell, A. M.; Li, J.; Han, J.; Meyyappan, M. 2002. Preparation of nucleic acid functionalized carbon nanotube arrays. *Nano Lett.* 2:1079–1081.

192. Li, J.; Ng, H. T.; Cassell, A.; Fan, W.; Chen, H.; Ye, Q.; Koehne, J.; Han, J.; Meyyappan, M. 2003. Carbon nanotube nanoelectrode array for ultrasensitive DNA detection. *Nano Lett.* 3:597–602.

193. Baker, S. E.; Cai, W.; Lasseter, T. L.; Weidkamp, K. P.; Hamers, R. J. 2002. Covalently bonded adducts of deoxyribonucleic acid (DNA) oligonucleotides with single-wall carbon nanotubes: Synthesis and hybridization. *Nano Lett.* 2:1413–1417.

194. Dwyer, C.; Guthold, M.; Falvo, M.; Washburn, S.; Superfine, R.; Erie, D. 2002. DNA-functionalized single-walled carbon nanotubes. *Nanotechnology* 13:601–604.

195. McKnight, T. E.; Melechko, A. V.; Hensley, D. K.; Mann, D. G. J.; Griffin, G. D.; Simpson, M. L. 2004. Tracking gene expression after DNA delivery using spatially indexed nanofiber arrays. *Nano Lett.* 4:1213–1219.

196. Boussif, O.; Lezoualc'h, F.; Zanta, M. A.; Mergny, M. D.; Scherman, D.; Demeneix, B.; Behr, J. P. 1995. A versatile vector for gene and oligonucleotide transfer into cells in culture and in vivo: Polyethylenimine. *Proc. Natl. Acad. Sci. USA* 92:7297–7301.

197. Gao, L. Z.; Nie, L.; Wang, T. H.; Qin, Y. J.; Guo, Z. X.; Yang, D. L.; Yan, X. Y. 2006. Carbon nanotube delivery of the GFP gene into mammalian cells. *ChemBioChem* 7:239–242.

198. Kam, N. W. S.; Liu, Z.; Dai, H. 2005. Functionalization of carbon nanotubes via cleavable disulfide bonds for efficient intracellular delivery of siRNA and potent gene silencing. *J. Am. Chem. Soc.* 127:12492–12493.

199. Liu, Z.; Winters, M.; Holodniy, M.; Dai, H. J. 2007. siRNA delivery into human T cells and primary cells with carbon nanotube transporters. *Angew. Chem. Int. Ed.* 46:2023–2027.

200. Langer, R. 1998. Drug delivery and targeting. *Nature* 392:5–10.

201. Moghimi, S. M.; Hunter, A. C.; Murray, J. C. 2001. Long-circulating and target-specific nanoparticles: Theory to practice. *Pharmacol. Rev.* 53:283–318.

202. Maeda, H.; Wu, J.; Sawa, T.; Matsumura, Y.; Hori, K. 2000. Tumor vascular permeability and the EPR effect in macromolecular therapeutics: A review. *J. Cont. Rel.* 65:271–284.

203. Gao, X. H.; Cui, Y. Y.; Levenson, R. M.; Chung, L. W. K.; Nie, S. M. 2004. *In vivo* cancer targeting and imaging with semiconductor quantum dots. *Nat. Biotechnol.* 22:969–976.

204. Iyer, A. K.; Khaled, G.; Fang, J.; Maeda, H. 2006. Exploiting the enhanced permeability and retention effect for tumor targeting. *Drug Discov. Today* 11:812–818.

205. Bartlett, D. W.; Su, H.; Hildebrandt, I. J.; Weber, W. A.; Davis, M. E. 2007. Impact of tumor-specific targeting on the biodistribution and efficacy of siRNA nanoparticles measured by multimodality in vivo imaging. *Proc. Natl. Acad. Sci. USA* 104:15549–15554.

206. Kam, N. W. S.; O'Connell, M.; Wisdom, J. A.; Dai, H. 2005. Carbon nanotubes as multifunctional biological transporters and near-infrared agents for selective cancer cell destruction. *Proc. Natl. Acad. Sci. USA* 102:11600–11605.

207. Chakravarty, P.; Marches, R.; Zimmerman, N. S.; Swafford, A. D.; Bajaj, P.; Musselman, I. H.; Pantano, P.; Draper, R. K.; Vitetta, E. S. 2008. Thermal ablation of tumor cells with antibody-functionalized single-walled carbon nanotubes. *Proc. Natl. Acad. Sci. USA* 105:8697–8702.

208. Zitzmann, S.; Ehemann, V.; Manfred, S. 2002. Arginine–glycine–aspartic acid (RGD)-peptide binds to both tumor and tumor-endothelial cells *in vivo*. *Cancer Res.* 62:5139–5143.

209. Liu, Z.; Cai, W. B.; He, L. N.; Nakayama, N.; Chen, K.; Sun, X. M.; Chen, X. Y.; Dai, H. J. 2007. *In vivo* biodistribution and highly efficient tumor targeting of carbon nanotubes in mice. *Nat. Nanotechnol.* 2:47–52.

210. McDevitt, M. R.; Chattopadhyay, D.; Kappel, B. J.; Jaggi, J. S.; Schiffman, S. R.; Antczak, C.; Njardarson, J. T.; Brentjens, R.; Scheinberg, D. A. 2007. Tumor targeting with antibody-functionalized, radiolabeled carbon nanotubes. *J. Nucl. Med.* 48:1180–1189.

211. Morin, G. B. 1989. The human telomere terminal transferase enzyme is a ribonucleoprotein that synthesizes TTAGGG repeats. *Cell* 59:521–529.

212. Sontheimer, E. J. 2005. Assembly and function of RNA silencing complexes. *Nat. Rev. Mol. Cell Biol.* 6:127–138.

213. Zhang, Z. H.; Yang, X. Y.; Zhang, Y.; Zeng, B.; Wang, Z. J.; Zhu, T. H.; Roden, R. B. S.; Chen, Y. S.; Yang, R. C. 2006. Delivery of telomerase reverse transcriptase small interfering RNA in complex with positively charged single-walled carbon nanotubes suppresses tumor growth. *Clin. Cancer Res.* 12:4933–4939.

214. Liu, Z.; Chen, K.; Davis, C.; Sherlock, S.; Cao, Q.; Chen, X.; Dai, H. 2008. Drug delivery with carbon nanotubes for *in vivo* cancer treatment. *Cancer Res.* 68:6652–6660.

215. Chen, J.; Chen, S.; Zhao, X.; Kuznetsova, L. V.; Wong, S. S.; Ojima, I. 2008. Functionalized single-walled carbon nanotubes as rationally designed vehicles for tumor-targeted drug delivery. *J. Am. Chem. Soc.* 130:16778–16785.

216. Barnes, K. R.; Kutikov, A.; Lippard, S. J. 2004. Synthesis, characterization, and cytotoxicity of a series of estrogen-tethered platinum(IV) complexes. *Chem. Biol.* 11:557–564.

217. Feazell, R. P.; Nakayama-Ratchford, N.; Dai, H.; Lippard, S. J. 2007. Soluble single-walled carbon nanotubes as longboat delivery systems for platinum(IV) anticancer drug design. *J. Am. Chem. Soc.* 129:8438–8349.

218. Dhar, S.; Liu, Z.; Thomale, J.; Dai, H.; Lippard, S. J. 2008. Targeted single-wall carbon nanotube-mediated Pt(IV) prodrug delivery using folate as a homing device. *J. Am. Chem. Soc.* 130:11467–11476.

219. Vreeburg, G.; Stell, P.; Holding, J.; Lindup, W. 1992. Cisplatin-albumin complex for treatment of cancer of the head and neck. *J. Laryngol. Otol.* 106:832–833.

220. Jongh, F.; Veen, R.; Veltman, S.; Wit, R.; Burg, M.; Bent, M.; Planting, A.; Graveland, W.; Stoter, G.; Verweij, J. 2003. Weekly high-dose cisplatin is a feasible treatment option: Analysis on prognostic factors for toxicity in 400 patients. *Br. J. Cancer* 88:1199–1206.

221. Bhirde, A. A.; Patel, V.; Gavard, J.; Zhang, G.; Sousa, A. A.; Masedunskas, A.; Leapman, R. D.; Weigert, R.; Gutkind, J. S.; James, F.; Rusling, J. F. 2009. Targeted killing of cancer cells *in vivo* and *in vitro* with EGF-directed carbon nanotube-based drug delivery. *ACS Nano* 3:307–316.

222. Zotchev, S. B. 2003. Polyene macrolide antibiotics and their applications in human therapy. *Curr. Med. Chem.* 10:211–223.

223. Zumbuehl, A.; Jeannerat, D.; Martin, S. E.; Sohrmann, M.; Stano, P.; Vigassy, T.; Clark, D. D.; et al. 2004. An amphotericin B-fluorescein conjugate as a powerful probe for biochemical studies of the membrane. *Angew. Chem. Int. Ed.* 43:5181–5185.

224. Wu, W.; Wieckowski, S.; Pastorin, G.; Benincasa, M.; Klumpp, C.; Briand, J. P.; Gennaro, R.; Prato, M.; Bianco, A. 2005. Targeted delivery of amphotericin B to cells by using functionalized carbon nanotubes. *Angew. Chem. Int. Ed.* 44:6358–6362.

6 Biocatalytic Nanosystems

Jaehong Lim and Su Seong Lee
Institute of Bioengineering and Nanotechnology

CONTENTS

6.1 INTRODUCTION

Enzymes endowed by nature are ubiquitous and versatile as catalysts that span some nanometers in size. Their paramount activity and specificity under mild and physiologically friendly conditions are most beneficial, which allow them to be applicable to various fields, including synthesis of chemicals and pharmaceuticals, integration to biosensors, biofuel cells, and many others. However, enzymes are inherently proteins that are sensitive, unstable, and incompatible in most cases with organic media. In order to make them more useful in industrial processes, a tremendous number of efforts has been dedicated to circumventing the drawbacks in stability and compatibility with various organic media. One traditional strategy is to immobilize them on solid supports comprising inorganic or organic materials. Through immobilization, their solubility and stability can be significantly improved and the catalytic reactions can be more precisely controlled to meet high standards and tricky regulations in industry. An additional advantage of their immobilization includes facile recovery of the catalytic system from the reaction mixture at the end of the reactions so that the recovered exorbitant enzymes can be reused in the next run. Enzyme immobilization was first reported on inorganic support materials through covalent linkage in 1969.[1] Obviously, it is the most important factor to consider for enzyme immobilization that support materials should be chemically and mechanically benign and stable in their repeated usage. To date, a number of synthetic scaffolds and support materials have been adopted to immobilize enzymes for various enzymatic reactions and other applications. The representative examples include gels,[2,3] macromolecules,[4–6] nanoparticles, nanoporous materials, carbon nanotubes (CNTs), nanofibers, microspheres,[7–9] and surface-anchored molecules.[10–14] The size matters in the case of porous material so that the pores should be large enough for substrates to diffuse freely throughout the particles.

In this chapter, various nanomaterials are explored in enzyme immobilizations for a variety of applications.

6.2　NANOMATERIALS FOR BIOCATALYST IMMOBILIZATION

Many types of nano-based advanced materials with unique nanostructures have been developed as promising resources for solid support, associated with the seminal progress of nanoscience since the 1990s. Nanoparticles, nanofibers, nanotubes, and nanoporous (mesoporous) materials are examples. Initially, enzymes were linked onto nanomaterials by using conventional immobilization methods such as simple physical adsorption, entrapment, and covalent bond formation. Toward immobilizing the enzymes, a suitable nanomaterial can be selected from a pool of nanomaterials depending on each application. The most impacting advantage of nanomaterials in most applications is their high surface area-to-volume ratio, which gives rise to highly facilitated enzyme loading. It can lead to enhanced enzymatic activity per unit mass or volume compared to both free enzymes and conventional supported enzymatic systems that resort to non-nanomaterials. It is therefore natural that the immobilization of enzymes on nanomaterials should attract wide interest for both fundamental and applied researches.[15]

Both physical and chemical characteristics are important in selecting the support materials in conjugation with those of enzymes to be immobilized. These characteristics include nanostructures such as particle shape, pore size and structure, and surface properties such as hydrophobicity, hydrophilicity, and charges. Inorganic materials are well known to have strong mechanical strength, high chemical resistance, and thermal stability. Various inorganic nanomaterials are available for the immobilization of enzymes along with significant progress in nanosciences. Organic nanomaterials such as polymeric materials have also been drawing broad attention as support materials due to their facile functionalization for enzyme immobilization. Recently, polymeric materials were used to make novel nanocomposites in combination with inorganic nanomaterials. To date, various novel strategies have been introduced for the immobilization of enzymes on nanomaterials toward the development of novel nano-enzymatic systems.

6.2.1　Nanoparticle Supports

Metallic and semiconductor nanoparticles are comparable in size to proteins, antibodies, and DNA, which makes them suitable for the formation of novel hybrid materials. It is thus natural to come up with an idea to integrate nanoparticles and biomolecules, hoping to create unique combined properties. The first use of nanoparticles in the immobilization of biomolecules traces back to the early 1980s[16–18] and a substantial amount of effort has been devoted so far to the development of nanoparticle–biomolecule conjugates for such applications as nano-enzymatic systems, biosensors, and nanodevices. The immobilization of enzymes on nanoparticles has particular advantages: (1) high enzyme loading due to the high surface area of nanoparticles, (2) no limitations in internal diffusion due to the use of exposed surface for immobilization, (3) enhancement of catalytic activity and stability,[19,20] and (4) changes in substrate specificity[21] compared to free enzymes as well as conventional supported enzymes. Whereas enzymes require high ionic strength and neutral pH for good catalytic viability,[22,23] nanoparticles will tend to aggregate under these conditions, resulting in the loss of their unique properties.[24] Interestingly, it is reported that enzymes and nanoparticles can be integrated to behave so synergistically that the former can improve the colloidal stability of the latter,[25] while the latter can enhance the stability of the former in enzyme–nanoparticle conjugates.[26] Wu and coworkers[27] studied how the size of nanoparticles can affect the catalytic behavior of enzyme–nanoparticle conjugates. The authors developed a shielding model to explain the correlation between the size effects and the kinetic responses. They found that the size of enzyme–nanoparticle conjugates is a controllable and efficient factor for adjusting the enzymatic activity. Representative examples of nanoparticles as enzyme support materials are introduced in this section.

Silica nanoparticles (SNPs) are highly useful materials for the immobilization of enzymes due to the abundance of reactive silanol groups on their surface, which can be easily functionalized by various compounds such as organosilanes. Kim and coworkers[28,29] demonstrated a successful immobilization on SNPs using an enzyme, *Mucor javanicus* lipase. First, SNPs were modified with ethylenediamine. Subsequently, glutaraldehyde and 1,4-phenylene diisothiocyanate were attached, resulting in remarkably increased loading of lipase. The immobilized lipase retained a high level of catalytic activity over a wide range of pH and showed an enhanced thermal stability compared to the free lipase. Glucose oxidase (GO_x) was successfully immobilized on SNPs by physical entrapment within photopolymerized hydrogels prepared from two different molecular weights (MWs; 575 and 8000 Da) of polyethylene glycol (PEG).[30] The hydrogel entrapment led to decrease in reaction rates and increase in apparent K_m values of SNP-immobilized GO_x. The hydrogel from the higher MW PEG minimized these negative effects due to enhanced mass transfer owing to higher water content and larger mesh size, which resulted in 100 times faster reaction than the hydrogel from the lower PEG. The long-term stability was greatly enhanced compared to non-entrapped SNP-immobilized GO_x and entrapped GO_x without SNP.

Ansari and coworkers[31,32] utilized ZnO nanoparticles (ZnO NPs) for the immobilization of *Aspergillus oryzae* β-galactosidase by simple bioaffinity-based adsorption. For the bioaffinity-based adsorption, concanavalin A (Con A) was attached to the ZnO NPs. The enzyme immobilized onto Con A-layered ZnO NP retained 84% of the enzymatic activity. The resulting immobilized enzyme retained 60% of activity at 60°C for 2 h, while the free enzyme lost 81% of activity under similar experimental conditions. In addition, the immobilized enzyme retained more than 80% of activity even after six repeated runs. The same authors also reported that ZnO NP-immobilized β-galactosidase showed 85% of activity, while native ZnO kept only 60% of β-galactosidase upon immobilization.[33] The ZnO NP-immobilized enzyme exhibited much greater thermal, storage, and operational stability compared to the native ZnO-immobilized enzyme. The NP-immobilized β-galactosidase also hydrolyzed a larger amount of lactose in milk than the native ZnO-immobilized β-galactosidase.

Gold nanoparticles (AuNPs) and magnetic nanoparticles (MNPs) are the two types of nanoparticles that have been most frequently used for enzyme immobilization. AuNPs have a high affinity for most biomolecules because amine groups[19,34,35] and cysteine residues in enzymes enable them to bind strongly to AuNPs, and the surface of gold is easily modified with compounds such as thiol or dithiocarbamate groups. The easy functionalization of AuNPs with thiol-containing compounds facilitates the immobilization of enzymes through covalent linkage, physical adsorption, and electrostatic interactions.[20,36–40] Enzymes could be immobilized on AuNPs without any surface modification, resulting in improved stability and significantly enhanced catalytic activity.[40] However, it is not easy to recycle the enzyme–AuNP conjugates from the reaction medium due to their physical characteristics even by a prolonged use of ultracentrifugation.[19,34,35] This problem can be overcome by tethering AuNPs to relatively larger microsized materials.[41] Phadtare and coworkers[10] immobilized pepsin on polyurethane microsphere–AuNP conjugates resulting in enhanced storage time and thermal stability. This approach also facilitated the separation of the immobilized enzyme from the reaction medium. The same authors reported the immobilization of fungal protease on AuNPs attached to amine-functionalized zeolite microspheres.[41] The assembly of AuNPs on the zeolite surface led to a core–shell structure and the relatively larger particles facilitated their separation from the reaction medium. It has also shown enhanced stability against pH and temperature. Xu and coworkers[42] assembled AuNPs on submicron-sized poly(N-isopropylacrylamide)/polyethyleneimine (PEI) core–shell microgels for the immobilization of horseradish peroxidase (HRP) and urease. The amino groups on the PEI were utilized to interact with AuNPs for the assembly. The assembled particles could be easily recovered from the reaction medium for reuse. The immobilized enzyme showed enhanced catalytic activity at lower enzyme concentration compared to the free analog. In addition, the HRP/nanogold/microgel systems showed higher activity at a variable range of pH and temperature, as well as improved storage stability.

One of the drawbacks of using nanoparticles for enzyme immobilization is that their dispersion in reaction media and recovery after the reaction are often troublesome as mentioned in AuNP-immobilized enzymes. Such small nanoparticles are nearly impossible to separate from a reaction mixture by conventional methods such as filtration. Efficient separation can be achieved by using MNPs that have been popularly used in the immobilization of various catalysts such as organometallic catalysts and biocatalysts due to the beneficial superparamagnetic property, which facilitates the recovery of supported catalysts from the reaction medium by simply applying a magnet on completing the reaction. MNPs also have an advantage of lower mass transfer resistance and less fouling.[43] The first example of using a magnetic support was reported by Matsunaga and coworkers in 1987.[17] MNPs with a diameter of ~100 nm were extracted from magnetotactic bacteria and used for the immobilization of an enzyme, GO_x. The loading amount of the enzyme was 25–80 times higher than that of bulk magnetite due to the much smaller size of the nanoparticles, and the enzymatic activity was enhanced by a factor of 30. In a recycling test, the catalyst retained 80% of the initial activity after five repeated runs. The same authors also demonstrated the use of synthetic Fe_3O_4 nanoparticles (10–15 nm in diameter), synthesized by a precipitation method in an aqueous medium for the immobilization of thermolysin.[44] These immobilized nanoparticles have been successfully recovered by an external magnetic field. To date, MNPs have been used to immobilize a vast number of enzymes including lipase, glucoamylase, amylase, penicillin G acylase, and GO_x.[45–52] Table 6.1 summarizes representative examples of MNP-supported enzymes. The use of MNPs as a support material for enzymatic reactions clearly showed the advantages in association with facile recovery and reuse of the catalytic system.

Semiconductor quantum dots (QDs) have unique properties such as size-dependent photophysical properties, excitation–emission features, large Stokes shifts, and outstanding photostability.[64–67] Nanosized enzymes and QDs have been expected to yield synergistically novel hybrid nanomaterials through a covalent conjugation. These conjugates aim to combine the unique optical and electrical properties of QDs with the specificity and catalytic abilities of enzymes for bioanalytical applications. There has been a tremendous number of studies on the utilization of QDs in biosensing and bioimaging in recent years.[68,69]

Another potential solid support in immobilizing an enzyme for biosensor applications is zirconia nanoparticles in conjunction with their high surface area; high thermal, mechanical, and chemical resistance; and excellent biocompatibility.[70–72] Several studies are found in the literature on adopting zirconia nanoparticles with or without

TABLE 6.1
Representative Examples of Enzymes Immobilized on MNPs

Enzyme	Enzyme Type	Support	Reference
Glucose oxidase	Oxidase	Fe_3O_4 from magnetotactic bacteria (100 nm)	17
Glucose oxidase, horseradish peroxidase	Oxidoreductase	Polystyrene/F_3O_4 composite	53
D-Amino acid oxidase	Oxidase	F_3O_4 (Cu^{2+} iminodiacetic acid surface)	54
D-Amino acid oxidase	Oxidase	F_3O_4 (20 nm, aldehyde surface)	55
Cholesterol oxidase	Oxidase	γ-Fe_2O_3 (10–20 nm)/SiO_2, aldehyde surface	56
Lipase	Esterase	γ-Fe_2O_3 (20 ± 10 nm)	57
Lipase (*Candida rugosa*)	Esterase	Fe_3O_4 (20 nm)	58
Lipase (*C. rugosa*)	Esterase	Fe_3O_4 (8–10 nm)/ionic liquid	59
Lipase (*C. rugosa*)	Esterase	Fe_3O_4 sol–gel	60
Lipase (*Arthrobacter* sp.)	Esterase	Fe_3O_4/SiO_2 sol–gel	61
Lipase (*Serratia marcescens*)	Esterase	Fe_3O_4 (50 nm)	62
Thermolysin	Hydrolase	Fe_3O_4 (10–15 nm)	51
β-Lactamase		Silica-coated γ-Fe_2O_3/Fe_3O_4 (8–13 nm)	63

surface functionalization. For example, Huckel and coworkers[73] reported the covalent immobilization of enzymes on a porous zirconia with its surface functionalized with 3-isothiocyanatopropyltriethoxysilane. By Bellezza and coworkers,[74] myoglobin was immobilized on phosphate and phosphonate-grafted zirconia nanoparticles through a physical adsorption approach. Reshmi and coworkers[75] immobilized amylase on zirconia through physical adsorption without surface modification, and Chen and coworkers[76] produced highly active, enantioselective, and reusable enzymes by immobilizing lipases on hydrophobically modified zirconia nanoparticles through physical adsorption.

Recently, nanodiamonds have attracted a broad range of interest as a potential material for developing various biological and analytical platform technologies.[77] Some studies have been performed by taking advantage of their hardness, durability, and biocompatibility.[78,79] Chang and coworkers[80] reported noncovalent immobilization of cytochrome *e* on nanodiamonds of variable sizes. Wei and coworkers[81] immobilized trypsin on detonation nanodiamond (3–10 nm) for highly efficient proteolysis. Peptide-*N*-glycosidase F (PNGase F) immobilized on detonation nanodiamonds exhibited faster sequential glycosidase digestion of glycopeptides.

As an alternative approach, nanoparticles can be assembled on zeolite or mesoporous materials. For example, pepsin and fungal protease were immobilized on AuNPs assembled on amine-functionalized zeolites. This approach enhanced thermal and pH stability of these enzymes.[46,82] Vinoba and coworkers[83] reported the immobilization of human carbonic anhydrase (hCA) on AuNPs assembled on amine/thiol-functionalized mesoporous Santa Barbara Amorphous-15 (SBA-15) in a way to capture carbon dioxide. The zeta potentials of the resulting materials indicated that the electronegative charges on Au/3-aminopropyltriethoxysilane (APTES)/SBA-15 and Au/3-mercaptopropyltriethoxysilane (MPTES)/SBA-15 were essential for electrostatic interactions with hCA. Compared to bare SBA-15, the loading amount of hCA on Au/SBA-15 was significantly higher due to the much facilitated bioconjugation of enzymes to AuNPs. In addition, the biocatalytic activities of hCA/Au/APTES/SBA-15 and hCA/Au/MPTES/SBA-15 for hydrolysis of *para*-nitrophenyl acetate showed enhanced catalytic activities in association with high K_m and K_{cat}/K_m values compared to HCA/SBA-15.

Dendritic polymers are ideal nanoparticles[84,85] for the immobilization of enzymes due to their unique chemical nature.[86,87] They have numerous surface functional groups, which facilitate high loading of enzymes. More importantly, the immobilized enzymes are fully accessible to reaction substrates. Ge and coworkers[88] reported the immobilization of lipase on dendritic aromatic polyamides that were synthesized from *p*-phenylenediamine and trimesic acid at up to 5–6 of enzyme to polymer molar ratio. The Michaelis–Menten constant K_m of the immobilized lipase was identical to that of its native counterpart, but the V_{max} was 20% higher, indicating the existence of an interfacial activation effect.[89] In addition, lipase immobilized onto the dendritic polymer exhibited significantly enhanced stability against high temperatures and organic solvents. This phenomenon seems to originate from the abundance of hydrophilic carboxylic acid groups on the polymer that create a favorable microenvironment for lipase to stay intact.

Polymeric nanoparticles are also good support materials for enzyme immobilizations due to their easy functionalization. Several groups reported a one-step method to immobilize cellulase on well-defined polymer, polymethyl methacrylate (PMMA).[90] The resulting catalyst consisted of a PMMA core and cellulase shell. The particle formation was strongly influenced by pH and cellulose-to-methyl methacrylate (MMA) weight ratio. Through optimizing the reaction conditions, spherical core–shell nanoparticles with a uniform coating of cellulase on the PMMA core were successfully produced. The diameter of the nanoparticles falls in the range of 80–120 nm with narrow size distribution, and the loading amount of cellulase was as high as 56 mg/g of PMMA. The cellulase on core–shell nanoenzyme particles showed improved thermal stability and extremely high catalytic activity at a broader range of pH compared to free cellulase. Eldin and coworkers[91] reported the synthesis of poly-acrylonitrile-co-MMA (PAN-co-MMA) nanospheres by a precipitation polymerization technique and then functionalization of PAN-co-MMA nanospheres by the reaction with ethylenediamine. The resulting nanospheres were used for the immobilization of β-galactosidase by covalent bonding with glutaraldehyde. The immobilized enzyme was found to have enhanced operational, thermal, and storage stabilities. Miletic and coworkers[92] reported the immobilization of lipase on polystyrene (PS) nanoparticles. The authors observed that the catalytic activity of the immobilized enzyme was significantly enhanced compared to free enzyme. Watanabe and coworkers[93] prepared polymer nanoparticles by combining a phospholipid polymer shell with a PS core. These nanoparticles were used for the immobilization of acetylcholinesterase, choline oxidase, and HRP-labeled IgG to facilitate sequential enzymatic reactions. Lipolytic enzymes were immobilized by Palocci and coworkers[94] on nanostructured PS and PMMA using hydrophobic interactions between enzymes and support materials. The immobilized lipases exhibited considerably improved activity and selectivity compared to lipases immobilized on non-nanostructured same support materials.

6.2.2 Nanofibers and Nanotubes

Nanofibers are one-dimensional nanomaterials, which include polymeric nanofibers and carbon nanofibers.[95] They have a high surface area-to-volume ratio, representing approximately two-thirds of that of nanoparticles of the same diameter based on an equal amount of material. Nanofibers have nevertheless many competitive advantages over nanoparticles. They are much easier to produce and handle. They can be applied in various forms such as coils, sheets, and dispersed fibers, and are easily attached to the surface of other materials or blended with them. These properties can offer more flexibility in designing bioreactors.[96] Jia and coworkers[95] reported the immobilization of α-chymotrypsin onto PS nanofibers 120 nm in diameter. While the immobilized enzyme retained 65% of its initial hydrolytic activity, the half-life of the immobilized enzyme in anhydrous methanol was enhanced 18-fold at 22°C. It is noteworthy that the transesterification activity of the immobilized enzyme was 5670-fold higher than that of the native enzyme in isooctane. This enhanced performance can be attributed to the facilitated transfer of hydrophobic substrates through the hydrophobic and porous architecture of the PS nanofiber. The glutaraldehyde-cross-linked α-chymotrypsin aggregates covalently attached to the PS nanofiber showed a ninefold increased activity compared to that obtained by coating a single layer of α-chymotrypsin.[97] An and coworkers[98] reported the immobilization of lipase on electrospun PS-poly(styrene-co-maleic anhydride) (PS-PSMA) nanofibers through an enzyme precipitate coating method. The coating was accomplished by a three-step process, which comprises covalent attachment, precipitation, and cross-linking of precipitated enzymes. Han and coworkers[99] utilized a coaxial electrospinning technique to prepare nanofibers that embed stabilized enzymes. The resulting core/sheath fibers contain diisopropylfluorophosphatase (DFPase) in the sheath and polymer in the core, which can be utilized for the production of mats and fabrics to decontaminate hazardous chemicals and protect people and equipments. Ghosh and coworkers[100] used polyaniline nanofiber for the immobilization of anti-leukemia enzyme L-asparaginase. The immobilized enzyme exhibited enhanced thermal and pH stability compared to free enzyme.

Among the various carbon nanomaterials, CNTs are one of the most popular materials for biological applications. CNTs are well-ordered and hollow graphitic nanomaterials with a high aspect ratio. Their length falls in the range of a few hundred nanometers to some micrometers with a few nanometers diameter. Asuri and coworkers[7] reported the immobilization of soybean protein peroxidase onto single-walled carbon nanotubes (SWNTs) by physical adsorption. The immobilized peroxidase was generated at the aqueous–organic interface in the presence of surfactants. The enzymatic activity was 3 times higher due to the facilitated mass transport in the biphasic system compared to the native enzyme. CNTs are more important emerging materials in the field of enzymatic biofuel cells, in conjunction with their large specific surface, excellent biocompatibility, antifouling properties, and high conductivity. Another example of immobilizing alkyl hydroperoxide reductase on functionalized SWNTs was reported by Wang and coworkers.[101] The SWNTs were modified with nitrilotriacetate group terminated with Co^{2+}, which was used for the noncovalent immobilization of His-tagged enzymes. The immobilized alkyl hydroperoxide reductase systems exhibited ~87% of the native enzymatic activity.

Dendrimer molecules can be used to modify CNTs for the immobilization of enzymes. Zhang and coworkers[102] used dendrimer-modified CNTs to immobilize trypsin for a novel on-plate digestion in combination with matrix-assisted laser desorption/ionization mass spectrometry (MALDI-MS). This system exhibits excellent digestion performance in a short period of time. Zhao and coworkers[103] reported the immobilization of glucoamylase on dendrimer-functionalized magnetic CNTs. In their studies, PAMAM was grafted on the surface of the nanotube and its amine functional groups were utilized for the enzyme immobilization through adsorption and covalent bond or metal–ion affinity interactions. Table 6.2 represents a few examples of enzymes immobilized on nanofibers or nanotubes.

TABLE 6.2
Several Examples for Enzymes Immobilized on Nanofibers and Nanotubes

Enzyme	Support	Immobilization Method	Reference
α-Chymotrypsin	Polystyrene nanofibers	Covalent	96
α-Chymotrypsin	Polystyrene nanofibers	Covalent, glutaraldehyde coupling of enzyme aggregates	97
Lipase	Peptide nanotube	Physical adsorption	104
Peroxidase	Single-walled carbon nanotube	Physical adsorption in the presence of surfactant	7

6.2.3 Nanoporous Materials

Toward enzyme immobilizations, silica gel is obviously one of the most popular solid supports due to its reactive surface silanol groups. These silanol groups can be easily functionalized for facile enzyme immobilization. However, the traditional silica gels suffer from the small pore size and non-open pore structure responsible for lower activity than free enzymes.

Since Mobil research group discovered the M41S family of mesoporous silicates (MPS), there have been numerous studies on mesoporous materials. Unlike sol–gel silica materials, mesoporous silicas have tunable and uniform pore size, high surface area with easy functionalization, and restricted nanospaces for enzyme immobilization. They possess a narrow distribution of pore size in the range of 2–30 nm. Table 6.3 shows various mesoporous silica materials that have been utilized for enzyme immobilization. The traditional mesoporous materials such as activated carbon or zeolites have already been utilized as a support material for the immobilization of enzymes. The resulting supported enzymes showed significantly improved stability presumably due to the confinement effect within nanopores with comparable size.

MPS materials are drawing a lot of attention in the immobilization of enzymes due to easy control of pore size as well as the high surface area as mentioned above. They are available in different pore size and shape. These pores can be further tailor-made and their surface can be easily functionalized with various organosilanes. Their well-defined pore structure and connectivity are advantageous for well-designed immobilization. It is important to select a suitable MPS with an appropriate pore size, surface properties (charges, hydrophilicity/hydrophobicity, surface functional

TABLE 6.3
A Summary of Typical Mesoporous Silica Materials for Enzyme Immobilization

Mesoporous Silica	Pore Structure	Pore Diameter (nm)	Reference
MCM-41	2D hexagonal, channel	2–10	105
MCM-48	Bicontinuous	2–4	106
FSM-16	2D hexagonal, channel	4	107
SBA-1	3D cubic mesostructure	2–3	108
SBA-15	2D hexagonal, channel	5–30	109
SBA-16	Spherical cages	5–30	110
FDU-12	3D cage	10–15	111
MCF	Cellular foam	10–50	112
HMS	Disordered mesostructure	2–10	113
MSU-X	Disordered mesostructure	2–15	114
IBN-X	Nanoparticle with nanopores	5–20	115
PMOs	2D/3D hexagonal	2–20	116
SMS	Sponge-like	3.3–4.7	117
BMS	Bimodal	10–40	118
Sibunit	Mesoporous carbon	18	119

groups), and spatial structure for effective immobilization of a target enzyme with specific molecular size, shape, and surface properties. In addition, MPS can facilitate mass transport of substrates and products through the rigid, open, and large pores.

Diaz and coworkers[120] reported for the first time on the immobilization of globular proteins such as cytochrome *c*, papain, and trypsin on MCM-41 in 1996. In most cases, time-dependent loss of enzymatic activity is closely related to conformational changes of the enzymes. Confining biocatalysts in nanopores of comparable size is expected to enhance the stability of enzymes in nanopores. These MPS materials have been utilized for better supported enzyme systems in combination with other immobilization methods. To date a variety of enzymes have been immobilized on many kinds of mesoporous materials. Table 6.4 lists up the examples of enzymes immobilized on mesoporous materials.

TABLE 6.4
Examples of Enzymes Immobilized on Mesoporous Materials

Enzyme	Mesoporous Materials	References
α-Amylase	MCM-41, MCF, SBA-15	121
Carbonic anhydrase	Modified MSN	122
Catalase	SBA-15	123
Cellulase	MSN, modified MSN	124
Cellulase	Modified FDU-12	125
Chloroperoxidase	SBA-16	126
Chloroperoxidase	SBA-15, SBA-16, MCM-41, AlMCM-41	127, 128
Chloroperoxidase, glucose oxidase	Modified SBA-15	129, 130
Chloroperoxidase	MCF	131
Conalbumin, cyctochrome *c*, β-lactoglobulin, myoglobin, ovalbumin, trypsin	SBA-15, thiol-modified SBA-15	132
Conalbumin	Modified MCF	133
Cytochrome *c*, trypsin, papain, HRP	MCM-41	120
Cytochrome *c*	MCM-48, SBA-15, Nb-TMS-1, Nb-TMS-4	134, 135
Cytochrome *c*	MCM-41, MPS-127	136–139
Cytochrome *c*	MCM-41, AlMCM-41, SBA-15, AlSBA-15. CMK-1, CMK-2, CMK-3	140, 141
Cytochrome *c*	Modified IBN4	142
Cytochrome *c*	Modified SBA-15	143
Cytochrome *c*, xylanase	SBA-15, PMO	144
Deoxyriboaldolase	Interparticle pore-type mesoporous silica (IMS)	145
Glucoamylase, invertase	Modified MCF	146
HRP, subtilisin Carlsberg	FSM-16, MCM-41, SBA-15	147, 148
HRP/anti-human IgG	Mesocellular carbon foam (MSU-F-C)	142
HRP	SBA-15	149
Human carbonic anhydrase	Modified SBA-15	150

(Continued)

TABLE 6.4 (continued)
Examples of Enzymes Immobilized on Mesoporous Materials

Enzyme	Mesoporous Materials	References
Human carbonic anhydrase	Gold nanoparticle assembled onto functionalized SBA-15	83
Laccase	Magnetic mesoporous silica spheres	151
Laccase	Magnetic mesoporous silica nanoparticles	152
Lipase	MTS	153
Lipase	Magnetic MCF	154
Lipase	FDU-12, KIT-6, SBA-16	155
Lipase	Modified commercial mesoporous silica	156
Lipase	MCM-41, sponge mesoposous silicas (SMS)	117
Lipase	Modified MCF	157
Lysozyme, trypsin	MCM-41, SBA-15	158–160
Lysozyme	Modified SBA-15	161
Lysozyme	MCM-41, SBA-15, AlMCM-41, AlSBA-15	162
Lysozyme	CMK-1, CMK-3	163
Microperoxidase-11	Mesoporous metal-organic frame work (MOE)	164
Organophosphorus hydrolase	Modified SBA-15	129
Penicillin acylase	MCM-41	165
Penicillin acylase	Modified SBA-15, KIT-6	166
Penicillin G acylase	SBA-15, MCF, modified SBA-15 and MCF	167
Porcine pancreatic lipase	SBA-15	168
Porcine pancreatic lipase	Modified short rod-shaped mesoporous silica (SRSMS)	169
Porcine pepsin	SBA-15	170
RNase A	MCM-48	171
Serine protease	Mesoporous carbon gel	172
Soybean peroxidase	Mesoporous ZnS nanorattles	167
Subtilisin	Mesoporous silica nanoparticle (MSN)	173
Superoxide dismutase	Modified KIT-6	174
Thrombin	MCF	175
Trypsin	MCM-41, MCF	176
Trypsin	Modified MCM-41	177
Bovine serum albumin	AlMCM-41	178
Urease	MCM-41	179

6.2.4 IMMOBILIZATION METHODS

Enzymes can be immobilized on nanomaterials by using conventional methods that have been used for enzyme immobilization on conventional solid support materials. Figure 6.1 illustrates the representative methods that enzyme immobilization on nanomaterials is based on. The interactions between enzymes and support materials as carrier should be considered during the course of the immobilization process. The functional groups on the surface of both enzyme and carrier are significant for

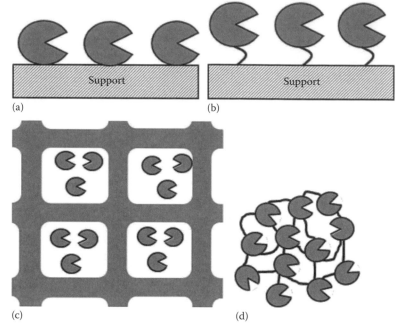

FIGURE 6.1 Conventional methods for the immobilization of enzymes on support materials: (a) physical adsorption, (b) covalent bonding, (c) entrapment, and (d) cross-linking.

the immobilization. The surface of the support material can be functionalized for effective immobilization in accordance with the surface properties of the enzyme.

Nanoparticles can be functionalized on a surface by two methods. One is postfunctionalization that is grafting of organic compounds with functional groups on the surface of nanoparticles.[180] The other method is *in situ* functionalization that is simultaneously modifying nanoparticles with organic compounds.[181–183] AuNPs are typically synthesized by the *in situ* functionalization method in the presence of thiolate compounds,[184–186] whereas nanoparticles such as MFe_2O_4 (M = Co, Mn, Fe)[187–189] and QDs[190] are synthesized in hydrophobic solvents of high boiling point at high temperature and modified with organic functional compounds[191,192] by the postfunctionalization method.

As mentioned in the previous section, MNPs are undoubtedly the most actively studied support material for enzyme immobilization due to their advantageous magnetic property, which greatly facilitates the separation of supported catalysts from the reaction mixture. However, the bare surface of MNPs lacks active functional groups for surface modification that is required for enzyme immobilization. One common method for the immobilization of enzymes on MNPs is to coat the nanoparticles with a silica layer. The silica layer contains a high coverage of silanol groups that can be functionalized by organosilanes with a variety of functional groups. Amine-functionalized MNPs are useful for biocatalysts to be immobilized, which makes many researchers take advantage of.[62,193–195] Amine functionalization was performed by coating 3-aminopropyltriethoxysilane on Fe_3O_4 nanoparticles activated through the treatment with sodium hydroxide. These amine groups can react with glutaraldehyde to generate aldehyde groups on the surface of the nanoparticles, which can be used for the immobilization of enzymes through the formation of Schiff bases.

Organic macromolecules provide other good moieties that functionalize MNPs to increase the biocatalyst loading amount and stability. They include glycidyl methacrylate (GMA), MMA, 2-hydroxyethyl methacrylate (HEMA), methacryloxyethyl trimethyl ammonium chloride (MATAC), and so on.[196–198] Liu and coworkers[199] reported the functionalization of Fe_3O_4 nanoparticles with a copolymer that consisted of HEMA and dimethyldiallylammonium chloride (DMDAAC). This copolymer coating gave rise to extremely high loading of *Candida rugosa* lipase due to the simultaneous use of two immobilization methods that were electrostatic adsorption and covalent bonding. Dendrimeric compounds can also be used for the functionalization of iron oxide nanoparticles. Uzun and coworkers[200] used polyamidoamine (PAMAM) dendrimer to functionalize superparamagnetic nanoparticles to immobilize invertase. They found out that the dendrimers played a role in increasing the enzyme loading. Superparamagnetic nanocomposites containing MNPs are another type of functionalization of MNPs. The Fe_3O_4@Clays nanocomposites were successfully prepared by a facile solvothermal process and the exposed surface of the clay was used to immobilize glucoamylase.[201] The resulting enzymes on the nanocomposites showed superior thermal stability and reusability. The authors also demonstrated the regeneration of supports at the expiry of the immobilized enzyme by wrapping the inactivated glucoamylase with fresh glucoamylase.

In the past several years, click chemistry has attracted great attention. It has been applied in organic synthesis, medicinal chemistry, polymers and material sciences, bioconjugates, and peptide chemistry. Functional enzyme–AuNP conjugates has been developed by that simple and versatile chemistry.[202] An acetylene-functionalized *Thermomyces lanuginosus* lipase was clicked with azidofunctionalized water-soluble AuNPs mediated by a catalytic amount of copper. The immobilized lipase well retained its original enzymatic activity.

The immobilization of enzymes on nanoporous materials also resorts to conventional methods. Usually, enzyme immobilizations have been conducted through surface functionalization of materials. Figures 6.2 and 6.3 show various functionalization methods for the enzyme immobilization onto MPS.[203] During the course of immobilization, the enzymes immobilized in the pores of mesoporous materials should retain the integrity of secondary and tertiary structures with intact active sites. Physical adsorption is one simple method. Under these immobilization conditions, the biocatalyst can sustain its activity because it has enough degree of freedom upon absorption, which secures its active site uncovered for transformations. This physical adsorption method utilizes relatively weak interactions such as hydrogen bonding, hydrophobic interactions, and van der Waals attractions through multiple interactions. Deere and coworkers[138] reported the effects of pore size and surface charge on the oxidative activity of immobilized cytochrome *c*. Kisler and coworkers[158] reported the separation of biological molecules by physical adsorption using MPS with different pore size. The adsorption rate depended on the sizes of both the molecules and the MPS pores. However, the immobilization through such weak physical interactions as van der Waals or dispersion forces can lead to leaching. The recovery rate of the adsorbed enzymes in subsequent reaction cycles is also reduced due to continual enzyme leaching.

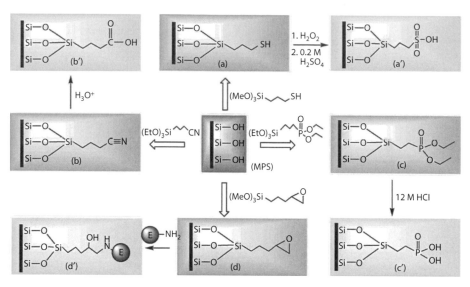

FIGURE 6.2 Examples of surface modification of MPS with different functional groups. (Reprinted from *Nano Today*, 4, Lee, C.-H., et al., Mesoporous materials for encapsulating enzymes, 165–179, Copyright 2009, with permission from Elsevier.)

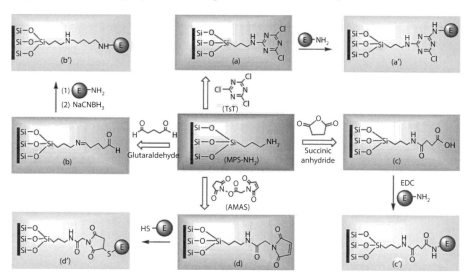

FIGURE 6.3 Methods for immobilization of enzymes on MPS materials via covalent bindings. (Reprinted from *Nano Today*, 4, Lee, C.-H., et al., Mesoporous materials for encapsulating enzymes, 165–179, Copyright 2009, with permission from Elsevier.)

This leaching problem can be overcome by immobilizing enzymes through strong electrostatic interactions. This is an easy method to immobilize enzymes by matching the zeta potential of MPS with average charges of enzymes. For example, aluminum atoms can be incorporated in the silica network of MPS to provide negative charges. Aluminosilicate surface offers suitable environments for the immobilization of positively charged enzymes through electrostatic interactions, while other metal ions are also available in accordance with the charges of the target enzyme.[128,204,205] Amine groups on the surface of MPS can enhance the binding of negatively charged enzymes, while carboxylate groups can increase the loading of positively charged enzymes. This tunable functionalization was successfully utilized for the immobilization of negatively charged GO_x and positively charged organophosphorus hydrolase in the nanochannels of the MPS such as SBA-15.[206,207] SBA-16 impregnated with Cs^+ ions was found to have an increased activity of immobilized chloroperoxidase (CPO) compared to a catalyst prepared by physical adsorption.[208] The charged state of an enzyme is determined by the isoelectric point (pI). At a pH below its pI, the enzyme will carry a net positive charge, while it figures a net negative charge above its pI. Vinu and coworkers[204] demonstrated that the immobilization of cytochrome c on different MPS materials largely depended on the pH of the solution. Takahashi and coworkers[147,148] also reported similar pH effects on the immobilization of HRP and subtilisin on FSM-16, MCM-41, and SBA-15.

Another simple and useful method to reduce leaching is to functionalize the surface of nanoporous materials, in particular, mesoporous silica. The functionalization can be performed by using various organosilanes.[209,210] The surface can be modified by two approaches: (1) co-condensation with organosilanes and (2) postmodification through grafting. Aliphatic hydrocarbons and thiol, vinyl, amine, and perfluoro groups can be incorporated on the surface of mesoporous silica materials. For example, the silica surface can be functionalized with primary amine groups, which can be utilized for covalent coupling of enzymes via amide bond formations.[211,212] In general, covalent bonding involves the functionalization of surface silanol groups by organosilanes with nucleophilic (amine, thiol) or electrophilic (alkyl halide) functional groups. Figure 6.3 shows a few covalent bonding methods. His-tagged enzymes can be immobilized by affinity toward metals, which results in the merits of high stability, activity, and reusability. The active center of immobilized enzyme should be less hindered from the modifications because the six contiguous histidines are attached to either the N- or C-terminus of the enzyme. The strong coordination of His-tagged enzymes to a single metal can stabilize the whole enzyme. Miyazaki and coworkers[213] reported the immobilization of His-tagged enzymes on the silica microchannel surface with nickel complexes through coordinate binding. This method was also applied to nanoparticles in the studies of Xu and coworkers[191] who reported the synthesis of FePt nanoparticles with nickel-terminated nitrilotriacetic acid. These nanoparticles showed high affinity and specificity to His-tagged proteins.

Another method to circumvent the leaching problem is to entrap enzymes in the pores of nanoporous materials. The pore gate of mesoporous silica can be reduced up to ~1 nm by silanation or coating with microporous silicas after enzyme immobilization, although the enzymatic activity after encapsulation is frequently decreased.[212] Postmodification following the encapsulation of enzyme on mesoporous silica also causes a decrease in catalytic activity due to partial compromise of the enzyme. Wang and coworkers[214] reported a novel method to encapsulate enzymes in the pores of mesoporous silica to overcome the leaching problem. In their studies, the enzymes were first immobilized in bimodal mesoporous silica (BMS) spheres and a nanocomposite shell was then formed on the surface of BMS by assembling polymer and

SNPs sequentially. Hydrophobic medication has been reported to be highly useful for the entrapment of lipases. Methyltrimethoxysilane, propyltrimethoxysilane, and polydimethylsiloxane have been used to modify the silica surface to be hydrophobic allowing for highly efficient entrapment of lipases in sol–gel silica matrix.[2,215] The resulting catalyst showed high esterification activity and enhanced stability.

An advanced approach is to combine the existing methods, such as physical adsorption, entrapment, and cross-linking. Cross-linked enzyme aggregates (CLEAs) were first reported by Sheldon and coworkers[216–221] Conventionally, cross-linking is performed in a two-step process. First, enzymes are absorbed inside the nanopores of MPS materials. Second, the absorbed enzymes are cross-linked by adding glutaraldehyde to yield highly CLEAs. Highly loaded, stable, and active enzyme aggregates can be obtained through this approach. Figure 6.4 illustrates this immobilization process.[222] Hyeon and coworkers reported on the cross-linked biocatalyst entrapped in the pores of hierarchically ordered mesocellular mesoporous silica materials (HMMS).[223] HMMS has two kinds of pores: a large mesocellular pore (37 nm) and a smaller channel pore (13 nm).[224] In this method, enzymes were immobilized on the surface of HMMS by a simple absorption method and then cross-linked with glutaraldehyde to give CLEAs entrapped in the mesocellular pores. Recently, Jung and coworkers[131] reported an optimized method to encapsulate CLEAs in the cell pores of mesocellular siliceous foams (MCFs). The authors successfully demonstrated that this approach was useful to immobilize sensitive biocatalysts such as CPO and GO_x and the resulting immobilized biocatalyst showed greatly enhanced catalytic activity and stability. The presence of CLEAs in the cell pores of the support was validated by small-angle neutron scattering (SANS) through perfluoropentane adsorption. Hyeon and coworkers further modified this immobilization approach by incorporating MNPs into HMMS during the formation of CLEAs, which resulted in easier magnetic recycling of the supported catalysts.[225] CLEAs combine covalent enzyme attachment on various nanomaterials leading to enhanced enzyme loading, enzymatic activity, and stability. CLEAs can form on the surface of electrospun polymer nanofibers. Enzymes are initially bound covalently to the surface of nanofibers and additional enzyme molecules are then attached to the bound ones through cross-linking that results in a CLEA coating on the fibers. This approach has been successfully applied to various nanomaterials, including nanofibers as introduced previously,[97,226,227] CNTs,[228] and MNPs.[229] Through the multilayer enzyme coating, the loading of enzymes on nanomaterials was increased by 1–2 orders of magnitude. The enzyme stability was also improved by multiple covalent linkages preventing the

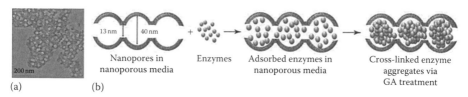

(a)   (b)

Nanopores in   Enzymes   Adsorbed enzymes in   Cross-linked enzyme
nanoporous media   nanoporous media   aggregates via
                                                               GA treatment

FIGURE 6.4 Immobilization of enzymes via the formation of CLEAs inside nanopores. (Reprinted from *Trends Biotechnol.*, 26, Kim, J., et al., Nanobiocatalysis and its potential applications, 639–646, Copyright 2008, with permission from Elsevier.)

denaturation of the enzymes. Therefore, these enzyme systems could be repeatedly recycled,[97,229] and thus have been successfully applied to continuous flow reactors over long periods of operation.[226,228]

To facilitate the recovery of supported enzymes, mesoporous materials can be endowed with magnetic properties by incorporating MNPs. Zhu and coworkers[151] reported the synthesis of magnetite-incorporated mesoporous silica spheres (Fe_3O_4@ MSS), and laccase was then immobilized on it via physical adsorption or covalent attachment to amine-functionalized Fe_3O_4@MSS. Zhang and coworkers also reported magnetite-incorporated MCM-41. Instead of direct synthesis of magnetite on support materials, magnetite nanocrystals were encapsulated in MCM-41 nanospheres through the packing and self-assembly of composite nanocrystal–surfactant micelles and the surfactant–silica complex.

Han and coworkers[230] introduced high pressure to efficiently entrap lipase in the cell pores of MCF. The hydrophobically modified MCF was first packed into a high-performance liquid chromatography (HPLC) column and the stock solution of lipase was circulated through the packed column for 2 h under high flow conditions in the presence of high back pressure. Compared to the conventional stirring method, this pressure-driven method resulted in significantly higher enzyme loading on MCF (up to 275 mg/g) in a shorter time. In addition, this method resulted in enhanced thermal stability and recyclability. Figure 6.5 shows the pressure-driven method for the immobilization of lipase and a continuous flow reaction system for kinetic resolution of 1-phenylethanol.

6.2.5 BIOCATALYTIC REACTIONS

Unlike large solid materials, nanoparticles dispersed in a solution move in Brownian motion. The mobility of catalysts is an important factor in the determination of catalytic activities explaining the high activity observed for biocatalysts attached to nanoparticles. Enzymes have been utilized in various catalytic reactions such as resolution of racemic mixture (kinetic resolution), hydrolysis, esterification, chemical building blocks from renewable sources, biomass refinement, biodegradation, oxidation reactions in organic synthesis, protein degradation, and many others.[231] In particular, biocatalysts have been drawing a great deal of attention as a manufacturing

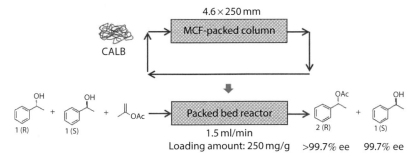

FIGURE 6.5 Pressure-driven method for the immobilization of lipase and a continuous flow reaction system for kinetic resolution of 1-phenylethanol.

system to produce chiral pharmaceuticals due to their high enantioselectivity and regioselectivity.[232–235] The catalytic efficiency is high enough under mild reaction conditions. Good regioselectivity can merge a multistep reaction into a single-step reaction by avoiding the typical and tedious protection and deprotection steps that are often essential in typical organic reactions. The nanosized and nonporous structure of nanoparticles provide large surface area for high enzyme loading minimizing mass transfer resistance. Table 6.5 lists various enzymatic reactions mediated by nanomaterial-supported enzymes.

TABLE 6.5
Enzymatic Reactions Mediated by Nanomaterial-Supported Enzymes

Enzyme	Microbial Source	Enzymatic Reactions
Alcohol dehydrogenase	Baker's yeast	Ethanol oxidation
Alginate lyase	*Streptomyces* sp.	Degradation of alginate: alginate oligosaccharides
α-Amylase	*Aspergillus oryzae*	Hydrolysis of starch
Chloroperoxidase	*Caldariomyces fumago*	Oxidation of 4,6-dimethyldibenzo-thiophene; oxidation of indole
α-Chymotrypsin	(Bovine) pancreas	Resolution of (±)-*trans*-4-methoxy-3-phenylglycidic acid methyl ester (esterification)
β-D-Galactosidase (lactase)	*A. oryzae*	Synthesis of galactooligosaccharides from lactose
Glucose amylase		Hydrolysis of dextrin
Glucose oxidase	*A. niger*	Oxidation of β-D-glucose
HAB mutase		Conversion of hydroxyaminobenzene to 2-aminophenol
HRP	Horseradish	Oxidation of 1,2-diaminobenzene
Laccase	*Trametes versicolor*	Oxidation of dibenzothiophene: biodegradation of benzo[α]pyrene (oxidation)
β-Lactamase	*Bacillus cereus*	Hydrolysis of phenoxymethyl penicillin (penicillin V)
L-Lactate dehydrogenase	Rabbit muscle	Enantioselective conversion of 2-*oxo* acid to (S)-2-hydroxy acid
Lipase	*Candida antarctica* B	Resolution of 1-phenylethanol (esterification)
	Pseudomonas cepacia	Hydrolysis of triacetin and tributyrin; acylation of 1-phenylethanol; resolution of (RS)-N-(2-ethyl-6-methylphenyl)alanine (hydrolysis)
	Pseudomonas sp.	Resolution of 2-octanol (esterification); transesterification of methyl (±)-mandelate and vinyl acetate

(Continued)

TABLE 6.5 (continued)
Enzymatic Reactions Mediated by Nanomaterial-Supported Enzymes

Enzyme	Microbial Source	Enzymatic Reactions
	Rhizomucor miehei	Conversion of caprylic acid into monocaprylin (esterification)
	Rhizopus oryzae, R. niveus, Mucor javanicus, Pseudomonas fluorescens, P. cepacia	Esterication of acetic acid with ethanol
	P. fluorescens	Ethanolysis sunflower oil (transesterification)
Manganese peroxide	*Phanerochaete chrysosporium*	Pulp bleaching; oxidation of Mn^{2+} to Mn^{3+}
Nitrilase	Recombinant from *Arabidopsis thaliana*	Hydrolysis of 3-cyanopyridine to nicotinic acid
Pepsin	Porcine gastric mucosa	Digestion of casein
Phamnulose-1-phosphate aldolase	Recombinant from *Escherichia coli*	Aldol addition between dihydroxyacetone phosphate and (S)-benzyloxycarbonyl (Cbz)-alaninal
Silicatein	Recombinant from *E. coli*	Polycondensation of tetraethoxysilane
Soybean peroxide	Soybean	Polymerization of 2-aminophenol to 2-aminophenoxazin-3-one (oxidation)
Trypsin	Bovine pancreas	Digestion of proteins (proteolysis)

6.2.6 OTHER APPLICATIONS

Along with the marvelous specificity of enzymes, nanomaterial-supported enzymes have been explored in various applications. In this section, the potential applications of nanobiocatalytic systems such as wastewater treatment and biofuel cells are briefly introduced.

At present, bioenergy is one of the most important renewable energy sources focusing on the replacement of fossil fuels.[236] Environmental technology is another emerging area in both researches and practical applications for the ecofriendly remediation of environmental contaminants. Many researchers have been exploring nanotechnology-based approaches for bioenergy and environmental remediation technology. Recently, Szamocki and coworkers[237] reported the immobilization of glutamate dehydrogenase (GDH) on porous gold electrodes. The resulting electrodes showed increased overall signals and potentially high power outputs on their application to biofuel cells. Wang and coworkers[238] reported on a packed bed reactor system with lipase–Fe_3O_4 nanoparticle biocomposite catalysts. This system was successfully utilized for effective and continuous biodiesel production based on methanolysis of soybean oil. Tran and coworkers[239] immobilized *Burkholderia* sp. lipase on silica-coated Fe_3O_4 nanoparticles that were functionalized with long alkyl groups. The immobilized lipase was used to catalyze the transesterification of olive oil with methanol to produce fatty acid methyl esters. Laccase immobilized on zinc tetraaminophthalocyanine–Fe_3O_4 nanoparticle composite can be used for the breakdown of lignin, which is one of the biomass-based feedstocks.[240,241] This immobilized laccase has good thermal, storage, and operational stability. Nanoporous gold-immobilized lignin peroxidase (LiP) could be used in the effective colorization of aromatic dye molecules such as fuchsine, rhodamine B, and pyrogallol red,[242] which show a potential to be used in the degradation of aromatic pollutants. Hommes and coworkers[243] immobilized laccase on fumed SNPs for biological wastewater treatment. The immobilized laccase exhibited increased enzymatic activity and long-term stability.

6.3 NOVEL NANOSYSTEMS FOR BIOCATALYSTS

Recently, various types of novel biocatalytic nanosystems have been explored for more efficient enzymatic reactions. In this section, biocatalytic nanosystems via self-assembly, nano-entrapment, single-enzyme nanoparticles (SENs), and biosensing are introduced.

6.3.1 NANOSYSTEMS BY SELF-ASSEMBLY

Well-designed nanostructures can be established through self-assembly using hydrophobic, electrostatic, or other types of molecular interactions among building blocks. Self-assembly is one kind of bottom-up approach. Surfactant-like enzyme–polymer amphiphiles can form catalytic molecular layers, nanowires, or nanoparticles under certain conditions via self-assembly. Block copolymer amphiphiles can form micelles to encapsulate enzymes. This self-assembly can lead to interfacial catalysis, multi-enzyme systems, and artificial cells. Surfactant-like enzyme–polymer molecules can be synthesized by covalent linkage of enzyme to polymers such as PS, PMMA, poly(L-lactic acid), and PEG. These giant molecules can form catalytic molecular layers at the interface of aqueous/organic biphasic systems. Both polymer coils and enzymes are of nanometer size, making the overall size of the conjugate small enough to be driven to the oil–water interface by affinity forces. While enzymes have interactions with water, polymers have interactions with oil as a complementary behavior. As a result, the conjugates lead to a unique biocatalyst system with interfaces for catalytic reactions.[244–246] Wang and coworkers found that CPO–PS conjugates assembled at the interface of oil and water. Velonia and coworkers[247] demonstrated that uniform amphiphilic lipase–PS conjugates formed well-defined micrometer-long fibers of 30 nm in diameter.[247] It is also reported that the well-defined HRP-PS amphiphiles formed micelles with diameters in the range of several hundred nanometers.[248,249]

Block copolymer amphiphiles can form nanoparticles/polymersomes that are similar to liposomes via self-assembly. Ishihara and coworkers reported the immobilization of acetylcholinesterase, choline oxidase, and HRP-labeled IgG on phospholipid polymer-assembled nanoparticles.[93] This three-enzyme system proceeded effectively in comparison with free enzyme in solution because the local concentration of each enzyme was higher and diffusion of newly produced substrates was more effective. Vriezema and coworkers demonstrated that HRP, GO$_x$, and lipase could be assembled in the polymersome formed by a rod–coil-type diblock copolymer PS-*b*-poly(lisocyanoalanine (2-thiophen-3-yl-ethyl)amide). HRP was mainly accommodated in the hydrophobic shell, GO$_x$ in the hydrophilic core, and lipase in the aqueous exterior of polymersome.[250]

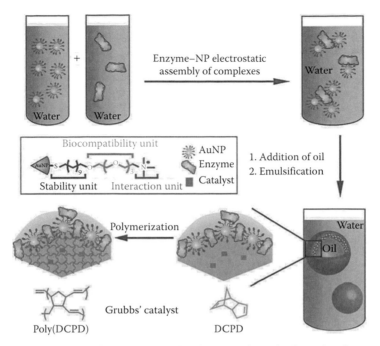

FIGURE 6.6 Formation of catalytic CLMPs via core polymerization using first-generation Grubbs catalyst. (Jeong, Y., et al. Reusable biocatalytic crosslinked microparticles self-assembled from enzyme-nanoparticle complexes. *Chem. Commun.*, 2011, 47: 12077–12079. Reproduced by permission of The Royal Society of Chemistry.)

This three-enzyme system showed high catalytic efficiency and also isolated each catalytic cycle to prevent interference by other compounds. This system approaches one step closer to the cellular environments, mimicking the conditions in living cells.

Recently, Jeong and coworkers[251] reported a versatile method to fabricate cross-linked microparticle (CLMP) scaffolds for enzyme immobilization, which was composed of enzymes, nanoparticles, and polymer cores. NP–enzyme complexes were formed by self-assembly through electrostatic interactions. Figure 6.6 illustrates the process of the enzyme immobilization. The immobilized enzymes exhibited enhanced stability, facile recovery of the catalyst, and improved compatibility with nonaqueous reaction media.

6.3.2 NANOENTRAPMENT

Nanoentrapment is a technique to make nanoparticles that contain enzymes. It is usually achieved by a water-in-oil microemulsion system that is also called reverse micelles. The entrapment of enzymes in nanoparticles is conducted through polymerization in the water phase or water–oil interface.[18,252–255] However, this approach should be optimized to tackle the two issues that are to control (1) the size of reverse micelles and (2) the number of enzymes within each micelle. These factors affect the final properties of the entrapped enzymes. Yang and coworkers[256] reported the entrapment of MNPs along with enzymes into spherical SNPs.

6.3.3 SINGLE-ENZYME NANOPARTICLE

The single-enzyme nanoparticle (SEN) has emerged as an innovative way of stabilizing enzymes because enzymes in a nanoparticle generally exhibit excellent stability even under relatively harsh conditions.[257,258] Yan and coworkers[257] reported a two-step procedure that includes surface acryloylation and *in situ* aqueous polymerization to encapsulate a single enzyme in nanogel. Figure 6.7 illustrates this two-step process. The aqueous polymerization simplified the enzyme encapsulation in nanostructured form compared with polymerization in organic solvents. HRP nanogels by this approach showed similar biocatalytic activity to free HRP. This method was also validated with carbonic anhydrase.[259] These enzyme nanogels displayed 80%–95% of the catalytic activity of their native counterpart. Slightly compromised activity might come from minor mass transfer restriction across the thin, porous, and flexible polymer shell. The multipoint linkages between the enzyme and the hydrophilic polyacrylamide shell resulted in significantly enhanced thermal stability in the presence of organic solvents. When incubated in anhydrous methanol at 50°C, free lipase was fully denatured within 30 min, while the lipase nanogel retained 80% of its initial activity. The polyacrylamide shell around the enzyme effectively prevented essential water from being replaced by the polar solvent, which resulted in higher tolerance to anhydrous hydrophilic organic solvents. Kim and coworkers[260,261] reported armored SENs, generated by surrounding each enzyme molecule with porous organic/inorganic composites of less than a few nanometers in thickness. This method has significantly stabilized chymotrypsin and trypsin, and enhanced mass transfer through a porous armor surrounding network. This SEN can be immobilized in the nanopores of MPS materials to stabilize enzymatic activity without limiting the substrate diffusion. Patil and coworkers[262] reported another method to create a nanostructure surrounding an enzyme molecule by wrapping each enzyme molecule with a thin layer of cationic organoclay oligomers through simple mixing of the enzymes with organoclays. These nanoparticles assembled and integrated into nanostructural materials. In addition, the entrapped enzymes showed enhanced thermal and chemical stability.

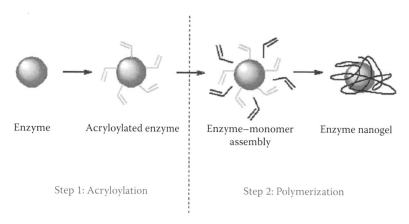

Enzyme   Acryloylated enzyme   Enzyme–monomer   Enzyme nanogel
                                            assembly

Step 1: Acryloylation   Step 2: Polymerization

FIGURE 6.7 Fabrication of single-enzyme nanogel (SEN) via a two-step process. (Reprinted from *Biochem. Eng. J.*, 44, Ge, J., et al., Recent advances in nanostructured biocatalysts, 53–59, Copyright 2009, with permission from Elsevier.)

6.3.4 BIOCATALYTIC NANOSYSTEMS FOR BIOSENSING

Nanostructured inorganic nanomaterials have many advantages for biosensors, including lower reagent consumption, minimized sample volume, lower energy consumption, less space requirement, and faster reaction kinetics.[263] There have been numerous applications of inorganic nanomaterials in the development of biosensors due to their high surface area-to-volume ratio and high electrical conductivity.[264–267]

QDs have great application potential in the development of biosensors due to their excellent optical property and large surface area. They have unique size-controlled optical properties. The electrostatic layer-by-layer (LBL) self-assembly method[268] provides an alternative method to produce novel nanocomposite biosensors.[269–275] The LBL method provides simplicity, economy, universality, and ecofriendly environments of film fabrication leading to increased uses. The optical, electrical, and electrochemical response of nanoparticles in the multilayer film can be tailored through the layer architecture.[276,277] Li and coworkers[278] developed a blood glucose sensor by generating multilayer films of CdTe QDs and GO_x by using the LBL technique. When the film is contacted with a glucose solution, the photoluminescence of the CdTe QDs in the film was quickly quenched through the formation of surface defects on QDs by hydrogen peroxide produced by the enzymatic reaction of GO_x and glucose.

Mesoporous material-supported enzymes can be used as biosensor. For example, cytochrome c was immobilized on highly ordered mesoporous niobium oxide films and then used as a biosensor for the electrocatalysis of hydrogen peroxide.[279] Cytochrome c absorbed on an electrode surface shows a pseudoperoxidase activity due to the presence of cytochrome heme. The absorbed enzymes retained their electrocatalytic activity and the biosensor showed 100% enhancement in sensitivity over the normal Nb_2O_5 electrode. Recently, Dai and coworkers[280] reported the immobilization of hemoglobin on a hexagonal mesoporous silica (HMS)-modified glassy carbon electrode. The direct electron transfer of the immobilized enzyme displayed two couples of redox peaks, which correspond to two immobilization states. The immobilized hemoglobin retained its biological activity and exhibited an excellent response to the reduction of both H_2O_2 and NO_2^-. This led to the development of a biosensor for the detection of both H_2O_2 and NO_2^-.

Zhu and coworkers[281] developed a sensitive enzyme-based biosensor for glucose detection by using dendrimer-encapsulated Pt nanoparticles via an LBL assembling method. PAMAM dendrimer molecules were used to covalently immobilize enzymes through carbodiimide coupling. Li and coworkers[282] also utilized PAMAM dendrimers to modify a gold electrode. AuNPs were attached to PAMAM for the immobilization of tyrosinase. A biosensor was developed by using this modified electrode to detect penicillamine with good sensitivity, operational stability, and good reproducibility.

REFERENCES

1. Chibata, I. 1978. *Immobilized Enzymes*. Wiley: New York.
2. Reetz, M., et al. 1995. Efficient heterogeneous biocatalysts by entrapment of lipases in hydrophobic sol-gel materials. *Angew. Chem. Int. Ed. Engl.* 34: 301–303.
3. Wang, Q., et al. 2008. Enzymatic hydrogelation to immobilize an enzyme for high activity and stability. *Soft Matter* 4: 550–553.

4. Helmsa, B., et al. 2006. The dendrimer effect in homogeneous catalysis. *Adv. Synth. Catal.* 348: 1125–1148.

5. Renner, C., et al. 2006. Arginine- and lysine-specific polymers for protein recognition and immobilization. *J. Am. Chem. Soc.* 128: 620–628.

6. Haag, R., et al. 2006. Polymer therapeutics: Concepts and applications. *Angew. Chem. Int. Ed.* 45: 1198–1215.

7. Asuri, P., et al. 2006. Directed assembly of carbon nanotubes at liquid–liquid interfaces: Nanoscale conveyors for interfacial biocatalysis. *J. Am. Chem. Soc.* 128: 1046–1047.

8. Nepal, D., et al. 2007. Proteins and carbon nanotubes: Close encounter in water. *Small* 3: 1259–1265.

9. Zhu, H., et al. 2005. Combined physical and chemical immobilization of glucose oxidase in alginate microspheres improves stability of encapsulation and activity. *Bioconjug. Chem.* 16: 1451–1458.

10. Phadtare, S., et al. 2003. Direct assembly of gold nanoparticle "shells" on polyurethane microsphere "cores" and their application as enzyme immobilization templates. *Chem. Mater.* 15: 1944–1949.

11. Alves, C.S., et al. 2009. Biomolecular characterization of CD44-fibrin(ogen) binding: Distinct molecular requirements mediate binding of standard and variant isoforms of CD44 to immobilized fibrin (OGEN). *J. Biol. Chem.* 284: 1177–1189.

12. DeLouise, L.A., et al. 2005. Enzyme immobilization in porous silicon: Quantitative analysis of the kinetic parameters for glutathione-S-transferases. *Anal. Chem.* 77: 1950–1956.

13. Cullen, S.P. 2008. Surface-anchored poly(2-vinyl-4,4-dimethyl azlactone) brushes as templates for enzyme immobilization. *Langmuir* 24: 13701–13709.

14. Bahshi, L., et al. 2008. Following the biocatalytic activities of glucose oxidase by electrochemically cross-linked enzyme–Pt nanoparticles composite electrodes. *Anal. Chem.* 80: 8253–8259.

15. You, C., et al. 2009. Affinity capturing for targeting proteins into micro and nanostructures. *Anal. Bioanal. Chem.* 393: 1563–1570.

16. Rembaum, A., et al. 1980. Immunomicrospheres: Reagents for cell labeling and separation. *Science* 208: 364.

17. Matsunaga, T., et al. 1987. Use of magnetic particles isolated from magnetotactic bacteria for enzyme immobilization. *Appl. Microbiol. Biotechnol.* 26: 328–332.

18. Khmelnitsky, Y.L., et al. 1989. Surface-modified polymeric nanogranules containing entrapped enzymes: A novel biocatalyst for use in organic media. *Biotechnol. Tech.* 3:275–280.

19. Gole, A., et al. 2001. Pepsin-gold colloid conjugates: Preparation, characterization, and enzymatic activity. *Langmuir* 17: 1674–1679.

20. Wu, C.-S., et al. 2008. An enzymatic kinetics investigation into the significantly enhanced activity of functionalized gold nanoparticles. *Chem. Commun.* 5327–5329.

21. You, C.-C., et al. 2006. Modulation of the catalytic behavior of α-chymotrypsin at monolayer-protected nanoparticle surfaces. *J. Am. Chem. Soc.* 128: 14612–14618.

22. Polgar, L. 1995. Effects of ionic strength on the catalysis and stability of prolyl oligopeptidase. *Biochem. J.* 312(Pt 1): 267–271.

23. Timasheff, S.N., et al. 1997. *Protein Structure: A Practical Approach*, 2nd ed. IRL Press: Oxford.

24. Mahl, D., et al. 2010. Gold nanoparticles: Dispersibility in biological media and cell biological effect. *J. Mater. Chem.* 20: 6176–6181.

25. Casals, E., et al. 2008. Distribution and potential toxicity of engineered inorganic nanoparticles and carbon nanostructures in biological systems. *TrAC. Trends Anal. Chem.* 27: 672–683.

26. Pandey, P., et al. 2007. Application of thiolated gold nanoparticles for the enhancement of glucose oxidase activity. *Langmuir* 23: 3333–3337.
27. Wu, C.-S., et al. 2011. Size-modulated catalytic activity of enzyme-nanoparticle conjugates: A combined kinetic and theoretical study. *Chem. Commun.* 47: 7446–7448.
28. Kim, J., et al. 2006. Nanostructures for enzyme stabilization. *Chem. Eng. Sci.* 61: 1017–1026.
29. Kim, M.I., et al. 2006. Immobilization of *Mucor javanicus* lipase on effectively functionalized silica nanoparticles. *J. Mol. Catal. B Enzym.* 39:62–68.
30. Jang, E., et al. 2010. Fabrication of polyethylene glycol-based hydrogels entrapping enzyme-immobilized silica nanoparticles. *Polym. Adv. Technol.* 21: 476–482.
31. Ansari, S.A., et al. 2011. Designing and surface modification of ZnO nanoparticles for biomedical applications. *Food Chem. Toxicol.* 49: 2107–2115.
32. Ansari, S.A., et al. 2011. Immobilization of *Kluyveromyces lactis* β galactosidase on concanavalin A layered aluminium oxide nanoparticles—Its future aspects in biosensor applications. *J. Mol. Catal. B Enzym.* 70: 119–126.
33. Husain, Q., et al. 2011. Immobilization of *Aspergillus oryzae* β galactosidase on zinc oxide nanoparticles via simple adsorption mechanism. *Int. J. Biol. Macromol.* 49: 37–43.
34. Gole, A., et al. 2001. On the preparation, characterization, and enzymatic activity of fungal protease-gold colloid bioconjugates. *Bioconjug. Chem.* 12: 684–690.
35. Gole, A., et al. 2002. Studies on the formation of bioconjugates of endoglucanase with colloidal gold. *Colloids Surf. B* 25: 129–138.
36. Laszlo, J.A., et al. 2007. Influence of self-assembled monolayer surface chemistry on *Candida antarctica* lipase B adsorption and specific activity. *J. Mol. Catal. B Enzym.* 48: 84–89.
37. Mazur, M., et al. 2007. Immobilization of laccase on gold, silver and indium tin oxide by zirconium–phosphonate–carboxylate (ZPC) coordination chemistry. *Bioelectrochemistry* 71: 15–22.
38. Reis, P., et al. 2006. Lipase-catalyzed reactions at different surfaces. *Langmuir* 22: 8169–8177.
39. Rusmini, F., et al. 2007. Protein immobilization strategies for protein biochips. *Biomacromolecules* 8: 1775–1789.
40. Villalonga, R., et al. 2007. Supramolecular chemistry of cyclodextrins in enzyme technology. *Chem. Rev.* 107: 3088–3116.
41. Phadtare, S., et al. 2004. Immobilization and biocatalytic activity of fungal protease on gold nanoparticle-loaded zeolite microspheres. *Biotechnol. Bioeng.* 85: 629 637.
42. Xu, J., et al. 2007. Gold nanoparticles bound on microgel particles and their application as an enzyme support. *Nanotechnology* 18: 265704.
43. Gardimalla, H.M.R., et al. 2005. Superparamagnetic nanoparticle-supported enzymatic resolution of racemic carboxylates. *Chem. Commun.* 4432–4434.
44. Kobayashi, H., et al. 1991. Amino-silane modified superparamagnetic particles with surface-immobilized enzyme. *J. Colloid. Interface Sci.* 141: 505–511.
45. Betancor, L., et al. 2005. Dextran aldehyde coating of glucose oxidase immobilized on magnetic nanoparticles prevents its inactivation by gas bubbles. *J. Mol. Catal. B Enzym.* 32: 97–101.
46. Huang, S.H., et al. 2003. Direct binding and characterization of lipase onto magnetic nanoparticles. *Biotechnol. Prog.* 19: 1095–1100.
47. Lei, H., et al. 2004. The preparation and catalytically active characterization of papain immobilized on magnetic composite microspheres. *Enzyme Microb. Technol.* 35: 15–21.
48. Jang, K.H., et al. 2001. Levan production by use of the recombinant levansucrase immobilized on titanium-activated magnetite. *Process Biochem.* 37: 339–343.
49. Wang, W., et al. 2007. Study of the epoxydized magnetic hydroxyl particles as a carrier for immobilizing penicillin G acylase. *Enzyme Microb. Technol.* 40: 255–261.

50. Namdeo, M., et al. 2009. Immobilization of α-amylase onto cellulose-coated magnetite (CCM) nanoparticles and preliminary starch degradation study. *J. Mol. Catal. B Enzym.* 59: 134–139.

51. Wang, F., et al. 2007. Reversible immobilization of glucoamylase by metal affinity adsorption on magnetic chelator particles. *J. Mol. Catal. B Enzym.* 48: 1–7.

52. Rossi, L.M., et al. 2004. Glucose oxidase-magnetite nanoparticle bioconjugate for glucose sensing. *Anal. Bioanal. Chem.* 380: 606–613.

53. Caruso, F., et al. 2000. Enzyme multilayers on colloid particles: Assembly, stability, and enzymatic activity. *Langmuir* 16: 9595–9603.

54. Chien, L.J., et al. 2008. Biosilicification of dual-fusion enzyme immobilized on magnetic nanoparticle. *Biotechnol. Bioeng.* 100: 223–230.

55. Hsieh, H.C., et al. 2009. Stabilization immobilization onto magnetic nanoparticles. *Biotechnol. Lett.* 31: 557–563.

56. Sulek, F., et al. 2010. Surface functionalization of silica-coated magnetic nanoparticles for covalent attachment of cholesterol oxidase. *J. Magn. Magn. Mater.* 322: 179–185.

57. Dyal, A., et al. 2003. Activity of *Candida rugosa* lipase immobilized on γ-Fe₂O₃ magnetic nanoparticles. *J. Am. Chem. Soc.* 125: 1684–1685.

58. Shu, B., et al. 2006. Resolution of (+/−)-menthol by immobilized *Candida rugosa* lipase on superparamagnetic nanoparticles. *Food Chem.* 96: 1–7.

59. Jiang, Y.Y., et al. 2009. Magnetic nanoparticles supported ionic liquids for lipase immobilization: Enzyme activity in catalyzing esterification. *J. Mol. Catal. B Enzym.* 58: 103–109.

60. Yilmaz, E., et al. 2011. Immobilization of *Candida rugosa* lipase on magnetic sol-gel composite supports for enzymatic resolution of (R,S)-Naproxen methyl ester. *J. Mol. Catal. B Enzym.* 69: 35–41.

61. Chaubey, A., et al. 2009. *Arthrobacter* sp. lipase immobilization on magnetic sol–gel composite supports for enantioselectivity improvement. *Process Biochem.* 44: 154–160.

62. Hu, B., et al. 2009. Immobilization of *Serratia marcescens* lipase onto amino-functionalized magnetic nanoparticles for repeated use in enzymatic synthesis of Diltiazem intermediate. *Process Biochem.* 44: 1019–1024.

63. Tsang, S.C., et al. 2006. Silica-encapsulated nanomagnetic particle as a new recoverable biocatalyst carrier. *J. Phys. Chem. B* 110: 16914–16922.

64. Alivisatos, A.P. 1996. Semiconductor clusters, nanocrystals, and quantum dots. *Science* 271: 933–937.

65. Nirmal, M., et al. 1999. Luminescence photophysics in semiconductor nanocrystals. *Acc. Chem. Res.* 32: 407–414.

66. Wu, X.Y., et al. 2003. Immunofluorescent labeling of cancer marker Her2 and other cellular targets with semiconductor quantum dots. *Nat. Biotechnol.* 21: 41–46.

67. Alivisatos, P. 2004. The use of nanocrystals in biological detection. *Nat. Biotechnol.* 22: 47–52.

68. Gill, R., et al. 2008. Semiconductor quantum dots for bioanalysis. *Angew. Chem. Int. Ed.* 47: 7602–7625.

69. Medintz, I.L., et al. 2005. Quantum dot bioconjugates for imaging, labelling and sensing. *Nat. Mater.* 4: 435–446.

70. Zong, S.Z., et al. 2007. Reagentless biosensor for hydrogen peroxide based on immobilization of protein in zirconia nanoparticles enhanced grafted collagen matrix. *Biosens. Bioelectron.* 22: 1776–1782.

71. Liu, B., et al. 2003. Amperometric biosensor based on a nanoporous ZrO₂ matrix. *Anal. Chim. Acta* 478: 59–66.

72. Zong, S.Z., et al. 2006. Zirconia nanoparticles enhanced grafted collagen tri-helix scaffold for unmediated biosensing of hydrogen peroxide. *Langmuir* 22: 8915–8919.

73. Huckel, M., et al. 1996. Porous zirconia: A new support material for enzyme immobilization. *J. Biochem. Biophys. Methods* 31, 165–179.
74. Bellezza, F., et al. 2005. Immobilization of myoglobin on phosphate and phosphonate grafted-zirconia nanoparticles. *Langmuir* 21: 11099–11104.
75. Reshmi, R., et al. 2007. Immobilization of α-amylase on zirconia: A heterogeneous biocatalyst for starch hydrolysis. *Catal. Commun.* 8: 393–399.
76. Chen, Y.Z., et al. 2008. Immobilization of lipases on hydrophobilized zirconia nanoparticles: Highly enantioselective and reusable biocatalysts. *Langmuir* 24: 8877–8884.
77. Mochalin, V.N., et al. 2012. The properties and applications of nanodiamonds. *Nat. Nanotech.* 7: 11–23.
78. Krueger, A. 2008. New carbon materials: Biological applications of functionalized nanodiamond materials. *Chem. Eur. J.* 14, 1382–1390.
79. Chow, E.K., et al. 2011. Nanodiamond therapeutic delivery agents mediate enhanced chemoresistant tumor treatment. *Sci. Transl. Med.* 3: 73ra21.
80. Chang, H.-C., et al. 2004. Adsorption and immobilization of cytochrome c on nanodiamonds. *Langmuir* 20: 5879–5884.
81. Wei, L., et al. 2009. Immobilization of enzyme on detonation nanodiamond for highly efficient proteolysis. *Talanta* 80: 1298–1304.
82. Mukhopadhyay, K., et al. 2003. Gold nanoparticles assembled on amine-functionalized Na–Y zeolite: A biocompatible surface for enzyme immobilization. *Langmuir* 19: 3858–3863.
83. Vinoba, M., et al. 2011. Immobilization of human carbonic anhydrase on gold nanoparticles assembled onto amine/thiol-functionalized mesoporous SBA-15 for biomimetic sequestration of CO_2. *Langmuir* 27: 6227–6234.
84. Crooks, R.M., et al. 2001. Dendrimer-encapsulated metal nanoparticles: Synthesis, characterization, and applications in catalysis. *Acc. Chem. Res.* 34: 181–190.
85. Wilson, O.M., et al. 2005. Synthesis, characterization, and structure-selective extraction of 1–3-nm diameter AuAg dendrimer-encapsulated bimetallic nanoparticles. *J. Am. Chem. Soc.* 127: 1015–1024.
86. Cosulich, M.E., et al. 2000. Performance evaluation of hyperbranched aramids as potential supports for protein immobilization. *Polymer* 41: 4951–4956.
87. Yemul, O., et al. 2005. Covalent-bonded immobilization of lipase on poly(phenylene sulfide) dendrimers and their hydrolysis ability. *Biomacromolecules* 6: 2809–2814.
88. Ge, J., et al. 2007. Hyperbranched polymer conjugated lipase with enhanced activity and stability. *Biochem. Eng. J.* 36: 93–99.
89. Verger, R. 1997. Interfacial activation of lipases: Facts and artifacts. *Trends Biotechnol.* 15: 32–38.
90. Ho, K.M., et al. 2008. Facile route to enzyme immobilization: Core–shell nanoenzyme particles consisting of well-defined poly(methyl methacrylate) cores and cellulase shells. *Langmuir* 24: 11036–11042.
91. Eldin, M.M.S., et al. 2010. Immobilization of β galactosidase onto copolymers nanoparticles of poly (acrylonitrile-co-methylmethacrylate): Characterization and application to whey hydrolysis. *Nanotech Conference & Expo 2010*, June 21–25, Anaheim, CA.
92. Miletic, N., et al. 2010. Immobilization of *Candida antarctica* lipase B on polystyrene nanoparticles. *Macromol. Rapid Commun.* 31:71–74.
93. Watanabe, J., et al. 2006. Sequential enzymatic reactions and stability of biomolecules immobilized onto phospholipid polymer nanoparticles. *Biomacromolecules* 7: 171–175.
94. Palocci, C., et al. 2007. Lipolytic enzymes with improved activity and selectivity upon adsorption on polymeric nanoparticles. *Biomacromolecules* 8: 3047–3053.
95. Jia, H., et al. 2002. Enzyme-carrying polymeric nanofibers prepared via electrospinning for use as unique biocatalysts. *Biotechnol. Prog.* 18: 1027–1032.

96. Herricks, T.E., et al. 2005. Direct fabrication of enzyme-carrying polymer nanofibers by electrospinning. *J. Mater. Chem.* 14: 3241–3245.

97. Kim, B.C., et al. 2005. Preparation of biocatalytic nanofibres with high activity and stability via enzyme aggregate coating on polymer nanofibres. *Nanotechnology* 16: S382–S388.

98. An, H.J., et al. 2011. Enzyme precipitate coating of lipase on polymer nanofibers. *Bioprocess Biosyst. Eng.* 34: 841–847.

99. Han, D., et al. 2011. Deactivating chemical agents using enzyme-coated nanofibers formed by electrospinning. *ACS Appl. Mater. Interfaces* 3: 4633–4639.

100. Ghosh, S., et al. 2012. Polyaniline nanofiber as a novel immobilization matrix for the anti-leukemia enzyme L-asparaginase. *J. Mol. Catal. B Enzym.* 74: 132–137.

101. Wang, L., et al. 2012. Nanoparticle-supported consecutive reactions catalyzed by alkyl hydroperoxide reductase. *J. Mol. Catal. B Enzym.* 76: 9–14.

102. Zhang, Y., et al. 2010, Immobilization of trypsin on water-soluble dendrimer-modified carbon nanotubes for on-plate proteolysis combined with MALDI-MS analysis. *Mol. Biosyst.* 1447–1449.

103. Zhao, G., et al. 2011. Reversible immobilization of glucoamylase onto magnetic carbon nanotubes functionalized with dendrimer. *Appl. Micobiol. Biotechnol.* 91: 591–601.

104. Yu, L., et al. 2005. Fabrication and application of enzyme-incorporated peptide nanotubes. *Bioconjug. Chem.* 16: 1484–1487.

105. Kresge, C.T., et al. 1992. Ordered mesoporous molecular sieves synthesized by a liquid-crystal template mechanism. *Nature* 359: 710–712.

106. Monnier, A., et al. 1993. Cooperative formation of inorganic-organic interfaces in the synthesis of silicate mesostructures. *Science* 261: 1299–1303.

107. Inagaki, S., et al. 1993. Synthesis of highly ordered mesoporous materials from a layered polysilicate. *J. Chem. Soc. Chem. Commun.* 680–682.

108. Huo, Q.S., et al. 1994. Generalized synthesis of periodic surfactant inorganic composite-materials. *Nature* 368: 317–321.

109. Zhao, D., et al. 1998. Triblock copolymer syntheses of mesoporous silica with periodic 50 to 300 Angstrom Pores. *Science* 279: 548–552.

110. Zhao, C., et al. 1998. Nonionic triblock and star diblock copolymer and oligomeric surfactant syntheses of highly ordered, hydrothermally stable, mesoporous silica structures. *J. Am. Chem. Soc* 120: 6024–6036.

111. Serra, E., et al. 2007. Lipase immobilization in ordered mesoporous materials. *Stud. Surf. Sci. Catal.* 165: 897–900.

112. Schmidt-Winkel, P., et al. 1999. Mesocellular siliceous foams with uniformly sized cells and windows. *J. Am. Chem. Soc.* 121: 254–255.

113. Tanev, P.T., et al. 1995. A neutral templating route to mesoporous molecular sieves. *Science* 267: 865–867.

114. Chen, C.Y., et al. 1993. Studies on mesoporous materials I: Synthesis and characterization of MCM-41. *Microporous Mater.* 2: 17–26. .

115. Han, Y., et al. 2005. Generalized fluorocarbon-surfactant-mediated synthesis of nanoparticles with various mesoporous structures. *Angew. Chem. Int. Ed.* 44: 288–292.

116. Hoffmann, F. 2006. Silica-based mesoporous organic-inorganic hybrid materials. *Angew. Chem. Int. Ed.* 45: 3216–3251.

117. Galarnea, A., et al. 2006. Immobilization of lipase on silicas. Relevance of textural and interfacial properties on activity and selectivity. *New J. Chem.* 30: 562–571.

118. Wang, Y., et al. 2004. Enzyme encapsulation in nanoporous silica spheres. *Chem. Commun.* 1528–1529.

119. Kovalenko, G.A., et al. 2008. Immobilization of glucoamylase by adsorption on carbon supports and its application for heterogeneous hydrolysis of dextrin. *Carbohydr. Res.* 343: 1202–1211.

120. Diaz, J.F., et al. 1996. Enzyme immobilization in MCM-41 molecular sieve. *J. Mol. Catal. B Enzym.* 2: 115–126.
121. Pandya, P.H., et al. 2005. Studies on the activity and stability of immobilized α-amylase in ordered mesoporous silicas. *Micropor. Mesopor. Mater.* 77: 67–77.
122. Méndez, J., et al. 2012. Stimulus-responsive controlled release system by covalent immobilization of an enzyme into mesoprous silica nanoparticles. *Bioconjug. Chem.* 23: 698–704.
123. Wang, Y., et al. 2005. Mesoporous silica spheres as supports for enzyme immobilization and encapsulation. *Chem. Mater.* 17: 953–961.
124. Chang, R.H.-Y., et al. 2011. Cellulase immobilized mesoporous silica nanocatalysts for efficient cellulose-to-glucose conversion. *Green Chem.* 13: 2844–2850.
125. Hartono, S.B., et al. 2010. Functionalized mesoporous silica with very large pores for cellulase immobilization. *J. Phys. Chem. C* 114: 8353–8362.
126. Hartmann, M., et al. 2006. Selective oxidation of indole by chloroperoxidase immobilized on the mesoporous molecular sieve SBA-15. *J. Porous Mater.* 13: 347–352.
127. Montiel, C., et al. 2007. Immobilization of chloroperoxidase on silica-based materials for 4,6-dimethyl dibenzothiophene oxidation. *J. Mol. Catal. B Enzym.* 48: 90–98.
128. Terrés, E., et al. 2008. Immobilization of chloroperoxidase on mesoporous materials for the oxidation of 4,6-dimethyldibenzothiophene, a recalcitrant organic sulfur compound present in petroleum fractions. *Biotechnol. Lett.* 30: 173–179.
129. Jung, D., et al. 2008. Oxidation of Indole with CPO and GO_x Immobilized on SBA-15. *Stud. Surf. Sci. Catal.* 174B: 1045–1050.
130. Jung, D., et al. 2008. Oxidation of indole using chloroperoxidase and glucose oxidase immobilized on SBA-15 as tandem biocatalyst. *Micropor. Mesopor. Mater.* 113: 523–529.
131. Jung D., et al. 2009. Formation of cross-linked chloroperoxidase aggregates in the pores of mesocellular foams: Characterization by SANS and catalytic properties. *ChemSusChem* 2: 161–164.
132. Humphrey, H.H.P., et al. 2001. Size selective protein adsorption on thiol-functionalised SBA-15 mesoporous molecular sieve. *Phys. Chem. Chem. Phys.* 2001, 3, 2983–2985.
133. Han, Y.J., et al. 1999. A mesoporous silicate sequestration and release of proteins. *J. Am. Chem. Soc.* 121: 9897–9898.
134. Gimon-Kinsel, M.E., et al. 1998. Mesoporous molecular sieve immobilized enzymes. *Stud. Surf. Sci. Catal.* 117: 373–380.
135. Washmon-Kriel, L., et al. 2000. Cytochrome c immobilization into mesoporous molecular sieves. *J. Mol. Catal. B Enzym.* 2000, 10: 453–469.
136. Deere, J., et al. 2001. Adsorption and activity of cytochrome c on mesoporous silicates. *Chem. Commun.* 465–466.
137. Deere, J., et al. 2001. Adsorption of cytochrome c onto ordered mesoporous silicates. *Stud. Surf. Sci. Catal.* 135: 233.
138. Deere, J., et al. 2002. Mechanistic and structural features of protein adsorption onto mesoporous silicates. *J. Phys. Chem. B* 106: 7340–7347.
139. Deere, J., et al. 2003. Adsorption and activity of proteins onto mesoporous silica. *Catal. Lett.* 85: 19–23.
140. Vinu, A., et al. 2004. Adsorption of cytochrome c on mesoporous molecular sieves: Influence of pH, pore diameter, and aluminum incorporation. *Chem. Mater.* 16: 3056–3065.
141. Vinu, A., et al. 2003. Adsorption of cytochrome C on new mesoporous carbon molecular sieves. *J. Phys. Chem. B* 107: 8297–8299.
142. Piao, Y., et al. 2009. High performance immunoassay using immobilized enzyme in nanoporous carbon. *Analyst* 134: 926–932.
143. Cheng, S.-H., et al. 2011. Site-specific immobilization of cytochrome c on mesoporous silica through metal affinity adsorption to enhance activity and stability. *New J. Chem.* 35: 1809–1816.

144. Hudson, S., et al. 2005. Methodology for the immobilization of enzymes onto mesoporous materials. *J. Phys. Chem. B* 109: 19496–19506.

145. Nara, T.Y., et al. 2011. Improvement of aldehyde tolerance and sequential aldol condensation activity of deoxyriboaldolase via immobilization on interparticle pore type mesoporous silica. *J. Mol. Catal. B Enzym.* 68: 181–186.

146. Szymanska, K., et al. 2007. Application and properties of siliceous mesostructured cellular foams as enzymes carriers to obtain efficient biocatalysts. *Micropor. Mesopor. Mater.* 2007; 99: 167–175.

147. Takahashi, H., et al. 2000. Catalytic activity in organic solvents and stability of immobilized enzymes depend on the pore size and surface characteristics of mesoporous silica. *Chem. Mater.* 12: 3301–3305.

148. Takahashi, H., et al. 2001. Immobilized enzymes in ordered mesoporous silica materials and improvement of their stability and catalytic activity in an organic solvent. *Micropor. Mesopor. Mater.* 44–45: 755–762.

149. Ikemoto, H., et al. 2010. Stability and catalytic kinetics of horseradish peroxidase confined in nanoporous SBA-15. *J. Phys. Chem. C* 114: 16174–16180.

150. Vinoba, M., et al. 2012. Carbonic anhydrase conjugated to nanosilver immobilized onto mesoporous SBA-15 for sequestration of CO_2. *J. Mol. Catal. B Emzym.* 75: 60–67.

151. Zhu, Y., et al. 2007. Immobilization of *Trametes versicolor* laccase on magnetically separable mesoporous silica spheres. *Chem. Mater.* 19: 6408–6413.

152. Wang, F., et al. 2010. Magnetic mesoporous silica nanoparticles: Fabrication and their laccase immobilization performance. *Bioresour. Technol.* 101: 8931–8935.

153. Mureseanu, M., et al. 2005. A new mesoporous micelle-templated silica route for enzyme encapsulation. *Langmuir* 21: 4648–4655.

154. Zhang, Y., et al. 2008. An efficient resolution of racemic secondary alcohols on magnetically separable biocatalyst. *Biochem. Biophys. Res. Commun.* 365: 609–613.

155. Serra, E., et al. 2008. Immobilization of lipase in ordered mesoporous materials: Effect of textural and structural parameters. *Micropor. Mesopor. Mater.* 114: 201–213.

156. Blanco, R.M., et al. 2004. Functionalization of mesoporous silica for lipase immobilization: Characterization of the support and the catalysts. *J. Mol. Catal. B Enzym.* 30: 83–93.

157. Jin, Q., et al. 2011. Hydrophobic surface induced activation of *Pseudomonas cepacia* lipase immobilized into mesoporous silica. *Langmuir* 27: 12016–12024.

158. Kisler, J.M., et al. 2001. Separation of biological molecules using mesoporous molecular sieves. *Micropor. Mesopor. Mater.* 44–45: 769–774.

159. Kisler, J.M., et al. 2001. Adsorption of proteins on mesoporous molecular sieves. *Mater. Phys. Mech.* 4: 89–93.

160. Yang, J., et al. 2003. Adsorption of lysozyme and trypsin onto mesoporous silica materials. *J. Stud. Surf. Sci. Catal.* 146: 775–778.

161. Fan, J., et al. 2003. Rapid and high-capacity immobilization of enzymes based on mesoporous silicas with controlled morphologies. *Chem. Commun.* 2140–2141.

162. Vinu, A., et al. 2004. Adsorption of lysozyme over mesoporous molecular sieves MCM-41 and SBA-15: Influence of pH and aluminum incorporation. *J. Phys. Chem. B* 108: 7323–7330.

163. Vinu, A., et al. 2005. Biomaterial immobilization in nanoporous carbon molecular sieves: Influence of solution pH, pore volume, and pore diameter. *J. Phys. Chem. B* 109: 6436–6441.

164. Lykourinou, V., et al. 2011. Immobilization of MP-11 into a mesoporous metal-organic framework, MP-11@mesoMOF: A new platform for enzymatic catalysis. *J. Am. Chem. Soc.* 133: 10382–10385.

165. He, J., et al. 2000. A new support for the immobilization of penicillin acylase. *J. Mol. Catal. B Enzym.* 11: 45–53.

166. Lü, Y., et al. 2008. Immobilized penicillin G acylase on mesoporous silica: The influence of pore size, pore volume and mesophases. *Micropor. Mesopor. Mater.* 114: 507–510.
167. Sun, H., et al. 2009. Immobilization of penicillin G acylase on oxirane-modified mesoporous silicas. *Langmuir* 25: 1807–1812.
168. He, J., et al. 2006. Formation of a mesoporous bioreactor based on SBA-15 and porcine pancreatic lipase by chemical modification following the uptake of enzymes. *J. Mater. Chem.* 16: 4307–4315.
169. Wang, C., et al. 2011. Porcine pancreatic lipase immobilized in amino-functionalized short rod-shaped mesoporous silica prepared using poly(ethylene glycol) and triblock copolymer as templates. *J. Phys. Chem. C* 115: 22191–22199.
170. Manyar, B.G., et al. 2008. Active biocatalysts based on pepsin immobilized in mesoporous SBA-15. *J. Phys. Chem. C* 112: 18110–18116.
171. Ravindra, R., et al. 2004. Protein encapsulation in mesoporous silicate: The effects of confinement on protein stability, hydration, and volumetric properties. *J. Am. Chem. Soc.* 126: 12224–12225.
172. Chaijitrsakoola, T., et al. 2008. Effects of pore characters of mesoporous resorcinol–formaldehyde carbon gels on enzyme immobilization. *J. Mol. Catal. B Enzym.* 55: 137–141.
173. Murai, K., et al. 2012. Enzyme structure and catalytic properties affected by the surface functional groups of mesoporous silica. *Catal. Sci. Technol.* 2: 310–315.
174. Falahati, M., et al. 2012. The effect of functionalization of mesoporous silica nanoparticles on the interaction and stability of confined enzyme. *Int. J. Biol. Macromol.* 50: 1048–1054.
175. Baker, S.E., et al. 2008. Blood clot initiation by mesocellular foams: Dependence on nanopore size and enzyme immobilization. *Langmuir* 24: 14254–14260.
176. Gomez, J.M., et al. 2003. Transesterification catalyzed by trypsin supported on MCM-41. *Catal. Lett.* 88: 183–186.
177. Goradia, D., et al. 2005. The adsorption characteristics, activity and stability of trypsin onto mesoporous silicates. *J. Mol. Catal. B Enzym.* 32: 231–239.
178. Ji, L., et al. 2004. Al-MCM-41 sorbents for bovine serum albumin: Relation between Al content and performance. *Micropor. Mesopor. Mater.* 75: 221–229.
179. Hossain, K.Z., et al. 2008. Adsorption of urease on PE-MCM-41 and its catalytic effect on hydrolysis of urea. *Colloids Surf. B Biointerfaces* 2008; 62: 42–50.
180. Baraton, M.-I. (Ed.) 2003. *Synthesis, Functionalization and Surface Treatment of Nanoparticles.* American Scientific Publishers: Stevenson Ranch, CA.
181. Sanchez, C., et al. 2001. Designed hybrid organic–inorganic nanocomposites from functional nanobuilding blocks. *Chem. Mater.* 13: 3061–3083.
182. Anderson, M., et al. 2002. Preparation of nanosize anatase and rutile TiO2 by hydrothermal treatment of microemulsions and their activity for photocatalytic wet oxidation of phenol. *J. Phys. Chem. B* 106: 10674–10679.
183. Yin, S., et al. 2005. Synthesis of excellent visible-light responsive TiO_2–xNy photocatalyst by a homogeneous precipitation-solvothermal process. *J. Mater. Chem.* 15: 674–682.
184. Brust, M., et al. 1994. Synthesis of thiol-derivatised gold nanoparticles in a two-phase liquid–liquid system. *J. Chem. Soc. Chem. Commun.* 801–802.
185. Bartz, M., et al. 1999. "Sticky" gold colloids through protection–deprotection and their use in complex metal–organic–inorganic architectures. *J. Chem. Soc. Chem. Commun.* 2085–2086.
186. Templeton, A.C., et al. 2000. Monolayer-protected cluster molecules. *Acc. Chem. Res.* 33: 27–36.
187. Hyeon, T., et al. 2001. Synthesis of highly crystalline and monodisperse maghemite nanocrystallites without a size-selection process. *J. Am. Chem. Soc.* 123: 12798–12801.

188. Park, J., et al. 2004. Ultra-large-scale syntheses of monodisperse nanocrystals. *Nat. Mater.* 3: 891–895.
189. Sun, S., et al. 2000. Monodisperse FePt nanoparticles and ferromagnetic FePt nanocrystal superlattices. *Science* 287: 1989–1992.
190. Gittins, D.I., et al. 2001. Spontaneous phase transfer of nanoparticulate metals from organic to aqueous media. *Angew. Chem. Int. Ed.* 40: 3001–3004.
191. Xu, C., et al. 2004. Nitrilotriacetic acid-modified magnetic nanoparticles as a general agent to bind histidine-tagged proteins. *J. Am. Chem. Soc.* 126: 3392–3393.
192. Hong, R., et al. 2005. Surface PEGylation and ligand exchange chemistry of FePt nanoparticles for biological applications. *Chem. Mater.* 17: 4617–4621.
193. Li, Y.G., et al. 2009. In situ magnetic separation and immobilization of dibenzothiophene-desulfurizing bacteria. *Bioresour. Technol.* 100: 5092–5096.
194. Yong, Y., et al. 2008. Characterization of *Candida rugosa* lipase immobilized onto magnetic microspheres with hydrophilicity. *Process Biochem.* 43: 1179–1185.
195. Zhu, H., et al. 2009. Immobilization of glycolate oxidase from *Medicago falcata* on magnetic nanoparticles for application in biosynthesis of glyoxylic acid. *J. Mol. Catal. B Enzym.* 61: 174–179.
196. Gulay, B., et al. 2007. Immobilization of β-galactosidase onto magnetic poly(GMA–MMA) beads for hydrolysis of lactose in bed reactor. *Catal. Commun.* 8: 1094–1101.
197. Bayramoglu, G., et al. 2008. Covalent immobilization of chloroperoxidase onto magnetic beads: Catalytic properties and stability. *Biochem. Eng. J.* 38: 180–188.
198. Yang, Y., et al. 2008. Preparation and application of polymer-grafted magnetic nanoparticles for lipase immobilization. *J. Magn. Magn. Mater.* 320: 2350–2355.
199. Liu, X., et al. 2011. Preparation of carriers based on magnetic nanoparticles grafted polymer and immobilization for lipase. *Biochem. Eng. J.* 56: 142–149.
200. Uzun, K., et al. 2010. Covalent immobilization of invertase on PAMAM-dendrimer modified superparamagnetic iron oxide nanoparticles. *J. Nanopart. Res.* 12: 3057–3067.
201. Zhao, G., et al. 2011. Enzymes immobilized on superparamagnetic Fe_3O_4@Clays nanocomposites: Preparation, characterization, and a new strategy for the regeneration of supports. *J. Phys. Chem. C* 115: 6350–6359.
202. Brennan, J.L., et al. 2006. Bionanoconjugation via click chemistry: The creation of functional hybrids of lipases and gold nanoparticles. *Bioconjug. Chem.* 17: 1373–1375.
203. Lee, C.-H., et al. 2009. Mesoporous materials for encapsulating enzymes. *Nano Today* 4: 165–179.
204. Vinu, S., et al. 2004. Adsorption of cytochrome c on mesoporous molecular sieves: Influence of pH, pore diameter, and aluminum incorporation. *Chem. Mater.* 16: 3056–3065.
205. Rosales Hernández, M.C., et al. 2005. Immobilization of cytochrome P-450 on MCM-41 with different silicon/aluminum ratios. *Micropor. Mesopor. Mater.* 80: 25–31.
206. Lei, C., et al. 2008. Enzyme specific activity in functionalized nanoporous supports. *Nanotechnology* 19: 125102.
207. Lei, C., et al. 2006. Characterization of functionalized nanoporous supports for protein confinement. *Nanotechnology* 17: 5531–5538.
208. Aburto, J., et al. 2005. Stability and catalytic properties of chloroperoxidase immobilized on SBA-16 mesoporous materials. *Micropor. Mesopor. Mater.* 83: 193–200.
209. Subramanian, A., et al. 1999. Comparison of techniques for enzyme immobilization on silicon supports. *Enzyme Microb. Technol.* 24: 26–34.
210. Impens, N.R.E.N., et al. 1999. Silylation of micro-, meso- and non-porous oxides: A review. *Micropor. Mesopor. Mater.* 28: 217–232.
211. Chong, A.S.M., et al. 2003. Functionalization of SBA-15 with APTES and characterization of functionalized materials. *J. Phys. Chem. B* 107: 12650–12657.

212. Yiu, H.H.P., et al. 2005. Enzymes supported on ordered mesoporous solids: A special case of an inorganic–organic hybrid. *J. Mater. Chem.* 15: 3690–3700.
213. Miyazaki, M., et al. 2006. Microchannel enzyme reactors and their applications for processing. *Trends Biotechnol.* 24: 463–470.
214. Wang, Y.J., et al. 2005. Enzyme multilayer-modified porous membranes as biocatalysts. *Chem. Mater.* 17: 171–175.
215. Reetz, M.T., et al. 1996. Efficient immobilization of lipases by entrapment in hydrophobic sol-gel materials. *Biotechnol. Bioeng.* 49: 527–534.
216. van Langen, L.M., et al. 2003. Penicillin acylase catalysed synthesis of ampicillin in hydrophilic organic solvents. *Adv. Synth. Catal.* 345: 797–801.
217. Lopez-Serrano, L.P., et al. 2002. Cross-linked enzyme aggregates with enhanced activity: Application to lipases. *Biotechnol. Lett.* 24: 1379–1383.
218. Hobbs, B., et al. 2006. Continuous kinetic resolution catalysed by cross-linked enzyme aggregates, "CLEAs", in supercritical CO_2. *Green Chem.* 8: 816–821.
219. Ruiz Toral, A., et al. 2007. Cross-linked *Candida antarctica* lipase B is active in denaturing ionic liquids. *Enzyme Microb. Technol.* 40: 1095–1099.
220. Cao, L., et al. 2000. Cross-linked enzyme aggregates: A simple and effective method for the immobilization of penicillin acylase. *Org. Lett.* 2: 1361–1364.
221. Cao, L., et al. 2001. Cross-linked aggregates of penicillin acylase: Robust catalysts for the synthesis of β-lactam antibiotics. *J. Mol. Catal. B Enzym.* 11: 665–670.
222. Kim, J., et al. 2008. Nanobiocatalysis and its potential applications. *Trends Biotechnol.* 26:639–646.
223. Lee, J., et al. 2005. Synthesis of hierarchically ordered mesocellular mesoporous silica materials hosting crosslinked enzyme aggregates. *Small* 1: 744–753.
224. Kim, M.I., et al. 2008. One-dimensional crosslinked enzyme aggregates in SBA-15: Superior catalytic behavior to conventional enzyme immobilization. *Micropor. Mesopor. Mater.* 111: 18–23.
225. Kim, J., et al. 2005. A magnetically separable, highly stable enzyme system based on nanocomposites of enzymes and magnetic nanoparticles shipped in hierarchically ordered, mesocellular, mesoporous silica. *Small* 1: 1203–1207.
226. Lee, J.H., et al. 2007. Stable and continuous long-term enzymatic reaction using an enzyme-nanofiber composite. *Appl. Microbiol. Biotechnol.* 75: 1301–1307.
227. Nair, S., et al. 2007. Improving biocatalytic activity of enzyme-loaded nanofibers by dispersing entangled nanofiber structure. *Biomacromolecules* 8: 1266–1270.
228. Fischback, M.B., et al. 2006. Miniature biofuel cells with improved stability under continuous operation. *Electroanalysis* 18: 2016–2022.
229. Lee, J., et al. 2008 Simple synthesis of functionalized superparamagnetic magnetite/silica core/shell nanoparticles and their application as magnetically separable high-performance biocatalysts. *Small* 4: 143–152.
230. Han, Y., et al. Pressure-driven enzyme entrapment in siliceous mesocellular foam. *Chem. Mater.* 18: 643–649.
231. Hartmann, M., et al. 2010. Biocatalysis with enzymes immobilized on mesoporous hosts: The status quo and future trends. *J. Mater. Chem.* 20:844–857.
232. Patel, R.N. 2004. Biocatalytic synthesis of chiral pharmaceutical intermediates. *Food Technol. Biotechnol.* 42: 305–325.
233. Thayer, A.M. 2006. Enzymes at work. *Chem. Eng. News* 84: 15–25.
234. Thayer, A.M. 2006. Biocatalysis helps reach a resolution. *Chem. Eng. News* 84: 29–31.
235. Hummel, W., et al. 1989. Dehydrogenases for the synthesis of chiral compounds. *Eur. J. Biochem.* 184: 1–13.
236. Yuan, J.S., et al. 2008. Plants to power: Bioenergy to fuel the future. *Trends Plant Sci.* 13: 421–429.

237. Szamocki, R., et al. 2007. Improved enzyme immobilization for enhanced bioelectro-catalytic activity of porous electrodes. *Electrochem. Commun.* 9: 2121–2127.
238. Wang, X., et al. 2011. Biodiesel production in packed-bed reactors using lipase-nanoparticle biocomposite. *Bioresour. Technol.* 102:6352–6355.
239. Tran, D.-T., et al. 2012. Immobilization of *Burkholderia* sp. lipase on a ferric silica nanocomposite for biodiesel production. *J. Biotechnol.* 158:112–119.
240. Huang, J., et al. 2007. Zinc tetraaminophthalocyanine-Fe$_3$O$_4$ nanoparticle composite for laccase immobilization. *Int. J. Nanomedicine* 2: 775–784.
241. Bugg, T.D.H., et al. 2010. The emerging role for bacteria in lignin degradation and bio-product formation. *Curr. Opin. Biotechnol.* 22: 1–7.
242. Chico, B., et al. 2009. Polyelectrostatic immobilization of gold nanoparticles-modified peroxidase on alginate-coated gold electrode for mediatorless biosensor construction. *J. Electroanal. Chem.* 629: 126–132.
243. Hommes, G., et al. 2012. Production of a robust nanobiocatalyst for municipal wastewater treatment. *Bioresour. Technol.* 115: 8–15.
244. Zhu, G., et al. 2004. Polymer–enzyme conjugates can self-assemble at oil/water inter-faces and effect interfacial biotransformations. *J. Am. Chem. Soc.* 126: 11132–11133.
245. Wang, L., et al. 2005. Self-assembling of polymer-enzyme conjugates at oil/water inter-faces. *Biotechnol. Prog.* 21: 1321–1328.
246. Zhu, G., et al. 2005. Novel interface-binding chloroperoxidase for interfacial epoxida-tion of styrene. *J. Biotechnol.* 117: 195–202.
247. Velonia, K., et al. 2002. Lipase polystyrene giant amphiphiles. *J. Am. Chem. Soc.* 124: 4224–4225.
248. Boerakker, M.J., et al. 2002. Giant amphiphiles by cofactor reconstitution. *Angew. Chem. Int. Ed.* 41: 4239–4241.
249. Reynhout, I.C., et al. 2007. Self-assembled architectures from biohybrid triblock copolymers. *J. Am. Chem. Soc.* 129: 2327–2332.
250. Vriezema, D.M., et al. 2007. Positional assembly of enzymes in polymersome nanoreac-tors for cascade reactions. *Angew. Chem. Int. Ed.* 46: 7378–7382.
251. Jeong, Y., et al. 2011. Reusable biocatalytic crosslinked microparticles self-assembled from enzyme-nanoparticle complexes. *Chem. Commun.* 47: 12077–12079.
252. Daubresse, C., et al. 1994. Enzyme immobilization in nanoparticles produced by inverse microemulsion polymerization. *J. Colloid Interface Sci.* 168: 222–229.
253. Jain, T.K., et al. 1998. Nanometer silica particles encapsulating active compounds: A novel ceramic drug carrier. *J. Am. Chem. Soc.* 120: 11092–11095.
254. Ma, D., et al. 2004. Fabrication of protein/silica core-shell nanoparticles by microemulsion-based molecular wrapping. *Adv. Mater.* 16: 1838–1841.
255. Munshi, N., et al. 1997. Size modulation of polymeric nanoparticles under controlled dynamics of microemulsion droplets. *J. Colloid Interface Sci.* 190: 387–391.
256. Yang, H.H., et al. 2004. Magnetite-containing spherical silica nanoparticles for bioca-talysis and bioseparations. *Anal. Chem.* 76: 1316–1321.
257. Yan, M., et al. 2006. Encapsulation of single enzyme in nanogel with enhanced biocata-lytic activity and stability. *J. Am. Chem. Soc.* 128: 11008–11009.
258. Hegedus, I., et al. 2009. Improvement of chymotrypsin enzyme stability as single enzyme nanoparticles. *Chem. Eng. Sci.* 64: 1053–1060.
259. Yan, M., et al. 2007. Fabrication of single carbonic anhydrase nanogel against denatur-ation and aggregation at high temperature. *Biomacromolecules* 8: 560–565.
260. Kim, J., et al. 2003. Single-enzyme nanoparticles armored by a nanometer-scale organic/inorganic network. *Nano Lett.* 3: 1219–1222.
261. Kim, J., et al. 2006. Single enzyme nanoparticles in nanoporous silica: A hierarchi-cal approach to enzyme stabilization and immobilization. *Enzyme Microb. Technol.* 39: 474–480.

262. Patil, A.J., et al. 2004. Synthesis and self-assembly of organoclay wrapped biomolecules. *Angew. Chem. Int. Ed. Engl.* 43: 4928–4933.

263. Libertino, S., et al. 2007. Experimental characterization of proteins immobilized on Si-based materials. *Microelectron. Eng.* 84: 468–473.

264. Zhang, Y., et al. 2009. An enzyme immobilization platform for biosensor designs of direct electrochemistry using flower-like ZnO crystals and nano-sized gold particles. *J. Electroanal. Chem.* 627: 9–14.

265. Crespilho, F.N., et al. 2006. A strategy for enzyme immobilization on layer-by-layer dendrimer gold nanoparticle electrocatalytic membrane incorporating redox mediator. *Electrochem. Commun.* 8: 1665–1670.

266. Delvaux, M., et al. 2003. Immobilisation of glucose oxidase within metallic nanotubes arrays for application to enzyme biosensors. *Biosens. Bioelectron.* 18: 943–951.

267. Knopp, D., et al. 2009. Bioanalytical applications of biomolecule-functionalized nanometer-sized doped silica particles. *Anal. Chim. Acta.* 647: 14–30.

268. Decher, G. 1997. Fuzzy nanoassemblies: Toward layered polymeric multicomposites. *Science* 277: 1232–1237.

269. Tang, Z., et al. 2006. Biomedical applications of layer-by-layer assembly: From biomimetics to tissue engineering. *Adv. Mater.* 18: 3203–3224.

270. Jiang, C., et al. 2006. Freestanding nanostructures via layer-by-layer assembly. *Adv. Mater.* 18: 829–840.

271. Constantine, C.A., et al. 2003. Layer-by-layer biosensor assembly incorporating functionalized quantum dots. *Langmuir* 19: 9863–9867.

272. Zhang, X., et al. 2007. Layer-by-layer assembly: From conventional to unconventional methods. *Chem. Commun.* 1395–1405.

273. Lisdat, F., et al. 2009. Self-assembly of electro-active protein architectures on electrodes for the construction of biomimetic signal chains. *Chem. Commun.* 274–283.

274. Dronov, R., et al. 2008. Communication in a protein stack: Electron transfer between cytochrome c and bilirubin oxidase within a polyelectrolyte multilayer. *Angew. Chem. Int. Ed.* 47: 3000–3003.

275. Dronov, R., et al. 2008. Layer-by-layer arrangement by protein–protein interaction of sulfite oxidase and cytochrome c catalyzing oxidation of sulfite. *J. Am. Chem. Soc.* 2008, 130, 1122–1123.

276. Liu, S., et al. 2002. Polyoxometalates as pH-sensitive probes in self-assembled multilayers. *Chem. Commun.* 976–977.

277. Wang, Y., et al. 2003. Multicolor luminescence patterning by photoactivation of semiconductor nanoparticle films. *J. Am. Chem. Soc.* 125: 2830–2831.

278. Li, X., et al. 2009. Glucose biosensor based on nanocomposite films of CdTe quantum dots and glucose oxidase. *Langmuir* 25: 6580–6586.

279. Xu, X., et al. 2003. Ordered mesoporous niobium oxide film: A novel matrix for assembling functional proteins for bioelectrochemical applications. *Adv. Mater.* 15, 1932–1936.

280. Dai, Z., et al. 2004. Direct electron transfer and enzymatic activity of hemoglobin in a hexagonal mesoporous silica matrix. *Biosens. Bioelectron.* 19: 861–867.

281. Zhu, Y., et al. 2007. Sensitive biosensors based on (dendrimer encapsulated Pt nanoparticles)/enzyme multilayers. *Electroanalysis* 19: 698–703.

282. Li, N.B., et al. 2007. A penicillamine biosensor based on tyrosinase immobilized on nano-Au/PAMAM dendrimer modified gold electrode. *Electroanalysis* 19: 2428–2436.

283. Ge, J., et al. 2009. Recent advances in nanostructured biocatalysts. *Biochem. Eng. J.* 44: 53–59.

7 Magnetically Induced Hyperthermia for Biomedical Applications

Michael Fardis, Ioannis Rabias,
Georgios Diamantopoulos, Eleni Karakosta,
Danai Tsitrouli, Vassilios Tzitzios,
and Georgios Papavassiliou
National Centre for Scientific Research "Demokritos"

CONTENTS

7.1   INTRODUCTION

Magnetically induced hyperthermia involves the heat dissipated by magnetic particles (usually in the form of colloidal suspensions) exposed to alternating magnetic fields and has been mainly utilized for applications in cancer treatment. It can be considered as one of the many manifestations of the interaction of electromagnetic radiation with matter. It is also called magnetic fluid hyperthemia [1] since it requires the utilization of magnetic fluids (ferromagnetic liquids or ferrofluids), which is defined as stable colloidal suspensions of ultrafine particles of a ferromagnet or ferrite in any ordinary liquid (e.g., water, liquid hydrocarbon, etc.). The greater sensitivity of cancer cells to hyperthermia compared to normal cells is the basic concept behind this biophysical treatment of cancer. Since the pioneering work of Gilchrist et al. in 1957 [2], magnetically induced hyperthermia has been the subject of considerable theoretical and experimental investigations for both *in vitro* and *in vivo* applications. The ultimate goal of these efforts was to increase the efficiency of the technique [quantified by the specific absorption rate (SAR)] by finding the optimum conditions for maximum heating. This required not only a search for correlation of the various structural, material, magnetic, and colloidal properties of magnetic fluids and their associated nanoparticles with hyperthermia performance but also theoretical understanding of the response of nanoparticle assemblies on the parameters of the alternating field.

There is a considerable number of monographs [3,4] and review articles [5–12] in which the physics and the applications of magnetically induced hyperthermia are described. This chapter does not intend to describe all the work performed in the field; nor does it seek only to summarize the most important. Instead, a connection between the fundamental properties of magnetic fluids and the mechanisms responsible for the occurrence of magnetic hyperthermia is attempted with reference made to the work that provides a correct understanding of the phenomenon.

Magnetic iron oxides are model systems for magnetic hyperthermia due to their exceptional biocompatibility compared to other magnetic materials, although in the search of materials with high magnetization (a prerequisite for efficient magnetic hyperthermia), many magnetic materials have been considered. For example, apart from the extensively studied Fe_3O_4 and γ-Fe_2O_3, many other substituted soft ferrites $Fe_{1-x}Mn_xFe_2O_4$ [13] and lanthanum manganates [14] have been considered due to their stability against oxidation and their ability to self-regulate the heating by tuning the Curie temperature by composition. High coercive cobalt ferrite [12,15–17] and FeCo [18] nanoparticles have also been investigated, but their biocompatibility issues must be further addressed. Quite recently, the high saturation magnetization of metallic iron nanoparticles was employed in order to increase the efficiency of magnetic hyperthermia of metallic iron nanocubes by a factor of 3 compared to optimized chemically synthesized iron oxide nanoparticles [19]. Nevertheless, in this system, problems with surface oxidation and toxicity must be further considered.

Of equal importance with magnetization is the size of the nanoparticles in magnetic hyperthermia performance. The research effort devoted to the study of the optimum size of nanoparticles in magnetic hyperthermia during the past decade has resulted in a very large literature on the subject (e.g., [20–40,41]). The size effect will be discussed in detail in Section 7.2.2 devoted to the principal physical mechanisms of magnetic hyperthermia.

The influence of the colloidal parameters of the magnetic fluids on the efficiency of magnetic hyperthermia has also been considered in the literature. The effect of the concentration of the particles in the magnetic fluid is closely associated with the interparticle dipole–dipole interactions and its effect on the magnetic heating is a rather complex issue [42]. The influence of solvent viscosity has also been examined by several authors [28,29,42].

Two fundamental parameters that externally influence the magnetic heating of nanoparticles are the frequency and the strength of the externally applied alternating magnetic field used to generate the induction heating. The dependence of heating on these parameters has also been the subject of intense investigation since it is directly related to the physiological response of human tissues to intense high-frequency magnetic fields (see, e.g., [24,28,43–45]). These dependences will not be considered in this chapter.

Finally, since the pioneering work of Rosensweig [46] on the physical formulation of induction heating in magnetic hyperthermia, a series of works on modeling the power generation from magnetic nanoparticles as well as tumor heating has been reported (for recent reports, see [47–53]).

7.2 HEAT DISSIPATION MECHANISMS IN MAGNETIC NANOPARTICLES—THE PHYSICAL ORIGIN OF MAGNETIC HYPERTHERMIA

As briefly mentioned in Section 7.1, magnetic fluids or ferrofluids consist of small, about 10 nm diameter, single-domain (SD) magnetic particles (of a ferromagnet or ferrite) dispersed in water or oil-based solvent forming a colloidal suspension. The main characteristic of a magnetic fluid, which is of fundamental and practical interest, is that it is a liquid with strong magnetic properties. In Section 7.2.1, we comment on some of the most important properties of a magnetic fluid pertinent to the heating power efficiency of the fluid in magnetic hyperthermia applications. In Section 7.2.2, we describe the relaxation mechanism of the magnetic fluids responsible for heat dissipation.

7.2.1 BASIC PROPERTIES OF MAGNETIC FLUIDS

7.2.1.1 Stability of Colloidal Systems

The stability of a colloidal dispersion against agglomeration and sedimentation is the first essential factor characterizing a magnetic fluid. The particles in suspension must be small enough that Brownian motion prevents particle agglomeration arising primarily from magnetic and van der Waals interactions between the particles. Agglomeration results in the development of domains within the magnetic fluid with high and low number densities of the nanoparticles and the approximation of noninteracting particles is no longer valid. A proper account of the interparticle interactions must be taken into account in order to study equilibrium properties—magnetization, magnetic susceptibility, specific heat, and surface tension—and phase transitions [54]. A popular synthetic method in order to prevent agglomeration in magnetic fluids is the coating of nanoparticles with appropriate nonmagnetic materials such as surfactants. Ferrofluids can also be electrostatically stabilized, forming ionic aqueous ferrofluids. In this case, surface charges lead to interparticle electrostatic repulsions that can overcome the van der Waals forces and magnetic attractions [55,56].

7.2.1.2   Static Magnetic Properties of Magnetic Fluids

The most fundamental property of a magnetic fluid is the magnetization arising from the magnetic moments that each particle possesses. Since the first reports on the synthesis and applicability of stable magnetic fluids (see, e.g., [57]), considerable research was devoted to improving the saturation magnetization of the magnetic fluids. As will be shown further, this is also the case for the magnetic hyperthermia experiments. As an example of the many efforts devoted to understanding the theoretical barriers in improving the saturation magnetization, in what follows we present the work of Scholten, who back in 1983 [58], posed the question: How magnetic can a magnetic fluid be? Taking into account the requirements of fluidity (which limits the volume fraction φ of solid material) and stability toward aggregation, the bulk magnetization of the particle material, and the chain length of the surfactant, Scholten [58] was able to theoretically calculate the magnetization limits as a function of the particle diameter d for magnetite particles composing a magnetic fluid. This is reproduced in Figure 7.1, where with the three limiting factors—namely, magnetic attraction, surfactant thickness δ, and van der Waals attraction—the areas above the curves are forbidden. This leaves the cross-hatched part as the accessible area for the attainable saturation magnetization M_s of a stable magnetic fluid (shown here for $\varphi = 0.5$).

From Figure 7.1, it is thus clear that the reason why most stable ferrofluids are also useful in many biomedical applications is because they have particles with diameters in the range of 8–20 nm.

In the presence of a magnetic field, a uniform and isotropic magnetic fluid responds as a paramagnet, and since the magnetic moments of the suspended particles usually exceed the moments of individual atoms by 4–5 orders of magnitude, the term superparamagnetism has been introduced (first by Bean [59]) to describe the magnetization of the magnetic fluids. Hence, assuming noninteracting, SD particles in the superparamagnetic (SP) state, the magnetization of a magnetic fluid is described by the Langevin function according to the classical theory of paramagnetism [60]. Since inevitably there will be a distribution of the sizes of the magnetic particles, it is a customary practice to introduce a distribution function of the magnetic moments in Langevin function [61].

7.2.2   Heat Dissipation Mechanisms in Magnetic Fluids

7.2.2.1   Mechanisms of Relaxation of Magnetization in the SP State

The magnetization of a magnetic fluid may relax after the removal of the applied magnetic field primarily by two fluctuation mechanisms known in the literature as the Brownian and Néel mechanisms [57,62]. In the Brownian mechanism, the particle magnetization may relax by rotation of the particles themselves with respect to

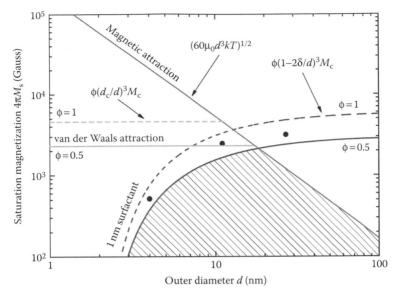

FIGURE 7.1 Theoretical magnetization limits as a function of outer particle diameter for magnetite particles. The circles are experimental data (unpublished). The sample with $d = 27$ nm was not stable nanoparticle dispersion. (Reprinted from *Journal of Magnetism and Magnetic Materials*, 39(1–2), Scholten, P.C., How magnetic can a magnetic fluid be?, 99–106, Copyright 1987, with permission from Elsevier.)

the liquid matrix. The mechanism is characterized by the Brownian rotational diffusion time τ_B given by

$$\tau_B = \frac{3V_H\eta}{k_B T} \tag{7.1}$$

where V_H is the hydrodynamic particle volume including the coating, η is the viscosity of the carrier liquid, k_B is Boltzmann's constant, and T is the absolute temperature.

In the Néel mechanism, the relaxation is determined by the rotation of the magnetic vector within the particle and is associated with the *magnetic anisotropy K* that couples—through the spin–orbit interaction—the magnetic moment with preferred crystal axes with a strength given by the anisotropy energy. Néel first pointed out that in subdomain particles, even in the absence of an external magnetic field, the magnetization can be reversed by thermal fluctuations over the energy barrier KV between different directions of easy magnetization. The efficiency of the disorientation action of the fluctuations depends on the ratio $\sigma = KV/k_B T$ of the magnetic anisotropy energy to the thermal energy. For the Néel process, in the asymptotic limit $\sigma \geq 2$, Brown [63] obtained the relaxation time of τ_N that characterizes this mechanism by

$$\tau_N = \tau_0 \left(\frac{KV_M}{k_BT} \right)^{-1/2} \exp\left(\frac{KV_M}{k_BT} \right) \qquad (7.2)$$

where K is the magnetic anisotropy constant, V_M is the volume of the magnetic core of the particle, and τ_0 is an electronic relaxation time associated with the regular precession of the magnetic moment around the easy direction of the magnetization at an energy minimum.

The above two fluctuation mechanisms determine the dynamics of magnetization of a suspension and are the principal factors in a magnetic hyperthermia experiment. As Shliomis points out, the mechanisms are physically different [62]: The Néel process is determined by the properties of the ferromagnet, whereas the Brownian process is determined with the viscosity of the liquid. On the other hand, both mechanisms may be viewed as a rotational diffusion of the magnetic moment in different matrices, within the particle or in the liquid. Hence, an effective relaxation time τ_{eff}, given by $1/\tau_{eff} = 1/\tau_B + 1/\tau_N$, may be defined and the shorter rotational diffusion time determines the most prevailing mechanism.

Other relaxation mechanisms leading to induction heating by eddy currents and ferromagnetic resonance will not be discussed since in this work we consider only small particles (<15 nm) and frequencies well below those in ferromagnetic resonance.

7.2.2.2 Power Dissipation in Magnetic Fluids: SP State

The physical formulation of induction heating of SP nanoparticles by alternating magnetic fields was given by Rosensweig [46]. Starting from first principles, Rosensweig established the conversion of magnetic work to internal energy when the magnetization of the magnetic fluid lags the applied magnetic field. He then expressed the magnetization in terms of the complex susceptibility $\chi = \chi' - i\chi''$, where χ' and χ'' are frequency dependent, a valid approach for low field strengths and minimal interactions between the particles. He subsequently derived the volumetric power dissipation of a magnetic fluid by an alternating magnetic field with strength H_0 and frequency $f = \omega/2\pi$, given by (in SI units)

$$P = \mu_0 \pi \chi'' f H_0^2 \qquad (7.3)$$

Rosensweig finally established the relationship between χ'' and the material parameters of the ferrofluid using the relaxation equations of Shliomis [62] that lead to a Debye model relation:

$$\chi'' = \frac{\omega\tau}{1 + \left(\omega\tau\right)^2} \chi_0 \qquad (7.4)$$

where χ_0 is the equilibrium susceptibility and τ the effective relaxation time due to the Brownian and Néel mechanisms described above. The power dissipation is then expressed as

$$P = \pi\mu_0\chi_0 fH_0^2 \frac{2\pi f\tau}{1 + \left(2\pi f\tau\right)^2} \tag{7.5}$$

The equilibrium susceptibility χ_0 is magnetic field dependent and may be related to the cord susceptibility of the Langevin equation through the expression:

$$\chi_0 = \chi_i \frac{3}{\xi}\left(\coth\xi - \frac{1}{\xi}\right) \tag{7.6}$$

where $\xi = \mu_0 M_d H V_M/k_B T$, M_d is the saturation magnetization, and χ_i is the initial susceptibility given by the initial slope of the magnetization curve.

As a first demonstration of the agreement of the Rosensweig model with available experimental data, we show in Figure 7.2 the SAR (in units of W g^{-1}), which is a measure of the power dissipation P, of various ferrofluids as a function of the initial susceptibility χ_i measured on dry particles as reported by Brusentsov et al. [20]. The measurements were performed at 0.88 MHz and 90 Oe peak magnetic field and the various ferrofluids covered a wide range of particle diameters, that is, from 3 up to 1000 nm.

The good correlation of the SAR value of various magnetic fluids of different diameters with the initial magnetization measured on the dry particles composing the fluids shows not only the validity of Equation 7.5 of the Rosensweig model but also the importance of magnetization in the induction heating of the magnetic fluids. In essence, the initial susceptibility is proportional to the volume of the particle [46]; therefore, the above linear relation between SAR and χ_i is valid for quite a large range of diameters.

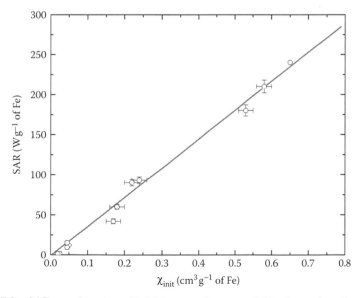

FIGURE 7.2 SAR as a function of initial magnetic susceptibility for various ferrofluids at $f = 0.88$ MHz and $H_0 = 90$ Oe. (Data from Brusentsov, N.A., et al., *Journal of Magnetism and Magnetic Materials*, 225(1–2), 113–117, 2001.)

7.2.2.3 Power Dissipation in Magnetic Fluids: Stable SD and Multidomain States

It is well accepted that the magnetic state of nanoparticles depends strongly on their size and shape. In this section, we consider the dependence of the power dissipation with the diameter of the nanoparticles.

In Figure 7.3a, we show the dependence of experimentally deduced SARs—in a reduced form—on the particle diameter for selected ferrofluids reported in the literature. The SAR values have been properly scaled by frequency and squared applied field $(f_0 H_0^2)$, in an effort to account for setups with different experimental conditions. Hence, according to Equation 7.5, the scaled quantity $SAR/f_0 H_0^2$ will reflect the diameter dependence of SAR through the dependence of χ_0 on diameter. It is tacitly assumed that the maximum heat dissipation P will occur only when $f\tau \approx 1$ (Equation 7.5).

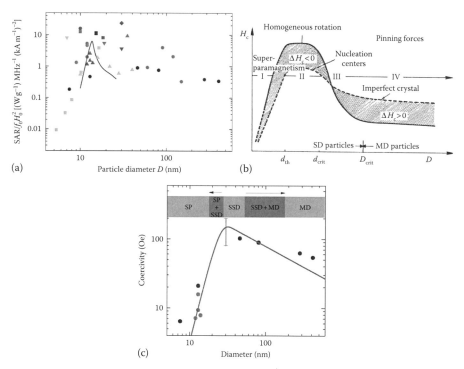

FIGURE 7.3 (See color insert.) (a) Reduced SAR (SAR/fH_0^2) as a function of particle diameter for various magnetic fluids. Data points are as follows: red circles (Data from Brusentsov, N.A., et al., *Journal of Magnetism and Magnetic Materials*, 225(1–2), 113–117, 2001.); black circles (From Ma, M., et al., *Journal of Magnetism and Magnetic Materials*, 268(1–2), 33–39, 2004.); blue circles (From Rabias, I., et al., *Biomicrofluidics*, 4(2), 024111 (1–8), 2010.); black squares (From Hergt, R., et al., *Journal of Magnetism and Magnetic Materials*, 270(3), 345–357, 2004.); blue squares (From Hergt, R., et al., *Journal of Magnetism and Magnetic Materials*, 280(2–3), 358–368, 2004.); green squares (From Fortin, J.P., et al., *Journal of the American Chemical Society*, 129(9), 2628–2635, 2007.); red squares (From Hilger, I., et al., *Radiology*, 218(2), 570–575, 2001.); blue triangles (From Hosono, T., et al., *Journal of Magnetism and*

It is observed in Figure 7.3a that despite the scatter of the experimental data, the reduced SAR values initially increase with increasing particle diameter, then reach a maximum in the size range 10–20 nm and subsequently gradually decrease. Theoretical calculations of SAR as a function of particle diameter have been performed by Rosensweig [46] based on Equation 7.5. These calculations show that an optimum particle size giving maximum heating rate exists, which is shown as line in Figure 7.3a for a particular set of experimental conditions taking into account the polydispersity of the samples. These calculations explain well the initial increase of SAR with diameter, reproduce the observed maximum but fall much more rapidly at larger sizes. This is due to the fact that Rosensweig's calculations assume SDSP particles. But it is well known that the magnetic state of the particles depends strongly on their size and shape. This state can be conveniently described by considering the coercive field H_c of the magnetic material through the different mechanisms involved in its magnetization process. Following closely the description and notation of Kronmüller, it is possible to distinguish four different regions for the coercive field as function of particle size D (Figure 7.3b) [64]. The first region (I) is the (unstable) SP region for particle diameters less than the critical diameter $D < d_{th}$ where the reversion of magnetization takes place by a thermally activated process. The second region (II) (homogeneous rotation in Figure 7.3b) represents particles with $d_{th} < D < d_{cr}$ where the reversion of magnetization is independent of size and takes place by a uniform rotation process. This

FIGURE 7.3 **(Continued)** *Magnetic Materials*, 321(19), 3019–3023, 2009.); red triangle (From Timko, M., et al., *Journal of Magnetism and Magnetic Materials*, 321(10), 1521–1524, 2009.); green triangles (From Levy, M., et al., *Journal of Physics—Condensed Matter*, 20(20), 2008.); green inverted triangle (From Jordan, A., et al., *Journal of Nanoparticle Research*, 5(5–6), 597–600, 2003.); red inverted triangle (Data from Zhang, L.Y., et al., *Journal of Magnetism and Magnetic Materials*, 311(1), 228–233, 2007.); blue inverted triangle (From Verges, M.A., et al., *Journal of Physics D—Applied Physics*, 41(13), 134003 (1–10), 2008.); diamond (From Hergt, R., et al., *Journal of Magnetism and Magnetic Materials*, 293(1), 80–86, 2005.). The line is a theoretical calculation (From Rosensweig, R.E., *Journal of Magnetism and Magnetic Materials*, 252(1–3), 370–374, 2002.) based on Equation 7.5 using a distribution of particle sizes. (b) Qualitative dependence of H_c on the particle diameter D. (With kind permission from Springer Science: *Science and Technology of Nanostructured Magnetic Materials*, Micromagnetism and magnetization processes in modern magnetic materials, 1991, p. 657, Kronmuller, H., Figure 7.3.) The behavior for perfect (solid line) and imperfect (dashed line) particles is shown. (c) Experimental values of coercivity H_c as a function of particle diameter for the same magnetic fluids as in Figure 7.3a (where applicable). Data points are as follows: black circles (From Ma, M., et al., *Journal of Magnetism and Magnetic Materials*, 268(1–2), 33–39, 2004.); red circles (From Hosono, T., et al., *Journal of Magnetism and Magnetic Materials*, 321(19), 3019–3023, 2009.); green line (From Alphandery, E., et al., *ACS Nano*, 3(6), 1539–1547, 2009.). The blue line is an approximate expression (From Hergt, R., S. Dutz, and M. Roder, *Journal of Physics—Condensed Matter*, 20(38), 2008.) (see text for details). On the top of Figure 7.3c, the critical sizes and ranges for the magnetic states of magnetite nanoparticles as calculated from Muxworthy and Williams are shown as shaded regions (From Muxworthy, A.R. and W. Williams, *Journal of the Royal Society Interface*, 6(41), 1207–1212, 2009.). The arrows indicate the variation of the regions of magnetic states with increasing interactions between the particles.

region is also referred to as stable SD (SSD) magnetic state [65]. The third region (III) represents particles with $d_{cr} < D < D_{crit}$ where an inhomogeneous rotation process (curling mode) with decreasing critical fields takes place. Finally in the fourth region (IV), for larger particles $D > D_{crit}$, the SD particles transform into multidomain (MD) particles where the reversion of magnetization takes place by domain wall displacements. It could then be argued that the maximum heating rate corresponds to particles being in the homogeneous rotation (SSD) state and the subsequent gradual decrease of the heating rate originates from the transition to the MD state. With respect to the above considerations, we also present in the top of Figure 7.3c (shaded areas) calculations of critical sizes performed by Muxworthy and Williams [65] of the critical SP to SSD size of elongated magnetite particles as well as the SD to MD critical sizes. These critical size calculations were performed as functions of the particle elongation axial ratio (short/long axis) including also the contribution of magnetic interactions [65]. Only the results for symmetrical particles (axial ratio = 1) are shown in Figure 7.3c. The arrows indicate the variation of the regions of magnetic states with increasing interactions between the particles. For lower axial ratios, the critical lengths significantly increase [65]. It is clear that the largest SAR values lie in the transition region between SP and SSD regions. This observation has also been noted by Hergt et al. [66] and Dutz et al. [67], but it was mainly based on *magnetic* measurements of hysteresis losses of magnetic nanoparticle powders. In particular, Dutz has found a good correlation between the hysteresis losses per cycle and the coercivity of the measured minor loops [67]. In this work, we have rather attempted to correlate the *calorimetrically* measured SAR with coercivity through their dependences on diameter. The strong magnetic signal of magnetosomes is exhibited in the SSD magnetic state [26,68]. Finally, in Figure 7.3c, we show the experimental values (where applicable) of the coercive field H_c as a function of particle diameter for the same experimental data of Figure 7.3a from which the SAR values were obtained. The solid line is the expression [66]:

$$H_c(D) = H_M \left(\frac{D}{D_1}\right)^{-0.6} \left[1 - \exp\left(-\frac{D}{D_1}\right)^5\right] \tag{7.7}$$

which can approximate experimental observations. The data of Figure 7.3c can well be approximated with Equation 7.7 using $D_1 = 25$ nm for the adjustable parameter.

The qualitative dependence of H_c on the particle diameter D—for this rather limited number of experimental data—is thus verified.

7.3 MATERIALS, INSTRUMENTATION, AND METHODS

7.3.1 SYNTHETIC METHODS FOR PREPARATION OF MAGNETIC FLUIDS

Since the first attempts to produce ferromagnetic liquids by dispersing ferromagnetic particles in a carrier fluid in 1779 and the first successful development of an ultrastable ferromagnetic liquid by Papell in 1965 for the National Aeronautics and Space Administration (NASA) [57], the synthetic methods (based primarily on wet chemistry methods) of magnetic fluids and associated magnetic nanoparticles have been the focus of intensive research [69,70]. In magnetic hyperthermia, magnetic fluids based on iron oxide nanoparticles are mostly preferred due to their biological compatibility.

In the following, a case study [71] is presented for the synthetic route of a dispersion of highly charged dextran-coated γ-Fe$_2$O$_3$ (maghemite) nanoparticles, which will be subsequently investigated for its magnetic hyperthermia performance both *in vitro* (Section 7.4) and *in vivo* (Section 7.5). The synthetic efforts of this study have focused on the optimization of the surface charge of the dextran coating, while keeping pH close to the physiological acidity value in the living organisms (pH ~7), which is a prerequisite for biological applications. The reason for synthesizing highly charged nanoparticles is to endure constant heating for several minutes at high temperatures and keep the colloidal stability of the magnetic fluid intact. In a colloidal suspension during magnetically induced radio frequency (rf) heating, the resulting temperature rise increases the average numbers of particle collisions. Hence, keeping nanoparticles as far as possible, by increasing electrostatic repulsion, it is possible to minimize the number of particle collisions (and thus prevent agglomeration that reduces the efficiency of the induction heating) for a long period of time.

The dispersion of γ-Fe$_2$O$_3$ (maghemite) nanoparticles is synthesized by the reaction of ferric chloride and ferrous chloride in the presence of KOH, using the co-precipitation method [55,72]. Three magnetic fluid suspensions are synthesized: one comprising uncoated maghemite nanoparticles and two comprising nanoparticles coated with dextran, a biocompatible macromolecule that easily adsorbs on the maghemite surface. The dextran molecule hinders cluster growth after nucleation due to the reaction between iron cations and hydroxide anions. The nominal molecular weight of the dextran coating used was 55,000 Da.

Specifically, maghemite nanoparticles (magnetic fluid samples S1, S2, S3) are prepared by co-precipitation mixing 100 ml acidic solutions of 0.66 M FeCl$_3$ and 0.33 M FeCl$_2$. In the case of S2 and S3 magnetic fluids, 1 wt.% of dextran is also added. A 100 ml alkaline solution of KOH (1 M) is then added dropwise over 5–10 min with stirring on a magnetic stirrer while maintaining constant temperature to prevent widening of nanoparticles' size distribution. The stirring continues for a short period of 20 min under a nitrogen gas atmosphere at 60°C—a longer period would introduce particle growth. The particles obtained are washed 3 times with ethanol and water using ultracentrifugation (5000 rpm for 10 min at 10°C) with nitrogen-purged water. The magnetic fluids are prepared at high pH and are constantly stirred during this fast one-step reaction to avoid the appearance of larger particles. The pH of the final magnetic fluid is decreased by carefully numbered titrations of 0.01 M HCl (three washes) to achieve neutrality. In the last titration, 0.1 wt.% of dextran is added for better dispersion. Last, and of extreme importance, continuous sonication for 10 min and repetitive filtering of the final colloid through a 0.2 µm porous membrane is performed. For comparison and optimization reasons, three magnetic fluids with different surface charge are investigated: an ionic one, with no coating (S1) and zeta potential value 8 mV, and two dextran-coated and zeta potential values 70 mV (S2) and 350 mV (S3), respectively. In the case of S1, nanoparticle agglomerations, with average size ~200 nm according to dynamic light scattering measurements, are formed right after the synthesis at neutral pH. The highest values of zeta potential for S1 (40 mV and −40 mV, respectively) are observed at low (<4) and high (>8) pH values, most likely due to the hydrodynamic forces introduced by sonication, which are strong enough to prevent the formation of weak bonds.

On the other hand, both dextran-coated S2 and S3 magnetic fluids exhibit positive zeta potential values at neutral pH and are nicely dispersed into the fluid, due to strong electrostatic and steric repulsion forces. In this way, zeta potential values as high as 350 mV (S3) at pH ~7 are achieved. The coated maghemite nanoparticle magnetic fluid (S3) yield, determined by weighing of the lyophilized sample of the preparation, is 20 mg/ml, a value that characterizes a dense colloidal suspension.

7.3.2　Glioma Cell Lines—Animals

Male Wistar rats weighing 250–350 g were used in this study [71]. The rats were fed *ad libitum* with standard laboratory food and water. They were individually housed in a controlled environment (18–22°C; 50%–75% relative humidity) and maintained under a 12-h dark cycle. All animal procedures adhered to standard principles of animal care and were approved by the local animal welfare committee.

C6 glioma cells were maintained in a Ham F12 minimum essential medium containing 10% fetal bovine serum and 1% penicillin/streptomycin. The cells were grown to confluency in a humidified atmosphere of 5% CO_2 at 37°C. Exponential growth cultures were harvested with a solution of 0.05% trypsin and 0.02% ethylenediaminetetraacetic acid (EDTA) and resuspended in a Ham F12 medium. C6 cells were washed in a Ham F12 medium and viable cells counted by a hemocytometer. Finally, cells were suspended in a Ham F12 minimum essential medium to a final concentration of 8×10^6 cells per 10 µl for inoculation.

Rats were anesthetized by intraperitoneal (IP) injection of 10 mg/kg xylazine (Bayer, Leverkusen, Germany) and 100 mg/kg ketamine (Parke-Davis, Courbevoie, France), in combination with 0.05 mg/kg atropine (Bayer, Leverkusen, Germany).

Tissue covering the skull was gently elevated and the bregma identified. Approximately 8×10^6 cells were inoculated in the area anterior of the bregma.

After 2 weeks, the development of a tumor was palpable and visible. On week 4, tumors had an average size of 5–10 mm and inoculation of nanoparticles took place. Rats were anesthetized as above.

7.3.3　Magnetic Hyperthermia Instrumentation

7.3.3.1　Induction Heating Instrumentation

In vitro magnetic hyperthermia experiments are usually performed using laboratory inductor setups consisting of a high-power rf generator, an rf power meter, an impedance matching network, and one or more induction coil applicators. In this way, usually only single-frequency measurements may be performed and recently frequency-adjustable applicators have been considered [73].

The *in vitro* and *in vivo* magnetic hyperthermia experiments in the case studies considered (Sections 7.4 and 7.5) were performed using a 10 kW induction heating machine (Termotek, by Termomacchine, Torino, Italy) connected to a homemade four-loop copper water-cooled coil, operating at a fixed rf of 150 kHz. This setup easily provides alternating magnetic field amplitudes of up to 30 kA/m.

The amplitude of the rf field at the sample was measured by monitoring the inductive root mean square value of voltage (V_{rms}) at the coil. Then the intensity of the rf field may be calculated using the formula:

$$B_{rf} = \frac{V_{rms}\sqrt{2}}{2N\pi^2 r^2 f}$$

where B_{rf} is the rf field in Tesla, N the number of turns of the coil, r the radius of the coil, and f the rf frequency.

7.3.3.2 Method for Temperature Measurements

In magnetic hyperthermia and related research and applications where subjects and models are being exposed to intense rf fields, conventional thermocouple or thermistor probes cannot be used for such measurements due to severe field distortions caused by the metallic leads of these devices, which are also subject to induction heating themselves.

The most reliable method used for temperature measurements in magnetic hyperthermia experiments is based on a fiberoptic thermometry system that allows users to measure temperature in extremely harsh electromagnetic environments. The technology involved is called fluoroptic thermometry (FOT) and is based on probes that are totally immune to electromagnetic interference and are of entirely nonmetallic construction. These qualities make FOT probes perfectly suited for measuring temperatures in harsh environments often encountered during biomedical research, such as (1) high static magnetic fields and kilohertz range switching gradients used in magnetic resonance imaging, and (2) alternating magnetic fields at the kilohertz range like induction heating devices.

High-resistance thermistors of special construction may also be used for the temperature measurement in magnetic hyperthermia experiments. Since the signals of such temperature sensors are very weak, care should be taken in the construction of the electronics driving the thermistor.

Finally, another temperature probe is the thermographic camera. The thermographic camera technique has the advantage that the SAR pattern is obtained in a plane rather than at a single point where the conventional probe is inserted. However, this technique has lower accuracy in the measurement of temperature compared to the thermistor or the fiberoptic sensor.

7.3.3.3 SAR Calorimetric Determination

The efficiency of the heating power of a magnetic fluid is described by the amount of energy converted into heat per unit of time and mass and is called the specific absorption rate (SAR), given by (see, e.g., [74]):

$$SAR = \frac{\Delta Q}{\Delta t m_{Fe}} = c \frac{m_f}{m_{Fe}} \frac{\Delta T}{\Delta t}$$

where c is the specific heat capacity of the ferrofluid, calculated as the mass-weighted mean value of the magnetic material and water; m_f the mass of the ferrofluid; m_{Fe} the mass of the iron in the ferrofluid; T the temperature; and t the time. The rate of temperature change $\Delta T / \Delta t$ is measured from the initial slopes of the experimental temperature versus time curves.

7.4   *IN VITRO* MAGNETIC HYPERTHERMIA IN MAGNETIC FLUIDS

An important factor for efficient magnetic heating, especially for magnetic fluids in microliter quantities, is the nanoparticle concentration in the aqueous solution. In principle, the denser the magnetic fluid (in our case study 20 mg/ml, see Section 7.3.1), the highest the obtained heating effect. On the other hand, in dense magnetic fluids, considerable magnetic interparticle interactions are present (Section 7.2.1), which result in particle clustering and subsequent strong reduction of the magnetic heating efficiency. In the following *in vitro* case study [71], we will show how high surface charges on the surface of maghemite nanoparticles may prohibit nanoparticle agglomeration, keep the colloidal stability of the magnetic fluid intact, and ensure constant heating during magnetic hyperthermia applications for several minutes at high temperatures.

Figure 7.4 shows visible and infrared photos of samples—one with water and the other with magnetic fluid in the rf heater apparatus (Section 7.3.3). One can observe in the infrared part (Figure 7.4b) that the magnetic fluid sample, when heated, changes color to red while the water sample is not visible.

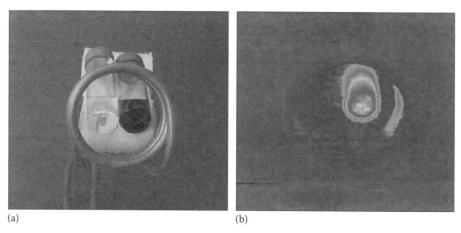

(a)   (b)

FIGURE 7.4   (See color insert.) (a) The copper coil of the magnetic heating apparatus used (Section 7.3.3) with an aqueous sample (left tube) and a dextran-coated maghemite magnetic fluid (right tube). (b) An infrared image of the samples during magnetic heating using a thermographic camera (Section 7.3.3). Heating is observed only in the magnetic fluid sample.

Figure 7.5 shows the temperature dependence as a function of the heating time for three magnetic fluids containing maghemite nanoparticles: S1 (uncoated particles, zeta potential 8 mV), S2 (dextran-coated particles, zeta potential 70 mV), and S3 (dextran-coated particles, zeta potential 350 mV), as described in Section 7.3.1 [71]. Heating is performed with a copper coil (inset in Figure 7.5b), which produces the moderate rf magnetic field with amplitude 11 kA/m and frequency 150 kHz, much lower than the typical value of 400–500 kHz commonly used. Samples are heated from room temperature to the maximum temperature value and then left to cool down to the initial conditions.

In Figure 7.5a, a strong effect of the zeta potential upon heating is observed: The S1 sample with the lowest zeta potential value does not produce any significant heating effect, and starts to flocculate right after heating. The S2 sample exhibits a respectable temperature rise, reaching 60°C within 10 min. Similarly, the S1 sample, S2, shows problems in stability and endurance, and it is instantly flocculated after the heating treatment. In contrast, the S3 sample exhibits an impressive heating effect, reaching 98°C within 3 min, with no traces of flocculation and a remarkable long-term stability, despite the fact that it almost reached water boiling temperature. The corresponding SAR is calculated at 286 W/g. This is among the highest SAR values obtained under the specific experimental conditions. Most spectacular, by scaling down the quantity of S3, an exceptional heating response is

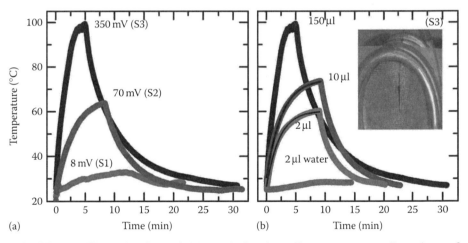

(a)   (b)   Time (min)

FIGURE 7.5   **(See color insert.)** Magnetic heating effect on aqueous dispersions of dextran-coated maghemite nanoparticles. (a) The influence of the zeta potential on 150 μl magnetic fluids S1 (green points), S2 (blue points), and S3 (black points). (b) The influence of the volume on 150 μl (black points), 10 μl (blue points), and 2 μl (red points) of magnetic fluid S3. The solid black lines refer to fitting of the experimental data. The green points correspond to the sample of 2 μl water, used as control sample. In the inset, the coil of the magnetic heating apparatus, with the 10 μl sample, and the optical fiber used for the temperature monitoring are shown, after removing the heat-insulating cover. (Reprinted with permission from Rabias, I., et al., Rapid magnetic heating treatment by highly charged maghemite nanoparticles on Wistar rats exocranial glioma tumors at microliter volume. *Biomicrofluidics*, 2010. 4(2): 024111 (1–8). Copyright 2010, American Institute of Physics.)

observed (Figure 7.5b): 2 µl of this magnetic fluid containing 40 µg of γ-Fe_2O_3 (red data points) exhibit a temperature rise of 33°C within 10 min.

The experimental data for sample S3 in Figure 7.5b have also been analyzed according to the expression $T(t) = T_{initial} + \Delta T_{max}\left[1 - \exp(-t/\tau)\right]$, where $T_{initial}$ is the initial temperature, ΔT_{max} the overall temperature change, and τ the time constant of heating [43,75]. The pertinent quantity in magnetic hyperthermia is the initial rate (dT/dt) $t = 0$ which in this case equals to $\Delta T_{max}/\tau$. The fits of the above equation to the experimental data during the heating process are shown as solid black lines in Figure 7.5b, and yield similar heating rates $\Delta T_{max}/\tau \approx 17$°C/min for the 2 and 10 µl samples. Reliable analysis of the 150 µl sample is not possible, due to the fast attainment of the boiling temperature of water. However, by fitting the experimental data during the cooling process, the same cooling rate $\Delta T_{max}/\tau \approx 12$°C/min is obtained for all three samples. This demonstrates the accuracy and reliability of the experiments. In addition, the 150 µl sample has not been physically or chemically destroyed by reaching the boiling temperature of water, a sign of the high stability of the synthesized nanodispersion.

Evidently, the principal factor that controls the heating effect in the colloid state is the prevention of agglomeration, that is, the elimination of interparticle interactions, provided that the size and magnetic properties of the maghemite core particles are "tuned" to maximum energy absorption. The *in vitro* experiments of these magnetic fluids markedly showed that it is the surface charge that prevents agglomeration during the heating stage of the magnetic fluid by minimizing the collisions between the nanoparticles. It is anticipated that strong interactions are present in the magnetic fluids due to the high concentration of maghemite in the suspensions (20 mg/ml), and it is the presence of the charged coating that prevents agglomeration and gives rise to the strong heating effect in the 350 mV S3 sample. Indeed, the less charged 70 mV S2 sample, which has the same high concentration (20 mg/ml) as the S3 sample, presents less magnetic heating than the S3 magnetic fluid (Figure 7.5a), due to the fact that the weak charge cannot compensate the large interparticle interactions and the S2 material exhibits flocculation and there is no colloidal stability during the magnetic heating process. Hence, this case study indicated that surface charge may play a pivotal role in the stability and magnetic heating efficiency of a magnetic fluid, especially at elevated temperatures for a long period of time.

7.5 *IN VIVO* MAGNETIC HYPERTHERMIA IN ANIMAL MODELS

Magnetic fluids for *in vivo* magnetic hyperthermia uses have specific constraints than those used for other applications. For *in vivo* magnetic hyperthermia applications, magnetic fluids require biocompatibility, must be capable of being functionalized, must retain their magnetic properties for a period of time in aqueous media with varying pH, must not be cleared too quickly from the bloodstream, and must form stable colloidal dispersions. If not, magnetic fluids introduced into the bloodstream are covered rapidly by components of the circulation, such as plasma proteins, in a process called *opsonization*. A significant fraction of the nanoparticles will be cleared from the circulation system in as little as 15 min.

Also one should consider that the efficacy of magnetic hyperthermia is balancing between the rates of thermal energy deposition with thermal dissipation. Tissue heating is complex due to factors affecting temperature change such as blood flow, tissue density, and fat. The dependence of temperature rise on distance is steep, and there are delays in heating and cooling after the field is applied or removed. Skull shield tissues produce inhomogeneous heating. Tumors in internal organs, such as the liver and kidney, have proven to be more difficult to heat due to high blood flow. Nonuniformity of tumors also poses a complication, as large tumors heat at a greater rate than small tumors due to poorer tissue cooling and differences in heat conduction in the necrotic regions of large tumors.

In this case study [71], one of the most significant challenges implementing colloidal magnetic nanoparticles in medicine—the efficient magnetic heating of microliter quantities—has been investigated. In particular, we examine the *in vivo* efficiency of the highly charged dextran-coated maghemite magnetic fluid (sample S3, Sections 7.3.1 and 7.4.1) in magnetic hyperthermia of small rat glioma tumors. Gliomas are a group of heterogeneous primary central nervous system tumors arising from the glial cells. A recent review of the application of magnetic hyperthermia in glioma treatment using iron oxide nanoparticles is given by Silva [76].

As described analytically in Sections 7.3 and 7.4, synthetic efforts have been focused on the optimization of the surface charge of the dextran coating, while keeping pH close to the physiological acidity value in the living organisms (pH ~7), which is a prerequisite for biological applications. The difference to previous synthetic attempts is the high charge of the dextran coating, which according to this study maintains the colloidal stability and good dispersion of the magnetic fluid during the magnetic heating stage. The ultimate goal is to accomplish nonsurgically the treatment of millimeter-sized tumors.

Specifically, 150 μl of magnetic fluid containing 3 mg of dextran-coated γ-Fe$_2$O$_3$ (sample S3) reached temperatures up to 99°C within 3 min with no indication of flocculation, when exposed to a moderate magnetic field with amplitude of 11 kA/m and frequency of 150 kHz; during *in vivo* treatment, by infusing the magnetic fluid in animal model (rat) glioma tumors for 20 min causes an impressive cancer tissue dissolution [71]. An infrared temperature image (upper inset in Figure 7.6b) shows the ability to heat a precise area of the glioma tumor. Following treatment, the rats were sacrificed, tumors were excised, and paraffin-embedded sections were stained to reveal the nuclei and cytoplasm of cells using hematoxylin and eosin, a standard staining protocol for examining tissue integrity.

As can be seen in Figure 7.6b and d, the treatment led to extensive tumor tissue damage and dissolution, indicating that the obtained temperatures are close to boiling temperatures. Control experiments included the infusion of S3 magnetic fluid without subsequent treatment, as well as exposure to magnetic hyperthermia in the absence of magnetic fluid (Figure 7.6a and c). No tumor tissue damage is observed in either case. Thus, the produced surface-charged coated magnetic fluid S3 performed excellently in the *in vivo* studies, due to the preservation of the good dispersion of the magnetic fluid within the tumor during the hyperthermia heating.

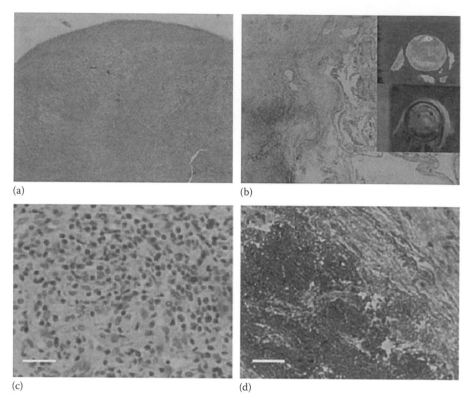

FIGURE 7.6 **(See color insert.)** For *in vivo* magnetic heating of small rat glioma tumors, 150 μl S3 magnetic fluid is infused into rat glioma tumors with size 5–10 mm, and subsequently subjected to magnetic hyperthermia treatment for 20 min. Panels (a) and (c) (low and high magnification, respectively) represent sections of control tumor tissue treated without nanoparticles. Panels (b) and (d) (low and high magnification, respectively) show extensive damage of the tumor tissue after treatment with magnetic fluid. White bars = 200 μm. The lower inset in panel (b) shows the experimental setup for *in vivo* magnetic heating. The upper inset is an infrared image, which demonstrates the ability of the magnetic fluid to produce strong localized heating at the tumor position. (Reprinted with permission from Rabias, I., et al., Rapid magnetic heating treatment by highly charged maghemite nanoparticles on Wistar rats exocranial glioma tumors at microliter volume. *Biomicrofluidics*, 2010. 4(2): 024111 (1–8). Copyright 2010, American Institute of Physics.)

7.6   CONCLUSION

Understanding the considerable interplay between the structural, magnetic, and colloidal parameters in a colloidal assembly of magnetic nanoparticles is an important challenge in the field of magnetic hyperthermia. It has implications at both a fundamental and an applied level. The most significant quantities pertinent to the physical mechanisms of the phenomenon include the size and distribution of the particles, their crystallinity, chemical composition, magnetic state, concentration, interparticle interactions, solvent viscosity, and stability of the fluid medium. In addition, external parameters such as the frequency and the amplitude of the alternating magnetic field directly influence the heating power of the particles.

In this chapter, the fundamental properties and relaxation mechanisms of magnetic nanoparticles are considered in connection with the efficiency of the associated magnetic fluids in magnetically induced hyperthermia. Two case studies (*in vitro* and *in vivo*) have also been presented. Initially, the colloidal stability and the magnetic properties of the magnetic fluid are briefly discussed. Then, the established heat dissipation mechanisms are reviewed. Particular emphasis is given in the dependences of the power dissipation (SAR) on some parameters characterizing the magnetic fluids such as the initial susceptibility and the diameter of the magnetic nanoparticles. An attempt has been made to correlate the calorimetrically measured SAR values with the magnetic state of the nanoparticles and particularly the transitions from the SP to the SSD and MD magnetic states. This was accomplished through the dependence of the SAR and the coercivity of the nanoparticles on their diameters using literature data.

In the first case study, the importance of the colloidal stability of the magnetic fluids in the efficiency of magnetic hyperthermia is demonstrated. In particular, in the *in vitro* study, it is shown that high surface charges on the surface of magnetic nanoparticles may prohibit nanoparticle agglomeration, keep the colloidal stability of the magnetic fluid intact, and ensure constant magnetic heating during magnetic hyperthermia applications for several minutes at high temperatures. The results of the *in vitro* study lead to the argument that a balance between density and charge is the key for an effective and stable magnetic fluid at elevated temperatures. The successful application of such magnetic fluids in magnetic hyperthermia in animal models is described in the *in vivo* study.

The final conclusion of this chapter is that a magnetic fluid with high colloidal stability (obtained, e.g., by surface charges) consisting of magnetic nanoparticles with diameters corresponding to the SSD magnetic state is expected to show exceptional heating ability in magnetic hyperthermia applications.

A relevant issue to be addressed in the field of magnetic hyperthermia is the detailed theoretical examination of the influence of the magnetic dipole–dipole interactions between the nanoparticles in the efficiency of the magnetic induction. This is a complex problem and quite recently has only been tackled numerically [77]. Since the interparticle dipole–dipole interaction is closely associated with the concentration of the nanoparticles, a peak of the SAR is expected at a given concentration [77]. Experimental data are rather scarce (however, see [33,42,78]) to support the theoretical predictions and more experimental efforts are consequently needed along this direction.

REFERENCES

1. Jordan, A., et al., Magnetic fluid hyperthermia (MFH): Cancer treatment with AC magnetic field induced excitation of biocompatible superparamagnetic nanoparticles. *Journal of Magnetism and Magnetic Materials*, 1999. 201: p. 413–419.
2. Gilchrist, R.K., et al., Selective inductive heating of lymph nodes. *Annals of Surgery*, 1957. 146(4): p. 596–606.
3. Hergt, R. and W. Andrä, Magnetic hyperthermia and thermoablation, in *Magnetism in Medicine: A Handbook*, 2nd ed, eds. W. Andrä and H. Nowak, 2007. Wiley-VCH Verlag GmbH & Co. KGaA: Weinheim, p. 550.

4. Baronzio, G.F. and E.D. Hager, *Hyperthermia in Cancer Treatment: A Primer*, 2006. Springer: New York.
5. Pankhurst, Q.A., et al., Progress in applications of magnetic nanoparticles in biomedicine. *Journal of Physics D—Applied Physics*, 2009. 42(22): 224001 (1–15).
6. Mornet, S., et al., Magnetic nanoparticle design for medical diagnosis and therapy. *Journal of Materials Chemistry*, 2004. 14(14): p. 2161–2175.
7. Neuberger, T., et al., Superparamagnetic nanoparticles for biomedical applications: Possibilities and limitations of a new drug delivery system. *Journal of Magnetism and Magnetic Materials*, 2005. 293(1): p. 483–496.
8. Hergt, R., et al., Magnetic particle hyperthermia: Nanoparticle magnetism and materials development for cancer therapy. *Journal of Physics—Condensed Matter*, 2006. 18(38): p. S2919–S2934.
9. Pankhurst, Q.A., et al., Applications of magnetic nanoparticles in biomedicine. *Journal of Physics D—Applied Physics*, 2003. 36(13): p. R167–R181.
10. Figuerola, A., et al., From iron oxide nanoparticles towards advanced iron-based inorganic materials designed for biomedical applications. *Pharmacological Research*, 2010. 62(2): p. 126–143.
11. Laurent, S., et al., Magnetic fluid hyperthermia: Focus on superparamagnetic iron oxide nanoparticles. *Advances in Colloid and Interface Science*, 2011. 166(1–2): p. 8–23.
12. Sharifi, I., H. Shokrollahi, and S. Amiri, Ferrite-based magnetic nanofluids used in hyperthermia applications. *Journal of Magnetism and Magnetic Materials*, 2012. 324(6): p. 903–915.
13. Giri, Y., et al., Preparation and investigation of potentiality of different soft ferrites for hyperthermia applications. *Journal of Applied Physics*, 2005. 97(10): 10Q916 (1–3).
14. Vasseur, S., et al., Lanthanum manganese perovskite nanoparticles as possible in vivo mediators for magnetic hyperthermia. *Journal of Magnetism and Magnetic Materials*, 2006. 302(2): p. 315–320.
15. Verde, E.L., et al., Magnetic hyperthermia investigation of cobalt ferrite nanoparticles: Comparison between experiment, linear response theory, and dynamic hysteresis simulations. *Journal of Applied Physics*, 2012. 111(12): 123902 (1–8).
16. Fortin, J.P., F. Gazeau, and C. Wilhelm, Intracellular heating of living cells through Neel relaxation of magnetic nanoparticles. *European Biophysics Journal with Biophysics Letters*, 2008. 37(2): p. 223–228.
17. Kashevsky, B.E., et al., Study of cobalt ferrite nanosuspensions for low-frequency ferromagnetic hyperthermia. *Particuology*, 2008. 6(5): p. 322–333.
18. Lacroix, L.M., et al., Magnetic hyperthermia in single-domain monodisperse FeCo nanoparticles: Evidences for Stoner–Wohlfarth behavior and large losses. *Journal of Applied Physics*, 2009. 105(2): 023911 (1–4).
19. Mehdaoui, B., et al., Large specific absorption rates in the magnetic hyperthermia properties of metallic iron nanocubes. *Journal of Magnetism and Magnetic Materials*, 2010. 322(19): p. L49–L52.
20. Brusentsov, N.A., et al., Evaluation of ferromagnetic fuids and suspensions for the site-specific radiofrequency-induced hyperthermia of MX11 sarcoma cells in vitro. *Journal of Magnetism and Magnetic Materials*, 2001. 225(1–2): p. 113–117.
21. Hilger, I., et al., Electromagnetic heating of breast tumors in interventional radiology: In vitro and in vivo studies in human cadavers and mice. *Radiology*, 2001. 218(2): p. 570–575.
22. Jordan, A., et al., Increase of the specific absorption rate (SAR) by magnetic fractionation of magnetic fluids. *Journal of Nanoparticle Research*, 2003. 5(5–6): p. 597–600.
23. Ma, M., et al., Size dependence of specific power absorption of Fe3O4 particles in AC magnetic field. *Journal of Magnetism and Magnetic Materials*, 2004. 268(1–2): p. 33–39.

24. Hergt, R., et al., Maghemite nanoparticles with very high AC-losses for application in RF-magnetic hyperthermia. *Journal of Magnetism and Magnetic Materials*, 2004. 270(3): p. 345–357.

25. Hergt, R., et al., Enhancement of AC-losses of magnetic nanoparticles for heating applications. *Journal of Magnetism and Magnetic Materials*, 2004. 280(2–3): p. 358–368.

26. Hergt, R., et al., Magnetic properties of bacterial magnetosomes as potential diagnostic and therapeutic tools. *Journal of Magnetism and Magnetic Materials*, 2005. 293(1): p. 80–86.

27. Okawa, K., et al., Heating ability of magnetite nanobeads with various sizes for magnetic hyperthermia at 120 kHz, a noninvasive frequency. *Journal of Applied Physics*, 2006. 99(8): 08H102 (1–3).

28. Fortin, J.P., et al., Size-sorted anionic iron oxide nanomagnets as colloidal mediators for magnetic hyperthermia. *Journal of the American Chemical Society*, 2007. 129(9): p. 2628–2635.

29. Zhang, L.Y., H.C. Gu, and X.M. Wang, Magnetite ferrofluid with high specific absorption rate for application in hyperthermia. *Journal of Magnetism and Magnetic Materials*, 2007. 311(1): p. 228–233.

30. Levy, M., et al., Magnetically induced hyperthermia: Size-dependent heating power of gamma-Fe(2)O(3) nanoparticles. *Journal of Physics—Condensed Matter*, 2008. 20(20): 204133 (1–5).

31. Goya, G.F., et al., Magnetic hyperthermia with Fe3O4 nanoparticles: The influence of particle size on energy absorption. *IEEE Transactions on Magnetics*, 2008. 44(11): p. 4444–4447.

32. Motoyama, J., et al., Size dependent heat generation of magnetite nanoparticles under AC magnetic field for cancer therapy. *Biomagnetic Research and Technology*, 2008. 6: p. 4.

33. Verges, M.A., et al., Uniform and water stable magnetite nanoparticles with diameters around the monodomain-multidomain limit. *Journal of Physics D—Applied Physics*, 2008. 41(13): 134003 (1–10).

34. Hosono, T., et al., Synthesis of magnetite nanoparticles for AC magnetic heating. *Journal of Magnetism and Magnetic Materials*, 2009. 321(19): p. 3019–3023.

35. Balakrishnan, S., M.J. Bonder, and G.C. Hadjipanayis, Particle size effect on phase and magnetic properties of polymer-coated magnetic nanoparticles. *Journal of Magnetism and Magnetic Materials*, 2009. 321(2): p. 117–122.

36. Joshi, H.M., et al., Effects of shape and size of cobalt ferrite nanostructures on their MRI contrast and thermal activation. *Journal of Physical Chemistry C*, 2009. 113(41): p. 17761–17767.

37. Gonzales-Weimuller, M., M. Zeisberger, and K.M. Krishnan, Size-dependent heating rates of iron oxide nanoparticles for magnetic fluid hyperthermia. *Journal of Magnetism and Magnetic Materials*, 2009. 321(13): p. 1947–1950.

38. Levy, M., et al., Correlating magneto-structural properties to hyperthermia performance of highly monodisperse iron oxide nanoparticles prepared by a seeded-growth route. *Chemistry of Materials*, 2011. 23(18): p. 4170–4180.

39. Mehdaoui, B., et al., Optimal size of nanoparticles for magnetic hyperthermia: A combined theoretical and experimental study. *Advanced Functional Materials*, 2011. 21(23): p. 4573–4581.

40. Jeun, M., et al., Physical limits of pure superparamagnetic Fe3O4 nanoparticles for a local hyperthermia agent in nanomedicine. *Applied Physics Letters*, 2012. 100(9): 092406 (1–4).

41. Timko, M., et al., Magnetic properties and heating effect in bacterial magnetic nanoparticles. *Journal of Magnetism and Magnetic Materials*, 2009. 321(10): p. 1521–1524.

42. Pineiro-Redondo, Y., et al., The influence of colloidal parameters on the specific power absorption of PAA-coated magnetite nanoparticles. *Nanoscale Research Letters*, 2011. 6(1): p. 383.

43. Bekovic, M. and A. Hamler, Determination of the heating effect of magnetic fluid in alternating magnetic field. *IEEE Transactions on Magnetics*, 2010. 46(2): p. 552–555.
44. Li, C.H., P. Hodgins, and G.P. Peterson, Experimental study of fundamental mechanisms in inductive heating of ferromagnetic nanoparticles suspension (Fe(3)O(4) iron oxide ferrofluid). *Journal of Applied Physics*, 2011. 110(5): 054303 (1–10).
45. Hiergeist, R., et al., Application of magnetite ferrofluids for hyperthermia. *Journal of Magnetism and Magnetic Materials*, 1999. 201: p. 420–422.
46. Rosensweig, R.E., Heating magnetic fluid with alternating magnetic field. *Journal of Magnetism and Magnetic Materials*, 2002. 252(1–3): p. 370–374.
47. Habib, A.H., et al., Evaluation of iron-cobalt/ferrite core-shell nanoparticles for cancer thermotherapy. *Journal of Applied Physics*, 2008. 103(7): 07A307 (1–3).
48. Ondeck, C.L., et al., Theory of magnetic fluid heating with an alternating magnetic field with temperature dependent materials properties for self-regulated heating. *Journal of Applied Physics*, 2009. 105(7): 07B324 (1–3).
49. Suto, M., et al., Heat dissipation mechanism of magnetite nanoparticles in magnetic fluid hyperthermia. *Journal of Magnetism and Magnetic Materials*, 2009. 321(10): p. 1493–1496.
50. Purushotham, S. and R.V. Ramanujan, Modeling the performance of magnetic nanoparticles in multimodal cancer therapy. *Journal of Applied Physics*, 2010. 107(11): 114701 (1–9).
51. Carrey, J., B. Mehdaoui, and M. Respaud, Simple models for dynamic hysteresis loop calculations of magnetic single-domain nanoparticles: Application to magnetic hyperthermia optimization. *Journal of Applied Physics*, 2011. 109(8): 083921 (1–17).
52. Mamiya, H. and B. Jeyadevan, Hyperthermic effects of dissipative structures of magnetic nanoparticles in large alternating magnetic fields. *Scientific Reports*, 2011. 1: p. 157.
53. Landi, G.T. and A.F. Bakuzis, On the energy conversion efficiency in magnetic hyperthermia applications: A new perspective to analyze the departure from the linear regime. *Journal of Applied Physics*, 2012. 111(8): 083915 (1–8).
54. Kalikmanov, V.I., Statistical thermodynamics of ferrofluids. *Physica A*, 1992. 183(1–2): p. 25–50.
55. Massart, R. and V. Cabuil, Effect of some parameters on the formation of colloidal magnetite in alkaline-medium—Yield and particle-size control. *Journal de Chimie Physique et de Physico—Chimie Biologique*, 1987. 84(7–8): p. 967–973.
56. Bacri, J.C., et al., Magnetic colloidal properties of ionic ferrofluids. *Journal of Magnetism and Magnetic Materials*, 1986. 62(1): p. 36–46.
57. Charles, S.W. and J. Popplewell, Ferromagnetic liquids, in *Ferromagnetic Materials*, ed. E.P. Wohlfarth, Vol. 2, 1980. North-Holland: Amsterdam, p. 509.
58. Scholten, P.C., How magnetic can a magnetic fluid be? *Journal of Magnetism and Magnetic Materials*, 1983. 39(1–2): p. 99–106.
59. Bean, C.P., Hysteresis loops of mixtures of ferromagnetic micropowders. *Journal of Applied Physics*, 1955. 26(11): p. 1381–1383.
60. Bean, C.P. and J.D. Livingston, Superparamagnetism. *Journal of Applied Physics*, 1959. 30(4): p. S120–S129.
61. Chantrell, R.W., J. Popplewell, and S.W. Charles, Measurements of particle-size distribution parameters in ferrofluids. *IEEE Transactions on Magnetics*, 1978. 14(5): p. 975–977.
62. Shliomis, M.I., Magnetic fluids. *Soviet Physics Uspekhi*, 1974. 17(2): p. 153–169.
63. Brown, W.F., Thermal fluctuations of a single-domain particle. *Physical Review*, 1963. 130(5): p. 1677–1686.
64. Kronmuller, H., Micromagnetism and magnetization processes in modern magnetic materials, in *Science and Technology of Nanostructured Magnetic Materials*, eds. G.C. Hadjipanayis and G.A. Prinz, 1991, NATO ASI Series B, Physics. Plenum Press: New York, p. 657.

65. Muxworthy, A.R. and W. Williams, Critical superparamagnetic/single-domain grain sizes in interacting magnetite particles: Implications for magnetosome crystals. *Journal of the Royal Society Interface*, 2009. 6(41): p. 1207–1212.
66. Hergt, R., S. Dutz, and M. Roder, Effects of size distribution on hysteresis losses of magnetic nanoparticles for hyperthermia. *Journal of Physics—Condensed Matter*, 2008. 20(38): 385214 (1–12).
67. Dutz, S., et al., Hysteresis losses of magnetic nanoparticle powders in the single domain size range. *Journal of Magnetism and Magnetic Materials*, 2007. 308(2): p. 305–312.
68. Alphandery, E., et al., Assemblies of aligned magnetotactic bacteria and extracted magnetosomes: What is the main factor responsible for the magnetic anisotropy? *ACS Nano*, 2009. 3(6): p. 1539–1547.
69. Tartaj, P., et al., The preparation of magnetic nanoparticles for applications in biomedicine. *Journal of Physics D—Applied Physics*, 2003. 36(13): p. R182–R197.
70. Gupta, A.K. and M. Gupta, Synthesis and surface engineering of iron oxide nanoparticles for biomedical applications. *Biomaterials*, 2005. 26(18): p. 3995–4021.
71. Rabias, I., et al., Rapid magnetic heating treatment by highly charged maghemite nanoparticles on Wistar rats exocranial glioma tumors at microliter volume. *Biomicrofluidics*, 2010. 4(2): 024111 (1–8).
72. Granqvist, C.G. and R.A. Buhrman, Ultrafine metal particles. *Journal of Applied Physics*, 1976. 47(5): p. 2200–2219.
73. Lacroix, L.-M., J. Carrey, and M. Respaud, A frequency-adjustable electromagnet for hyperthermia measurements on magnetic nanoparticles. *Review of Scientific Instruments*, 2008. 79(9): 093909 (1–5).
74. Hilger, I., et al., Heating potential of iron oxides for therapeutic purposes in interventional radiology. *Academic Radiology*, 2002. 9(2): p. 198–202.
75. Jozefczak, A. and A. Skumiel, Study of heating effect and acoustic properties of dextran stabilized magnetic fluid. *Journal of Magnetism and Magnetic Materials*, 2007. 311(1): p. 193–196.
76. Silva, A.C., et al., Application of hyperthermia induced by superparamagnetic iron oxide nanoparticles in glioma treatment. *International Journal of Nanomedicine*, 2011. 6: p. 591–603.
77. Haase, C. and U. Nowak, Role of dipole-dipole interactions for hyperthermia heating of magnetic nanoparticle ensembles. *Physical Review B*, 2012. 85(4): 045435 (1–5).
78. Jeun, M., et al., Effects of particle dipole interaction on the ac magnetically induced heating characteristics of ferrite nanoparticles for hyperthermia. *Applied Physics Letters*, 2009. 95(8): 082501 (1–3).

Part II

*Soft Block Nanobuilding:
New Preparation Routes
of Soft Nanomaterials
Using Biomolecules*

8 Engineered Biomolecules as Nanomaterials

Yun Jung Lee
Hanyang University

Ki Tae Nam
Seoul National University

CONTENTS

8.1 INTRODUCTION

Fabrication of advanced nanomaterials with multiple components, complex structure, and integrated functionality has become a trend in materials design for nanotechnology. The use of biological materials is advantageous over traditional top-down processing to produce these advanced nanomaterials in terms of exquisite spatial control at the nanometer scale and parallel self-assembly of multiple components, generating hierarchical structures to provide multifunctionality. These remarkable features have stimulated investigation into biomimetic approaches for the design of materials recently. Biomimetics is the emerging field of nanobiotechnology that adopts problem-solving methods inspired by nature's functions and structures. Use of nature's approach for control over small dimensions is based on building structures from the molecular level as nature does, "from the bottom up."[1]

Protein is one of the most fascinating nanostructured biomolecules that continues to inspire us to design new materials. Thus, design and synthesis of protein-like materials is one of the biggest challenges in nanoscience. Protein is a three-dimensionally defined nanostructure at the atomic level. The synthetic development of a three-dimensional

(3D) nanostructure can enable us to design a new device that functions as a biological system. Additionally, it can provide a new paradigm to evolve a totally new concept of electrochemical, optical, and electronic devices. In nature, protein is rich in information that is encoded with sequences of amino acids. Sequences are the arrangement of amino acids that determine the secondary structures of protein. Then, further folding includes the 3D architecture that is directly related to functions. This phenomenon is the best example of how the encoded information can translate into performance of the nanomaterial. This natural process has inspired many materials scientists to apply the underlying principle to the design and synthesis of nanomaterials. Previous studies suggest that small peptide fragments among the full sequence of proteins play a critical and independent role in assembly and folding. Therefore, many investigations have focused on identifying the important motif to drive the assembly of peptides. Protein has a specific structure determined by each tertiary structure via intramolecular interaction, whereas peptides, which are of quite short chain, are composed of 2–30 amino acids. Such a short length of chain gives them the ability to predict a specific structure that allows them to control synthetically.

Protein aggregation and assembly were first observed in nature. For example, prion and Alzheimer's diseases are directly related to the irreversible and filamentous aggregations of proteins. Investigations have revealed that the important determinant in protein assembly is the short peptide sequences. For the first time, in 1993, Shuguang Zhang at MIT observed the spontaneous assembly of the alternating sequence of hydrophobic and hydrophilic residues into the two-dimensional (2D) macrofilms. The sequence is (Ala-Glu-Ala-Glu-Ala-Lys-Ala-Lys)$_2$ (EAK16), which was found in zuotin, a yeast protein. The formation of beta-sheet-like structures was confirmed by circular dichroism and optical microscopy. This pioneering study has triggered many approaches to synthesize nanomaterials based on the short peptide sequences. Proteins and peptides can be assembled into various structures of zero-dimensional (0D), one-dimensional (1D), 2D, and 3D structures. The important lesson that we can learn from protein and peptide-based assembly is that the sequence controls the behavior. By controlling the sequence precisely, the morphology can be tuned and functionalities can be provided selectively. Although there are many advantages to these approaches, the control of the assembled structures is still challenging. Therefore, as a starting effort, preorganized structures have been tried first. Instead of utilizing the assembly behavior, biological molecules have been used as a template.

Biotemplating is a technique that produces material with controlled morphologies and structures by employing biomaterials as templates for material synthesis. In nature, proteins from bones, shells, diatoms, and magnetotactic bacteria play a crucial role in nucleating and regulating the crystal structure of inorganic materials such as calcium carbonate, silica, and magnetic materials, thus templating these materials.[2–5] Biotemplating in nanomaterial synthesis thus refers to the efforts in extending nature-based biological templating systems to the technologically important functional materials that have not yet been explored by nature. A variety of biological matter from individual biomolecules [deoxyribonucleic acid (DNA), peptides, proteins, etc.] to biological entities (virus, bacteria, fungi, etc.) have been utilized as biotemplates for guided formation of nanostructured materials. This chapter demonstrates the use of viruses, the most heavily studied biological entity for biotemplating, as biological tools for hybrid nanomaterial design.

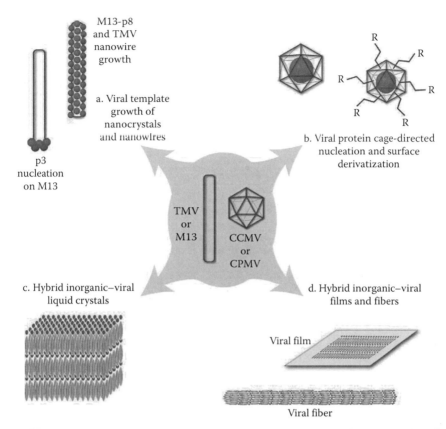

FIGURE 8.1 Illustration showing some routes for biohybrid materials synthesis using viruses, both rod-shaped such as M13 or TMV and spherical cage viruses such as CCMV or CPMV. (Reprinted from *Acta Materialia*, 51, Flynn, C. E., Lee, S. W., Peelle, B. R., and Belcher, A. M., Viruses as vehicles for growth, organization and assembly of materials, 5867–80, Copyright 2003, with permission from Elsevier.)

Exploiting viruses for the fabrication of biohybrid materials is based on the use of highly ordered crystalline templates from which to nucleate and assemble materials (Figure 8.1).[6] Viruses are particles of submicroscopic dimension ranging from 20 to 800 nm. They are normally composed of protective protein coats, called capsids, encasing infectious genomic materials such as DNA or ribonucleic acid (RNA). Capsid protein shells are self-assembled from a number of identical sub-unit proteins in precise 3D hierarchical structures. Viruses do not have their own metabolism and reproduce by infecting a host organism. Depending on the type of host for replication, they are categorized as plant viruses, animal viruses, and bacteriophages. (Bacteriophages are viruses that infect bacteria.) From a materials design perspective, however, classification based on their morphological feature is more useful. Viruses roughly assume four types of morphology: rod-shaped or filamentous, spherical or near-spherical (icosahedral), enveloped, and complex structure. Rod-shaped and spherical viruses have been mostly utilized as templates for materials design in nanotechnology. The most widely investigated viruses as viral scaffolds for nanomaterials designs are M13 virus, tobacco mosaic virus (TMV), cowpea mosaic virus (CPMV), and cowpea chlorotic mottle virus (CCMV). M13 and TMV are rod-shaped, and CPMV and CCMV are spherical.

The functional usefulness of viruses as templating scaffolds lies in their inherent morphological features, programmable coat proteins, and possible mass production. Viruses are well equipped with some characteristics that are suitable for nanofabrication. (1) Viruses have inherent nanodimensions ranging from a few tens to several hundred nanometers, in the same range of the nanomaterials to be generated.[7] (2) The structure and dimensions of viruses are exquisitely precise and uniform. (3) Genetic and chemical modifications of constituent protein units are easily attainable using basic molecular biology and chemistry. Specifically, a small number of viral genes and proteins makes them easily programmable for expression of novel peptides through genetic modification.[6] (4) Mass production is possible by proliferation in the respective hosts, which is a requirement for use in engineering applications.[8]

8.2 TYPES OF VIRUSES FOR NANOMATERIALS DESIGN

8.2.1 Rod-Shaped or Filamentous Viruses

8.2.1.1 M13 Virus

The M13 virus is a rod-shaped bacteriophage that infects bacteria. It is composed of a circular single-stranded DNA molecule of approximately 6407 nucleotides long.[9] The wild-type filamentous the M13 virus has a high aspect ratio with approximately a 6.5-nm diameter and an 880-nm length. The length of the cylinder reflects the length of the packaged single-stranded DNA genome. Viral DNA is encased in a flexible cylinder covered by the major coat protein p8. Roughly 2700 copies of p8 coat protein self-assemble into the capsid in a repeating helical array, resulting in a fivefold symmetry along the length of the virus. Computational simulation of M13 virus shows that the closest distance of p8 protein neighbors is around 3 nm.[10] At one end of the M13 virus, there are approximately five molecules each of p7 and p9. The other end has about five molecules each of p3 and p6, totaling 10–16 nm in length. Each subunit protein is modifiable through chemical or genetic engineering to generate multifunctional viruses highly decorated with heterofunctional proteins at a different location of the virus.

The expression of peptide-based functionalities on their surfaces, mass production in large quantities through bacterial amplification, and self-assembly into precisely ordered nanorod structures make the M13 virus attractive building blocks for use in nanotechnology. Although unmodified, wild-type viruses can also serve as a template for nanomaterial growth, controlled synthesis is often difficult to achieve since the surfaces of wild-type viruses are usually not ideal for the synthesis of materials for which nature has not yet had a chance to control. The weak interactions between the wild-type virus and the materials result in inhomogeneous coating of nanoparticles, and even easy detachment from the viral template. Therefore, modification or engineering is sometimes inevitable for the fabrication of elaborately controlled nanostructured materials. The surface proteins of viruses are programmable functional moieties inscribed as amino acids. Genetic engineering could modify these surface functional groups on the virus with affinities to new functional materials and/or facilitation of nucleation of growth of materials. The beauty of using the M13 virus for the generation of nanohybrid materials lies in the availability of the combinatorial approach that mimics an evolutionary cycle for materials recognition in nature. In a natural organism, directed templating from organic matrices such as protein has nucleated and assembled inorganic materials with precise alignment, orientation, and shape. Magnetotactic bacteria nucleate and align magnetic iron oxide (IO) particles using vesicles to respond to the geomagnetic field for the purpose of navigation.[2] Abalone shell and silica sponge have evolved specific protein–inorganic interfaces to control the mechanism of inorganic formation.[3–5] These interactions not only facilitate nucleation of inorganic materials, but can also control crystal phase and preferential growth of specific crystal surface and size, and even stabilize metastable crystalline form.[4,5] The combinatorial approach, or so-called phage display technique, is analogous to natural selection since it identifies and selects specific peptides that have an affinity or interaction to target materials of interest as nature does. Combinatorial M13 phage libraries are initially constructed by engineering the native M13 genome to display ~1 × 10^9 different random peptide sequences fused to the N-terminus of the p3 protein at the proximal end of M13 virus, and they are commercially available now (New England BioLabs, Beverly, MA, USA). This library is called the type 3 library. The viral libraries are exposed to targets, and positive target recognition viruses that have binding affinity to targets are isolated from the 10^9 different viruses. (Each virus has a different peptide insert on p3.) DNA sequencing of the screened viruses identifies the peptide sequence inserted responsible for binding to the targets. The overall process is called phage display or biopanning. For the selection of specific peptide motifs, this technique was traditionally used in the pharmaceutical industry with organic targets.[9,11] Belcher and coworkers pioneered the use of the phage display technique to the identification of specific interactions of viral-displayed peptide libraries with inorganic targets to select peptide recognition specific to inorganic materials. Successful identification of specific interaction between expressed peptide and inorganic materials was demonstrated using III–V semiconductor materials such as GaAs and InP.[12] The clone selected for GaAs[100] target preferentially bound to GaAs[100] but not to Si[100]. Material-specific peptides not only discriminated chemical differences but also sensed crystallographic orientation of the target surface. The peptide screened for GaAs[100] surface had a 10^3 times higher affinity for [100] substrate compared to its affinity for GaAs[111]A or [111]B substrates. Moreover, the GaAs-specific clone was substrate-specific for GaAs over AlGaAs, showing its ability to recognize atomic substitution. The ability of peptides expressed on the M13 virus in recognizing specific structure could be further extended to biomolecular recognition of crystal defects.[13] Phage display was used to find a polypeptide that shows binding affinity for surface defects and threading dislocations in (100) germanium grown heteroepitaxially on silicon substrate.

The protein that recognized a molecular imprint, identified through combinatorial biopanning, could be used to template and synthesize materials in an analogous way that abalone shells do in nature. The M13 virus with material-specific peptide displayed only on the p3 end of the virus was used in the first M13-based nanocrystal growth study. Two virus-bound peptide sequences were identified to have affinity to ZnS, named Z8, and A7.[14,15] These two peptide sequences were shown to control ZnS particle size and shape at room temperature under aqueous conditions. Crystals grown in the presence of the Z8 clone were ~4 nm in size with zinc blend structure, while the A7 clone templated the growth of 4 nm by 2 nm wurtzite crystal. In the control experiments, particles grown without ZnS-specific virus clone or with wild-type virus clone were noncrystalline and were much larger (>100–500 nm) in size on distribution. Given that A7 and Z8 peptides had different structures (cyclic vs. linear), both peptide sequence and structure controlled the nucleation of crystal phase.

To fabricate a 1D virus–inorganic hybrid nanostructure, material-specific peptide sequences were genetically engineered into the p8 helical major coat protein. Highly crystalline ZnS and CdS nanocrystals were nucleated along the length of viruses that have ZnS-specific peptides fused to the p8 capsids. Discrete nanoparticles formed quasi-continuous 1D semiconductor nanowire.[14,16] Single-crystalline ZnS nanowire was obtained using thermal annealing.[10] To form single-crystalline nanowires, the template should be removed to eliminate the blocking effects of nucleating peptides. ZnS nanowires were preferentially oriented in the [001] direction perpendicular to the wire length direction before annealing. Upon thermal annealing at 350°C, discrete polycrystalline particles were assembled onto the single-crystalline nanowire. Ordering of nanoparticles with regard to preferred crystallographic orientation along the length of the virus could be a result of the stability of peptide fusion and the symmetry of the virus coat. The ordering of nanoparticles nucleated on the viral template promoted the single-crystal nature of the annealed nanowires. The control of crystallization of nanoparticles with the specifically binding virus (with displayed peptides) was also applied to magnetic nanoparticles.[10,17,18] Amine-rich peptide, which is known to be an excellent ligand for Pt, was fused to the coat protein of M13 virus. This viral template facilitated nucleation of $L1_0$-phase FePt ferromagnetic particles.

While a specific binding motif serves for highly specific single material growth, nonspecific electrostatic interactions can also be utilized for general material synthesis using biotemplates. The wild-type M13 viruses are negatively charged and the electrostatic interaction between cationic aqueous metal complexes and the anionic carboxylic groups of the p8 protein of M13 virus could generate metal nanowires of Rh, Ru, and Pd.[19] Metal precursors such as $PdCl_2$, K_2PdCl_4, $RuCl_3$, and K_3RhCl_6 yield neutral and cationic complexes in neutral aqueous environment, for example, $Rh\left(H_2O\right)_6^{3+}$, $Pd\left(H_2O\right)_6^{2+}$, and $Ru\left(H_2O\right)_6^{3+}$. Incubation of these precursors with wild-type M13 virus, followed by borohydride reduction, produced metallic nanowires. In contrast, typical Pt and Au metal precursors such as K_2PtCl_6 and $HAuCl_4$ yield anionic complexes in water. Therefore, Au and Pt systems do not show nanoparticles templating on M13 virus. To enhance electrostatic interaction between the M13 virus template and the cationic species, M13 virus has been genetically engineered to have tetraglutamate (-EEEE) fused to the N-terminus of each molecule of p8 major coat protein. This modified virus is termed E4 virus. The presence of extra carboxylic acid groups, compared with wild-type M13 virus, enabled increased ionic interaction between cation and E4 virus. Therefore, E4 virus was considered as efficient versatile template for material growth.[20] Through the interaction of E4 virus and Co^{2+} ions, Co_3O_4 nanowire was produced at room temperature.[21] Co^{2+} ions conjugated with E4 virus template were first reduced by $NaBH_4$-reducing agent and spontaneous oxidation to Co_3O_4 followed in aqueous environment. Single-crystalline

Ag nanowire was also fabricated on the general E4 virus template.[22] Ag+ ions from Ag(CH₃COO) precursor were photoreduced to metallic silver in the presence of carboxylic group containing peptides on the E4 virus under ambient light. The formation of single crystal is associated with the high density of incorporated peptide (the nearest-neighbor separation of peptide on the capsid of M13 virus was calculated as ~3 nm[10]) allowing the nucleated silver to grow in the thermodynamically most favorable single-crystalline form without postannealing on the scaffold.

Inherent self-assembling property of the virus can be used to assemble inorganic nanomaterials along with the self-assembly of the viral particles. Shape anisotropy of rod-shaped M13 virus leads to liquid crystalline alignment at very high virus concentrations. Liquid crystalline behaviors are controlled by factors such as concentration of the virus suspension, ionic strength of the solution, and external fields.[15] M13 virus building block formed viral films with chiral smectic C structures, a conformation arising from the helical structure of the M13 virus. Using M13 virus with ZnS-binding peptide motif on p3 end, a viral-ZnS nanocrystal liquid crystalline suspension was formed through one-pot synthesis route: a high concentration of engineered viruses were suspended in a ZnS nanocrystal precursor solution and directly formed viral-ZnS nanocrystal liquid crystalline suspension. Despite attached nanoparticles, the formation of liquid crystalline suspension was directed by long, rod-shaped virus. When dried on various substrates in high concentration, the functionalized viral–liquid crystalline system evolved a self-supporting hybrid film material that was ordered on nanoscale (Figure 8.2c). While the approach described above utilized specific interaction between nanomaterials and the virus for the fabrication

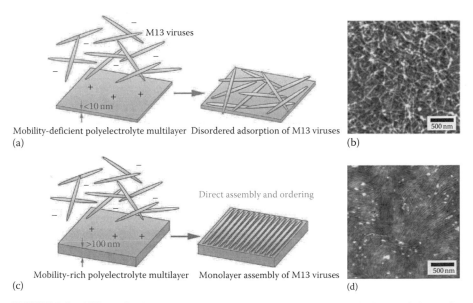

FIGURE 8.2 Effect of polyelectrolyte multilayer mobility on virus ordering. (a) Scheme for random virus absorption. (b) AFM image for (a). (c) Scheme for direct dense ordering of viral monolayer. (d) AFM image for (c). (Reprinted with permission from Yoo, P. J., et al., 2008, 1081–89. Copyright 2008 American Chemical Society.)

of hybrid liquid crystalline films, streptavidin/anti-streptavidin interaction has been implemented between the virus and the nanoparticles to develop universal handles for nanomaterials in the self-assembly of viruses and viral-based films.[23] Anti-streptavidin M13 virus with peptide on its p3 end having specific binding affinity to streptavidin protein was first selected through biopanning. Using the streptavidin-specific virus and streptavidin-coated nanoparticles, various nanoparticles such as 10 nm gold nanoparticles, organic fluorescent dyes (fluorescein), and biological molecules (R-phycoerythrin) could be aligned in viral films. Long, rod-shaped viruses can also be used for the fabrication of 1D fiber-like structures by imitating the spinning process of the silk spider. Extrusion of liquid crystalline virus suspension through capillary tubes into the cross-linking solutions such as glutaraldehyde (wet spinning) or under influence of high electric field (electrospinning) generated M13 virus-based micro- and nanofibers.[24] The resulting fibers showed nematic ordered morphologies due to flowing forces.

Rod-shaped TMV and M13 viruses are suitable macromolecules for flow-induced alignment due to their uniformity and rigidity. Since the liquid crystalline transition (isotropic–nematic transition) occurs above a certain critical concentration, ordered patterns with fibers and strips were formed on the substrates as the meniscus receded when the droplets of M13 virus suspension were allowed to evaporate.[25] However, the generated pattern was not uniform and showed radial distribution from the center of the film. To generate thin films with aligned nanogrooves, convective assembly was used as shown in Figure 8.3. The convective assembly mechanism depends on the evaporation of water at the substrate–solution–air three-phase interface. The viruses are ordered at the three-point interfaces as solvent evaporates. Virus concentration, surface wettability, and the meniscus withdrawal rate are the key parameters for the control of thickness, orientation, and packing of the anisotropic viruses.[26] The viruses are oriented perpendicular to the drying front due to the rotational diffusion of rod-shaped virus in a linear flow created by solvent convection to the drying front.

Evaporation-induced self-assembly was extended to produce biomimetic, self-templating assembly of M13 virus into long-range, ordered, supramolecular

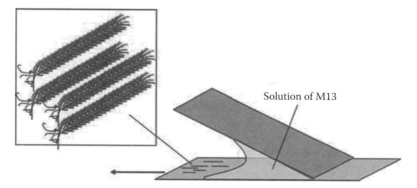

Solution of M13

FIGURE 8.3 Schematic representation of the convective assembly apparatus system used to deposit aligned viruses. (Rong, J. H., Lee, L. A., Li, K., et al., 2008. Oriented cell growth on self-assembled bacteriophage M13 thin films. *Chemical Communications* 41: 5184–87. Reproduced by permission of The Royal Society of Chemistry.)

films showing multiply hierarchical organization and helical twist.[27] The process consists of dipping of glass substrates into the virus suspension and pulling at a precisely controlled speed. Varying parameters that control the kinetics and thermodynamics of assembly such as virus concentration, pulling speed, ionic concentration, virus surface chemistry, and substrate surface properties allowed tunable supramolecular structures. Three distinct structures were created by this approach: nematic orthogonal twist, cholesteric helical ribbons, and smectic helicoidal nanofilaments (Figure 8.4). Liquid crystalline phase transition and competing interfacial forces at the interface appeared to be critical in determining morphologies of the supramolecular structures during assembly. The resulting films displayed structure-dependent distinctive optical and photonic properties showing potential as a chiral reflector/filter and structural color matrices.

Along with the liquid crystalline behavior, shape anisotropy combined with the surface charge of the M13 virus enabled ordering of the M13 virus on the polymer surface. M13 viruses self-assembled into a liquid crystalline 2D layer on a polymer surface, which is a polyelectrolyte multilayer grown by the layer-by-layer (LBL) technique,[28] which uses electrostatic interactions between charged species allowing absorption of multiply charged species to create nanometer-scale films. M13 viruses generally have negative surface charges; thus, they were included in the LBL process to incorporate M13 virus particles in cohesive thin films. The virus was randomly deposited on the oppositely charged polyelectrolyte (polycations) surface first. When the deposited M13 layer was exposed to the negatively charged polyelectrolyte (polyanions) that have stronger electrostatic interaction with polycations, the stronger negative charges forced virus macromolecules to "float" to the surface. The liquid crystalline behavior of virus particles finally induced a spontaneous ordering on the surface of cohesive polyelectrolyte multilayer, resulting in an ordered viral monolayer. Since the interaction is electrostatic in this assembly process, the virus binding, floating behavior, and density of viral monolayer were controlled by pH, which influences the surface charge of the virus (Figure 8.5).[29] This two-dimensionally ordered virus scaffold could be used as a template for nanoparticle nucleation or binding, enabling the assembly of dense, highly ordered, and nanostructured hybrid monolayers even on free-standing polymer films. Since the ordering is driven by interdiffusion of polyelectrolyte, the mobility of the polyelectrolyte influences the assembly of the virus on the top surface (Figure 8.2).[29,30] Specifically, the diffusive lateral mobility of underlying polycations can be transferred to the surface-adsorbed viruses leading to a highly packed structure. The electrostatically assembled viruses on the polyelectrolyte multilayer were further patterned by solvent-assisted capillary molding to fabricate micrometer-scale dense polyelectrolyte multilayer patterns with a virus monolayer on top.[30]

Various nanoarchitectures have been fabricated using engineered multifunctional M13 virus as template. The concept of multifunctionality was first incorporated to create nanoring structures.[31] A virus was bifunctionally engineered with anti-streptavidin peptide on p3 end and hexa-histidine peptide at the opposite end of the virus, p9 (Figure 8.6a). To be paired with this bifunctional virus, a heterobifunctional linker molecule consisting of streptavidin conjugated with nitrilotriacetic acid (Ni-NTA) was synthesized (Figure 8.6b). Addition of a linker molecule triggered the ring reaction and the reversible formation of a virus-based nanoring with circumference

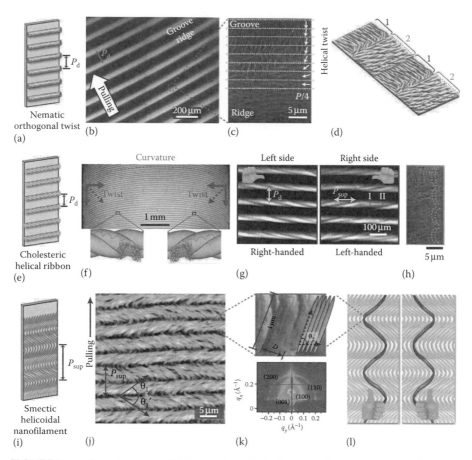

FIGURE 8.4 **(See color insert.)** Self-templated helical supramolecular structures. (a–d) The nematic orthogonal twist structure. (a) Diagram. (b) Scanning electron microscopy (SEM) image. (c) AFM image depicting left-handed rotation of virus fiber bundles. (d) Diagram of alternating nematic grooves and cholesteric ridges. (e–h) The cholesteric helical ribbon (CHR) structure. (e) Diagram. (f) Photograph of CHR structures showing the curved menis-cuses. (g) SEM image of the CHR structure on the left and right sides, which shows right and left handedness. (h) AFM image showing that CHR is composed of twisted cholesteric phage. (i–l) The smectic helicoidal nanofilament (SHN) structure. (i) Diagram. (j) AFM image of the SHN structure. (k) (upper) Enlarged AFM showing SHN structure, which is composed of smectic C bundles. (Lower) Grazing-incidence small-angle x-ray scattering measurement showing pseudohexagonal packed structures within the SHN. (l) Proposed model of the SHN structure composed of left-handed and right-handed helicoidal nanofilaments. (Reprinted by permission from Macmillan Publishers Ltd. *Nature*, Chung, W. J., et al., 2011, copyright 2011.)

corresponding to the lengths of the packaged DNA has been confirmed by atomic force microscopy (AFM) (Figure 8.7).

Programmable assembly of a complex nanostructure has been enabled genetically by using an M13 virus template. The M13 virus genome has been rationally engineered to produce viral particles with distinct substrate-specific peptides expressed on the

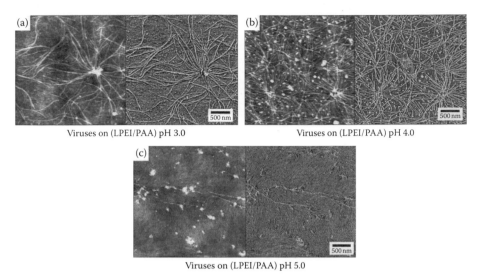

FIGURE 8.5 Effect of deposition pH on the virus assembly in LBL multilayer. (a) Disordered and aggregated virus assembly at pH 3.0. (b) Scattered viral assembly at pH 4.0. (c) Ordered dense monolayer of viruses at pH 5.0. LPEI, linear poly(ethylene imine); PAA, poly(acrylic acid). (Reprinted with permission from Yoo, P. J., et al., 2008, 561–71. Copyright 2008 American Chemical Society.)

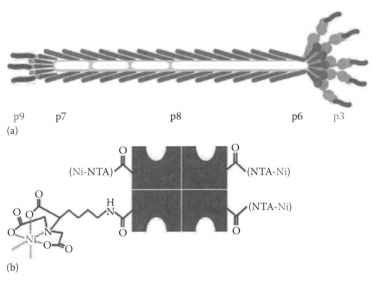

FIGURE 8.6 (a) Schematic representation of bifunctionally engineered M13 virus. His6 peptide displayed as p9 fusion, whereas anti-streptavidin peptide displayed as p3 fusion. (b) Tetrameric streptavidin conjugated with four nickel-nitrilotriacetic acid (Ni-NTA) groups. (Reprinted with permission from Nam, K. T., et al., 2004, 23–27. Copyright 2004 American Chemical Society.)

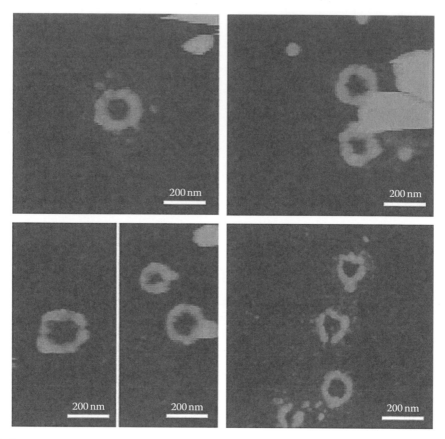

FIGURE 8.7 M13 virus-based ring structures observed by AFM on mica surface. (Reprinted with permission from Nam, K. T., et al., 2004, 23–27. Copyright 2004 American Chemical Society.)

capsid and the ends.[32] The M13 virus was highly engineered with desired modifications on both p3 and p8 proteins, termed type 8–3 clone. To select a suitable peptide motif for each protein group, phage libraries were employed. Once the specific binding motifs for targeted substrates are identified, a type 8–3 phage can be produced with different binding motifs on both p3 and p8 proteins by simultaneously modifying genes 3 and 8 insertions in a single viral genome (Figure 8.8). The type 3 library is the most commonly used screening pool and commercially available; however, a peptide motif selected from the type 3 library cannot be directly translated to p8 proteins because p3 and p8 proteins have their distinct structure information. Fusing peptide motifs from the type 3 library to p8 proteins may cause malfunctionality of the displayed motif. To select desirable peptide motifs for p8 proteins, the type 8 library with random 8-mer peptide displayed on the p8 protein surface was exploited. This engineered phage could further enable template assembly of various nanoarchitectures. A virus template engineered to have a gold-binding peptide sequence on the major coat protein p8 while simultaneously displaying streptavidin-binding peptide on the p3 end was

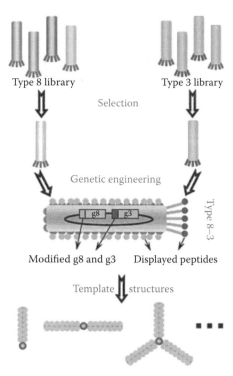

Type 8 library   Type 3 library

Selection

Genetic engineering

Type 8–3

Modified g8 and g3   Displayed peptides

Template structures

FIGURE 8.8 Scheme for engineering the type 8–3 phage. The genome of the engineered bacteriophage bears insertions in g8 and g3, which leads to motif expression on p8 and p3 proteins, respectively. (Reprinted with permission from Huang, Y., et al., 2005, 1429–37. Copyright 2004 American Chemical Society.)

used to assemble Au and CdSe nanocrystals. Au nanoparticles were assembled along the length of the virus and streptavidin-coated nanocrystals (CdSe) were conjugated with the p3 end of the virus. The assembled structures were ordered 1D arrays and other more complex geometries depending on the interaction mode (Figure 8.9).

To extend biological self-assembly from nanoscale into practical use, it is important to develop the ability to hierarchically organize inorganic and biological materials. Highly specific antibody interactions are useful toolkits for the macroscopic patterning virus. A biocompatible macroscopic positioning method such as microcontact printing was explored for the patterned transfer of antibodies from solution to substrate.[33] To overcome the limitation in feature size and pitch associated with the mechanical properties of the elastomer, a subtractive printing technique was applied. Subtractive printing used featureless elastomer and after inking antibody monolayer from the solution, the unwanted area was subtracted from the elastomer surface using a prefabricated nanoplate. The remaining antibodies were printed onto a blank substrate and subsequent M13 virus binding onto the macroscopic antibody patterns generated large-scale arrays of aligned virus.

Recent research of M13 virus-based hybrid nanomaterials has been driven to practical applications in electrochemical energy devices such as lithium

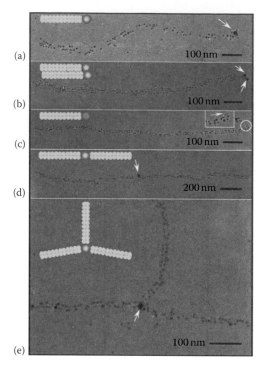

FIGURE 8.9 (a)–(e) TEM images of various nanoarchitectures templated on type 8–3 virus with gold-binding peptides on p8 and anti-streptavidin motif on p3. Arrows highlight the streptavidin-coated nanoparticles on p3 proteins. The insets show the assembly mode of observed structures. White dot, Au nanoparticles; light gray dot, CdSe nanocrystals; dark gray halo, streptavidin coating around nanoparticles. (Reprinted with permission from Huang, Y., et al., 2005, 1429–37. Copyright 2004 American Chemical Society.)

batteries,[20,21,34,35] solar cells,[36] water splitting,[37] and hydrogen generation.[38] Both electrochemically active materials and catalysts were templated. With the help of multifunctionality of the viral particle, the M13 virus can control the nanostructure and multifunctionality of the hybrid functional nanomaterials at the molecular level. The superior performances of biotemplated materials in practical applications are rooted in this ability to co-assemble multiple functional components at the molecular level.

The delicate nanostructure fabricated with the M13 virus template influenced the electrochemically induced transformation at the nanoscale. Co_3O_4 nanowires synthesized and assembled with the E4 virus clone was the first virus-based material system applied as lithium ion battery anodes.[21] Although viral-Co_3O_4 was synthesized at room temperature with mild chemistry, the cell assembled with this material performed similar to the high-temperature Co_3O_4 materials fabricated at a temperature above 500°C. Structural integrity and dense packing of virus capsid as well as uniform-sized nanomaterials with favorable crystallinity were counted as the electrochemical advantages of this system. To further improve capacity, a new hybrid electrode material was designed with additional genetic engineering. A gold-binding motif was incorporated into the major coat p8 protein of E4 virus. This hybrid clone, named AuE4 virus, has a gold-binding peptide motif spatially interspersed within p8 protein capsid fused with tetraglutamate, E4. Hybrid Au–Co_3O_4 wires with 5 nm Au nanoparticles showed superior electrochemical performances. Au nanoparticles could improve electronic conductivity or catalyze the reaction. When these nanowires were extended to controlled 2D liquid crystalline assembly on the polyelectrolyte multilayer, lightweight, flexible, and transparent electrodes with substrate multilayers (acting as a solid electrolyte) were constructed as free-standing films.

The nanoscale biological assembly and microscale nonbiological assembly can be synergistically combined to fabricate and spatially position the electrode component for small-scale power sources. Microbattery electrodes were stamped onto the platinum microband current collector using a microcontact printing technique.[39] The stamping ink was made of polyelectrolyte multilayers with self-assembled 2D liquid crystalline layer of viral-Co_3O_4 nanowires on the top surface. When stamped onto the Pt microband, Co_3O_4 nanowires served as the active anode material and polyelectrolyte multilayers as the solid electrolyte (Figure 8.10). This approach combined assembly technique at multiple length scale: biological self-assembly (liquid crystalline ordering), polymer electrostatic assembly (LBL), and soft-lithographic technique (microcontact printing). This new-electrode positioning method allowed a platform for integrating complex architectures into high-performance microbatteries. The fabricated electrode arrays showed full electrochemical functionality as a lithium–ion battery electrode.

The first M13 virus-designed cathode materials for lithium–ion batteries were demonstrated by templating amorphous iron phosphate (a-$FePO_4$).[20,34] The M13 virus template enabled elaborate nanostructure design and environmentally benign synthesis for the nanometer-sized a-$FePO_4$ formation for 3 V lithium–ion battery cathodes. Using the versatility of E4 virus template, a heterostructure was formed along the single virus scaffold with uniformly distributed silver nanoparticles through the whole system. The superiority of uniformly distributed Ag nanoparticles over the locally limited Ag nanowire networks in enhancing overall electronic conductivity of the composite electrode was experimentally demonstrated. The specific capacity was further improved by dehydration of the structural water. The biological template and synthetic chemistry were synergistically combined for producing anhydrous a-$FePO_4$ without thermal treatment via low temperature and eco-efficient chemistry. The electrochemical performances of this virus-designed material were comparable to the best reported values for a-$FePO_4$ synthesized at high temperature.

To develop materials that deliver more energy at a high rate, high-power lithium–ion battery cathodes were fabricated using the concept of biological multifunctionality.[20] The M13 virus was multiply engineered to have peptide groups with binding affinity to single-walled carbon nanotubes (SWNTs) on one part and peptides capable of nucleating a-$FePO_4$ at another location of the virus. Specific SWNT-binding peptides were isolated from biopanning. By manipulating two genes, the viruses were equipped with SWNT-binding peptides on the p3 end and a-$FePO_4$ nucleating peptides fused to the major coat protein of the virus. To electrically address electrode materials with poor electronic conductivity, the specific affinity between active materials and conducting materials was implemented in this way. The traditional wiring tools were simply functionalized for a single component, either active materials

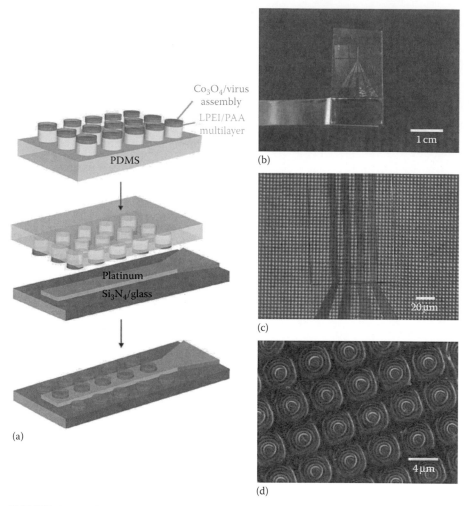

Co₃O₄/virus assembly
LPEI/PAA multilayer
PDMS
Platinum
Si₃N₄/glass

(a)

(b)

1 cm

(c)

20 μm

(d)

4 μm

FIGURE 8.10 **(See color insert.)** (a) Schematic procedure for constructing virus-based microbattery electrode. (b) Image of microbatteries on the Pt current collector. (c) Optical microscopy image of the microbattery electrode (4 μm diameter) on four Pt micro-bands (10 μm width). (d) SEM image of the stamped microbattery electrode. (Nam, K. T., Wartena, R., Yoo, P. J., et al., 2008. Stamped microbattery electrodes based on self-assembled M13 viruses. *Proceedings of the National Academy of Sciences of the United States of America* 105: 17227–31. Copyright 2008 National Academy of Sciences, U.S.A.)

or conducting materials, and the wiring depended on the random contact between the components. By developing a two-gene system with a universal handle to pick up electrically conducting carbon nanotubes, a novel multifunctional wiring platform was devised using basic biological principles. Through the biomolecular recognition and attachment of a-FePO₄-templated virus to SWNT networks, the active materials were wired electrically at the true nanoscale (Figure 8.11). The virus clone with the greatest affinity toward SWNTs enabled power performances of a-FePO₄

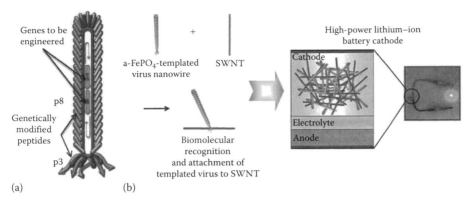

Genes to be engineered

p8

Genetically modified peptides

p3

(a)

a-FePO₄-templated virus nanowire

+

SWNT

Biomolecular recognition and attachment of templated virus to SWNT

(b)

High-power lithium–ion battery cathode

Cathode

Electrolyte

Anode

FIGURE 8.11 Biological toolkits: genetic engineering and biomolecular recognition. (a) A schematic presentation of multifunctional M13 virus with the proteins genetically engineered. (b) A schematic diagram for fabricating genetically engineered high-power lithium–ion battery cathodes using multifunctional two-gene system viruses and a photograph of the actually assembled battery used to power green LED of 105 mW. (From Lee, Y. J., Yi, H., Kim, W. J., et al., 2009. Fabricating genetically engineered high-power lithium-ion batteries using multiple virus genes. *Science* 324: 1051–55. Reprinted with permission of AAAS.)

comparable to that of crystalline lithium iron phosphate (c-LiFePO₄) and showed excellent capacity retention upon cycling.

Silver, gold, and their alloy nanowires were synthesized by using multiple clones and showed electrochemical activity as anodes for lithium–ion batteries[35] (Figure 8.12). Silver and gold belong to the alloy-forming anodes for lithium–ion batteries since they have several alloy phases with lithium and react with lithium at very low potential. However, little is known about their electrochemical response with lithium. Because Ag and Au react poorly with lithium at the micrometer scale, fundamental study of their electrochemical behavior has been limited. The absence of a nanoscale platform suppressed the electrochemical activation of these materials. The two M13 virus clones, genetically engineered for specificity (gold-binding virus) and versatility (E4 virus) served as a template for the synthesis of Au, Ag, and Au-rich AuAg alloy nanowires with diameters below 50 nm and a high aspect ratio. With the synergistic combination of biological building block and synthetic chemistry, this facile and high-yield synthesis conferred controls over particle size, morphology, and compositions. The biologically derived noble metal alloy nanowires showed electrochemical activities even when the electrodes were fabricated from bulk power forms. Improvement in capacity retention was achieved by alloy formation and surface stabilization. These noble metal nanowires served as a great model system in identifying important parameters that can induce stable electrochemical transformation at the nanoscale. Reducing materials dimension proved to be effective in decreasing mechanical stress; however, other factors such as surface characteristics and reaction/phase homogeneity appeared to influence more in maintaining structural stability and electrochemical performances at the nanoscale with diameters below 50 nm. Given the demonstration of electrochemical activity of noble metal alloy nanowires with various compositions,

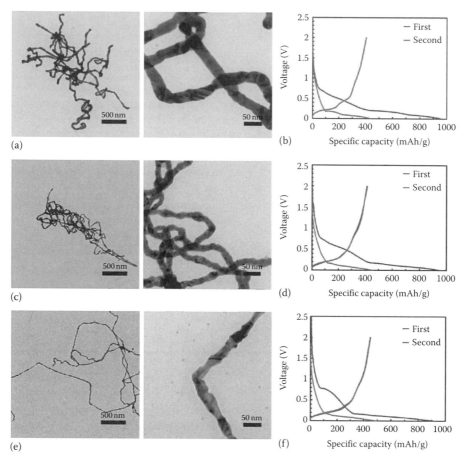

FIGURE 8.12 **(See color insert.)** Characterization of cetyltrimethylammonium bromide (CTAB)-stabilized Au_xAg_{1-x} alloy nanowires. (a and b) $x = 0.9$. (a) TEM images. (b) First two discharge/charge curves. (c and d) $x = 0.67$. (c) TEM images. (d) First two discharge/charge curves. (e and f) $x = 0.5$. (e) TEM images. (f) First two discharge/charge curves. (Reprinted with permission from Lee, Y. J., et al., 2010, 2433–40. Copyright 2010 American Chemical Society.)

the M13 biological toolkit extended its utility for the study of basic electrochemical properties of materials.

The M13 virus can serve as a template directing nanoscale organization of photoactive pigments into light-harvesting antenna. A model pigment zinc porphyrin (ZnDPEG) was conjugated with the major coat protein p8 via chemical linkage.[40] The pendant carboxylic groups of ZnDPEG chemically reacted with the primary amine of the p8 protein by the well-known carbodiimide coupling reaction. This chemical modification of the M13 virus is straightforward because of the exposed N-terminus and lysine residue on the viral surface. The close distances between primary amines on the viral surface were expected to allow the energy transfer between neighboring pigments on the virus template. The flexible N-terminus of p8 may further allow considerable orientational freedom for the attached pigments, thereby facilitating interactions between pigments. The photons absorbed actually traveled along the pigments on the virus and the energy transfer of the assembled pigments was controlled by genetic modification of amino acids on p8.

The nanoscale coassembly of ZnDPEG pigments and iridium oxide (IrO_2) catalysts on the single M13 virus template enabled the application of this biologically templated nanostructure to photochemical systems such as visible light-driven water oxidation systems.[37] An artificial light-driven water oxidation system is analogous to the natural photosystems such as cyanobacteria and plants.[41] In these natural systems, oxidation of water with an oxygen-evolving catalyst [the reaction center photosystem II (PSII)] is driven by light energy. Photons are captured in light-harvesting antenna complexes by chlorophyll pigments. This energy is efficiently transferred to the reaction center where it is transformed into a pair of spatially separated charge carriers. Transfer of electron and hole from the photosensitizer to electron acceptors and catalyst drives water splitting. The distances between the functional components are critically important in the transfer process. Therefore, the nanoscale co-assembly of photosensitizer and the reaction center catalyst could allow the successful modeling of the water oxidation systems on photosynthesis. In M13 virus-based water splitting systems, ZnDPEG pigment was adopted as a light-harvesting antenna and IrO_2 as a water-oxidation catalyst based on its well-known catalytic activity and stability under oxidizing conditions. A ZnDPEG photosensitizer was chemically conjugated with M13 virus carrying IrO_2-binding peptide on the major coat protein, identified through biopanning against IrO_2. IrO_2 was deposited on the ZnDPEG-conjugated virus. Immobilization of the virus scaffold into a porous polymer microgel matrix improved structural durability by preventing nanowire aggregation, allowing the materials to be recycled. M13 virus-templated nanoscale assembly of functional components remarkably enhanced the photocatalytic activity.

Catalysts supported on the surface of the M13 virus also outperformed traditional composite nanoparticle catalyst in converting ethanol to hydrogen fuel.[38] Extremely small nanocrystalline catalysts composed of ceria with rhodium and nickel were deposited on the E4 virus. The surface area of a M13-templated catalyst was higher than that of the untemplated catalyst of identical composition and resulted in smaller pores with narrower pore size distribution. The biotemplated catalysts showed better catalytic activity and thermal/long-term stability because the use of M13 virus template resulted in improvement of resistance to surface deactivation and less phase segregation.

SWNTs–TiO_2 core–shell nanocomposites rationally designed using M13 virus templates were applied to photovoltaic devices.[36] This nanoarchitecture was designed to increase power conversion efficiency of the dye-sensitized solar cells by improving photocollection efficiency. To efficiently collect photogenerated electrons, high electron mobility photoanodes should be developed. SWNTs have been considered as promising components of nanocomposite photoanodes because of their excellent electron mobility and 1D character. Efficient electron transfer from TiO_2 electron acceptors to SWNTs is expected to occur by forming core–shell structures with maximized contacts between SWNTs and TiO_2. The core–shell structure was fabricated using M13 virus template. M13 virus with SWNT-binding peptide motif on p8 major coat protein was selected through biopanning against SWNT films. Virus–SWNT complexes were first generated and TiO_2 nanocrystals were then biomineralized onto the complexes. The complexation of SWNTs with M13 virus enhanced colloidal stability of SWNTs and decreased bundling. Part of the SWNT surface is exposed to water, making direct contact with the biomineralized TiO_2. While surfactant-stabilized SWNTs could not efficiently template TiO_2, virus-stabilized SWNTs generated a core–shell platform. However, metallic SWNTs in the as-produced SWNTs provided short-circuit paths negating benefits from the semiconducting SWNTs that can provide efficient electron-diffusion path without recombination. Use of a metallic SWNTs–TiO_2 core–shell actually decreased power conversion efficiency compared to that of TiO_2-only photoanodes. The critical importance of the electronic type and degree of bundling of nanotubes was demonstrated. With semiconducting SWNTs and optimized amount of virus templates, power conversion efficiency of 10.6% was achieved.

The M13 virus has been widely applied to the biomedical field such as in tumor targeting, imaging, and therapy. M13 virus-derived filamentous phage with chimeric M13-adenosine-associated virus (AAV) gene cassette and displaying RGD peptide that binds to integrin overexpressed in tumor cells showed promising solid tumor-targeting performances after systemic administration in mice.[42] A targeted antibiotic drug-carrying M13 virus has also been demonstrated.[43] A genetically modified M13 virus with targeting moiety on the p8 body protein (selected using biopanning) or p3 [immunoglobulin G (IgG)-like] was loaded with chloramphenicol antibiotics via chemical conjugation. Controlled release of drug demonstrated the potential of using M13 virus for the targeted drug carrier.

Use of M13 virus templates as tissue-regenerating scaffolds has recently been explored.[44] M13 viruses were genetically engineered to express a high density of cell-signaling peptides on their major coat proteins. Signaling motifs of RGD, a cell adhesion integrin-binding motif, and IKVAV, a laminin motif known to promote neural cell adhesion, were chosen. Expressing these peptides on the major coat protein of the M13 virus was not straightforward since both peptides add an extra positive charge to the N-terminus of p8 proteins. Since p8 proteins constitute the main body of M13 virus, both the structure and the charge affect the ability of the virus to be packaged from the bacterial host. Direct insertion of these motifs could disrupt p8 body protein assembly because negative surface charges are favored in natural assembly of M13 coat proteins. To select peptide sequence bearing the cell signaling motifs but not disrupting major coat protein assembly, a partial library (framing RGD or IKVAV) cloning approach was tried. In the partial library, the random peptides have RGD or IKVAV sequence in their octamer sequence. The selected viruses self-assembled into directionally organized liquid crystalline-like materials due to their long rod shape and monodispersity. The constructed viral nanofiber scaffolds were able to support neural progenitor cell proliferation and differentiation as well as their growth in three dimensions. Oriented cell growth on self-assembled M13 virus films has also been accomplished with the convective assembly method.[25] Chemical grafting of RGD motif, which can bind to integrin receptors of all mammalian cells, to the virus surface enabled the oriented growth of NIH-3T3 cells on this substrate.

Multifunctional M13 virus has been assembled with fluorescent SWNTs and ligands simultaneously for targeted fluorescence imaging of tumors.[45] SWNTs stabilized by genetically engineered M13 virus with ligands for targeting tumors on p3 proximal ends can be successfully used as an efficient *in vivo* fluorescent imaging probe. For this purpose, M13 virus with SWNT-binding peptide motif on the p8 major coat protein was identified through biopanning with p8 library and subsequently incorporated with specific ligands on p3 ends by genetic means. Spatial separation of the functionalities could be advantageous for constructing targeted and fluorescent imaging probe complexes without compromising the fluorescence of SWNTs. With this approach, SWNTs have been successfully utilized for second near-infrared (NIR) window fluorescent imaging of molecularly targeted tumors for the first time.

8.2.1.2 Tobacco Mosaic Virus

TMV is a tubular virus created by the self-assembly of 2130 identical protein subunits that are arranged in a right-handed helical manner around the central viral RNA. The wild-type TMV is 300 nm in length, has a 18 nm outer diameter, and possesses a central open cavity with a diameter of 4 nm. Figure 8.13 demonstrates the schematic structure of the TMV particle.[46] TMV is remarkably robust and stable at temperatures as high as 60°C and pH range of 2–10 without disrupting its structure. Both the inner and outer surfaces of TMV are charged due to the presence of charged amino acids, which is favorable for mineralization. The charged surface can induce directed nucleation and growth of materials. Mineralization at the inner cavity can be used to generate nanowires and the outer surface can be used for nanotube formation upon removal of the virus template.

The relatively high thermal and chemical stability of TMV renders the wild-type TMV as a versatile template for materials synthesis. Various materials were generated

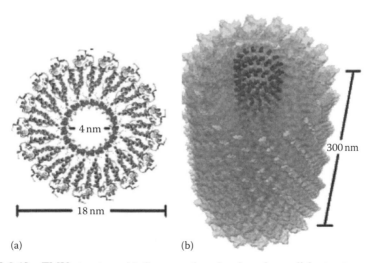

FIGURE 8.13 TMV structure. (a) Cross section showing planar disk structure and (b) a fully assembled capsid. (Reprinted with permission from Schlick, T. L., et al., 2005, 3718–23. Copyright 2005 American Chemical Society.)

at different pH conditions.[47] Metal sulfides such as CdS and PbS were deposited on the outer surface of the wild-type TMV at pH 5.0 and 7.0. The cationic metal precursor Cd^{2+} and Pb^{2+} electrostatically interacted with the negative charges of the TMV outer surface. Subsequent mineralization with H_2S resulted in metal sulfide nanotubes. IO-coated TMV nanocylinder was produced at higher pH of 9.0. Since TMV is also stable in an ethanol-rich environment as well as a harsh pH condition, TMV templates are compatible with the sol–gel deposition method using metal alkoxide precursors for several metal oxide depositions. Silica coating on wild-type TMV in alkaline ethanol was performed with tetraethoxyorthosilicate (TEOS) precursors.[48] However, unmodified wild-type TMV could only template very thin (<1 nm) silica layers. Pretreatment of TMV with aniline appeared effective in enhancing silica deposition to thick coating (>20 nm).[49] An aniline coating on TMV resulted in the alignment of TMV particles in micrometer-long threads probably because of the shielding of the charged groups on the TMV surface. Masking of charges and hydrophobic nature of aniline produced a uniform and attractive surface for silica formation. Titania layers were also produced on the wild-type TMV surface by a similar method.[50]

The inner cavity of TMV was exploited as a nanoreactor to grow thin nanowires with very high aspect ratios by electroless deposition.[51] The internal surface of the channel should be first activated with palladium or platinum ions. Ni and Co nanowires were then selectively formed inside the channel by electroless deposition (Figure 8.14). The spatial selectivity was given by the amino residue of the internal cavity. The amine groups at the inner surface of TMV can form complexes with $PdCl_4^{2-}$ and $PtCl_4^{2-}$. The exterior surface of TMV lacks amines, so it cannot be activated.

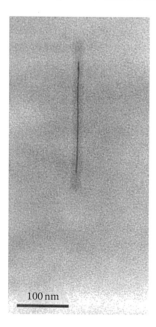

100 nm

FIGURE 8.14 TEM image of TMV after Pd(II) activation, followed by electroless deposition of Co. (Reprinted with permission from Knez, M., et al., 2003, 1079–81. Copyright 2003 American Chemical Society.)

Chemical control of surface charge was utilized for the control of spatial selectivity between exterior and interior surfaces of the wild-type TMV.[52] Some wild-type TMVs have basic amino acids on the outer surface and acidic amino acid in the cavity wall. Under acidic conditions, interactions of $AuCl_4^-$ or $PtCl_6^{2-}$ and the positively charged lysine and arginine residues on the outer surface are favored, selectively decorating metallic nanoparticles on the external surface of TMV. At pH neutral or higher, positive charges on the outer surface decrease and negative charges of acidic amino acids such as glutamate and aspartate in the cavity wall increase. Selective interaction of Ag^+ ions with the acidic groups produced regularly spaced spherical nanoparticles with a diameter of less than 5 nm inside the cavity along the axis of TMV rods. Similar experiments using a mutant TMV with reduced negative charge along the central cavity gave no nanoparticles associated with TMV rods, confirming that the negative charges were involved in the site-specific deposition. The pH was a useful chemical handle in controlling spatial selectivity.

Although wild-type viruses could be used as templates for mineralization, the weak interaction of wild-type virus with nanoparticles has had limited success. The biotemplating with wild-type virus resulted in inhomogeneous coating of nanoparticles, and even easy detachment from the viral template. Enhanced affinity of viruses to the functional nanomaterials has been accomplished through modification or engineering of viruses. A TMV rod was genetically engineered to express additional cysteines on the capsid protein.[53] In an aqueous solution, cysteine side chains exposed on the TMV surface can form thiol–metal complexes by covalently reacting with metal precursor ions. One or two cysteines were inserted at the amino-terminus of the coat protein through site-directed mutagenesis. Insertion of amino acid residues at this location did not significantly affect the virus assembly or stability. Cysteine insertion generated high density of metal-binding sites on the TMV outer surface providing more nucleation sites compared to the wild-type TMV. Based on the crystal structure of TMV coat proteins (TMVPs), the nearest neighbor distances between thiol groups were calculated as 2.3 nm axially and 3.5 nm radially. Densely deposited Au, Ag, and Pd clusters were synthesized on the cysteine-inserted TMV through in situ chemical reduction. Metal deposition on engineered TMV was relatively insensitive to pH, confirming that the metal binding is primarily driven by chemical association but not by electrostatic interaction. The enhanced interaction with metal cations through cysteine insertion was confirmed by analyzing metal ion uptake on the engineered TMV.[54] The results confirmed that the extra cysteines on the modified TMV template enhanced the total biosorption of metal ions and the sorption amount was dependent on the type of metal ions.

While most metallization processes use reducing agents, cysteine-modified TMV could reduce Pd ions without the presence of external reducing agent.[55] The reducing agent-free Pd mineralization on Cys-mutated TMV created uniform and dense metal nanowires, whereas only incomplete and irregular-shaped coating of Pd on the same TMV clone was produced under the same condition but with a dimethylamine-borane (DMAB) reducing agent (Figure 8.15). The thiol groups showed superior Pd precursor uptake over amine and hydroxyl groups under the same conditions as those used to coat Pd on TMV. This result suggests that high-density conjugation of metal ion–surface functionalities could catalyze self-mineralization on the

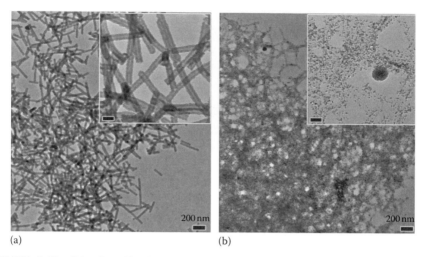

(a)   (b)

FIGURE 8.15 Pd mineralization on Cys-mutant TMV by self-mineralization process (a) without any reducing agent and by adding external reducing agent (DMAB) (b). Scale bar = 50 nm. (Reprinted with permission from Lim, J. S., et al., 2010, 3863–67. Copyright 2010 American Chemical Society.)

functional moiety sites. The self-mineralization mechanism elucidated that $PdCl_x(H_2O)_y$ precursors complexed with the surface functionalities are mineralized by oxidizing Cl^- to release HClO. The formation of HClO in the reaction medium was confirmed by solution acidification and UV–Vis absorption data.

Alignment or patterning of TMV largely depends on the shape anisotropy and inherent self-assembly of the rodlike TMV particles. TMV often shows a reversible head-to-tail higher order self-assembly.[47] Nanowires templated on these assembled TMV particles were several times the length of individual TMV particles. This assembly is attributed to complementary hydrophobic interaction between the dipolar ends of the helical structure. The head-to-tail aggregation is favored under acidic conditions because the mutual repulsion between acidic residues (glutamate and aspartate) is minimized by protonation.

In the absence of biological recognition, interfacial forces such as electrostatic, hydrophobic, and capillary forces have been applied to align virus particles. The convective assembly applied to TMV suspension generated aligned viral films with all the rods aligned parallel to the direction of assembly.[26] In this convective assembly, linear shear was generated by coating slides. The viruses were oriented parallel to the assembly direction or perpendicular to the drying front. The propensity for parallel alignment is consistent with rotational diffusion of a rod in a linear fluid flow created by solvent convection to the drying point. The virus concentration, substrate surface energy, and meniscus withdrawal speed are key factors for the thickness, orientation, and surface coverage of the viruses. These lined patterns of TMV can be transferred to flat, hydrophilic surface by microcontact printing. Controlled evaporation has also been exploited to create dynamic self-assembled structures. When the drying of a virus solution is conducted in a confined space such as glass capillary tubes[56] and between two glass slides,[57] the triple phase contact line (air–solution–substrate interface) was confined and the receding meniscus generated dynamic ordered patterns of virus. Glass capillary tube not only provides a confined space, but also creates a curved surface with multiple forces at the contact line to control the self-assembly process.[56] The fabricated hierarchical structure was determined by the preferred orientation of TMV at the air–liquid interface as well as the pinning–depinning process. The concentration of TMV particles was the most critical factor in controlling the orientation of the TMV in the resulting pattern. At low concentration with salts, strip patterns were produced around the interior of the capillary tubes and the distance between the two pinning lines gradually decreased deeper within the capillary due to the reduced water evaporation rate. TMV is oriented parallel to the plane of contact line (perpendicular to the long axis of the tube) to maximize the interfacial coverage per particle. The TMV concentration determines the amount of particles supplied to the strip-growing region, thus controlling the width and the thickness of the strips. As the TMV concentration increased, the entire capillary was covered with TMV without any strip patterns. The orientation of TMV also changed from perpendicular to the long axis of the tube to zigzag patterns. If the ionic strength of the solution was lowered by salt removal, the assembly behavior dramatically changed. At low ionic strength, the overall negative charges of TMV particles were not screened and TMV particles repelled each other. As a result, some TMVs were deposited at the contact line and other viruses were repelled. No regular patterns were observed at low concentration. At very high TMV concentration, the volume fraction of TMV at the interface increased, leading to enhanced dipole–dipole repulsion between TMV rods. The TMV particles were forced to orient perpendicular to the air–liquid interface, generating continuous thin films with TMV oriented perpendicular to the contact line but parallel to the long axis of the capillary tube. The patterned structure in the capillary tube was applied to guide the growth orientation of the smooth muscle cells to mimic the blood vessel structures. When the drying process was conducted between two glass slides, ordered strips could be patterned on a flat surface.[57] The resulting patterned surface could be applied to control surface hydrophobicity and direct the growth of the bone marrow stromal cells.

A solution of rod-shaped TMV particles was evaporated in a confined space between two glass slides to create large-scale strip patterns.[57] A controlled evaporation method was applied to regulate the height and width of the TMV strips. Strip patterns thus obtained can be used to control surface hydrophobicity and guide the directionality of cell adhesion and spreading in the cell growth on the TMV pattern. The capillary force alignment of TMV was further used in selective spacing of aligned TMV at the base of all protruding relief features of the stamp.[58] The selective placement was ascribed to discontinuous de-wetting, caused by selective wetting of the recesses by solvents that de-wet on the stamp surface. The highly regular virus strips can be printed on the flat surfaces without the use of any lithographic techniques.[59] The key step for the regularly spaced strip is the prealignment of the virus ink on the stamp. Wrinkled patterns of different wavelengths were used as stamps to control the interline distance of the virus patterns. The virus ink resides in the grooves of the relief structure and not on the top. This preferential arrangement is a consequence of a de-wetting process as described above. The defined virus strings with controllable spacing were produced with this low-cost and simple method.

The remarkable rigidity of TMV enabled vertical alignment of this rod-shaped particle.[60] This vertical alignment of biological entities can serve as a versatile platform for the fabrication of high-surface-area 1D functional materials.[61] Controlling molecular interaction at the interface is a key factor in aligning virus particles. TMV demonstrated preferred orientational alignment depending on the TMV concentration and ionic strength of the bulk solution.[60] At low TMV concentration, TMVs were aligned parallel to the oil–water interfaces, mediating the interfacial interactions at the greatest extent per particle. At high concentrations of TMV, the rods were oriented vertically to the interface, minimizing interrod electrostatic repulsion. The electrostatic repulsive forces between TMVs dominate interfacial assembly; thus, controlling ionic strength may play a key role in vertical alignment of the virus. To align TMV vertically on a solid substrate, cysteine-modified TMV was used in combination with controlling ionic concentration. Cysteine-modified TMV particles were aligned vertically on a gold surface via gold–thiol interactions.[61] The cysteine on the two ends of a TMV would be sufficiently exposed to make direct contact with the gold surface, while the recessed position of cysteine on the major coat protein may inhibit direct contact with the gold surface. This could contribute to the vertical positioning of viral rods on the gold surface.

In addition to the interfacial forces and chemical modification, specific recognition of biomolecules was also explored for patterning viral nanotemplates. To pattern TMV, hybridization of specific nucleic acid pairs was utilized.[62] Cysteine-modified TMV labeled with fluorescent markers was selectively immobilized on the predefined patterns via hybridization with probe DNA linked to electrodeposited chitosan. Labeled viruses were partially disassembled to expose RNA sequences complementary to DNA probe. The scheme of virus alignment through RNA hybridization is given in Figure 8.16. Nucleic acid hybridization-based assembly was further extended to construct TMV microarrays.[63] TMV nanotemplates were programmed with linker DNAs containing sequence-specific addresses. When glass substrate patterned with address-specific capture DNA (complementary to the addresses in linker DNA) was exposed to the programmed TMV, TMV microarray patterns were accomplished by direct hybridization between linker DNA and capture DNA. Since the nucleic acid hybridization was performed in an aqueous solution, it might be combined with microfluidic technique to generate hierarchically assembled TMV structures.[64] The hierarchical assembly of TMVs has been demonstrated with encoded hydrogel microparticles via nucleic acid hybridization. Microparticles encoded with capture DNA were produced in a microfluidic device. The microparticles consisted of spatially discrete regions including encoded identity information, an internal control, and capture DNA. TMVs were partially disassembled and programmed with linker DNA whose sequences are complementary to both TMV viral RNA and a capture DNA. A facile assembly of programmed TMVs onto microparticles was confirmed with high spatial and sequence selectivity. Direct embedding of functionalized TMV viral nanotemplates into polymer hydrogel matrix was demonstrated using microfluidic technique.[65] Functionalized TMVs were TMVs either covalently labeled with fluorescent markers or

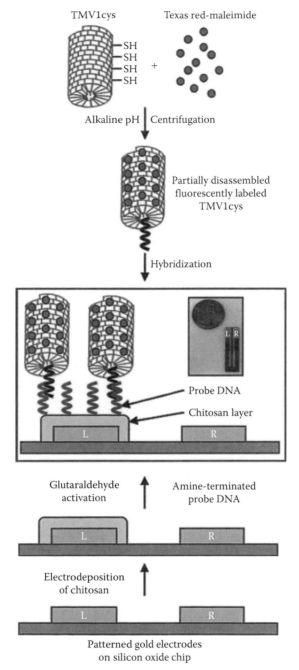

FIGURE 8.16 Diagram for the DNA probe-directed assembly of cysteine-modified TMV onto a readily addressable site. L and R represent left and right electrodes, respectively. The inset shows an actual chip. (Reprinted with permission from Yi, H. M., et al., 2005, 1931–36. Copyright 2005 American Chemical Society.)

metalized with Pd nanoparticles. These functionalized TMVs were suspended in a poly(ethylene glycol) (PEG)-based solution. Upon photopolymerization with UV light, microparticles with uniformly distributed TMV nanotemplates were formed. This microgel scaffolds offer highly porous 3D networks for immobilizing functionalized viral assemblies while maintaining the function and structure of the hybrid nanostructures. Janus microparticles with magnetic nanoparticles embedded on one side and functional TMV nanotemplates on the other side were also demonstrated for the facile separation of microgels from the bulk solution.

As for the practical application, TMVs coated with metal nanoparticles were first examined as electrical conductors. The cysteine-modified TMV could produce a continuous Pt layer with the increased nucleation site. This Pt nanowire templated on TMV showed ohmic electrical conductance.[66] A much thicker Pt coating on the TMV templates (~13 nm thick) improved electrical conductivity; however, the measured resistivity was still 10–100 times higher than bulk values. This was attributed to the polycrystallinity of the templated metal, the quality of the metal coating, and nanoscale dimensions of the structure.[67]

Pt nanoparticles incorporated into TMV capsids exhibited a novel electronic memory effect.[68] The memory effect is based on conductance switching with on/off ratio larger than 3 orders of magnitude. The conduction appeared to be related to the presence of Pt nanoparticles on the TMV template. The guanine base in viral RNA can be a charge donor with its aromatic ring, and electron tunneling from guanine to Pt nanoparticles through the insulating protein shell of TMV is responsible for conduction. Therefore, the mechanism of each process is ascribed to the charge trapping in the Pt nanoparticle for the data storage process and a tunneling for the high conductance state. The unique structure of the Pt–TMV complexes in which Pt nanoparticles are separated from viral RNA with an insulating protein shell is responsible for the conductance switching behavior with charge transfer and charge traps in the Pt nanoparticles.

Electron transfer through the TMV virion coat proteins was also found in TMV-templated ZnO field-effect transistors (FETs).[69] ZnO was deposited on Pd-activated TMV via electroless deposition (Figure 8.17a). To fabricate FETs by virus-directed self-assembly of mineralized ZnO, TMVs were immobilized on silicon substrates from aqueous solution with silicon dioxide as dielectric layer and prepatterned gold electrodes (Figure 8.17b). Divalent cations were added as a bridge to enhance adhesion between negatively charged TMV and silicon substrate. The FET performance of TMV/ZnO films showed remarkable differences to ZnO deposited on other templates such as self-assembled monolayers (SAMs) with carboxylate termination or DNAs under identical deposition conditions. TMV/ZnO showed 2 orders of magnitude higher charge carrier mobilities and drastically lower threshold voltage than those obtained with SAM/ZnO. DNA/ZnO films were even inferior to SAM/ZnO. This superior electronic performance was attributed to the electron injection capability of TMV templates. TMV not only functioned as a structural template but also obviously affected the properties of semiconducting layer.

The vertically aligned TMVs were applied to nickel–zinc batteries as high surface area electrodes.[61] TMV was genetically engineered to express cysteine residue and vertically aligned onto gold surface via gold–thiol interactions. Electroless deposition

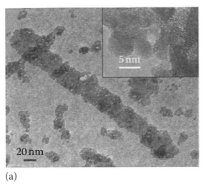
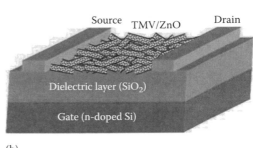

(a)   (b)

FIGURE 8.17 (a) TEM and high-resolution TEM (HRTEM) (inset) images of TMV-templated ZnO. (b) Schematic setup of the FET. (From Atanasova, P., Rothenstein, D., Schneider, J. J., et al. Virus-templated synthesis of ZnO nanostructures and formation of field-effect transistors. *Adv. Mater.*, 2011, 23, 4918–22. Copyright Wiley-VCH Verlag GmbH & Co. KGaA. Reproduced with permission.)

from nickel ion precursor in aqueous conditions resulted in coating layers composed of NiO, Ni(OH)$_2$, and Ni. Vertically oriented nanowires showed more than 10-fold increases in surface area. When tested within Ni–Zn battery systems after additional ambient oxidation, the viral electrodes increased the total capacity by more than double. The vertical virus alignment was structurally stable under prolonged battery tests. No noticeable loss in the structure of the coated viruses was observed after 30 charge–discharge cycles.

The vertically patterned TMV could serve as a novel 3D platform for the fabrication of high surface area functional electrode systems. The nickel metal coatings on patterned 3D TMV templates were used as a substrate for the subsequent deposition of silicon anode materials for lithium–ion batteries.[70] The resulting multilayered nanoscale 3D silicon anodes with the internal Ni metal layer functioning as a current collector have additional advantages from the processing perspective. Direct fabrication of nanostructured silicon rendered every silicon nanowire to be connected to the patterned current collector, eliminating the need for binders or conducting additives. The cysteine-modified TMV templates were 3D patterned onto stainless steel substrates. Metallization on this vertically aligned TMV was accomplished via electroless deposition of Ni. Silicon active anode materials were deposited via the physical vapor deposition (PVD) sputtering method. Most TMV tethered on the stainless steel surface vertically or near-vertically (Figure 8.18a). The resulting composite anodes exhibited high capacities and excellent charge–discharge cycling stability benefited from the unique structures with TMV biotemplates. A sponge-like silicon structure formed after repeated battery cycles appeared to enhance both reaction kinetics and anode stability (Figure 8.18b).

Self-assembling of TMVP monomers offers an attractive way for the construction of arrays of regularly spaced light-harvesting chromophores as natural light-harvesting systems.[71] Self-assembly of functionalized protein subunits into disk- and rod-shaped particles allowed efficient energy transfer between chromophores. The thiol-reactive organic donor and acceptor chromophores were reacted

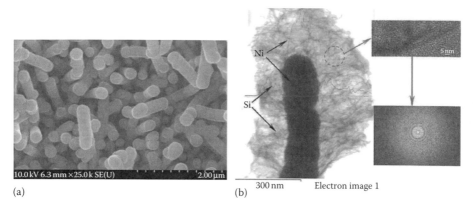

FIGURE 8.18 (a) SEM image of vertical TMV/Ni/Si nanowires. (b) Occurrence of a sponge-like silicon morphology upon cycling. TEM image with EDS spectra for Ni and Si after 75 cycles at 1C rate. Inset: HRTEM and fast Fourier transform (FFT) images of Si. (Reprinted with permission from Chen, X. L., et al., 2010, 5366–72. Copyright 2010 American Chemical Society.)

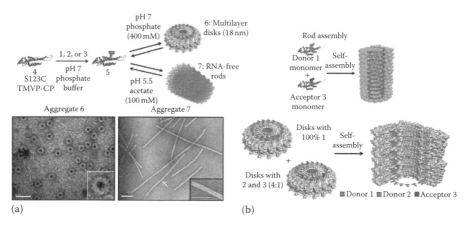

FIGURE 8.19 (a) Self-assembly of modified TMV coat protein into disk and rod structures and TEM images of disk (aggregate 6) and rod (aggregate 7). (b) Self-assembly of different light-harvesting structures with mixtures of monomers. (Reprinted with permission from Miller, R. A., et al., 2007, 3104–09. Copyright 2007 American Chemical Society.)

with cysteine-mutant TMVP monomers. These chromophore-functionalized TMVP monomers self-assembled into disk- and rod-shaped particles, and shape control was achieved by simple adjustments in pH and ionic strength of the buffer solutions (Figure 8.19a). Three chromophore systems were prepared by coassembly of monomers, functionalized with different chromophores, for broad spectrum light collection (Figure 8.19b). The systems thus prepared achieved highly efficient light energy transfer. Light energy transfer efficiency has been further enhanced by positioning donors and acceptors at specified locations with the engineered capsid proteins.[72] Circular permutant of the TMV capsid protein that repositions the N- and C-termini to the center of the assemblies could self-assemble into light-harvesting rods.

The new position of the N-terminus allows functional groups to be attached in the inner pore of the assembled particles, providing geometries reminiscent of the natural photosynthetic reaction center, which is surrounded by the light-harvesting chromophores. To construct similar light-harvesting systems, light-absorbing donor was conjugated to cysteine residue of the TMVP monomer and acceptor was subsequently conjugated to the N-termini of the same monomer. Monomer self-assembly into disk-installed centralized acceptor groups in the inner pore surrounded by the ring of donor chromophores. The resulting geometries enabled efficient energy transfer.

TMV-templated palladium nanoparticles have been examined as catalysts for promoting redox reactions.[73,74] Nanostructured Pd particles immobilized on TMV functioned as catalysts for chemical reactions such as dichromate reduction[73] and Suzuki coupling reaction.[74] Cysteine modification is not only for tunable and selective loading of noble metal catalysts on TMV template but also for immobilization of TMV template on gold substrate for easy catalyst recovery.

8.2.2 Spherical or Near-Spherical Viruses

8.2.2.1 Cowpea Chlorotic Mosaic Virus

Cowpea chlorotic mosaic virus (CCMV) is an icosahedral plant virus with 28 nm outer diameter. The capsid of CCMV is composed of 180 identical proteins that self-assembled into an empty protein cage. The protein shell defines an inner cavity with 18 nm diameter (Figure 8.20).[75] The native CCMV has genomic RNA encapsulated in the capsids. The CCMV genome consists of three unique single-stranded, anionic RNA. The viral capsid undergoes a pH-dependent reversible swelling behavior.[76] When placed in the medium of pH higher than 6.5, the capsid dimension increases by 10% in volume compared to the nonswollen form. At the same time, 60 separate pores in the viral capsid are opened to a size of 2 nm diameter. Therefore,

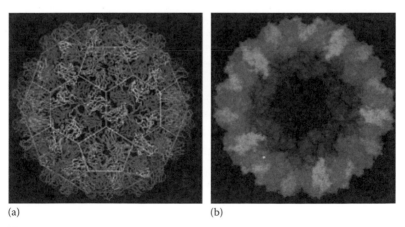

(a)   (b)

FIGURE 8.20 Ribbon diagram of the 180-subunit protein cage of CCMV (a) and cutaway view showing the central cavity of the protein cage (b). (From Douglas, T., Strable, E., Willits, D., et al. Protein engineering of a viral cage for constrained nanomaterials synthesis. *Adv. Mater.*, 2002, 14, 415–18. Copyright Wiley-VCH Verlag GmbH & Co. KGaA. Reproduced with permission.)

CCMV capsid in its swollen state allows substance exchange with surroundings, while no obvious substance exchange is observed with the closed structure at pH under 6.5. This reversible structural transition in turn enables the release or entrapment of molecules of interests. Selective trapping and deposition of materials can be possible by controlling the solution pH. The empty CCMV cage can be obtained by extracting the viral RNA at pH >6.5 when the capsid is disassembled. The empty CCMV cage can serve as a nanoreactor for size-constrained nanoparticle synthesis. The inner surface of the CCMV capsid is highly positively charged because the N-termini of protein subunits have nine basic amino acid residues projecting at the interior. The positive interior promotes anionic molecular precursor accumulation within the cavity via enhanced electrostatic interactions inducing selective nucleation of minerals in the CCMV cage.

The CCMV capsid without an RNA chain was exposed to polymetalate precursors such as tungstate, vanadate, and molybdate in its swollen form.[77] Oxometalate anions flowed in and were accumulated at the positive interior. The capsid was then closed by lowering the pH of the solution and nanocrystals were mineralized simultaneously. The nanocrystals were not generated without CCMV capsid under the same growth conditions, demonstrating the importance of local confinement by a cationic inner wall. The capsid acted as a nucleation catalyst as well as a reaction vessel for size and shape control. The electrostatic aspect of the precursor–template interaction was further investigated by pH-dependent encapsulation of anionic organic polymers. The positive inner wall of the native CCMV capsid could also be used for TiO_2 nanoparticle synthesis.[78] Two negatively charged Ti(IV) complexes were used for the formation of pH-controlled precipitation of titania-based materials. The choice of precursor has a profound impact on the structure of the final products. Use of sodium metatitanate ($Na_2Ti_3O_7$) produced amorphous nanoparticles, while crystalline β-TiO_2 was generated with Ti(IV) bis(ammonium lactate)dihydroxide (Ti-BALDHI). A similar approach was applied for the synthesis of monodispersed Prussian blue (PB) nanoparticles.[79] PB precursors employed were negatively charged iron complexes. The positively charged inner surface of native CCMV attracted and accumulated the precursors and subsequent polymerization by a photo-initiated stepwise reaction formed PB clusters. Monodispersed PB nanoparticles with ~18 nm in diameter were produced within the CCMV cage.

The electrostatic properties of the CCMV capsid surface can be altered by genetic engineering. The highly basic N-termini of native CCMV interior surface are required to package and condense the anionic RNA viral genome. However, the positive charges are not essential for the self-assembly of an empty protein cage *in vitro*. Therefore, the interior surface of CCMV can be engineered to carry negative charges to attract positively charged precursors. The nine basic amino acid residues of the N-terminus of the coat protein could be replaced with the glutamates (Glu), which provided negative charges to the inner wall of CCMV capsid without disrupting overall architecture of the cage.[75] The engineered CCMV capsid captured Fe^{2+} ions and catalyzed the mineralization of IO nanoparticles within the cage.

The interior of CCMV capsids also provides an ideal platform to study enzymatic reactions in a confined space. In a natural environment, enzymes are present in a confined reaction space, but most enzyme studies are carried out in a bulk aqueous solution. To bridge this gap between the experimental and real situations and properly study the enzymatic activity, single-enzyme experiments were designed in the restricted spatial environment of the CCMV capsid.[80] Individual horseradish peroxidase (HRP) enzymes were incorporated in the inner cavity of CCMVs. The number of encapsulated proteins could be controlled by the starting protein concentrations. The viral capsid allows the diffusion of substrate and product of the enzymatic reaction, and the permeability was changed with pH. The diffusion rate showed a discontinuity at pH 5.7, which corresponds to the structural transition of CCMV to the swollen state with large pores.

The reversible structural transition of RNA-free CCMV capsids enabled the encapsulation of various molecules, but only at low pH <6.5. At pH 7.5, the native virus is in a swollen state, but without the stabilizing interaction with RNA, the capsid disassembles into 90 capsid dimers. This special property has limited the widespread use of RNA-free CCMV capsid as a nanoreactor especially for encapsulating proteins and enzymes at physiological pH. It is possible to stabilize the RNA-free capsid at pH 7.5 by negatively charged polyelectrolytes or negatively charged particles, but these bulky matters fill the interior of the capsid, leaving virtually no space for other functional target molecules. This limitation has been overcome with the histidine-tag-modified capsid stabilized with metal ions.[81] The N-terminus of CCMV capsid proteins was modified with His-tag consisting of six histidines. Nickel and other metal ions were able to induce and stabilize capsid and capsid-like particles at neutral pH. This behavior was attributed to the interaction between His-tag and metal salts. This method could greatly expand the scope of the CCMV capsid as a nanoreactor to encapsulate functional molecules such as proteins and enzymes in physiological conditions.

The conjugation of organic substances with CCMV has been realized on the exterior surface of the proteins.[82] Native CCMV presents surface-exposed amine (lysine) and carboxylic acid (glutamate and aspartate on which functionalized fluorophores can be conjugated). Functionalized fluorophores were chemically conjugated on the external surface of CCMV via carbodiimide chemistry. CCMV engineered with cysteine residues on the exterior was utilized to attach a 24-amino-acid peptide by oxidative coupling of cysteine thiol to the free thiol of the peptide.

Ordered assembly of CCMVs into 2D layers can be accomplished through LBL techniques using both electrostatic and biomolecular recognition interactions.[83] LBL methods conventionally depend on the electrostatic interactions between differently charged polymeric species. In the first-type films incorporating CCMVs, these ionic interactions between negatively charged CCMVs and positively charged polylysine were employed (Figure 8.21a). In the second-type films, specific complementary biological interactions were introduced to the LBL techniques, expanding the scope of LBL technique beyond electrostatic interactions. For this purpose, CCMVs were biotinylated (CCMV-B) and repeated deposition of streptavidin and CCMV-B constituted the LBL cycle (Figure 8.21b). Streptavidin–biotin coupling reaction was adopted as a complementary biological interaction.

Electrostatic interaction was further utilized for the fabrication of hierarchical dendron–virus complexes.[84] CCMVs could be self-assembled into well-defined micrometer-sized object using photosensitive dendrons. Amine-functionalized

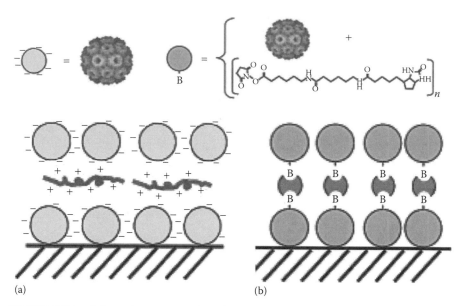

FIGURE 8.21 Schematic representation of multilayer films. CCMV cryo-reconstruction is shown above. (a) Polylysine interlayer between adlayers of CCMV. (b) Streptavidin interlayer between adlayers of CCMV-B. (Reprinted with permission from Suci, P. A., et al., 2006, 8891–96. Copyright 2006 American Chemical Society.)

dendrons can bind on the negatively charged CCMV surface through multivalent interactions acting as molecular glues between viruses. At least four cationic amines were required for the efficient complexation with virus.[85] The assembly size could be controlled by adjusting the generation and concentration of the dendron as well as the salt concentration. Disassembly was triggered by a short optical stimulus. Photochemical degradation of dendron led to the release of virus particles. While oppositely charged polyelectrolyte complexes are considered to be kinetically frozen systems, the optically triggered destruction of multivalent binding interactions was used as a tool to release the protein cages from their complexes. This electrostatic assembly between negatively charged CCMVs and amine-functionalized polymers was further extended for the large-scale assembly of PB nanoparticles.[85] The CCMV capsids loaded with PB nanoparticles can also be assembled, demonstrating the possibility of controlling large-scale assembly of various nanomaterials by controlling the virus assembly.

Practical application of CCMV to nanobiotechnology has not yet been actively pursued; however, biomedical application to MRI imaging[86] and targeted antimicrobial photodynamic therapy[87] have been reported. Magnetic resonance imaging (MRI) contrast agents have been developed by decorating CCMV with gadolinium. Gd^{3+} ions can bind at a specific metal-binding site of the CCMV surface. The large surface area of CCMVs allowed a large number of Gd^{3+} ion decorations showing high relaxivity values.[86] Sensitivity of antimicrobial photodynamic therapy has been enhanced by coupling the photosensitizer to a targeting nanoplatform. The genetic contruct of the CCMV nanoplatform facilitated the dual functionalization with the photosensitizer

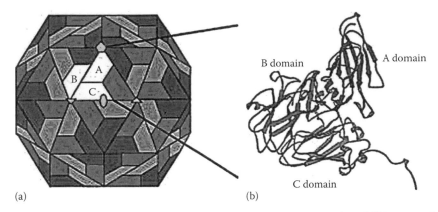

(a)   (b)

FIGURE 8.22 Structure of the CPMV. (a) A diagrammatic representation of CPMV showing the distribution of the two subunits that comprise the asymmetric unit. (b) The folds of the two subunits. (From Wang, Q., Lin, T. W., Tang, L., Johnson, J. E., and Finn, M. G. Icosahedral virus particles as addressable nanoscale building blocks. *Angew. Chem. Int. Ed.*, 2002, 41, 456–62. Copyright Wiley-VCH Verlag GmbH & Co. KGaA. Reproduced with permission.)

and targeting ligand. The designed versatile vesicles showed feasibility for selective photodynamic inactivation of pathogenic bacterium.[87]

8.2.2.2 Cowpea Mosaic Virus

Cowpea mosaic virus (CPMV) is an icosahedral plant virus whose structure is known at atomic resolution. The central two single-stranded RNAs are encapsulated by an icosahedral capsid with a dimension of ~30 nm outer diameter. The CPMV capsid comprises 60 copies of an asymmetric unit that contains two protein subunits: a small subunit with one domain, the A domain, and a large subunit with two domains, the B + C domains. The three domains together form the asymmetric unit (Figure 8.22).[88] CPMV has good thermal and chemical stability: the capsid is stable to moderately high temperature up to 60°C for at least 1 h, in a wide pH range of 3.5–9 at room temperature for a considerable period of time and even in some organic solvent–water mixture.[88]

The superior stability of CCMV allows a wide range of materials to be conjugated with this versatile template. A broad range of chemical and biological groups can be loaded to the numerous binding sites of the CPMV capsid surface. The external surface of the CPMV capsid provides addressable lysines, carboxylates, and tyrosines. For example, the wild-type CPMV possesses 60 lysines per virus particles with enhanced reactivity. Moreover, external modification of the CPMV capsid has been actively explored for additional functionalities. A CPMV mutant was prepared to create cysteine residue on the outer surface since native CPMV has no free sulfhydryl group exposed on the outer surface. Sulfhydryl group of cysteine reacts with maleimide, which is a great platform for bioconjugation with organic materials. Maleimidofluorescein organic dyes or monomaleimido-nanogold could be attached to the CPMV outer capsid via thiol functionalities on the protein surface.[88] High local concentration of fluorescein bound on the CPMV template exhibited strong fluorescence emission under UV light exposure. Dye molecule loading to CPMV template was also achieved using CPMV modified with azide–alkyne groups.[89] The exterior surface of CPMV coat protein was decorated with azides or alkynes at either reactive lysine or cysteine residues. Fluorescein derivatives containing complementary groups for the desired copper-catalyzed cycloaddition reaction efficiently coupled with the azides or alkynes on the CPMV.

Various kinds of cysteine-modified CPMV mutants have been used to demonstrate specific binding of gold nanoparticles to cysteines through gold–thiol interaction. Cysteine residues were engineered to the exterior surface of CPMV at different locations generating different mutants (Figure 8.21).[90] Unstained transmission electron microscopy (TEM) images of gold nanoparticles showed patterns that match the known locations of the inserted cysteine groups on the capsid (Figure 8.23). The proper positioning of cysteine insertion into capsid conferred the controlled gold nanoparticle attachment. These different mutants of

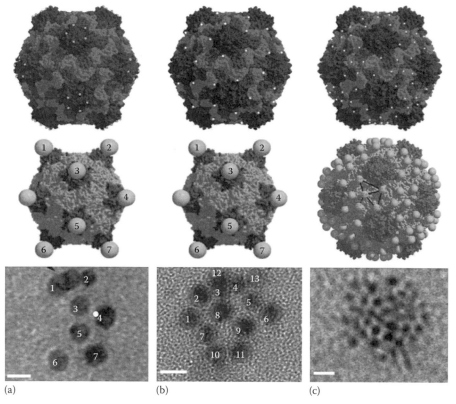

(a)   (b)   (c)

FIGURE 8.23 (a) BC mutant. (b) EF mutant. (c) DM mutant. (Top) Location of inserted cysteines for different mutants. Cysteines in white. (Middle) model of mutant with gold nanoparticles bound to cysteines. (Bottom) Unstained TEM image of gold nanoparticles bound to CPMV. Gold nanoparticles of 5 nm size for BC and EF mutants and gold nanoparticles of 2 nm size for DM mutant are used. Scale bar = 5 nm. (Reprinted with permission from Blum, A. S., et al., 2004, 867–70. Copyright 2004 American Chemical Society.)

CPMV served as scaffolds for gold nanoparticle assembly to produce a specific interparticle distance.

Quantum dots (QDs) were also decorated on the external surface of CPMV using histidine–QD binding.[91] Histidine can bind QDs through complexation to zinc in a ZnS coating. Short, histidine-containing peptides were conjugated to the lysine residues on the external surface of CPMV via chemical carbodiimide coupling reaction. Water-soluble QDs were bound to the CPMV external surface through the reaction with the histidine-containing peptide linker. A very high local concentration of QDs was generated on the viral scaffolds without inducing self-quenching among QDs. The CPMV–QD complexes enhanced quantum efficiency by 15%. Enhancement of signal with the increased local concentration of active materials on the viral scaffolds was also demonstrated using IO magnetic nanoparticles.[92] Cysteine inserted CPMV-T184C mutant displays five solvent-exposed lysines per subunit protein on the exterior surface. IO can be linked to the amine group of lysine residue by forming peptide bonds via carbodiimide coupling chemistry. Stepwise assembly process was employed to integrate monodispersed CPMV–IO hybrids on a substrate. CPMV-T184C anchored to an SAM on gold substrate using cysteine residue and IO linkage followed for CPMV–IO hybrid formation. By employing this stepwise assembly process, CPMV–IO hybrid bound to a substrate created local enhancement of magnetic field strength and showed possibilities for enhanced MRI.

Decoration of CPMV with redox-active organometallic complexes has been accomplished using addressable surface lysines[93] and carboxylates.[94] On the solvent-exposed outer surface of the CPMV capsid are five lysine groups per asymmetric subunit. Ferrocenecarboxylate was selectively coupled to the surface-exposed amine groups of lysines by forming peptide bonds.[93] Ferrocenecarboxylate having 600 molar excess was used to ensure maximum amine labeling. CPMV viral particles maintained integrity with the decorated redox-active complexes, and an electrochemical study revealed the presence of redox-active nanoparticles on the viral capsid. Electroactive viologen derivatives were attached to the surface-exposed carboxylate groups of CPMV capsid.[94] The accessible surface profile of CPMV indicates seven solvent-exposed carboxlyate groups from glutamate and aspartate on the surface. Methly(aminopropyl)viologen (MAV) was covalently attached to the carboxlyate groups by the standard protocol for peptide bond formation. The electrochemical analysis on the CPMV–viologen hybrid showed them to be redox-active nanoparticles. The virus could be decorated with 180 viologen derivatives. This corresponds to the three carboxlyates per asymmetric subunit being covalently functionalized with the viologen derivatives. At least 30% of the available carboxlyate on the surface was utilized. The display of multiple redox centers on the virus particle surface that are noninteracting could serve as a multielectron reservoir. This novel system may lead to the development of nanoscale electron-transfer mediators for redox catalysis, biosensors, and nanoelectronic devices.

Besides providing attachment sites for the conjugation of external substances, the outer surface of CPMV can be used as a scaffold for the controlled deposition and nucleation of inorganic materials. CPMV was genetically engineered to express a specific peptide sequence (YSDQPTQSSQRP) on the external surface of the capsid.[95] This peptide sequence was previously identified by phage display technique to have specific binding affinity to silica and used for favored mineralization.[96] This short peptide was inserted into the S protein of the capsid subunit; thus, totally 60 copies of peptide insert were displayed on the CPMV surface. Silication on the engineered CPMV was achieved by a sol–gel process with tetraethoxysilane (TEOS) and aminopropyltriethoxysilane precursors in aqueous buffer solution. Monodispersed silica nanoparticles of ~30 nm diameter were templated on the CPMV outer surface. Similar strategy was applied for the preparation of monodispersed, hollow FePt nanoparticles of ~30 nm diameter.[97] Again, chimeric virus technology that allows the presentation of foreign peptides on the particle surface has been used. The viral capsid surface of CPMV was genetically modified to include a certain short peptide sequence that templates the formation of FePt metals on the capsid surface. Dodecapeptide sequence HNKHLPSTQPLA, previously selected for FePt by phage display technique, was inserted into the small subunit of CPMV. FePt deposition on the CPMV surface was done under ambient environmental conditions in aqueous solvent. This method suggests an environmentally benign route for the fabrication of monodispersed nanoparticles of ~30 nm diameter.

Although genetic engineering is a convenient method for producing massive population of viruses with desired functionality, the genetic modification is not a requirement for equipping a virus with desired functionality. In some cases, it is sufficient or even required to chemically conjugate the appropriate peptide to the virus surface before mineralization.[98] Not all peptide sequences can be expressed on the surface of CPMV; when the insert is not well tolerated, the amplification yield can be low and there can be a problem with the stability of a chimera virus. Specifically, a chimera virus that includes peptides with affinity to ZnS cannot be produced at all. The peptides promoting mineralization of CoPt, FePt, and ZnS were chemically coupled to amino acid residues on the surface of wild-type CPMV.[98] Peptide sequences identified through an evolutionary screening process were synthesized with amine-terminus protected by caboxybenzyl. The carboxyl-terminus of the relevant peptide was chemically conjugated to the surface-exposed amines of lysines on the external surface of CPMV. Subsequent mineralization of CPMV-peptide with corresponding precursors produced monodispersed nanoparticles of ~30 nm diameter coated with CoPt, FePt, and ZnS.

Genetic or chemical modification of CPMV surface with material-specific peptides produces specific templates suitable for the mineralization of the corresponding material. Therefore, only a limited number of materials that have relevant peptides identified can be templated on the viral scaffolds. To complement the material-specific templates and prepare a wide range of materials, strategies for developing general templates that could mineralize a variety of materials have been explored. Preactivation of a capsid with palladium(II) and following electroless deposition allowed the metallization of wild-type CPMV with various metallic nanoparticles such as Co, Ni, Fe, Pt, CoPt, and NiFe at room temperature.[99] Anionic palladium ions were electrostatically bound to lysine amine side chains on the outer surface of the viral capsid and reduced to palladium clusters. Palladium clusters acted as nucleation sites for the subsequent metallic nanoparticle deposition by the electroless deposition. Metallic nanoparticles were fabricated on CPMV templates without any prior genetic or chemical modification and the need of nucleating peptides. Other methods of preparing general templates involved charge modification of the CPMV external surface.[100,101] Surface charge modification of CPMV appeared sufficient to promote the templated mineralization of various materials. To interact with cationic precursors, surface negative charge was increased by chemical conjugation of succinamate on the lysine group of CPMV surface.[100] When attacked by nucleophile amine, the cyclic structure of succinic anhydride changes to linear, with one end forming a peptide bond with the amine group and free carboxlyate group at the other end. Chemical modification of CPMV with succinic anhydride thus creates a surface carboxlyate group at the lysine site of the CPMV external surface. Maximum coverage of at least 240 addressable surface lysines with the carboxlyate group was achieved, increasing surface negative charge. Cationic cobalt ions and ferrous/ferric ions were attracted toward negatively charged CPMVs, and subsequent mineralization produced monodispersed cobalt and IO nanoparticles coated on the CPMV templates. On the other hand, positive charge was induced on the CPMV surface to promote adsorption of anionic precursor complexes.[101] Native CPMVs are anionic macromolecules at neutral pH with an isoelectric point (pI) of about pH 4.3 and do not efficiently interact with anionic complexes. The cationic polyelectrolyte poly(allylamine hydrochloride) (PAH) was electrostatically bound to the external surface of the CPMV capsid reversing the surface charge from negative to positive. Anionic gold complex was electrostatically adsorbed onto the cationic surface of polyelectrolyte-modified CPMV and then reduced under mild conditions to give metallic gold at the surface. Templated synthesis of narrowly dispersed gold nanoparticles was demonstrated with the method developed.

While the external surface of CPMV has been intensively exploited as a scaffold for mineralization, the internal cavity of CPMV has not been used to encapsulate materials since, unlike CCMV, it has been very difficult to obtain CPMV empty (RNA-free) virus-like particles (eVLPs). Recent discovery of producing large quantities of CPMV eVLP activated the internal cavity for material encapsulation.[102] Biotemplating inside the CPMV cavity is similar to that using CCMV, except that no pH-dependent structural transition has been reported for CPMV. The materials diffuse into its cavity via channels at the viral capsid. Cobalt and IO were successfully mineralized internally in the cavity of CPMV eVLP producing monodispersed nanoparticles of ~26 nm by environmentally benign process.[103] The integrity of CPMV was maintained upon internal mineralization, and the external surface of cobalt-containing VLP was still amenable for further chemical modification. The solvent-exposed lysines on the external surface of cobalt-VLP were functionalized with succinimide ester-activated biotin, and the biotinlyated cobalt-VLP could readily bind to streptavidin-coated substrates.

Assembling CPMV programmable building blocks into addressable layers has been demonstrated by combining nanolithographic techniques with cysteine-modified virus.[104] Chemoselective protein-to-surface linkers were adopted for the precise positioning of CPMV on the nanometric chemical templates. Amine-terminated alkanethiol linker molecule was patterned on the gold substrate first by dip-pen nanolithography (DPN). Long-chain aliphatic thiol formed high-density SAMs on the gold surface. The pattern dimension was close to the diameter of the cysteine-mutated CPMV. Highly selective reaction between maleimide attached to the amine group of the linker and the sulfhydryl of the cysteine on the CPMV surface immobilized the CPMV onto preformed pattern of the gold substrate. Cysteine-modified CPMV itself can bind to a gold surface to give a monolayer by gold–thiol interaction.[105] In contrast, no binding by wild-type CPMV was observed under the same reaction conditions. One disadvantage of working with cysteine-expressed CPMV is its tendency to aggregate by disulfide linkage between surface-exposed cysteine on different viruses. This limitation has been addressed by the introduction of *N*-succinimidyl *S*-acetylthiopropionate, acetate-protected thiol groups, and chemical conjugation to the surface-exposed lysine of CPMV. These protected thiol groups can be readily deprotected by deacetylation.[106]

While the aggregation phenomenon can be circumvented by the use of protected thiol groups, alternative ways for assembling CPMV particles are available. The widely investigated molecular recognition between streptavidin and biotin has been used for this purpose.[105] CPMV was biotinylated at solvent-exposed lysine sites. The biotin-functionalized CPMV can be readily deposited on the streptavidin-treated gold substrate. A bottom-up, LBL approach produced multilayers using this streptavidin–biotin recognition chemistry. Highly selective molecular recognition was also used for reversible assembly and disassembly of CPMV particles.[107] Complementary oligonucleotides were attached to CPMV scaffolds either at lysine residue or at genetically inserted cysteines on the outer surface of CPMV. The mixing of CPMVs carrying complementary oligonucleotides resulted in immediate aggregation by duplex base-pairing, and they were reversibly disassembled upon the addition of a competing oligonucleotide.

Biologically active CPMV-based thin films were constructed by electrostatic LBL assembly.[108] Since the p*I* of CPMV is ~5.5, the CPMV particle can be regarded as an anionic macromolecule. With cationic polyelectrolyte poly(diallyldimethylammonium chloride) (PDDA), CPMV particles were assembled into films by LBL. The fabricated CPMV-based films were biologically active for cell culture and the use of viral films as a novel support for cell adhesion and proliferation was explored. Cell attachment and growth behavior could be controlled by the coating density and surface coverage of the virus.

Unique raspberry-like nanocomposites of virus–polymer hybrid, potentially applicable to drug delivery, photovoltaics, catalysis, and optics, were generated by a controlled assembly based on noncovalent interactions between the polymers and CPMV viral particles.[109] Poly(4-vinylpyridine) (P4VP) was employed for this purpose because of the well-known ability of P4VP and block copolymers comprising P4VP to assemble with other polymers or nanoparticles to form various morphologies. There is very good coverage of CPMV particles on the surface of polymeric sphere-shaped raspberry-like nanocomposites (Figure 8.24).

The practical application of CPMV viral nanoparticles (VNPs) and virus-like particles (VLPs) mainly focuses on biomedical fields such as imaging, targeted delivery, and therapy. In the biomedical application of CPMV, immunogenicity is of particular importance. To shield VNPs from the immune system, the most popular approach is the PEGylation of VNPs. Attaching PEG chains to the external surface of CPMV appeared as an effective strategy to reduce biospecific interactions between biomolecules and cells or tissues resulting in marked increase in plasma

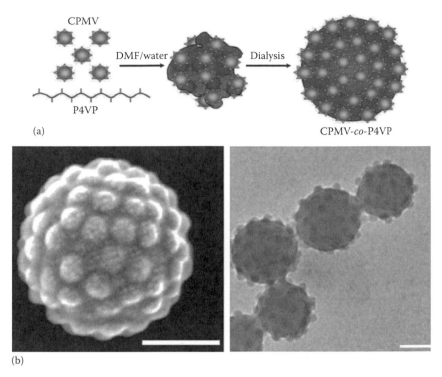

CPMV

DMF/water → Dialysis →

P4VP

(a)

CPMV-*co*-P4VP

(b)

FIGURE 8.24 (a) Schematics of CPMV-*co*-P4VP raspberry-like nanocomposite formation through noncovalent interaction. (b) Representative field emission SEM (FESEM) and TEM images of CPMV-*co*-P4VP raspberry-like nanocomposite. Scale bar = 100 nm. (From Li, T., Niu, Z. W., Emrick, T., Russell, T. R., and Wang, Q. Core/shell biocomposites from the hierarchical assembly of bionanoparticles and polymer. *Small*, 2008, 4, 1624–29. Copyright Wiley-VCH Verlag GmbH & Co. KGaA. Reproduced with permission.)

half-life.[110,111] PEGylating CPMV was indeed effective to eliminate the interaction of CPMVs with mammalian tumor cells and tissues.[110]

PEGlyation along with fluorescent labeling of CPMV also allowed noninvasive *in vivo* vascular imaging.[112] CPMVs were conjugated with Alexa Fluor dyes at the lysine sites of the external surface and subsequently coated with PEG. The resulting CPMV could be used to visualize the vascular and blood flow in living mouse and chick embryos to a depth of up to 500 μm. PEG coating minimized molecular interaction increasing half-life in the circulation of blood-borne agents and also completely inhibited the internalization by chick embryo endothelial cells *in vivo*. In imaging tumors with surface vimentine, specific interaction of CPMV with vimentin was exploited.[113,114] Vimentin is a type III intermediate filament predominantly surface expressed on cells involved in inflammation, but the function remains unknown. Cell-surface-expressed vimentin was found to mediate the internalization of CPMV into endothelial cells and other cells. The specific interaction of the fluorescent-labeled CPMV with vimentin protein allows the imaging of vascular structure and intravital vascular mapping in the developmental and tumor angiogenesis.[114]

In vivo tumor targeting and cell imaging has been recently demonstrated with CPMV particles multivalently functionalized with peptides.[112] For simultaneously targeting and imaging tumors, the external surface of CPMV was multivalently functionalized by F56 peptides and fluorescent PEGylated peptides. Efficient hydrazine ligation chemistry was applied for the functionalization. F56 peptides bind specifically to vascular endothelial growth factor receptor 1 (VEGFR-1) as was found through phage display technique. Tumors overexpressing VEGFR-1 could be targeted with F56 peptide ligands and imaged with fluorescent dyes with improved plasma circulation time via PEGylation. Multivalent display of targeting peptides or proteins on the surface of CPMV enabled enhanced binding or targeting ability. The developed CPMV-based multivalent platform has also been applied to *in vivo* targeting and imaging of human prostate cancer.[115] Stepwise synthesis of functional VNPs started with the functionalization of CPMV outer surface with NIR dye Alexa Fluor 647 at the lysine sites. Bombesin peptide ligands targeting gastrin-releasing peptide (GRP) receptors were attached at the outer ends of the PEG chains and this PEG-bombesin ligand was anchored on the CPMV external surface by copper(I)-catalyzed azide–alkyne cycloaddition chemistry. This methodology was adopted to maximize the conjugation efficiency of hydrophobic ligands such as bombesin. Prostate cancer cells with GRP receptors overexpressed were efficiently targeted and imaged using the multivalent CPMV scaffolds.

CPMV nanoparticles can also be used for therapeutic purposes. For photodynamic tumor therapy, photosensitizer C_{60} fullerene was conjugated to the multivalent attachment sites in the solvent-exposed amino acids of the CPMV capsid.[116] The CPMVs were decorated with PEG-C_{60} derivatives via azide–alkyne cycloaddition click reaction. The highly efficient covalent linkage between fullerene and protein nanoparticles lends structural, spectroscopic, and biological properties. The cellular uptake of dye-labeled VNP–PEG-C_{60} complexes in the human cancer cell was evaluated and these water-soluble and biocompatible VNP–PEG-C_{60} scaffolds served as vehicles for C_{60} delivery into cells.

Biosensors are the other mainstream application of CPMVs in the biomedical area. Genetically engineered CPMV particles were explored for the detection of DNA and toxins in several detection platforms.[117,118] The immobilized CPMV patterns served as a fluorescence signal enhancement platform.[118] Fluorescent dye molecules are often used in a microarray-based assay for the detection of target biological substances. When loaded onto a CPMV capsid at the organized spatial position, fluorescence quenching was effectively obviated and energy transfer from the virus to the dye molecule amplified the fluorescence signal for the detection of DNA–DNA hybridization. DNA hybridization was detected by CPMV using specific recognition between biotinylated DNA and avidin proteins. Cysteine groups inserted into the outer surface of CPMV were used to couple NeutrAvidin (NA) and fluorescent dyes (Cy5). The resulting NA-Cy5-CPMV acted as both a fluorescent signal-generating element (Cy5) and a recognition element (NA).

Signal enhancement on the CPMV scaffolds was also demonstrated in direct and sandwich immunoassay using antibody.[119] CPMVs showed capability as a simultaneous carrier for different types of molecules. A single virus capsid was labeled with two types of antibodies: chicken IgG and mouse IgG along with the Alexa Fluor 647 fluorescent dye. Such a modified virus could serve as a tracer in biosensors capable of multianalyte recognition. CPMVs were also modified with one type of antibody and dye. In sandwich immunoassays for staphylococcal enterotoxin B (SEB) detection, Alexa647–CPMV–anti-SEB complex produced a stronger signal than the mole equivalent of Alexa647-anti-SEB control, thereby improving the detection limit of SEB in sandwich immunoassay. Gliding assays were also employed where the capture antibody was coupled to gliding microtubules (MTs) using CPMV tracer scaffolds.[117] The kinesin-MT nanomachinery was used for detection of SEB using sandwich immunoassay-type construction. Kinesin is an ATP-dependent motor protein and travels along MTs, which are hollow tubular assemblies with 25 nm diameter. Gliding MTs carry an antigen-specific "capture" antibody, and the bound analyte is detected using fluorescent CPMV viral scaffold as the tracer (Figure 8.25). Use of the viral scaffold lowered the limit of detection down to 0.5 ng/mL on gliding MTs and 1 ng/mL on a static surface. Control experiments using anti-SEB dye as the tracer did not show any detection, possibly due to the small number of dyes in the control tracer. The advantage of CPMV as a nanoscaffold to couple active biomolecules and a larger number of reporter dye molecules on the same capsid for the detection of toxin was thus demonstrated.

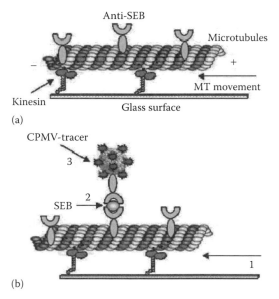

FIGURE 8.25 (a) Gliding assay: kinesin is immobilized on a glass surface inside a flow chamber. Kinesin heads bind to the MT and move toward the positive (+) end of the MT. The MTs have antigen-specific "capture" antibodies coupled (anti-SEB). (b) Immunoassay sandwich assay on a gliding MT: (1) anti-SEB-MTs are moved by kinesin; (2) a known amount of SEB is added to the microfluidic chamber where it binds to the corresponding site at the anti-SEB-MTs, followed by a wash to remove any unbound SEB; and (3) Cys5-CPMV-anti-SEB tracer is introduced, which binds to the SEB–anti-SEB-MT complex. (Reprinted with permission from Soto, C. M., et al., 2008, 5433–40. Copyright 2008 American Chemical Society.)

Application of CPMV viral template to the conductive electronic devices has not been widely investigated since the icosahedral viruses are too small to construct conventional microelectronic devices. Conductive networks on the nanoscale using CPMV as a template for the self-assembly were constructed and the electrical conductivity was examined using scanning tunneling microscopy.[120] Cysteine-modified CPMVs were decorated with gold nanoparticles at selected positions. Subsequently, the nearest-neighbor Au nanoparticles were interconnected with conducting molecular wires such as oligo(phenylene vinylene) (OPV) to create 3D molecular networks with suitable choice of the cysteine-modified mutant and the size of Au nanoparticles (Figure 8.26a). This gold–OPV–CPMV hybrid exhibited ohmic behavior and the resistance depended on the position of gold nanoparticles on the CPMV scaffolds (Figure 8.26c). When the 3D molecular network was constructed with thiol-terminated conjugated organic molecules having two stable conductance states, a switchable molecular network was realized with CPMV scaffolds.[121] Such bistable molecules allowed the formation of voltage-controlled molecular switches that could be used in nanoscale memory circuits. The resulting CPMV-based memory devices have a theoretical density of 1 petabit/cm^2,

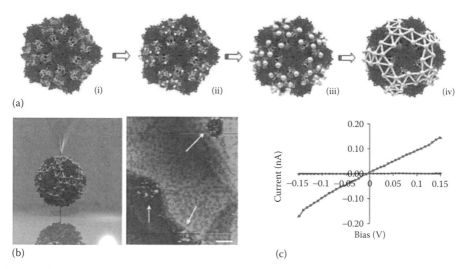

FIGURE 8.26 (a) Schematic of the procedure used to create molecular networks on the surface of the virus capsid: (i) CPMV capsid and (ii) DM mutant with two cysteines per subunit. The four nearest-neighbor cysteine-to-cysteine distances are 3.2, 4.0, 4.0, and 4.2 nm. (iii) DM with 2 nm gold nanoparticles bound to the inserted cysteines. (iv) DM with the 2 nm gold nanoparticles interconnected with OPV molecules. (b) Schematic of an STM experiment, which shows isolated conductive virus attached to gold substrate through a conducting molecule (left). STM image showing three EF mutants with 5 nm gold nanoparticles. Arrows point to the virus. (c) Typical *I–V* measurements of an EF mutant decorated with 5 nm gold nanoparticles before (dark gray) and after (light gray) assembly of OPV. (From Blum, A. S., Soto, C. M., Wilson, C. D., et al. An engineered virus as a scaffold for three-dimensional self-assembly on the nanoscale. *Small*, 2005, 1, 702–06. Copyright Wiley-VCH Verlag GmbH & Co. KGaA. Reproduced with permission.)

and increased storage density is expected with more than two conductance states available on each virus.

Nanoscale digital memory application of CPMV templates was also demonstrated with QD-coated CPMVs.[122] Aggregation issues were avoided using substrates to anchor cysteine-modified CPMV mutants via SAM linker on Au, followed by a stepwise functionalization with QDs. Two different color-emitting CdSe/ZnS core/shell QDs (QD_{red} and QD_{green}) were covalently coupled on the viral capsid. Organic soluble red- and green-emitting QDs were hydrophilized by carboxylation or amination for facile aqueous-based conjugation to engineered CPMV. Carboxylated green-emitting QDs were covalently attached to solvent-exposed lysine sites of CPMV surface. Amine-functionalized red-emitting QDs were addressed with heterobifunctional linker containing both carboxlyate and maleimide groups and conjugated to the remaining cysteines of the QD_{green}-modified CPMV particles. These QDs–CPMV hybrids showed reversible bistable electrical behavior during repeated writing–reading–erasing processes showing promise for future digital memory applications at the nanoscale.

8.3 CONCLUSION

In this chapter, we overview the virus-based nanotechnologies that have been developed recently. In conventional thought, the virus has been regarded as a harmful entity for human beings. But recent progresses using viruses, especially in nanoscience, demonstrate many of promising applications. One advantage of virus-based approaches is the ease of genetic engineering that allows for specific and targeted functionalization. In addition, the uniform size and homogeneous morphology make viruses useful as a biotemplate to grow various kinds of materials. Spherical or rodlike shapes can be used to synthesize 0D or 1D nanomaterials. Inorganic or metallic materials can be attached or grown. Additionally, organic molecules can be conjugated. Viruses truly provide new opportunities in the understanding of biology and nanomaterials and pave the way toward bio-based hybrid nanomaterials. Biological functionality and synthetic capability can be combined to make a new concept of hybrid materials. This approach will lead to many applications including use in electrochemical devices, such as hybrid catalysts, imaging agents, and drug delivery vehicles. We believe that it is just a new start in the matter of synthesis and assembly of nanomaterials. The virus can be a model system to realize bio-based manufacturing for nanoscale machine and multifunctional systems that could not be possible with the conventional approach.

ACKNOWLEDGMENTS

This research was supported by Basic Science Research Program through the National Research Foundation of Korea (NRF) funded by the Ministry of Education, Science and Technology (MEST; grant nos. 2012R1A1A1009029 and 2012R1A1A2021678). K. T. Nam also appreciates the support from Basic Science Research Program through the NRF funded by the MEST (grant no. 0417-20110030) and the NRF grant funded by the Korea government (MEST) (grant no. 2011-0031574).

REFERENCES

1. Seeman, N. C. and Belcher, A. M. 2002. Emulating biology: Building nanostructures from the bottom up. *Proceedings of the National Academy of Sciences of the United States of America* 99: 6451–55.
2. Mann, S. 1996. *Biomimietic Materials Chemistry*. New York: VCH.
3. Cha, J. N., Shimizu, K., Zhou, Y., et al. 1999. Silicate in filaments and subunits from a marine sponge direct the polymerization of silica and silicones in vitro. *Proceedings of the National Academy of Sciences of the United States of America* 96: 361–65.
4. Belcher, A. M., Wu, X. H., Christensen, R. J., et al. 1996. Control of crystal phase switching and orientation by soluble mollusc-shell proteins. *Nature* 381: 56–58.
5. Aizenberg, J., Tkachenko, A., Weiner, S., Addadi, L., and Hendler, G. 2001. Calcitic microlenses as part of the photoreceptor system in brittlestars. *Nature* 412: 819–22.
6. Flynn, C. E., Lee, S. W., Peelle, B. R., and Belcher, A. M. 2003. Viruses as vehicles for growth, organization and assembly of materials. *Acta Materialia* 51: 5867–80.
7. Douglas, T. and Young, M. 2006. Viruses: Making friends with old foes. *Science* 312: 873–75.
8. Steinmetz, N. F. and Evans, D. J. 2007. Utilisation of plant viruses in bionanotechnology. *Organic & Biomolecular Chemistry* 5: 2891–902.
9. Kay, B. K., Winter, J., and McCafferty, J. 1996. *Phage Display of Peptides and Proteins: A Laboratory Manual*. San Diego: Academic Press.
10. Mao, C. B., Solis, D. J., Reiss, B. D., et al. 2004. Virus-based toolkit for the directed synthesis of magnetic and semiconducting nanowires. *Science* 303: 213–17.
11. Smith, G. P. 1988. *Filamentous Phage as Cloning Vectors*. Boston: Butterworth.
12. Whaley, S. R., English, D. S., Hu, E. L., Barbara, P. F., and Belcher, A. M. 2000. Selection of peptides with semiconductor binding specificity for directed nanocrystal assembly. *Nature* 405: 665–68.
13. Sinensky, A. K. and Belcher, A. M. 2006. Biomolecular recognition of crystal defects: A diffuse-selection approach. *Advanced Materials* 18: 991–96.
14. Flynn, C. E., Mao, C. B., Hayhurst, A., et al. 2003. Synthesis and organization of nanoscale II-VI semiconductor materials using evolved peptide specificity and viral capsid assembly. *Journal of Materials Chemistry* 13: 2414–21.
15. Lee, S. W., Mao, C. B., Flynn, C. E., and Belcher, A. M. 2002. Ordering of quantum dots using genetically engineered viruses. *Science* 296: 892–95.
16. Mao, C. B., Flynn, C. E., Hayhurst, A., et al. 2003. Viral assembly of oriented quantum dot nanowires. *Proceedings of the National Academy of Sciences of the United States of America* 100: 6946–51.
17. Reiss, B. D., Mao, C. B., Solis, D. J., et al. 2004. Biological routes to metal alloy ferromagnetic nanostructures. *Nano Letters* 4: 1127–32.
18. Lee, S. K., Yun, D. S., and Belcher, A. M. 2006. Cobalt ion mediated self-assembly of genetically engineered bacteriophage for biomimetic Co-Pt hybrid material. *Biomacromolecules* 7: 14–17.
19. Avery, K. N., Schaak, J. E., and Schaak, R. E. 2009. M13 Bacteriophage as a biological scaffold for magnetically-recoverable metal nanowire catalysts: Combining specific and nonspecific interactions to design multifunctional nanocomposites. *Chemistry of Materials* 21: 2176–78.
20. Lee, Y. J., Yi, H., Kim, W. J., et al. 2009. Fabricating genetically engineered high-power lithium-ion batteries using multiple virus genes. *Science* 324: 1051–55.
21. Nam, K. T., Kim, D. W., Yoo, P. J., et al. 2006. Virus-enabled synthesis and assembly of nanowires for lithium ion battery electrodes. *Science* 312: 885–88.

22. Nam, K. T., Lee, Y. J., Krauland, E. M., Kottmann, S. T., and Belcher, A. M. 2008. Peptide-mediated reduction of silver ions on engineered biological scaffolds. *ACS Nano* 2: 1480–86.

23. Lee, S. W., Lee, S. K., and Belcher, A. M. 2003. Virus-based alignment of inorganic, organic, and biological nanosized materials. *Advanced Materials* 15: 689–92.

24. Lee, S. W. and Belcher, A. M. 2004. Virus-based fabrication of micro- and nanofibers using electrospinning. *Nano Letters* 4: 387–90.

25. Rong, J. H., Lee, L. A., Li, K., et al. 2008. Oriented cell growth on self-assembled bacteriophage M13 thin films. *Chemical Communications* 41: 5185–87.

26. Wargacki, S. P., Pate, B., and Vaia, R. A. 2008. Fabrication of 2D ordered films of tobacco mosaic virus (TMV): Processing morphology correlations for convective assembly. *Langmuir* 24: 5439–44.

27. Chung, W. J., Oh, J. W., Kwak, K., et al. 2011. Biomimetic self-templating supramolecular structures. *Nature* 478: 364–68.

28. Yoo, P. J., Nam, K. T., Qi, J. F., et al. 2006. Spontaneous assembly of viruses on multilayered polymer surfaces. *Nature Materials* 5: 234–40.

29. Yoo, P. J., Zacharia, N. S., Doh, J., et al. 2008. Controlling surface mobility in interdiffusing polyelectrolyte multilayers. *ACS Nano* 2: 561–71.

30. Yoo, P. J., Nam, K. T., Belchert, A. M., and Hammond, P. T. 2008. Solvent-assisted patterning of polyelectrolyte multilayers and selective deposition of virus assemblies. *Nano Letters* 8: 1081–89.

31. Nam, K. T., Peelle, B. R., Lee, S. W., and Belcher, A. M. 2004. Genetically driven assembly of nanorings based on the M13 virus. *Nano Letters* 4: 23–27.

32. Huang, Y., Chiang, C. Y., Lee, S. K., et al. 2005. Programmable assembly of nanoarchitectures using genetically engineered viruses. *Nano Letters* 5: 1429–34.

33. Solis, D. J., Coyer, S. R., Garcia, A. J., and Delamarche, E. 2010. Large-scale arrays of aligned single viruses. *Advanced Materials* 22: 111–14.

34. Lee, Y. J. and Belcher, A. M. 2011. Nanostructure design of amorphous FePO(4) facilitated by a virus for 3 V lithium ion battery cathodes. *Journal of Materials Chemistry* 21: 1033–39.

35. Lee, Y. J., Lee, Y., Oh, D., et al. 2010. Biologically activated noble metal alloys at the nanoscale: For lithium ion battery anodes. *Nano Letters* 10: 2433–40.

36. Dang, X. N., Yi, H. J., Ham, M. H., et al. 2011. Virus-templated self-assembled single-walled carbon nanotubes for highly efficient electron collection in photovoltaic devices. *Nature Nanotechnology* 6: 377–84.

37. Nam, Y. S., Magyar, A. P., Lee, D., et al. 2010. Biologically templated photocatalytic nanostructures for sustained light-driven water oxidation. *Nature Nanotechnology* 5: 340–44.

38. Neltner, B., Peddie, B., Xu, A., et al. 2010. Production of hydrogen using nanocrystalline protein-templated catalysts on M13 phage. *ACS Nano* 4: 3227–35.

39. Nam, K. T., Wartena, R., Yoo, P. J., et al. 2008. Stamped microbattery electrodes based on self-assembled M13 viruses. *Proceedings of the National Academy of Sciences of the United States of America* 105: 17227–31.

40. Nam, Y. S., Shin, T., Park, H., et al. 2010. Virus-templated assembly of porphyrins into light-harvesting nanoantennae. *Journal of the American Chemical Society* 132: 1462–63.

41. Ferreira, K. N., Iverson, T. M., Maghlaoui, K., Barber, J., and Iwata, S. 2004. Architecture of the photosynthetic oxygen-evolving center. *Science* 303: 1831–38.

42. Hajitou, A., Trepel, M., Lilley, C. E., et al. 2006. A hybrid vector for ligand-directed tumor targeting and molecular imaging. *Cell* 125: 385–98.

43. Yacoby, I., Shamis, M., Bar, H., Shabat, D., and Benhar, I. 2006. Targeting antibacterial agents by using drug-carrying filamentous bacteriophages. *Antimicrobial Agents and Chemotherapy* 50: 2087–97.

44. Merzlyak, A., Indrakanti, S., and Lee, S. W. 2009. Genetically engineered nanofiber-like viruses for tissue regenerating materials. *Nano Letters* 9: 846–52.
45. Yi, H. J., Ghosh, D., Ham, M. H., et al. 2012. M13 phage-functionalized single-walled carbon nanotubes as nanoprobes for second near-infrared window fluorescence imaging of targeted tumors. *Nano Letters* 12: 1176–83.
46. Schlick, T. L., Ding, Z. B., Kovacs, E. W., and Francis, M. B. 2005. Dual-surface modification of the tobacco mosaic virus. *Journal of the American Chemical Society* 127: 3718–23.
47. Shenton, W., Douglas, T., Young, M., Stubbs, G., and Mann, S. 1999. Inorganic-organic nanotube composites from template mineralization of tobacco mosaic virus. *Advanced Materials* 11: 253–56.
48. Royston, E., Lee, S. Y., Culver, J. N., and Harris, M. T. 2006. Characterization of silica-coated tobacco mosaic virus. *Journal of Colloid and Interface Science* 298: 706–12.
49. Royston, E. S., Brown, A. D., Harris, M. T., and Culver, J. N. 2009. Preparation of silica stabilized Tobacco mosaic virus templates for the production of metal and layered nanoparticles. *Journal of Colloid and Interface Science* 332: 402–07.
50. Fujikawa, S. and Kunitake, T. 2003. Surface fabrication of hollow nanoarchitectures of ultrathin titania layers from assembled latex particles and tobacco mosaic viruses as templates. *Langmuir* 19: 6545–52.
51. Knez, M., Bittner, A. M., Boes, F., et al. 2003. Biotemplate synthesis of 3-nm nickel and cobalt nanowires. *Nano Letters* 3: 1079–82.
52. Dujardin, E., Peet, C., Stubbs, G., Culver, J. N., and Mann, S. 2003. Organization of metallic nanoparticles using tobacco mosaic virus templates. *Nano Letters* 3: 413–17.
53. Lee, S. Y., Royston, E., Culver, J. N., and Harris, M. T. 2005. Improved metal cluster deposition on a genetically engineered tobacco mosaic virus template. *Nanotechnology* 16: S435–S441.
54. Lim, J. S., Kim, S. M., Lee, S. Y., et al. 2010. Formation of Au/Pd alloy nanoparticles on TMV. *Journal of Nanomaterials* Article ID 620505.
55. Lim, J. S., Kim, S. M., Lee, S. Y., et al. 2010. Biotemplated aqueous-phase palladium crystallization in the absence of external reducing agents. *Nano Letters* 10: 3863–67.
56. Lin, Y., Balizan, E., Lee, L. A., Niu, Z. W., and Wang, Q. 2010. Self-assembly of rod-like bio-nanoparticles in capillary tubes. *Angewandte Chemie International Edition* 49: 868–72.
57. Lin, Y. A., Su, Z. H., Xiao, G. H., et al. 2011. Self-assembly of virus particles on flat surfaces via controlled evaporation. *Langmuir* 27: 1398–402.
58. Balci, S., Leinberger, D. M., Knez, M., et al. 2008. Printing and aligning mesoscale patterns of tobacco mosaic virus on surfaces. *Advanced Materials* 20: 2195–200.
59. Horn, A., Hiltl, S., Fery, A., and Boker, A. 2010. Ordering and printing virus arrays: A straightforward way to functionalize surfaces. *Small* 6: 2122–25.
60. He, J. B., Niu, Z. W., Tangirala, R., et al. 2009. Self-assembly of tobacco mosaic virus at oil/water interfaces. *Langmuir* 25: 4979–87.
61. Royston, E., Ghosh, A., Kofinas, P., Harris, M. T., and Culver, J. N. 2008. Self-assembly of virus-structured high surface area nanomaterials and their application as battery electrodes. *Langmuir* 24: 906–12.
62. Yi, H. M., Nisar, S., Lee, S. Y., et al. 2005. Patterned assembly of genetically modified viral nanotemplates via nucleic acid hybridization. *Nano Letters* 5: 1931–36.
63. Yi, H., Rubloff, G. W., and Culver, J. N. 2007. TMV microarrays: Hybridization-based assembly of DNA-programmed viral nanotemplates. *Langmuir* 23: 2663–67.
64. Tan, W. S., Lewis, C. L., Horelik, N. E., et al. 2008. Hierarchical assembly of viral nanotemplates with encoded microparticles via nucleic acid hybridization. *Langmuir* 24: 12483–88.
65. Lewis, C. L., Lin, Y., Yang, C. X., et al. 2010. Microfluidic fabrication of hydrogel microparticles containing functionalized viral nanotemplates. *Langmuir* 26: 13436–41.

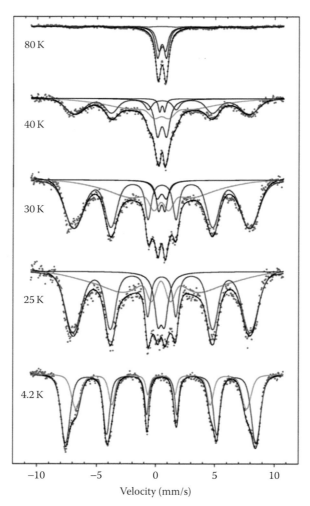

FIGURE 1.22 Mössbauer spectra of lyophilized *in vitro* reconstituted HoSF to 1500 ^{57}Fe atoms per protein. Solid lines through the experimental points are least square fits to a superposition of two types of iron subsites, including hyperfine field distributions. Subspectra are shown above the experimental data (see text and Table 1.1). (From Papaefthymiou, G. C., et al. Electronic and magnetic characterization of in vivo produced vs. in vitro reconstituted horse spleen ferritin. *Nanophase and Nanocomposite Materials V,* S. Komarneni, K. Kaneko, J. C. Parker, and P. O'Brien, eds., HH03-27, 2007. Copyright Materials Research Society. Reproduced with permission.)

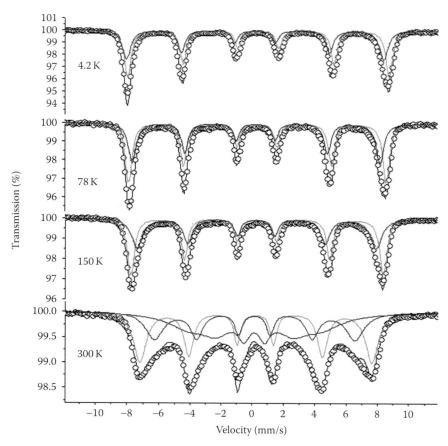

FIGURE 1.29 Mössbauer spectra of sample A at various temperatures. The spectra are fit to the superposition of two iron sites, the tetrahedral and octahedral coordination sites of the spinel crystallographic structure, with an additional intermediate relaxation component at 300 K. (Reprinted with permission from Papaefthymiou, G. C., et al., Interparticle interactions in magnetic core/shell nanoarchitectures, *Phys. Rev. B*, 80, 024406-1–024406-10, 2009. Copyright 2009 by the American Physical Society.)

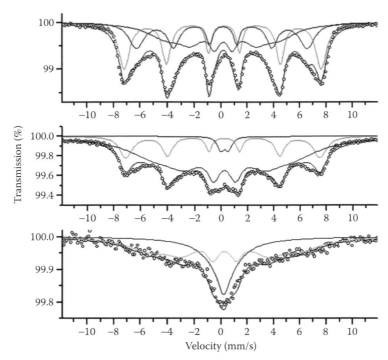

FIGURE 1.30 Room-temperature Mössbauer spectra of samples A, B, and C. With increasing magnetic core separation, spin relaxation increases, collapsing the magnetic spectral signature. (Reprinted with permission from Papaefthymiou, G. C., et al., Interparticle interactions in magnetic core/shell nanoarchitectures, *Phys. Rev. B*, 80, 024406-1–024406-10, 2009. Copyright 2009 by the American Physical Society.)

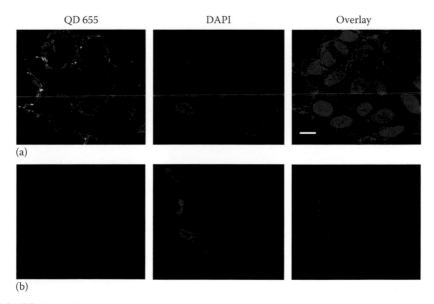

FIGURE 2.19 Confocal microscopy images of MCF7/HER2 cells stained with anti-HER2 iQD 655 (a) and mock-conjugated QD 655 (b). Scale bar: 20 μm. (Reprinted with permission from Barat, B., et al., 2009, 1474–81. Copyright 2009 American Chemical Society.)

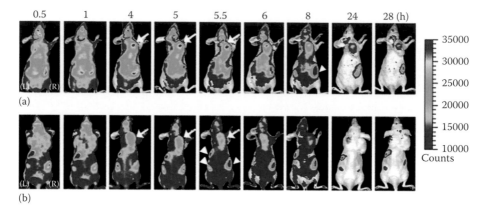

FIGURE 2.21 *In vivo* NIR fluorescence imaging. The dorsal images of SKOV3 tumor-bearing (arrows) mice (L, left side; R, right side) injected with QD710-Dendorn–RGD2 (200 pmol) (a) and QD710-Dendron (200 pmol) (b) at 0.5, 1, 4, 5, 5.5, 6, 8, 24, and 28 h, respectively. The incidental high fluorescent signals in other body parts (arrowheads) might have originated from regular rodent food in stomach and feces in intestine. (Reprinted with permission from Gao, J., et al., 2012, 281–6. Copyright 2012 American Chemical Society.)

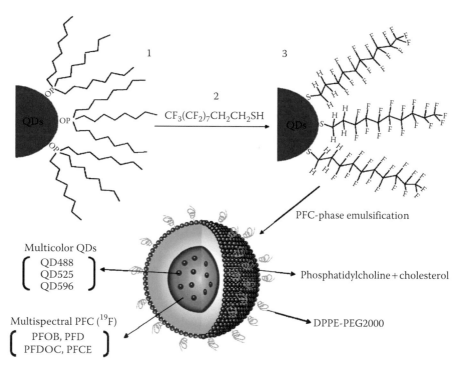

SCHEME 2.2 Schematic illustration of the preparation of bimodal imaging nanoprobes having both ^{19}F-based multispectral MR and QD-based multicolor optical imaging capabilities. (Reprinted with permission from Lim, Y.T., et al., 2009, 17145–54. Copyright 2009 American Chemical Society.)

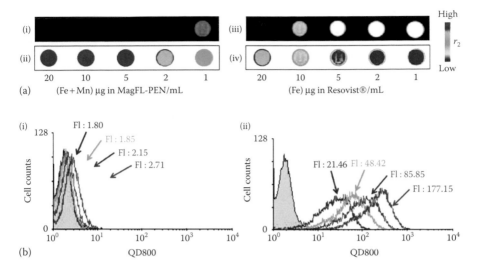

FIGURE 2.29 High-performance MR/NIR dual-modality imaging properties of MagFL-PEN. (a) T_2-weighted MR images of HeLa cells treated with MagFL-PEN (i and ii) and Resovist (iii and iv); parts (i) and (iii) are in white and black and (ii) and (iv) in pseudo color. (b) Fluorescence-activated cell sorting (FACS) analysis of HeLa cells labeled with various concentrations of QD800 (COOH) and MagFL-PEN [i, QD800 (COOH); ii, MagFL-PEN] at 12.5 (red), 25 (green), 50 (blue), and 100 pM (purple). (Reprinted with permission from Kim, H.M., et al., 2011, 8230–40. Copyright 2011 American Chemical Society.)

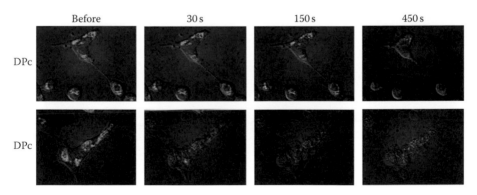

FIGURE 3.7 Time-dependent morphological changes of A549 cells treated with free DPc or DPc-loaded PIC micelle during photoirradiation. A549 cells were incubated with free DPc or DPc-loaded PIC micelle for 24 h at a 99% growth inhibitory concentration (IC99). After the medium replacement, the morphological changes in the cells during photoirradiation by the light source of a time-lapse sectioning fluorescent microscope were continuously monitored using the microscope's differential interference contrast (DIC) mode. The fluorescent images from DPc (red) and Rhodamine 123 (Rh123) (green), a dye that specifically stains mitochondria, were monitored. (Reprinted from *J. Control. Release*, 133, Nishiyama, M., et al., Enhanced photodynamic cancer treatment by supramolecular nanocarriers charged with dendrimer phthalocyanine, 245–251, Copyright 2009, with permission from Elsevier.)

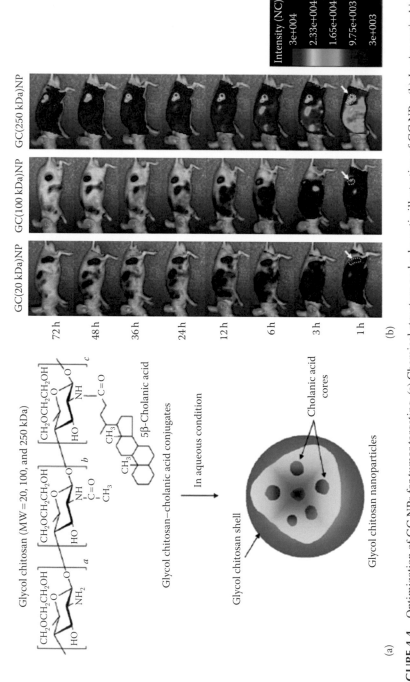

FIGURE 4.4 Optimization of GC NPs for tumor targeting. (a) Chemical structure and schematic illustration of GC NPs. (b) *In vivo* optical images of tumor-bearing mice models after intravenous injection of GC NPs with different molecular weights. (Reprinted from *Journal of Controlled Release*, 122, Park, K., J.-H. Kim, Y. S. Nam, S. Lee, H. Y. Nam, K. Kim, J. H. Park, et al., Effect of polymer molecular weight on the tumor targeting characteristics of self-assembled glycol chitosan nanoparticles, 305–14, Copyright 2007, with permission from Elsevier.)

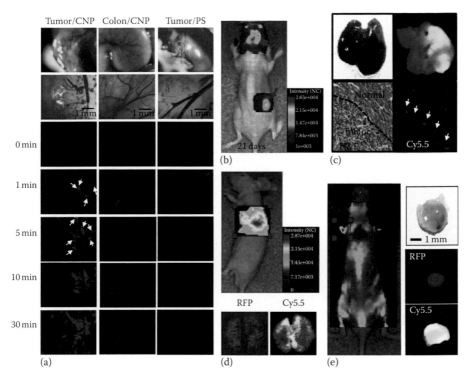

FIGURE 4.6 Biodistribution of GC NPs in various tumor models. (a) Live imaging of vascular structures after NP injection. (b) GC NPs in brain tumor model. (c) Distribution of GC NPs in liver tumor. (d) GC NPs in lung metastasis model. (e) Unintended second metastasis tumor on forearm and the accumulation of GC NPs. CNP, chitosan nanoparticle; PS, polystyrene beads; RFP, red fluorescence protein. (Reprinted from *Biomaterials*, 32, Na, J. H., H. Koo, S. Lee, K. H. Min, K. Park, H. Yoo, S. H. Lee, et al., Real-time and non-invasive optical imaging of tumor-targeting glycol chitosan nanoparticles in various tumor models, 5252–61, Copyright 2011, with permission from Elsevier.)

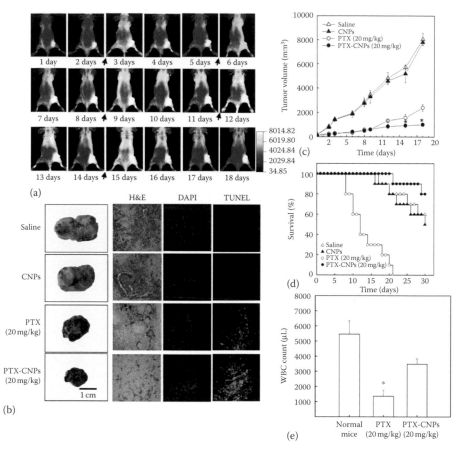

FIGURE 4.7 Tumor therapy with paclitaxel-loaded GC NPs. (a) Determination of injection interval based on *in vivo* optical imaging data. (b) Analysis of excised tumors after therapy. (c) Tumor growth data. (d) Survival rates of mice models and (e) the concentration of WBCs after tumor therapy with paclitaxel-loaded GC NPs. CNP, chitosan nanoparticle; DAPI, 4',6-diamidino-2-phenylindole. (Reprinted from *Journal of Controlled Release*, 146, Kim, K., J. H. Kim, H. Park, Y.-S. Kim, K. Park, H. Nam, S. Lee, et al., Tumor-homing multifunctional nanoparticles for cancer theragnosis: Simultaneous diagnosis, drug delivery, and therapeutic monitoring, 219–27, Copyright 2010, with permission from Elsevier.)

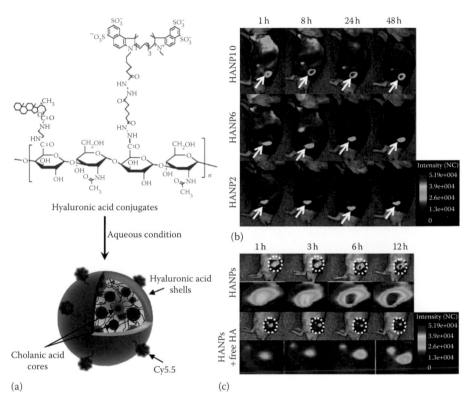

FIGURE 4.8 Development of HANPs. (a) Chemical structure and schematic illustration of HANPs. (b) *In vivo* tumor accumulation of HANPs with different 5β-cholanic acid ratios. (c) *In vivo* tumor accumulation of HANPs after pretreatment of hyaluronic acids. (Reprinted from *Biomaterials*, 31, Choi, K. Y., H. Chung, K. H. Min, H. Y. Yoon, K. Kim, J. H. Park, I. C. Kwon, and S. Y. Jeong, Self-assembled hyaluronic acid nanoparticles for active tumor targeting, 106–14, Copyright 2010, with permission from Elsevier.)

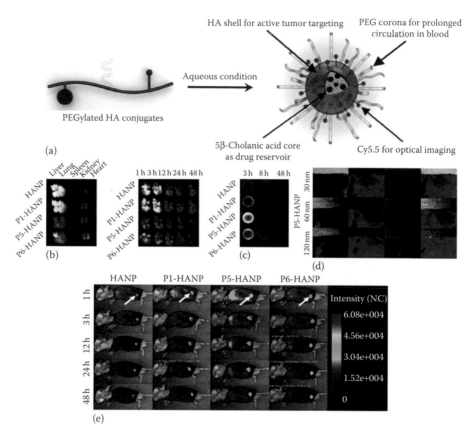

FIGURE 4.9 PEGylation of HANPs. (a) Schematic illustration of PEGylated HANPs and their self-assembly in aqueous condition. (b) *Ex vivo* organ images. (c) Fluorescence intensity of blood samples. (d) Intravital live image. (e) Whole-body images of mice models treated with PEGylated HANPs. (Reprinted from *Biomaterials*, 32, Choi, K. Y., K. H. Min, H. Y. Yoon, K. Kim, J. H. Park, I. C. Kwon, K. Choi, and S. Y. Jeong, PEGylation of hyaluronic acid nanoparticles improves tumor targetability in vivo, 1880–89, Copyright 2011, with permission from Elsevier.)

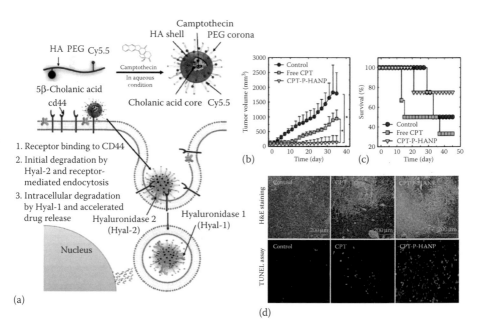

FIGURE 4.10 Tumor-targeted drug delivery with HANPs. (a) Schematic illustration of drug loading into HANPs and their cellular uptake. (b) Tumor growth data. (c) Survival rates. (d) Histological analysis of tumor-bearing mice models after treatment with camptothecin-loaded HANPs. (Reprinted with permission from Choi, K. Y., et al., 2011, 8591–99. Copyright 2011 American Chemical Society.)

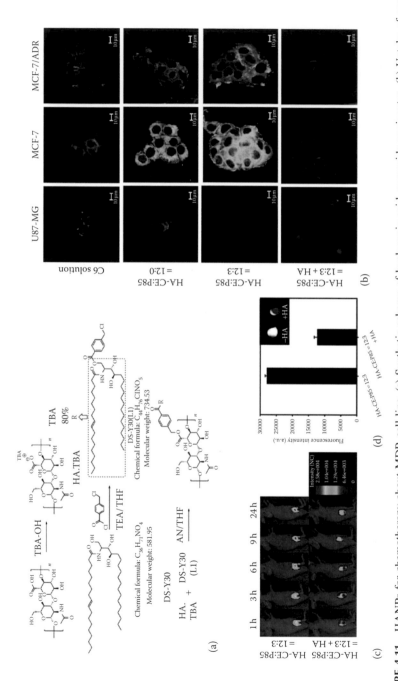

FIGURE 4.11 HANPs for chemotherapy about MDR cell line. (a) Synthetic scheme of hyaluronic acid–ceramide conjugates. (b) Uptake of coumarin 6-loaded HANPs in MDR cells. (d) *Ex vivo* tumor images of HANPs. (c) Whole-body images. (d) *Ex vivo* tumor images of MDR tumor-bearing mice models after intravenous injection of HANPs. AN, acetonitrile; TBA, tetra-*n*-butylammonium hydroxide; TEA, triethylamine; THF, tetrahydrofuran. (Reprinted from *Biomaterials*, 32, Cho, H.-J., H. Y. Yoon, H. Koo, S.-H. Ko, J.-S. Shim, J.-H. Lee, K. Kim, I. C. Kwon, and D.-D. Kim, Self-assembled nanoparticles based on hyaluronic acid–ceramide (HA-CE) and Pluronic® for tumor-targeted delivery of docetaxel, 7181–90, Copyright 2011, with permission from Elsevier.)

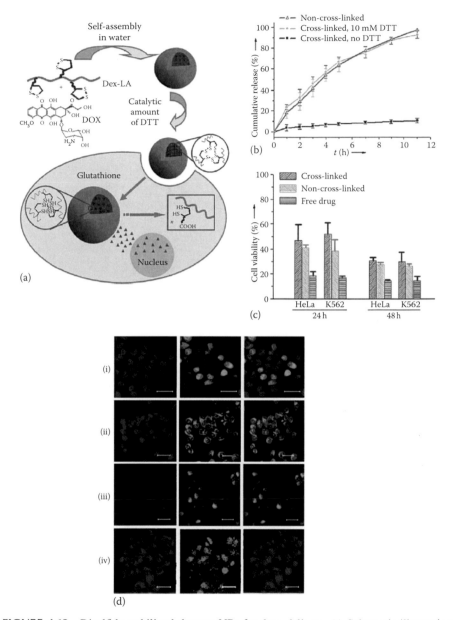

FIGURE 4.12 Disulfide-stabilized dextran NPs for drug delivery. (a) Schematic illustration of disulfide-stabilized dextran NPs and triggered release in cell cytosol. (b) Triggered release of DXR from dextran NPs. (c) Cell viability. (d) Cellular uptake of DXR-loaded dextran NPs: (i) DXR-loaded dextran NPs (0.5-h incubation); (ii) DXR-loaded dextran NPs (2-h incubation); (iii) Free DXR (0.5-h incubation); (iv) Free DXR (2-h incubation). (From Li, Y.-L., Zhu, L., Liu, Z., Cheng, R., Meng, F., Cui, J.-H., Ji, S.-J., and Zhong, Z., Reversibly stabilized multifunctional dextran nanoparticles efficiently deliver doxorubicin into the nuclei of cancer cells. *Angew. Chem. Int. Ed.*, 2009, 48, 9914–18. Copyright Wiley-VCH Verlag GmbH & Co. KGaA. Reproduced with permission.)

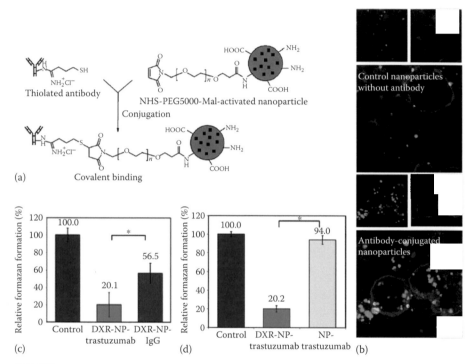

FIGURE 4.15 Antibody-conjugated albumin NPs. (a) Schematic illustration of antibody-conjugated albumin NPs. Cellular uptake (b) and cell viability assay (c and d) of antibody-conjugated albumin NPs. *The two samples are significantly different ($P < 0.01$; two-tailed Mann–Whitney U-test equivalent to the Wilcoxon rank-sum test). (Reprinted with permission from Anhorn, M. G., et al., 2008, 2321–31. Copyright 2008 American Chemical Society.)

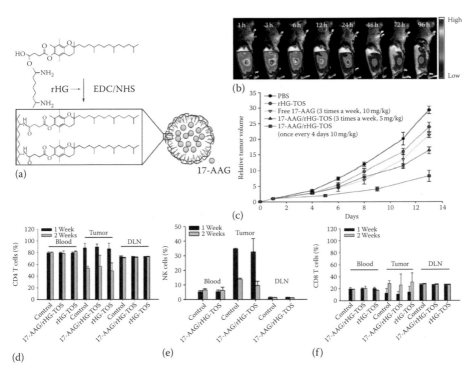

FIGURE 4.16 α-Tocopherol-conjugated gelatin NPs for 17-AAG delivery. (a) Schematic illustration of α-tocopherol-conjugated gelatin NPs and 17-AAG loading. (b) *In vivo* whole-body distribution of gelatin NPs. (c) Tumor growth data and percentages of CD4 T (d), NK (e), and CD8 T (f) cells in tumor-bearing mice models after intravenous injection of 17-AAG-loaded gelatin NPs. DLN, draining lymph node; EDC, 1-ethyl-3-(3-dimethylamino-propyl)carbodiimide hydrochloride; NHS, *N*-hydroxysuccinimide; rHG, recombinant human gelatin. (Reprinted with permission from Won, Y.-W., et al., 2011, 3839–48. Copyright 2011 American Chemical Society.)

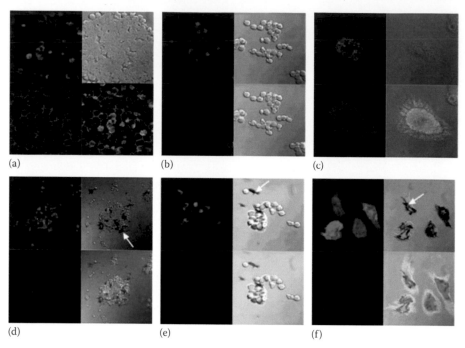

(a)　　　　　　　　(b)　　　　　　　　(c)

(d)　　　　　　　　(e)　　　　　　　　(f)

FIGURE 5.29　Confocal microscopy images. *f*-CNTs **34** and **36** localize inside B and T lymphocytes as well as macrophages. Three major immune cell populations, that is, B lymphocytes (a and d), T lymphocytes (b and e), and macrophages (c and f), were isolated from the spleen, lymph nodes, and peritoneal cavity of mice, respectively. They were then incubated with either *f*-CNT **34** (a–c) or **36** (d–f) (green fluorescence). The white arrows indicate the bundles of *f*-CNT **36** that are located outside lymphocytes (d and e) but inside the cytoplasm of macrophages (f). (Reprinted with permission from Dumortier, H., et al., 2006, 1522–1528. Copyright 2006 American Chemical Society.)

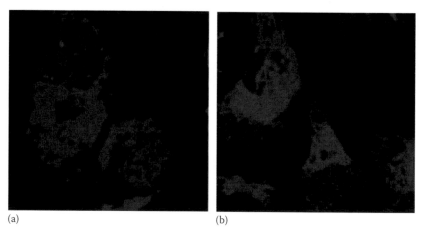

(a)　　　　　　　　　　　　　　(b)

FIGURE 5.45　Confocal fluorescence images of HeLa cells (nucleus stained with blue by Draq 5) after incubation in **49** (a) and **50** (b). Red color surrounding the nucleus corresponds to Cy3-labeled DNA molecules transported inside cells by SWNT carriers. (Reprinted with permission from Kam, N. W. S., et al., 2005, 12492–12493. Copyright 2005 American Chemical Society.)

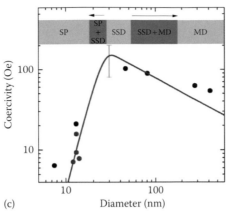

(c)

FIGURE 7.3 (c) Experimental values of coercivity H_c as a function of particle diameter for the same magnetic fluids as in Figure 7.3a (where applicable). Data points are as follows: black circles (From Ma, M., et al., *Journal of Magnetism and Magnetic Materials*, 268(1–2), 33–39, 2004.); red circles (From Hosono, T., et al., *Journal of Magnetism and Magnetic Materials*, 321(19), 3019–3023, 2009.); green line (From Alphandery, E., et al., *ACS Nano*, 3(6), 1539–1547, 2009.). The blue line is an approximate expression (From Hergt, R., S. Dutz, and M. Roder, *Journal of Physics—Condensed Matter*, 20(38), 2008.) (see text for details). On the top of Figure 7.3c, the critical sizes and ranges for the magnetic states of magnetite nanoparticles as calculated from Muxworthy and Williams are shown as shaded regions (From Muxworthy, A.R. and W. Williams, *Journal of the Royal Society Interface*, 6(41), 1207–1212, 2009.). The arrows indicate the variation of the regions of magnetic states with increasing interactions between the particles.

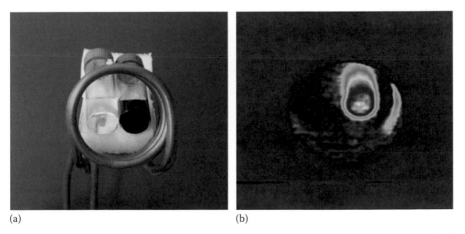

(a)　　　　　　　　　　　　　　　　　　(b)

FIGURE 7.4 (a) The copper coil of the magnetic heating apparatus used (Section 7.3.3) with an aqueous sample (left tube) and a dextran-coated maghemite magnetic fluid (right tube). (b) An infrared image of the samples during magnetic heating using a thermographic camera (Section 7.3.3). Heating is observed only in the magnetic fluid sample.

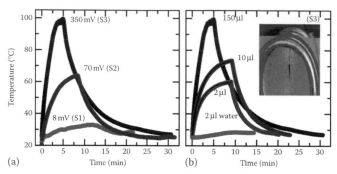

FIGURE 7.5 Magnetic heating effect on aqueous dispersions of dextran-coated maghemite nanoparticles. (a) The influence of the zeta potential on 150 µl magnetic fluids S1 (green points), S2 (blue points), and S3 (black points). (b) The influence of the volume on 150 µl (black points), 10 µl (blue points), and 2 µl (red points) of magnetic fluid S3. The solid black lines refer to fitting of the experimental data. The green points correspond to the sample of 2 µl water, used as control sample. In the inset, the coil of the magnetic heating apparatus, with the 10 µl sample, and the optical fiber used for the temperature monitoring are shown, after removing the heat-insulating cover. (Reprinted with permission from Rabias, I., et al., Rapid magnetic heating treatment by highly charged maghemite nanoparticles on Wistar rats exocranial glioma tumors at microliter volume. *Biomicrofluidics*, 2010. 4(2): 024111 (1–8). Copyright 2010, American Institute of Physics.)

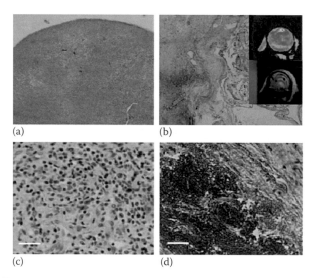

FIGURE 7.6 For *in vivo* magnetic heating of small rat glioma tumors, 150 µl S3 magnetic fluid is infused into rat glioma tumors with size 5–10 mm, and subsequently subjected to magnetic hyperthermia treatment for 20 min. Panels (a) and (c) (low and high magnification, respectively) represent sections of control tumor tissue treated without nanoparticles. Panels (b) and (d) (low and high magnification, respectively) show extensive damage of the tumor tissue after treatment with magnetic fluid. White bars = 200 µm. The lower inset in panel (b) shows the experimental setup for *in vivo* magnetic heating. The upper inset is an infrared image, which demonstrates the ability of the magnetic fluid to produce strong localized heating at the tumor position. (Reprinted with permission from Rabias, I., et al., Rapid magnetic heating treatment by highly charged maghemite nanoparticles on Wistar rats exocranial glioma tumors at microliter volume. *Biomicrofluidics*, 2010. 4(2): 024111 (1–8). Copyright 2010, American Institute of Physics.)

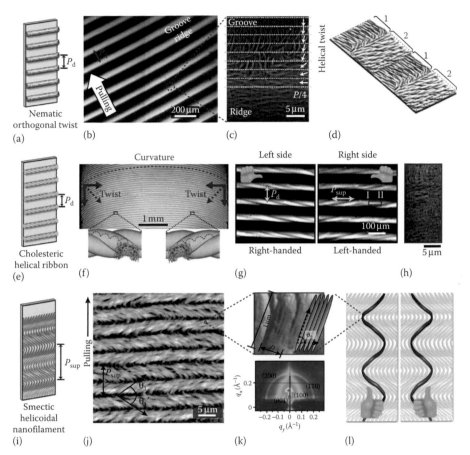

FIGURE 8.4 Self-templated helical supramolecular structures. (a–d) The nematic orthogonal twist structure. (a) Diagram. (b) Scanning electron microscopy (SEM) image. (c) AFM image depicting left-handed rotation of virus fiber bundles. (d) Diagram of alternating nematic grooves and cholesteric ridges. (e–h) The cholesteric helical ribbon (CHR) structure. (e) Diagram. (f) Photograph of CHR structures showing the curved meniscuses. (g) SEM image of the CHR structure on the left and right sides, which shows right and left handedness. (h) AFM image showing that CHR is composed of twisted cholesteric phage. (i–l) The smectic helicoidal nanofilament (SHN) structure. (i) Diagram. (j) AFM image of the SHN structure. (k) (upper) Enlarged AFM showing SHN structure, which is composed of smectic C bundles. (Lower) Grazing-incidence small-angle x-ray scattering measurement showing pseudohexagonal packed structures within the SHN. (l) Proposed model of the SHN structure composed of left-handed and right-handed helicoidal nanofilaments. (Reprinted by permission from Macmillan Publishers Ltd. *Nature*, Chung, W. J., et al., 2011, copyright 2011.)

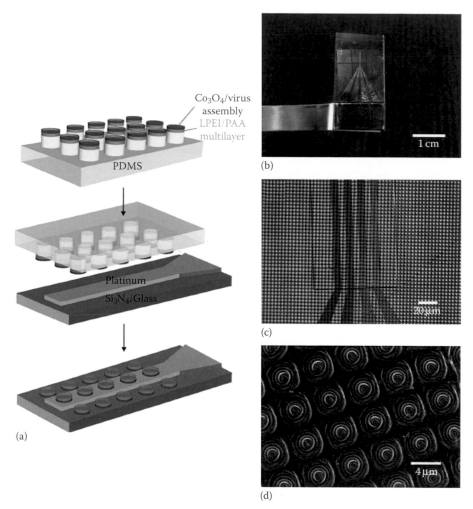

FIGURE 8.10 (a) Schematic procedure for constructing virus-based microbattery electrode. (b) Image of microbatteries on the Pt current collector. (c) Optical microscopy image of the microbattery electrode (4 μm diameter) on four Pt microbands (10 μm width). (d) SEM image of the stamped microbattery electrode. (Nam, K. T., Wartena, R., Yoo, P. J., et al., 2008. Stamped microbattery electrodes based on self-assembled M13 viruses. *Proceedings of the National Academy of Sciences of the United States of America* 105: 17227–31. Copyright 2008 National Academy of Sciences, U.S.A.)

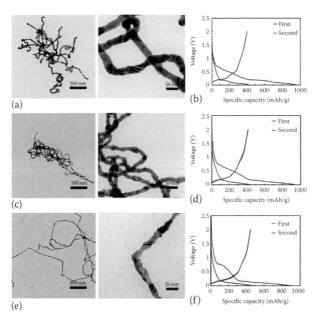

(a)

(b)

(c)

(d)

(e)

(f)

FIGURE 8.12 Characterization of cetyltrimethylammonium bromide (CTAB)-stabilized Au_xAg_{1-x} alloy nanowires. (a and b) $x = 0.9$. (a) TEM images. (b) First two discharge/charge curves. (c and d) $x = 0.67$. (c) TEM images. (d) First two discharge/charge curves. (e and f) $x = 0.5$. (e) TEM images. (f) First two discharge/charge curves. (Reprinted with permission from Lee, Y. J., et al., 2010, 2433–40. Copyright 2010 American Chemical Society.)

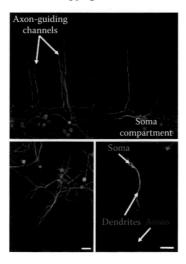

FIGURE 9.3 Immunocytochemistry images of neurons at 2 weeks in culture demonstrate that axons grew from the soma compartment into the axon/glia compartment through the arrays of axon-guiding microchannels, but dendrites and neuronal soma could not reach into the axon/glia compartment due to the length of the microchannels (200–800 µm long) and the height of the microchannels (2.5 µm). Axons were immunostained for neurofilament (NF) (red) and dendrite for microtubule-associated protein 2 (MAP2) (green). Scale bars = 20 µm. (With kind permission from Springer Science+Business Media: *Biomed. Microdevices*, Microfluidic compartmentalized co-culture platform for CNS axon myelination research, 11, 2009, 1145–1153, Park, J., Koito, H., Li, J., and Han, A., Figure 9.3.)

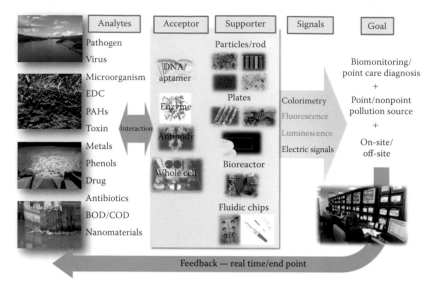

FIGURE 11.5 Flowchart for composition of environmental biosensors in environmental monitoring. BOD, biological oxygen demand; COD, chemical oxygen demand; EDC, endocrine-disrupting chemical.

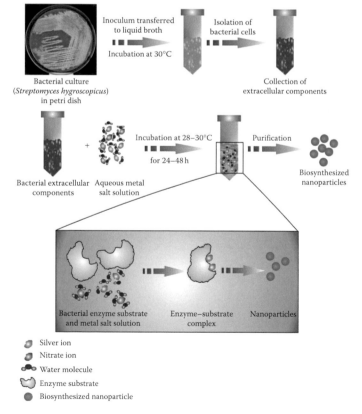

FIGURE 12.1 Schematic representation shows an example of biosynthetic pathway for preparation of AgNPs.

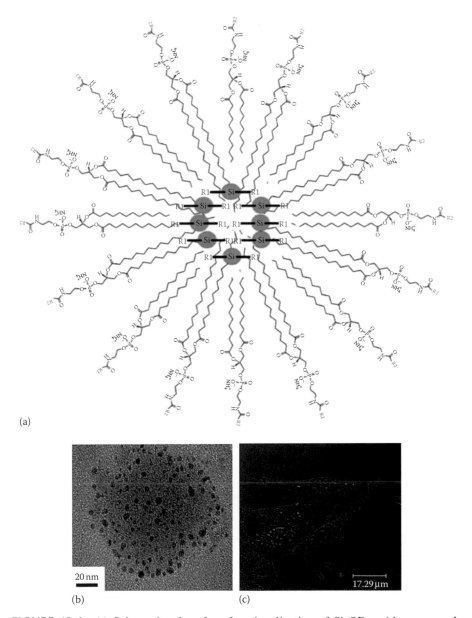

(a)

20 nm

17.29 μm

(b)   (c)

FIGURE 12.4 (a) Schematic of surface functionalization of Si QDs with compounds R1 (styrene, octadecene, or ethyl undecylenate) followed by encapsulation with phospholipid micelles that were terminated by the functional groups R2 (methoxy PEG, carboxyl, folate, or biotin). (b) TEM image of Si QDs encapsulated in several micelles. (c) Confocal microscopic visualization of live pancreatic cancer cells treated with amine-terminated micelle-encapsulated Si QDs. Scale bar = 17.29 μm. (Reprinted with permission from Erogbogbo et al., 2008, 873–878. Copyright 2008 American Chemical Society.)

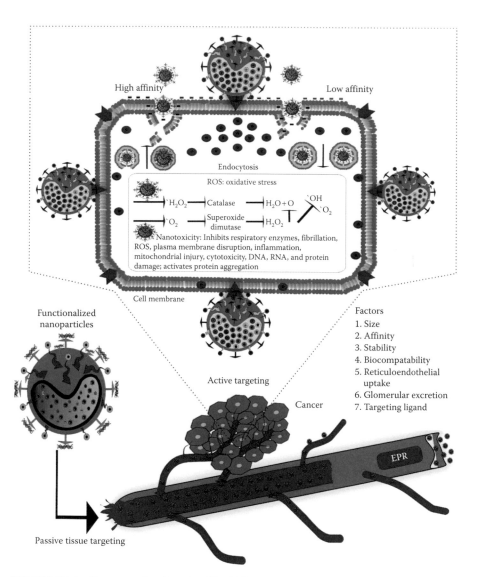

FIGURE 12.6 Programming functionalized NPs for specific tissue delivery using targeting ligand. Cancer cell-specific targeting through both passive (enhanced permeability and retention effect) and active pathways. Cationic charged functionalized NPs are more likely to have an increased affinity toward the cell membrane compared to anionic NPs. Factors influencing functionalized NPs are based on drug delivery and possible toxicity of functionalized NPs with the example of ROS mechanism of cell death.

66. Lee, S. Y., Choi, J. W., Royston, E., et al. 2006. Deposition of platinum clusters on surface-modified tobacco mosaic virus. *Journal of Nanoscience and Nanotechnology* 6: 974–81.

67. Gorzny, M. L., Walton, A. S., Wnek, M., Stockley, P. G., and Evans, S. D. 2008. Four-probe electrical characterization of Pt-coated TMV-based nanostructures. *Nanotechnology* 19: 165704.

68. Tseng, R. J., Tsai, C. L., Ma, L. P., and Ouyang, J. Y. 2006. Digital memory device based on tobacco mosaic virus conjugated with nanoparticles. *Nature Nanotechnology* 1: 72–77.

69. Atanasova, P., Rothenstein, D., Schneider, J. J., et al. 2011. Virus-templated synthesis of ZnO nanostructures and formation of field-effect transistors. *Advanced Materials* 23: 4918–22.

70. Chen, X. L., Gerasopoulos, K., Guo, J. C., et al. 2010. Virus-enabled silicon anode for lithium-ion batteries. *ACS Nano* 4: 5366–72.

71. Miller, R. A., Presley, A. D., and Francis, M. B. 2007. Self-assembling light-harvesting systems from synthetically modified tobacco mosaic virus coat proteins. *Journal of the American Chemical Society* 129: 3104–09.

72. Dedeo, M. T., Duderstadt, K. E., Berger, J. M., and Francis, M. B. 2010. Nanoscale protein assemblies from a circular permutant of the tobacco mosaic virus. *Nano Letters* 10: 181–86.

73. Yang, C. X. and Yi, H. M. 2010. Facile approaches to control catalytic activity of viral-templated palladium nanocatalysts for dichromate reduction. *Biochemical Engineering Journal* 52: 160–67.

74. Yang, C. X., Manocchi, A. K., Lee, B., and Yi, H. M. 2011. Viral-templated palladium nanocatalysts for Suzuki coupling reaction. *Journal of Materials Chemistry* 21: 187–94.

75. Douglas, T., Strable, E., Willits, D., et al. 2002. Protein engineering of a viral cage for constrained nanomaterials synthesis. *Advanced Materials* 14: 415–18.

76. Douglas, T. and Young, M. 1998. Host-guest encapsulation of materials by assembled virus protein cages. *Nature* 393: 152–55.

77. Douglas, T. and Young, M. 1999. Virus particles as templates for materials synthesis. *Advanced Materials* 11: 679–81.

78. Klem, M. T., Young, M., and Douglas, T. 2008. Biomimetic synthesis of beta-TiO(2) inside a viral capsid. *Journal of Materials Chemistry* 18: 3821–23.

79. de la Escosura, A., Verwegen, M., Sikkema, F. D., et al. 2008. Viral capsids as templates for the production of monodisperse Prussian blue nanoparticles. *Chemical Communications* (13): 1542–44.

80. Comellas-Aragones, M., Engelkamp, H., Claessen, V. I., et al. 2007. A virus-based single-enzyme nanoreactor. *Nature Nanotechnology* 2: 635–39.

81. Minten, I. J., Wilke, K. D. M., Hendriks, L. J. A., et al. 2011. Metal-ion-induced formation and stabilization of protein cages based on the cowpea chlorotic mottle virus. *Small* 7: 911–19.

82. Gillitzer, E., Willits, D., Young, M., and Douglas, T. 2002. Chemical modification of a viral cage for multivalent presentation. *Chemical Communications* (20): 2390–91.

83. Suci, P. A., Klem, M. T., Arce, F. T., Douglas, T., and Young, M. 2006. Assembly of multilayer films incorporating a viral protein cage architecture. *Langmuir* 22: 8891–96.

84. Kostiainen, M. A., Kasyutich, O., Cornelissen, J., and Nolte, R. J. M. 2010. Self-assembly and optically triggered disassembly of hierarchical dendron-virus complexes. *Nature Chemistry* 2: 394–99.

85. Kostiainen, M. A., Hiekkataipale, P., de la Torre, J. A., Nolte, R. J. M., and Cornelissen, J. 2011. Electrostatic self-assembly of virus-polymer complexes. *Journal of Materials Chemistry* 21: 2112–17.

86. Allen, M., Bulte, J. W. M., Liepold, L., et al. 2005. Paramagnetic viral nanoparticles as potential high-relaxivity magnetic resonance contrast agents. *Magnetic Resonance in Medicine* 54: 807–12.

87. Suci, P. A., Varpness, Z., Gillitzer, E., Douglas, T., and Young, M. 2007. Targeting and photodynamic killing of a microbial pathogen using protein cage Architectures functionalized with a photosensitizer. *Langmuir* 23: 12280–86.
88. Wang, Q., Lin, T. W., Tang, L., Johnson, J. E., and Finn, M. G. 2002. Icosahedral virus particles as addressable nanoscale building blocks. *Angewandte Chemie International Edition* 41: 459–62.
89. Wang, Q., Chan, T. R., Hilgraf, R., et al. 2003. Bioconjugation by copper(I)-catalyzed azide-alkyne 3+2 cycloaddition. *Journal of the American Chemical Society* 125: 3192–93.
90. Blum, A. S., Soto, C. M., Wilson, C. D., et al. 2004. Cowpea mosaic virus as a scaffold for 3-D patterning of gold nanoparticles. *Nano Letters* 4: 867–70.
91. Blum, A. S., Soto, C. M., Wilson, C. D., et al. 2006. Templated self-assembly of quantum dots from aqueous solution using protein scaffolds. *Nanotechnology* 17: 5073–79.
92. Martinez-Morales, A. A., Portney, N. G., Zhang, Y., et al. 2008. Synthesis and characterization of iron oxide derivatized mutant cowpea mosaic virus hybrid nanoparticles. *Advanced Materials* 20: 4816–20.
93. Steinmetz, N. F., Lomonossoff, G. P., and Evans, D. J. 2006. Decoration of Cowpea mosaic virus with multiple, redox-active, organometallic complexes. *Small* 2: 530–33.
94. Steinmetz, N. F., Lomonossoff, G. P., and Evans, D. J. 2006. Cowpea mosaic virus for material fabrication: Addressable carboxylate groups on a programmable nanoscaffold. *Langmuir* 22: 3488–90.
95. Steinmetz, N. F., Shah, S. N., Barclay, J. E., et al. 2009. Virus-templated silica nanoparticles. *Small* 5: 813–16.
96. Sarikaya, M., Tamerler, C., Schwartz, D. T., and Baneyx, F. O. 2004. Materials assembly and formation using engineered polypeptides. *Annual Review of Materials Research* 34: 373–408.
97. Shah, S. N., Steinmetz, N. F., Aljabali, A. A. A., Lomonossoff, G. P., and Evans, D. J. 2009. Environmentally benign synthesis of virus-templated, monodisperse, iron-platinum nanoparticles. *Dalton Transactions* (40): 8479–80.
98. Aljabali, A. A. A., Shah, S. N., Evans-Gowing, R., Lomonossoff, G. P., and Evans, D. J. 2011. Chemically-coupled-peptide-promoted virus nanoparticle templated mineralization. *Integrative Biology* 3: 119–25.
99. Aljabali, A. A. A., Barclay, J. E., Lomonossoff, G. P., and Evans, D. J. 2010. Virus templated metallic nanoparticles. *Nanoscale* 2: 2596–600.
100. Aljabali, A. A. A., Barclay, J. E., Cespedes, O., et al. 2011. Charge modified cowpea mosaic virus particles for templated mineralization. *Advanced Functional Materials* 21: 4137–42.
101. Aljabali, A. A. A., Lomonossoff, G. P., and Evans, D. J. 2011. CPMV-polyelectrolyte-templated gold nanoparticles. *Biomacromolecules* 12: 2723–28.
102. Saunders, K., Sainsbury, F., and Lomonossoff, G. P. 2009. Efficient generation of cowpea mosaic virus empty virus-like particles by the proteolytic processing of precursors in insect cells and plants. *Virology* 393: 329–37.
103. Aljabali, A. A. A., Sainsbury, F., Lomonossoff, G. P., and Evans, D. J. 2010. Cowpea mosaic virus unmodified empty viruslike particles loaded with metal and metal oxide. *Small* 6: 818–21.
104. Cheung, C. L., Camarero, J. A., Woods, B. W., et al. 2003. Fabrication of assembled virus nanostructures on templates of chemoselective linkers formed by scanning probe nanolithography. *Journal of the American Chemical Society* 125: 6848–49.
105. Steinmetz, N. F., Calder, G., Lomonossoff, G. P., and Evans, D. J. 2006. Plant viral capsids as nanobuilding blocks: Construction of arrays on solid supports. *Langmuir* 22: 10032–37.
106. Steinmetz, N. F., Evans, D. J., and Lomonossoff, G. P. 2007. Chemical introduction of reactive thiols into a viral nanoscaffold: A method that avoids virus aggregation. *Chembiochem* 8: 1131–36.

107. Strable, E., Johnson, J. E., and Finn, M. G. 2004. Natural nanochemical building blocks: Icosahedral virus particles organized by attached oligonucleotides. *Nano Letters* 4: 1385–89.
108. Lin, Y., Su, Z., Niu, Z., et al. 2008. Layer-by-layer assembly of viral capsid for cell adhesion. *Acta Biomaterialia* 4: 838–43.
109. Li, T., Niu, Z. W., Emrick, T., Russell, T. R., and Wang, Q. 2008. Core/shell biocomposites from the hierarchical assembly of bionanoparticles and polymer. *Small* 4: 1624–29.
110. Steinmetz, N. F. and Manchester, M. 2009. PEGylated viral nanoparticles for biomedicine: The impact of PEG chain length on VNP cell interactions in vitro and ex vivo. *Biomacromolecules* 10: 784–92.
111. Brunel, F. M., Lewis, J. D., Destito, G., et al. 2010. Hydrazone ligation strategy to assemble multifunctional viral nanoparticles for cell imaging and tumor targeting. *Nano Letters* 10: 1093–97.
112. Lewis, J. D., Destito, G., Zijlstra, A., et al. 2006. Viral nanoparticles as tools for intravital vascular imaging. *Nature Medicine* 12: 354–60.
113. Steinmetz, N. F., Cho, C. F., Ablack, A., Lewis, J. D., and Manchester, M. 2011. Cowpea mosaic virus nanoparticles target surface vimentin on cancer cells. *Nanomedicine* 6: 351–64.
114. Leong, H. S., Steinmetz, N. F., Ablack, A., et al. 2010. Intravital imaging of embryonic and tumor neovasculature using viral nanoparticles. *Nature Protocols* 5: 1406–17.
115. Steinmetz, N. F., Ablack, A. L., Hickey, J. L., et al. 2011. Intravital imaging of human prostate cancer using viral nanoparticles targeted to gastrin-releasing peptide receptors. *Small* 7: 1664–72.
116. Steinmetz, N. F., Hong, V., Spoerke, E. D., et al. 2009. Buckyballs meet viral nanoparticles: Candidates for biomedicine. *Journal of the American Chemical Society* 131: 17093–95.
117. Soto, C. M., Martin, B. D., Sapsford, K. E., Blum, A. S., and Ratna, B. R. 2008. Toward single molecule detection of staphylococcal enterotoxin B: Mobile sandwich immunoassay on gliding microtubules. *Analytical Chemistry* 80: 5433–40.
118. Soto, C. M., Blum, A. S., Vora, G. J., et al. 2006. Fluorescent signal amplification of carbocyanine dyes using engineered viral nanoparticles. *Journal of the American Chemical Society* 128: 5184–89.
119. Sapsford, K. E., Soto, C. M., Blum, A. S., et al. 2006. A cowpea mosaic virus nanoscaffold for multiplexed antibody conjugation: Application as an immunoassay tracer. *Biosensors & Bioelectronics* 21: 1668–73.
120. Blum, A. S., Soto, C. M., Wilson, C. D., et al. 2005. An engineered virus as a scaffold for three-dimensional self-assembly on the nanoscale. *Small* 1: 702–06.
121. Blum, A. S., Soto, C. M., Wilson, C. D., et al. 2007. Electronic properties of molecular memory circuits on a nanoscale scaffold. *IEEE Transactions on NanoBioscience* 6: 270–74.
122. Portney, N. G., Martinez-Morales, A. A., and Ozkan, M. 2008. Nanoscale memory characterization of virus-templated semiconducting quantum dots. *ACS Nano* 2: 191–96.

Part III

---

*Nanomaterials and Bio-MEMS:
Nano- and Microscale
Hybridization of Materials
and Applications*

9 Microfluidic-Based Polymer Scaffold Design for Tissue Engineering

Mohana Marimuthu and Sanghyo Kim
Gachon University

CONTENTS

9.1 INTRODUCTION

Langer and Vacanti defined and summarized the term, tissue engineering, as "an interdisciplinary field that applies the principles of engineering and life sciences toward the development of biological substitutes for the repair or regeneration of tissue or organ functions" in National Science Foundation (NSF)-sponsored meetings in 1988 and 1993.[1] Until now, the field of tissue engineering has been playing intrinsic and potential roles in replacing or restoring physiological functions of diseased and/or damaged organs. Products of tissue engineering can be of two types: one is a completely functional *ex vivo* developed organ to be implanted and the other is a combination of scaffold with cells that becomes functional tissue/organ after implantation.[2] In either of the types of tissue-engineered products, cells are the potential component for the treatment of diseased tissues where it plays significant roles such as proliferation, differentiation, cellular signaling, development of extracellular matrix, and most importantly, protein production.[3] There have been several tissues such as skin, blood vessels, bone, cartilage, kidney, and heart,[4] developed based on tissue engineering techniques and utilized for tissue regeneration that proves the success of tissue engineers.

The cells that are incorporated into scaffold can become functional tissue only when the scaffold can facilitate cellular development through several factors such as mechanical support, sufficient room for nutrient supply and excretion of cellular waste, gaseous transport, and protein/growth factor supplement. Researchers in earlier days used several porous scaffold fabrication methods such as solvent casting and particulate leaching where the pores are expected to facilitate nutrient supply for the cells in them.[5,6] However, due to lack of controlled internal polymer architecture, these methods were replaced with the rapid prototyping technique by which the three-dimensional (3D) scaffold with spatially controlled porous architecture can be developed using a computer-aided design (CAD) program.[7] Methods based on heat for 3D scaffold fabrication include lamination technique,[8] soft lithography,[9] fused deposition modeling,[10] selective laser sintering,[11] and 3D plotting technology,[12] where the polymeric sheets or particles are fused or deposited to form 3D scaffold with the application of heat and pressure. Similarly, light has been used to initiate the polymerization and solidification of polymeric solutions into a scaffold termed as the photopolymerization technique, which includes stereolithography, photopatterning, and photolithography.[13,14] Table 9.1 describes the advantages, disadvantages, and applications of various scaffold fabrication techniques.[15] The limitation of acellular scaffold fabrication techniques on multicellular engraftment leads to the development of 3D

TABLE 9.1
Advantages, Disadvantages, and Applications of Various Scaffold Fabrication Techniques

Fabrication Technique	Advantages	Disadvantages	Applications
Thermally induced phase separation	Can control the porosity and pore morphology	Achievable sizes range from only 10 to 2000 μm in diameter	Proteins and drug delivery and higher drug encapsulation efficiency
Solvent casting and particulate leaching	Simple operation, control of the pore size, and porosity by selecting the particle size and the amount of salt particles	Distribution of salt particles is often not uniform within the polymer solution, and the degree of direct contact between the salt particles is not well controlled, interconnectivity of pores in a final scaffold cannot be well controlled, limited membrane thickness, lack of mechanical strength, problems with residual solvent, residual porogens	Cardiac and vascular tissue engineering applications
Solid freeform fabrication techniques	Customized design, computer-controlled fabrication, anisotrophic scaffold microstructures, processing conditions	Lack of mechanical strength, limited to small pore sizes	Production of scale replicas of human bones and body organs to advanced customized drug delivery devices

(Continued)

TABLE 9.1 (continued)
Advantages, Disadvantages, and Applications of Various Scaffold Fabrication Techniques

Fabrication Technique	Advantages	Disadvantages	Applications
Phase separation	Allows incorporation of bioactive agents, highly porous structures	Lack of control over microarchitecture, problems with residual solvent, limited range of pore sizes	Drug release and protein delivery applications
Electrospinning	Easy process, high porosity, high surface area-to-volume ratio	Limited range of polymers, lack of mechanical strength, problems with residual solvent, lack of control over microarchitecture	Bone, skin, nerve, and cardiac tissue engineering

Source: Ravichandran, R., Sundarrajan, S., Venugopal, J. R., Mukherjee, S., and Ramakrishna, S. Advances in polymeric systems for tissue engineering and biomedical applications. *Macromol. Biosci.*, 2012, 12, 286–311. Copyright Wiley-VCH Verlag GmbH & Co. KGaA. Reproduced with permission.

assembly of cell sheets.[16] Although both the acellular and cellular scaffolds can provide mechanical support and heterogeneous cell engraftment, the main challenge to regenerate an organ is to provide a vascular architecture that plays a vital role in nutrient supply and metabolite transport.

The microfluidics technique has the ability to develop vascular-like flow patterns as small as capillaries of physiological vasculature with controlled flow rate mimicking *in vivo* conditions.[17] The microfluidics technique can also be used as a cell culture platform for controlling cellular microenvironment for multicellular interactions. It is possible using microfluidics to pattern biomolecules or cells three-dimensionally to generate completely functional tissues. The combined use of microfluidic and molding techniques was employed for the patterning of a cell–collagen matrix.[18] Microchannels under perfusion have been extensively studied as a microbioreactor system for the analysis of various cellular biology such as understanding axonal outgrowth[19] or hepatocyte development.[20] The study of multicellular interaction has also been carried out using a microfluidic platform that includes micropatterning of hepatocytes and fibroblasts,[21] and multicellular culture for mimicking blood vessels.[22] This chapter focuses on various types of polymeric scaffolds that are utilized for tissue regeneration and the role of microfluidics for designing these polymeric scaffolds, the role of a monoculture or multiculture, and the role of a microbioreactor.

9.2   POLYMERIC SCAFFOLDS FOR TISSUE ENGINEERING

Selection of polymeric materials suitable for specific tissue regeneration is an important challenge in the fabrication of scaffolds. These polymeric materials should be safe, biocompatible, mechanically stable, nonimmunogenic, and biodegradable, and their degradation products should remain nontoxic until elimination.[23] Polymers utilized for scaffold fabrication can be characterized depending on their source such as natural, synthetic, or hybrid of both with or without inorganic materials. To obtain a completely functional specific phenotype, polymeric scaffolds that are utilized for tissue engineering should possess the characteristics to incorporate biomolecules such as proteins, growth factors, and cells. Biomolecule- or cell-embedded scaffolds could regulate signaling mechanisms for various biological pathways and initiate cellular adhesion, migration, differentiation, and proliferation for generation of biomimetic functional tissue. Based on the type of biomolecules or cells to be incorporated, the scaffold materials can be differentiated. Among the scaffolds made of natural polymers, protein-based polymers such as collagen, gelatin, fibrin, and elastin, and polysaccharide-based polymers such as chitosan, alginate, hyaluronic acid, chondroitin sulfate, dextran, and agarose were widely studied for biomolecule or cell delivery. Collagen-based bone morphogenetic protein (BMP) carriers called INFUSE® Bone Graft (Medtronic, Minneapolis, MI) sponges have been developed and are commercially available in the market for treatment of spinal fusion.[24] Similarly, Surgifoam® (Ethicon, Inc., Somerville, NJ) is a commercially available porous gelatin disk that carries transforming growth factor beta-1 (TGF-β1) for cartilage tissue engineering.[25] Small interference RNA (siRNA) delivery through cationized gelatin was researched for silencing the TGF-h receptor gene for renal tissue engineering.[26] Chitosan- and alginate-based scaffolds were studied for delivery of TGF-β1 and BMP, respectively, for bone and cartilage tissue regeneration.[27,28] Hyaluronic acid microsphere and chondroitin sulfate scaffold were used for the delivery of DNA and vascular endothelial growth factor (VEGF), respectively, for vascular tissue engineering.[29,30]

For two decades, the poor mechanical strength and poor versatility in scaffold fabrication of natural polymers led to the high-order shift of research interest over synthetic polymers where several physical properties can be altered such as hydrophilicity to hydrophobicity or even to amphiphilicity. Among the synthetic polymers, poly(α-hydroxy acid)s such as poly(L-lactic acid) (PLLA), poly(glycolic acid), poly(ε-caprolactone), and/or poly(lactic-co-glycolic) acid (PLGA) are widely studied for tissue engineering and drug delivery applications. Indeed, two different PLGA-based scaffolds have been commercially available in the market in the name of Dermagraft and TransCyte (Advanced BioHealing, Inc., La Jolla, CA) for skin tissue engineering.[31] Recently, PLGA polymer has also been utilized for plasmid-encoding basic fibroblast growth factor delivery through a porous scaffold.[32] With the help of a modern electrospinning technique, PLLA polymer was electrospun into 0 scaffold incorporating platelet-derived growth factor-BB for complex tissue regneneration.[33] Several other synthetic polymers utilized for fabrication of scaffold include polypyrrole,[34] polyethylene glycol (PEG),[35] poly(carbonate-urea) urethane,[36] poly(propylene fumarate),[37] and polyphosphazenes.[38] Polypyrrole and poly(3,4-ethylenedioxythiophene) are unique polymers possessing conductive and semiconducting properties, which make them extremely appropriate for electrically active tissue regeneration, especially neurite outgrowth that was found to be enhanced further upon incorporation of biomolecules such as neurotrophin 3 and brain-derived neurotrophic factor.[39,40] Among all synthetic polymers, a widely studied polymer for gene delivery system is PEG or PEG-derived copolymers. For instance, a PEG graft polymerized with polyethylene imine was successfully used for DNA delivery in order to obtain extended gene expression in the spinal cord.[41] Elaborate discussions have taken place on a wide range of gene and growth factors incorporated into polymeric scaffolds for tissue regeneration.[23,42–45]

Stimuli-responsive polymers are currently in great demand for scaffold fabrication as their response behavior is similar to the physiological system to some extent. Responses given by these polymers are governed by such change in physical and/or chemical properties as conformational change, solubility change, and the change of hydrophilicity to hydrophobicity and vice versa.[15] The property change of the polymers could be caused by either the formation or breakdown of weak/secondary linkages such as hydrogen bond, hydrophobic interaction, electrostatic force, or acid–base reactions of polymers, or the difference in osmotic pressure.[46] Stimuli-responsive polymers have been characterized based on the types of stimuli which include internal stimuli such as pH or temperature and external stimuli such as magnetic or electric field, light, or ultrasound.[15] Every organ and tissue in the human body possesses a unique pH that increases the interest of study on pH-sensitive polymer-based scaffold for tissue regeneration. The polymers containing functional groups of weak acids such as carboxylic acids, phosphoric acid, and weak bases such as amines tend to either accept or donate protons, thereby changing the polymer's ionization state depending on environmental pH. Therefore, the polymers with a pK_a value of 3–10 are considered as pH-sensitive polymers.

Similarly, polymers that are sensitive to temperature respond by changing their hydration degree under aqueous environment. For instance, a temperature-sensitive polymer swells up and de-swells below and above its transition temperature, respectively, in order to equilibrate the hydration degree. The above transition process is generally reversible, which allows the use of these temperature-sensitive polymers as an on–off system depending on the presence/absence of stimuli.[13] Critically, transition temperature between 20°C and 40°C is optimum for temperature-sensitive polymers, although several factors including solvent type, salt concentration, and their molecular weight govern their transition process.[13] Transition between room temperature and body temperature and vice versa is the widely used phenomenon of making biodegradable and injectable scaffolds for biomedical applications. For instance, a pH-sensitive polymer, sulfamethazine oligomer has been bound to the extreme ends of a thermosensitive block copolymer, poly(ε-caprolactone-co-lactide)-poly(ethylene glycol)-poly(ε-caprolactone-co-lactide) (PCLA-PEG-PCLA), which formed pH- and thermo-sensitive hydrogel for bone tissue engineering.[47] This pH- or thermosensitive polymer remains in the solution under pH 8 and 37°C, whereas upon injection it becomes a hydrogel scaffold at physiological pH 7.4 and 37°C. Delivery of human mesenchymal stem cells and recombinant human BMP-2 was studied on this pH- or thermosensitive injectable scaffold for autologous bone regeneration.[47] Similar to pH and temperature, photosensitive polymers that undergo structural transformations through the change of functional groups of polymer backbone can be induced by a light of a specific wavelength.[48] Polymers that are prone to change their temporary shape to a permanent shape upon any of the stimuli, such as temperature, pH, light, electric/magnetic field, or enzyme, are termed as shape memory polymers. Hydroxylapatite, together with poly(D,L-lactide), is such an example of shape memory polymer, which has been examined by Zheng et al.[49] for hard tissue engineering. Extended discussion on stimuli-responsive polymers and their biomedical applications was found elsewhere.[15,50] Several other stimuli-responsive polymers that were studied for applications along with tissue regeneration, including clinical diagnostics, drug delivery, and sensing, are summarized in Table 9.2.

TABLE 9.2
Various Stimuli-Responsive Polymers and Their Properties and Applications

Functional Polymer	Examples	Properties	Applications
Conducting polymer	PEDOT, PPy, PANI	Possesses high electronic and ionic conductivities	Nerve and cardiac tissue engineering
Glucose-responsive polymer	PBA acid groups	Responses to the by-products that result from the enzymatic oxidation of glucose	Glusoce sensing and insulin delivery
pH-responsive polymer	Poly(acrylamide), poly(acrylic acid), poly(methacrylic acid), PDEAEMA, PDMAEMA	Exhibits a change in the ionization state upon variation of the pH leading to conformational change	Insulin delivery and drug delivery
Enzyme-responsive polymer	Genetically engineered variant of spider dragline silk	Undergoes macroscopic property changes when triggered by selective enzymatic reactions	Drug delivery
Temperature-responsive polymer	PNIPAM	Undergoes a conformational change upon the change in temperature	Cardiac tissue engineering and drug release
Antigen-responsive polymer	NSA, poly(acrylamide)	Antigen–antibody interactions	Biosensors and drug release
Redox/thiol-responsive polymer	Polymers containing disulfide-functional dimethacrylate	Responds to the interconversion of thiols and disulfides	Bioengineering and drug delivery
Shape memory polymer	Poly(D,L-lactide)	Can rapidly change its shape from temporary to permanent under appropriate stimulus	Biomedical applications
Electro-responsive polymer	Polyacrylamide gels, chondroitin sulfate, hyaluronic acid	Responds to either the presence or the absence of magnetic fields	Soft biomimetic actuators, sensors, cancer therapy agents, artificial muscles

(Continued)

TABLE 9.2 (continued)
Various Stimuli-Responsive Polymers and Their Properties and Applications

Functional Polymer	Examples	Properties	Applications
Ultrasound-responsive polymer	Polyglycolides, polylactides, and poly-[bis(p-carboxyphenoxy)] alkane anhydrides with sebacic acid and ethylene vinyl acetate copolymers	Responds to cavitation that results from high- and low-pressure waves generated by ultrasound energy	Medical treatment and diagnostics
Photoresponsive polymer	Azobenzene and spiropyran-containing polymer	Macromolecules that change their properties when irradiated with light of appropriate wavelength	Biological applications
Photoluminescent polymer	Chromophores attached to polyesters, polyamides, polyimides, polyurethanes	Polymers with emissive properties	Biosensors and medical diagnostics

NSA, N-succinimidylacrylate; PANI, poly(aniline); PBA, phenylboronic acid; PDEAEMA, poly(diethyl-aminoethyl methacrylate); PDMAEMA, poly(dimethylaminoethyl methacrylate); PEDOT, poly(3,4-ethylenedioxythiophene); PNIPAM, poly(N-isopropylacrylamide); PPy, polypyrrole.

Source: Ravichandran, R., Sundarrajan, S., Venugopal, J. R., Mukherjee, S., and Ramakrishna, S. Advances in polymeric systems for tissue engineering and biomedical applications. *Macromol. Biosci.*, 2012, 12, 286–311. Copyright Wiley-VCH Verlag GmbH & Co. KGaA. Reproduced with permission.

In some cases, physical and/or chemical modifications without altering inherent bulk properties of polymer or polymer scaffold would behave biomimetically for enhancing the cellular attachment, proliferation, and differentiation into a desired tissue. Polymer or polymer scaffold surface modification can be carried out using several techniques which include plasma treatment, ion sputtering, oxidation/reduction reactions, and corona discharge.[15] It is possible to change the functional group of the polymer surface to carboxylic or amine groups depending on the type of plasma chosen such as oxygen, ammonia, or air.[51] Appropriate plasma selection modifies the polymer surface chemically, through which various desired physical properties can be obtained such as hydrophilicity, refractive index, hardness, surface energy, biocompatibility, and even topographical changes.[52] Plasma-modified polymer surfaces can be further treated with various extracellular matrix components such as collagen, elastin, gelatin, and fibronectin for obtaining successful cellular functions.[53] For instance, plasma-treated nanofibrous scaffold of a complex PLLA-*co*-poly(ε-caprolactone)/gelatin was found to be highly biocompatible for attachment and proliferation of human foreskin fibroblasts for skin tissue engineering.[54]

9.3 MICROFLUIDICS AND POLYMERIC SCAFFOLD FABRICATIONS

Successful tissue regeneration highly depends on the execution of balance between the physiological and synthetic scaffold functions. Two-dimensional and 3D polymeric scaffolds are of great interest in the field of tissue engineering that can be achieved by integrated assembly of tubes, fibers, or micro- or nanoparticles of polymeric materials. Fibers or tubes as 3D scaffolds were conventionally fabricated using extrusion, casting, and layering techniques.[55,56] However, microfluidics has been studied as a cost-effective method for the continuous extrusion of microfibers and microtubes, overcoming most of the limitations of conventional methods. "On the fly" photopolymerization under microfluidic flow condition was the first microfluidic-based fiber fabrication technique introduced by Lee's group in which a mixture of photopolymerizable polymers was composed of 4-hydroxybutyl acrylate, acylic acid, ethyleneglycol dimethacrylate, and 2,2'-dimethoxy-2-phenyl-aceto-nephenone.[57] Lee's group also examined other microfluidic fiber fabrication mechanisms such as diffusion-controlled ionic cross-linking and phase inversion utilizing polymers such as sodium alginate and PLGA.[58,59] Recently, Mohana et al. developed microfluidic device for porous fiber formation utilizing the mechanisms of immersion precipitation and solvent evaporation of an ABA triblock copolymer poly(p-dioxanone-co-caprolactone)-block-poly(ethylene oxide)-block-poly(p-dioxanone-co-caprolactone) having both hydrophilic and hydrophobic segments for the delivery of biomolecules with lipophobic and lipophilic properties.[60] To some extent, polymeric particles also have an important role in tissue engineering applications. For instance, several research groups examined the scaffolds made of functional aggregation of polymeric microspheres.[61,62] The basic principle involved in developing such a 3D particle-based porous scaffold is packing of microparticles randomly and either physically or chemically inducing agglomeration.[63] Particle synthesis using microfluidic technology can be characterized as droplet-based method, multiphase flow method, photolithography-based method, and supraparticle synthesis using assembly of colloids described elaborately elsewhere.[64] For instance, Chung and coworkers developed a "railed microfluidics" method by which self-assembly of polymeric microstructures inside fluidic channels was demonstrated for tissue engineering applications.[65] In physiological condition, the exchange of nutrients and oxygen takes place throughout the 3D spaces with the help of vascular networks containing highly branched fractal-like morphologies. Recently, Ugaz and coworkers developed bio-inspired 3D microfluidic vascular networks using a microfabrication process in which electron beam irradiation was used to implant electric charge inside the polymer, poly(methyl methacrylate), and followed by controlled discharge of accumulated energy to produce a treelike vascular microchannel of ~10 μm in diameter.[66] Figure 9.1 shows the construction mechanism of biomimetic 3D microvascular networks. This new method acts as a new tool to embed 3D microchannel networks within the scaffold materials for supporting cell culture with larger volumes directing successful tissue regeneration.

In spite of using microfluidics as a platform for polymeric scaffold fabrication, some polymers with an embedded microfluidic structure itself act as scaffolds. Such polymers should possess several unique properties such as mechanical stability, biocompatibility,

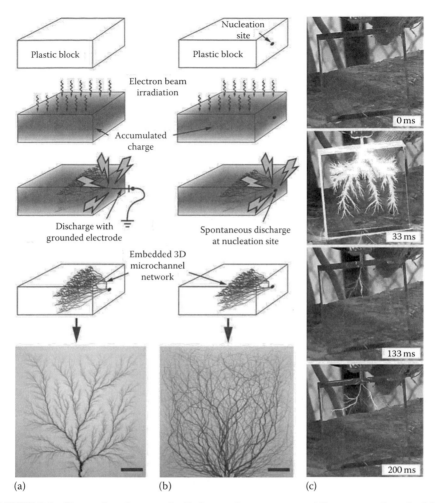

(a)   (b)   (c)

FIGURE 9.1 Harnessing electrostatic discharge phenomena to rapidly construct branched 3D microvascular networks. (a) In the grounded contact method, electron beam irradiation is used to implant a high level of internal electric charge inside a dielectric substrate. A grounded electrode is then brought into contact with the substrate surface, initiating sudden energy release that locally vaporizes the surrounding material leaving behind a treelike branched microchannel network. (b) In the spontaneous discharge method, a defect (e.g., small hole) is first created on the substrate surface prior to irradiation. When the internal electric charge exceeds a critical level upon exposure to the electron beam, the defect acts as a nucleation site for spontaneous energy release. The grounded contact method yields a more "treelike" morphology, while microchannels produced by spontaneous discharge permeate the substrate more uniformly. (c) Image sequence from a video recording of discharge by the grounded contact method shows that energy release is nearly instantaneous with subsequent weaker discharges persisting over longer timescales. All photographs depict microchannel networks in 1 inch × 3 inch × 3 inch polished acrylic blocks. Note that all networks extend in 3D throughout the volume of the blocks. Scale bars = 1 cm. (From Huang, J., Kim, J., Agrawal, N., Sudarsan, A. P., Maxim, J. E., Jayaraman, A., and Ugaz, V. M. Rapid fabrication of bio-inspired 3D microfluidic vascular networks. *Adv. Mater.* 2009, 21, 3567–3571. Copyright Wiley-VCH Verlag GmbH & Co. KGaA. Reproduced with permission.)

microstructural replicability, ability to bind into an air-tight fluidic network, diffusibility or permeability for small and large molecules, stability under physiological conditions (such as pH, temperature, and osmolarity) and be relatively inexpensive.[67] For instance, a PLGA-based highly branched multilayer microfluidic network was demonstrated as an analog to physiological microvascular network for tissue engineering applications.[68] Likewise, the calcium alginate is another example of a hydrogel with an embedded microfluidic network studied for controlled soluble species concentration and incorporation of multiple cell types within a 3D gel scaffold.[69] It is essential to develop a cell-seeded microfluidic scaffold for obtaining accurate biomimetic environment to direct the specific tissue regeneration. Biopolymer obtained from the *Bombyx mori* silkworm has also been applied for the fabrication of microfluidic scaffold.[70] A biodegradable elastomer, poly(glycerol sebacate), another polymer with excellent chemical and mechanical properties, was fabricated into an endothelialized microfluidic scaffold, an analog to microvasculature.[71] Recently, a new biomaterial, poly(1,3-diamino-2-hydroxypropane-*co*-polyol sebacate) was found to be a biodegradable microfluidic device which possesses a significantly longer degradation profile than other polymer (PLGA or silk fibroin)-based microfluidic scaffolds.[72] A detailed summary on biomaterials-based microfluidic systems was offered by Bettinger and Borenstein.[73]

9.4 MICROFLUIDIC CELL CULTURE SYSTEMS FOR TISSUE REGENERATION

A microfluidic system cell culture platform can deliver several types of substances such as growth factors, enzymes, fluorescent dyes, or drug materials with specific targets to single or multiple cells without disturbing them. Multiple streams of laminar flow in parallel with each other combined into a single stream without mixing of each fluid, except the diffusion in the interface. With the help of specifically designed geometries and structures, a microfluidic perfusion culture can mimic *in vivo* physiological conditions by producing fluidic shear stress[74] or interstitial fluid flow.[75] One important feature of a microfluidic cell culture system is surface area-to-volume (SAV) ratio. When this SAV ratio increases, diffusion of gas in the microfluidic system occurs efficiently. Indeed, efficient gas exchangeable design is significant for cells to maintain their metabolic activities.[76] For instance, microfluidic cell culture devices are well known for their high SAV ratio, and therefore enhance diffusion of gases such as oxygen for cell culture without the need of external oxygenation structure.[77] Likewise, maintaining specific temperature for cell culture plays an important role in obtaining unique cell physiology.[78,79] Due to the characteristics of heat transfer, cell culture under precisely controlled gaseous and temperature environments is significantly attainable with a microfluidic cell culture platform.[80] These characteristics of a microfluidic system make it unique as a cell culture platform for the studies of cell biology, cell–cell interaction, drug–cell interaction, and tissue regeneration. One of the promising roles of a microfluidic cell culture platform is to develop 3D tissue models for the exploration of drug sensitivity, drug toxicity analysis, drug therapeutic property studies, and cellular response related to concentration of drugs. A 3D liver tissue model for drug study has been developed by the co-culture of hepatocytes and endothelial cells in a photosensitive polymer-based microfluidic cell culture platform.[81] Similarly, a 3D HepaTox Chip has been developed by the Institute of Bioengineering and Nanotechnology, Singapore. It is a microfluidic-based multiplexed hepatocyte culture chip that generates linear concentration gradient for the study of drug toxicity.[82] Micropillars were designed at the middle of each culture platform to culture hepatocyte cells, where microchannels on either side allow medium perfusion. Such a design provided a 3D microenvironment for hepatocytes to behave phenotypically as a functional liver for the analysis of drug toxicity.[82] Several other microfluidic co-culture designs for *in vitro* models of liver tissue regeneration were studied elaborately by biomedical engineers.[83,84] In addition to vascular and liver tissue development, neuronal tissue regeneration is highly challengeable for tissue engineers to develop a competent multicell culture platform for facilitating cell–cell interactions, which is significantly vital for metabolic coupling of neuronal cells with astrocytes.[85–87] Varieties of worthwhile approaches based on a microfluidic neural co-culture platform for axon–glial interactions were developed.[88–90] *In vitro* neural tissue regeneration highly involves myelination that helps in the conduction of nerve impulses. *In vitro* myelination can be obtained when axons and oligodendrocytes or Schwann cells are co-cultured to initiate signaling between them.[91,92] Recently, two compartmentalized co-cultures of neurons and oligodendrocytes were studied based on a microfluidic system.[93] Microfluidic channels of two compartments were designed circularly as shown in Figure 9.2 to guide the axonal outgrowth and promote the myelination process. The microchannels of this device physically isolate the axons from cell bodies and dendrites (Figure 9.3), which is believed to facilitate the long-term co-culture of cells and enhanced axon-glia signaling.[93] A detailed review on microfluidic-based cell culture platforms for tissue engineering applications can be found elsewhere.[94]

9.5 MICROFLUIDIC BIOREACTORS FOR TISSUE ENGINEERING APPLICATIONS

Obtaining higher cell density while a cell culture is *in vitro* is an important factor in tissue engineering applications. To achieve this aspiration, continuous perfusion of nutrition and oxygen to the cells and continuous removal of metabolic waste from cultured cells should be ensured. Such a continuous perfusion culture is attainable using specifically designed microfluidic bioreactor systems. Along with continuous perfusion, some tissues such as blood vessels, cardiac muscles, and cartilage are in need of compression, shear stresses, and pulsative flow for improving mechanical properties; those characterics can also be afforded by microfluidic bioreactor designs.[2,95] A multilayered polydimethylsiloxane (PDMS)-based microfluidic perfusion bioreactor system with an oxygen chamber for the mammalian cell culture has been successfully demonstrated by high cell densities.[96] A bioreactor design with continuous perfusion has been examined to obtain a morphogenetically biomimetic 3D liver tissue model.[97] Powers and coworkers[97] revealed that such a continuous perfusion bioreactor system permits hepatocellular aggregate generation much similar to physiological structure, hepatic acinus. In addition, a bioreactor perfusion platform for a neuron–astrocyte co-culture has been inspected for 3D cell–cell and cell–matrix interactions to obtain high-density multicell population

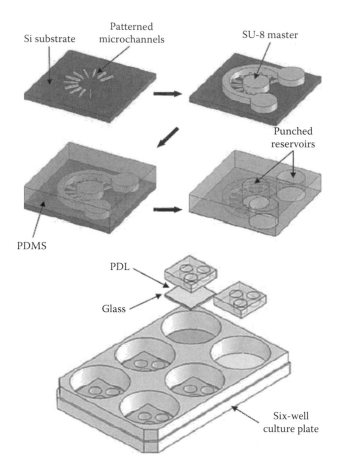

FIGURE 9.2 Fabrication and assembly steps for the microfluidic co-culture device. Two SU-8TM layers with different thicknesses were patterned on the top of a silicon substrate to form the axon-guiding microchannel array and the two cell culture compartments (soma and axon/glia). PDMS devices were replicated from the SU-8TM master using soft lithography process and 7-mm diameter reservoirs were punched out followed by sterilization in 70% ethanol for 30 min and bonding onto poly(D-lysine) (PDL) or Matrigel™-coated substrates (BD Biosciences, San Jose, CA). Each device fits into one-well of a conventional six-well polystyrene culture plate. (With kind permission from Springer Science+Business Media: *Biomed. Microdevices*, Microfluidic compartmentalized co-culture platform for CNS axon myelination research, 11, 2009, 1145–1153, Park, J., Koito, H., Li, J., and Han, A., Figure 9.2.)

for brain tissue regeneration applications.[98] A microbioreactor has been designed significantly for long-term culture of human foreskin fibroblast cells under constant perfusion of culture medium.[99] In addition, a bioreactor perfusion system has also been used for the seeding of human dermal fibroblast cells into porous electrospun poly(ε-caprolactone) nanofibrous mats for the study of skin tissue engineering.[100] Recently, a unique flow perfusion bioreactor embedded with PLLA–collagen scaffold as shown in Figure 9.4 was studied for the repair of defects in a complex abdominal wall.[101] It was demonstrated that the culture of dermal fibroblasts under perfusion conditions enhances

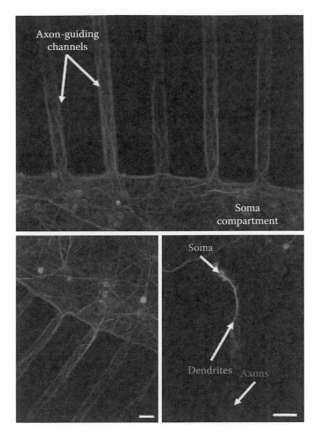

FIGURE 9.3   (See color insert.) Immunocytochemistry images of neurons at 2 weeks in culture demonstrate that axons grew from the soma compartment into the axon/glia compartment through the arrays of axon-guiding microchannels, but dendrites and neuronal soma could not reach into the axon/glia compartment due to the length of the microchannels (200–800 μm long) and the height of the microchannels (2.5 μm). Axons were immunostained for neurofilament (NF) (red) and dendrite for microtubule-associated protein 2 (MAP2) (green). Scale bars = 20 μm. (With kind permission from Springer Science+Business Media: *Biomed. Microdevices*, Microfluidic compartmentalized co-culture platform for CNS axon myelination research, 11, 2009, 1145–1153, Park, J., Koito, H., Li, J., and Han, A., Figure 9.3.)

cell proliferation and distribution within the PLLA–collagen scaffolds. A construct with high cellular density was observed within 7 days of dermal cell culture under perfusion and found increased cellularity by 28th day of culture period. *In vitro* perfusion ensured that a highly cellularized and matured construct was implanted, and its significant survival rate of cells with expression of extracellular protein collagen types I and III was examined. Furthermore, an electrospun poly(ε-caprolactone) microfiber scaffold was also studied after coating with cartilaginous extracellular matrix for cartilage tissue engineering under a flow perfusion bioreactor system.[102] These studies prove the efficiency of a microfluidic perfusion bioreactor system for the reconstruction of functional large, complex, and/or hard tissues.

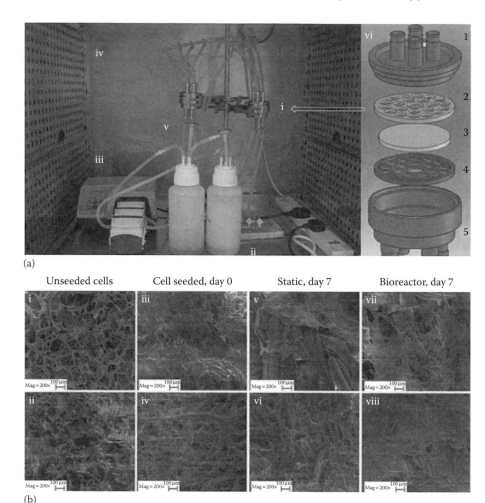

(a)

(b)

FIGURE 9.4 (a) Perfusion bioreactor system consisting of (i) a flow chamber that has a scaffold holder and four media flow channel; (ii) a media container; (iii) a multichannel peristaltic pump (Watson-Marlow 323 series; Watson-Marlow Ltd., Falmouth, UK). (iv) The whole system is housed in a humidified CO_2 incubator, allowing gaseous exchange to occur through the silicone rubber tubing, connected to (v) a 0.2-mm sterile filter. The media was pumped through the chamber and continuously perfused around the cell-loaded scaffold from underneath at a flow rate of 6 mL/min for up to 4 weeks. (vi) Schematic representation of 3D model of the bioreactor, indicating (1) screwing top part, (2) top guiding holder, (3) scaffold, (4) bottom guiding holder, and (5) screwing bottom part. (b) scanning electron microscopy (SEM) of cell-loaded scaffolds: scaffold without cell seeding (i and ii), cell-seeded for 2 h only (iii and iv), cell-loaded scaffolds in static condition for 7 days (v and vi), and cell-loaded scaffolds in perfusion bioreactor for 7 days (vii and viii). (Reprinted from *Biomaterials*, 31, Pu, F., Rhodes, N. P., Bayon, Y., Chen, R., Brans, G., Benne, R., and Hunt, J. A., The use of flow perfusion culture and subcutaneous implantation with fibroblast-seeded PLLA-collagen 3D scaffolds for abdominal wall repair, 4330–4340, Copyright 2010, with permission from Elsevier.)

9.6 CONCLUSION

The challenge for constructing the functional biomimetic artificial organs *in vitro* paves the way for the inventions of several microfabrication technologies such as microfluidics. The most important limitations in developing artificial tissues are allowing hierarchical multicell interactions three-dimensionally under perfusion culture for nutrient supply and waste removal mimicking the physiological environment. By combining biology with bio-MEMS techniques, it is highly possible to overcome the above-mentioned limitations to provide a suitable environment for cells to grow and interact *in vitro* and mimic living systems. One bio-MEMS technique is microfluidics, which has high potential for tissue engineering applications. Microfluidics has been utilized to understand fundamental biological functions such as factors influencing cellular proliferation, differentiation or apoptosis, migration, and gene expressions. These understandings help design a suitable culture platform providing physiological microenvironments such as cell–cell interactions, cell–extracellular matrix interactions, soluble signaling phenomena, and mechanical forces for tissue regeneration. Indeed, several researchers are investigating a variety of biodegradable polymeric functional scaffolds together with microfluidics for biomimetic tissue development. Microfluidic-based *in vitro*-developed tissue models were employed not only for regeneration applications but also in drug research such as toxicity analysis, therapeutic activity analysis, and dose analysis. However, utilization of a microfluidic cell culture platform for tissue regeneration applications or drug research is still in the developmental stage, although it is one of the highly emerging fields of interest. In spite of its huge application areas, some technical issues such as complex operation procedure to carry out the experiments or reading out the data in a simple understandable format with an equal or higher level of accuracy than conventional methods should be addressed. To overcome these hurdles, microfluidic chip designers should have a healthy understanding with biologists or users, and therefore, microfluidic scaffolding design and culture platforms would make several steps forward to be commercialized in the near future.

REFERENCES

1. Langer, R., and Vacanti, J. 1993. Tissue engineering. *Science* 260:920–926.
2. Andersson, H., and Berg, A. V. D. 2004. Microfabrication and microfluidics for tissue engineering: State of the art and future opportunities. *Lab Chip* 4:98–103.
3. Ochoa, E., and Vancanti, J. 2002. An overview of the pathology and approaches to tissue engineering. *Ann. N.Y. Acad. Sci.* 979:10–26.
4. Marler, J., Upton, J., Langer, R., and Vacanti, J. 1998. Transplantation of cells in matrices for tissue generation. *Adv. Drug Deliv. Rev.* 33:165–182.
5. Liao, C., Chen, C., Chen, J., Chiang, S., Lin, Y., and Chang, K. 2002. Fabrication of porous biodegradable polymer scaffolds using a solvent merging/particulate leaching method. *J. Biomed. Mater. Res.* 59:676–681.
6. Oh, S. H., Kang, S. G., Kim, E. S., Cho, S. H., and Lee, J. H. 2003. Fabrication and characterization of hydrophilic poly(lactic-*co*-glycolic acid)/poly(vinyl alcohol) blend cell scaffolds by melt-molding particulate-leaching method. *Biomaterials* 24:4011–4021.

7. Yang, S., Leong, K. F., Du, Z., and Chua, C. K. 2002. The design of scaffolds for use in tissue engineering: Part II. Rapid prototyping techniques. *Tissue Eng.* 8:1–11.
8. Borenstein, J. T., Terai, H., King, K. R., Weinberg, E. J., Kaazempur-Mofrad, M. R., and Vacanti, J. P. 2002. Microfabrication technology for vascularized tissue engineering. *Biomed. Microdevices* 4:167–175.
9. Vozzi, G., Flaim, C., Ahluwalia, A., and Bhatia, S. 2003. Fabrication of PLGA scaffolds using soft lithography and microsyringe deposition. *Biomaterials* 24:2533–2540.
10. Zein, I., Hutmacher, D. W., Tan, K. C., and Teoh, S. H. 2002. Fused deposition modeling of novel scaffold architectures for tissue engineering applications. *Biomaterials* 23:1169–1185.
11. Lee, G., Barlow, J., Fox, W., and Aufdermorte, T. 1996. Biocompatibility of SLS-formed calcium phosphate implants. *Proceedings of Solid Freeform Fabrication Symposium,* Austin, TX, August 12–14.
12. Landers, R., Hubner, U., Schmelzeisen, R., and Mulhaupt, R. 2002. Rapid prototyping of scaffolds derived from thermoreversible hydrogels and tailored for applications in tissue engineering. *Biomaterials* 23:4437–4447.
13. Cooke, M. N., Fisher, J. P., Dean, D., Rimnac, C., and Mikos, A. G. 2003. Use of stereolithography to manufacture critical-sized 3D biodegradable scaffolds for bone in growth. *J. Biomed. Mater. Res. B* 64B:65–69.
14. Yu, T., Chiellini, F., Schmaljohann, D., Solaro, R., and Ober, C. K. 2000. Microfabrication of hydrogels as polymer scaffolds for tissue engineering applications. *Polym. Prepr.* 41:1699–1700.
15. Ravichandran, R., Sundarrajan, S., Venugopal, J. R., Mukherjee, S., and Ramakrishna, S. 2012. Advances in polymeric systems for tissue engineering and biomedical applications. *Macromol. Biosci.* 12:286–311.
16. Shimizu, T., Yamato, M., Kikuchi, A., and Okano, T. 2003. Cell sheet engineering for myocardial tissue reconstruction. *Biomaterials* 24:2309–2316.
17. El-Ali, J., Sorger, P. K., and Jensen, K. F. 2006. Cells on chips. *Nature* 442:403–411.
18. Tan, W., and Desai, T. A. 2003. Microfluidic patterning of cells in extracellular matrix biopolymers: Effects of channel size, cell type, and matrix composition on pattern integrity. *Tissue Eng.* 9:255–267.
19. Taylor, A. M., Blurton-Jones, M., Rhee, S. W., Cribbs, D. H., Cotman, C. W., and Jeon, N. L. 2005. A microfluidic culture platform for CNS axonal injury, regeneration and transport. *Nat. Methods* 2:599–605.
20. Leclerc, E., Sakai, Y., and Fujii, T. 2004. Perfusion culture of fetal human hepatocytes in microfluidic environments. *Biochem. Eng. J.* 20:143–148.
21. Kane, B. J., Zinner, M. J., Yarmush, M. L., and Toner, M. 2006. Liver-specific functional studies in a microfluidic array of primary mammalian hepatocytes. *Anal. Chem.* 78:4291–4298.
22. Tan, W., and Desai, T. A. 2004. Microscale multilayer coculture for biomimetic blood vessels. *J. Biomed. Mater. Res. A* 72:146–160.
23. Marimuthu, M., and Kim, S. 2009. Survey of the state of the art in biomaterials, cells, genes and proteins integrated into micro- and nanoscaffolds for tissue regeneration. *Curr. Nanosci.* 5:189–203.
24. Chevallay, B., and Herbage, D. 2000. Collagen-based biomaterials as 3D scaffolds for cell cultures: Application for tissue engineering and gene therapy. *Med. Biol. Eng. Comput.* 38:211–218.
25. Awad, H. A., Quinn, W. M., Leddy, H. A., Gimble, J. M., and Guilak, F. 2004. Chondrogenic differentiation of adipose-derived adult stem cells in agarose, alginate, and gelatin scaffolds. *Biomaterials.* 25:3211–3222.
26. Barquinero, J., Eixarch, H., and Perez-Melgosa, M. 2004. Retroviral vectors: New applications for an old tool. *Gene Ther.* 1:S3–S9.

27. Zhang, Y., Cheng, X., Wang, J., Wang, Y., Shi, B., Huang, C., Yang, X., and Liu, T. 2006. Novel chitosan/collagen scaffold containing transforming growth factor-beta1 DNA for periodontal tissue engineering. *Biochem. Biophys. Res. Commun.* 344:362–369.

28. Grunder, T., Gaissmaier, C., Fritz, J., Stoop, R., Hortschansky, P., and Mollenhauer, J. 2004. Bone morphogenetic protein-2 enhances the expression of type II collagen and aggrecan in chondrocytes embedded in alginate beads. *Osteoarthr. Cartil.* 12:559–567.

29. Yun, Y. H., Goetz, D. J., Yellen, P., and Chen, W. L. 2004. Hyaluronan microspheres for sustained gene delivery and site-specific targeting. *Biomaterials* 25:147–157.

30. Liu, Y., Yang, H., Otaka, K., Takatsuki, H., and Sakanishi, A. 2005. Effects of vascular endothelial growth factor (VEGF) and chondroitin sulfate A on human monocytic THP-1 cell migration. *Colloids Surf. B* 43:216–220.

31. Jiang, W. G., and Harding, K. G. 1998. Enhancement of wound tissue expansion and angiogenesis by matrix-embedded fibroblast (Dermagraft), a role of hepatocyte growth factor scatter factor. *Int. J. Mol. Med.* 2:203–210.

32. Rives, C. B., Rieux, A. D., Zelivyanskaya, M., Stock, S. R., Lowe, W. L., and Shea, L. D. 2009. Layered PLG scaffolds for in vivo plasmid delivery. *Biomaterials* 30:394–401.

33. Wei, G., Jin, Q., Giannobile, W. V., and Ma, P. X. 2006. Nano-fibrous scaffold for controlled delivery of recombinant human PDGF-BB. *J. Control. Release* 112:103–110.

34. Stauffera, W. R., and Cuia, X. T. 2006. Polypyrrole doped with 2 peptide sequences from laminin. *Biomaterials* 27:2405–2413.

35. Park, H., Temenoff, J. S., Tabata, Y., Capland, A. I., and Mikos, A. G. 2007. Injectable biodegradable hydrogel composites for rabbit marrow mesenchymal stem cell and growth factor delivery for cartilage tissue engineering. *Biomaterials* 28:3217–3227.

36. Rashid, S. T., Salacinski, H. J., Button, M. J. C., Fuller, B., Hamilton, G., and Seifalian, A. M. 2004. Cellular engineering of conduits for coronary and lower limb bypass surgery: Role of cell attachment peptides and pre-conditioning in optimizing smooth muscle cells (SMC) adherence to compliant poly(carbonate-urea)urethane (MyoLinke) scaffolds. *Eur. J. Vasc. Endovasc. Surg.* 27:608–616.

37. Fisher, J. P., Vehof, J. W. M., Dean, D., van der Waerden, J., Holland, T. A., Mikos, A. G., and Jansen, J. A. 2002. Soft and hard tissue response to photocrosslinked poly(propylene fumarate) scaffolds in a rabbit model. *J. Biomed. Mater. Res.* 59:547–556.

38. Conconi, M. T., Lora, S., Menti, A. M., Carampin, P., and Parnigotto, P. P. 2006. In vitro evaluation of poly[bis(ethyl alanato)phosphazene] as a scaffold for bone tissue engineering. *Tissue Eng.* 12:811–819.

39. Abidian, M. R., Corey, J. M., Kipke, D. R., and Martin, D. C. 2010. Conducting-polymer nanotubes improve electrical properties, mechanical adhesion, neural attachment, and neurite outgrowth of neural electrodes. *Small* 6:421–429.

40. Thompson, B. C., Richardson, R. T., Moulton, S. E., Evans, A. J., Stephen, O., Clark, G. M., and Wallace, G. C. 2010. Conducting polymers, dual neurotrophins and pulsed electrical stimulation—Dramatic effects on neurite outgrowth. *J. Control. Release* 141:161–167.

41. Shi, L., Tang, G. P., Gao, S. J., Ma, Y. X., Liu, B. H., Li, Y., Zeng, J. M., Ng, Y. K., Leong, K.,W., and Wang, S. 2003. Repeated intrathecal administration of plasmid DNA complexed with polyethylene glycol-grafted polyethylenimine led to prolonged transgene expression in the spinal cord. *Gene Ther.* 10:1179–1188.

42. Liu, X., Holzwarth, J. M., and Ma, P. X. 2012. Functionalized synthetic biodegradable polymer scaffolds for tissue engineering. *Macromol. Biosci.* 2012, doi:10.1002/mabi.201100466.

43. Bettinger, C. J. 2011. Biodegradable elastomers for tissue engineering and cell–biomaterial interactions. *Macromol. Biosci.* 11:467–482.

44. Jia, X., and Kiick, K. L. 2009. Hybrid multicomponent hydrogels for tissue engineering. *Macromol. Biosci.* 9:140–156.

45. Ravichandran, R., Venugopal, J. R., Sundarrajan, S., Mukherjee, S., and Ramakrishna, S. 2010. Applications of conducting polymers and their issues in biomedical engineering. *J. R. Soc. Interface* 7:559–579.
46. Schmajljohann, B. 2006. Thermo- and pH-responsive polymers in drug delivery. *Adv. Drug. Deliv. Rev.* 58:1655–1670.
47. Kim, H. K, Shim, W. S., Kim, S. E., Lee, K. H., Kang, E., Kim, J. H., Kim, K., Kwon, I. C., and Lee, D. S. 2009. Injectable in situ-forming pH/thermo-sensitive hydrogel for bone tissue engineering. *Tissue Eng. A* 15:923–933.
48. Dai, S., Ravi, P., and Tam, K. C. 2009. Thermo- and photo-responsive polymeric systems. *Soft Matter* 5:2513–2533.
49. Zheng, X., Zhou, S., Li, X., and Weng, J. 2006. Shape memory properties of poly(D,L-lactide)/hydroxyapatite composites. *Biomaterials* 27:4288–4295.
50. Stuart, M. A. C., Huck, W. T. S., Genzer, J., Müller, M., Ober, C., Stamm, M., Sukhorukov, G. B., et al. 2010. Emerging applications of stimuli-responsive polymer materials. *Nat. Mater.* 9:101–113.
51. Park, H., Lee, K. Y., Lee, S. J., Park, K. E., and Park, W. H. 2007. Plasma-treated poly(lactic-co-glycolic acid) nanofibers for tissue engineering. *Macromol. Res.* 15:238–243.
52. Wan, Y., Qu, X., Lu, J., Zhu, C., Wan, L., and Yang, J. 2004. Characterization of surface property of poly(lactide-co-glycolide) after oxygen plasma treatment. *Biomaterials* 25:4777–4783.
53. Shen, H., Hu, X., Bei, J., and Wang, S. 2008. The immobilization of basic fibroblast growth factor on plasma-treated poly(lactide-co-glycolide). *Biomaterials* 29:2388–2399.
54. Chandrasekaran, A. R., Venugopal, J., Sundarrajan, S., and Ramakrishna, S. 2011. Fabrication of a nanofibrous scaffold with improved bioactivity for culture of human dermal fibroblasts for skin regeneration. *Biomed. Mater.* 6:015001.
55. Dalton, P. D., Flynn, L., and Shoichet, S. C. 2002. Manufacture of poly(2-hydroxyethyl methacrylate-co-methyl methacrylate) hydrogel tubes for use as nerve guidance channels. *Biomaterials* 22:3843–3851.
56. Chou, S. Y., Krauss, P. R., and Renstrom, P. J. 1996. Imprint lithography with 25-nanometer resolution. *Science* 272:85–87.
57. Jeong, W., Kim, J., Kim, S., Lee, S., Mensinge, G., and Beebe, D. J. 2004. Hydrodynamic microfabrication via "on the fly" photopolymerization of microscale fibers and tubes. *Lab Chip* 4:576–580.
58. Shin, S., Park, J., Lee, J., Park, H., Park, Y., Lee, K., Whang, C., and Lee, S. 2007. "On the fly" continuous generation of alginate fibers using a microfluidic device. *Langmuir* 23:9104–9108.
59. Hwang, C. M., Khademhosseini, A., Park, Y., Sun, K., and Lee, S. 2008. Microfluidic chip-based fabrication of PLGA microfiber scaffolds for tissue engineering. *Langmuir* 24:6845–6851.
60. Marimuthu, M., Kim, S., and An, J. 2010. Amphiphilic triblock copolymer and a microfluidic device for porous microfiber fabrication. *Soft Matter* 6:2200–2207.
61. Borden, M., El-Amin, S. F., Attawia, M., and Laurencin, C. T. 2003. Structural and human cellular assessment of a novel microsphere-based tissue engineered scaffold for bone repair. *Biomaterials* 24:597–609.
62. Borden, M., Attawia M., and Laurencin, C. T. 2002. The sintered microsphere matrix for bone tissue engineering: In vitro osteoconductivity studies. *J. Biomed. Mater. Res.* 61:421–429.
63. Malafaya, P. B., Pedro, A. J., Peterbauer, A., Gabriel, C., Redl, H., and Reis, R. L. 2005. Chitosan particles agglomerated scaffolds for cartilage and osteochondral tissue engineering approaches with adipose tissue derived stem cells. *J. Mater. Sci. Mater. Med.* 16:1077–1085.

64. Dendukuri, D., and Doyle, P. S. 2009. The synthesis and assembly of polymeric microparticles using microfluidics. *Adv. Mater.* 21:4071–4086.
65. Chung, S. E., Park, W., Shin, S., Lee, S. A., and Kwon, S. 2008. Guided and fluidic self-assembly of microstructures using railed microfluidic channels. *Nat. Mater.* 7:581–587.
66. Huang, J., Kim, J., Agrawal, N., Sudarsan, A. P., Maxim, J. E., Jayaraman, A., and Ugaz, V. M. 2009. Rapid fabrication of bio-inspired 3D microfluidic vascular networks. *Adv. Mater.* 21:3567–3571.
67. Cabodi, M., Choi, N. W., Gleghorn, J. P., Lee, C. S. D., Bonassar, L. J., and Stroock, A. D. 2005. A microfluidic biomaterial. *J. Am. Chem. Soc.* 127:13788–13789.
68. King, K. R., Wang, C. C. J., Kaazempur-Mofrad, M. R., Vacanti, J. P., and Borenstein, J. T. 2004. Biodegradable microfluidics. *Adv. Mater.* 16:2007–2012.
69. Choi, N. W., Cabodi, M., Held, B., Gleghorn, J. P., Bonassar, L. J., and Stroock, A. D. 2007. Microfluidic scaffolds for tissue engineering. *Nat. Mater.* 6:908–915.
70. Bettinger, C. J., Cyr, K. M., Matsumoto, A., Langer, R., Borenstein, J. T., and Kaplan, D. L. 2007. Silk fibroin microfluidic devices. *Adv. Mater.* 19:2847–2850.
71. Fidkowski, C., Kaazempur-Mofrad, M. R., Borenstein, J. T., Vacanti, J. P., Langer, R., and Wang, Y. D. 2005. Endothelialized microvasculature based on a biodegradable elastomer. *Tissue Eng.* 11:302–309.
72. Wang, J., Bettinger, C. J., Langer, R. S., and Borenstein, J. T. 2010. Biodegradable microfluidic scaffolds for tissue engineering from amino alcohol-based poly(ester amide) elastomers. *Organogenesis* 6:212–216.
73. Bettinger, C. J., and Borenstein, J. T. 2010. Biomaterials-based microfluidics for engineered tissue constructs. *Soft Matter* 6:4999–5015.
74. Vickerman, V., Blundo, J., Chung, S., and Kamm, R. D. 2008. Design, fabrication and implementation of a novel multi-parameter control microfluidic platform for three-dimensional cell culture and real-time imaging. *Lab Chip* 8:1468–1477.
75. Ng, C. P., and Pun, S. H. 2008. A perfusable 3D cell–matrix tissue culture chamber for in situ evaluation of nanoparticle vehicle penetration and transport. *Biotechnol. Bioeng.* 99.1490–1501.
76. Wu, M., Huang, S., and Lee, G. 2010. Microfluidic cell culture systems for drug research. *Lab Chip* 10:939–956.
77. Prokop, A., Prokop, Z., Schaffer, D., Kozlov, E., Wikswo, J., Cliffel, D., and Baudenbacher, F. 2004. NanoLiterBioReactor: Long-term mammalian cell culture at nanofabricated scale. *Biomed. Microdevices* 6:325–339.
78. Chong, S. L., Mou, D. G., Ali, A. M., Lim, S. H., and Tey, B. T. 2008. Cell growth, cell-cycle progress, and antibody production in hybridoma cells cultivated under mild hypothermic conditions. *Hybridoma* 27:107–111.
79. Brandam, C., Castro-Martínez, C., Délia, M. L., Ramón-Portugal, F., and Strehaiano, P. 2008. Effect of temperature on *Brettanomyces bruxellensis*: Metabolic and kinetic aspects. *Can. J. Microbiol.* 54:11–18.
80. Huang, C. W., and Lee, G. B. 2007. A microfluidic system for automatic cell culture. *J. Micromech. Microeng.* 17:1266–1274.
81. Leclerc, E., Miyata, F., Furukawa, K. S., Ushida, T., Sakai, Y., and Fujii, T. 2004. Effect on liver cells of stepwise microstructures fabricated in a photosensitive biodegradable polymer by soft lithography. *Mater. Sci. Eng. C* 24:349–354.
82. Toh, Y. C., Lim, T. C., Tai, D., Xiao, G., van Noort, D., and Yu, H. 2009. A microfluidic 3D hepatocyte chip for drug toxicity testing. *Lab Chip* 9:2026–2035.
83. Toh, Y. C., Zhang, C., Zhang, J., Khong, Y. M., Chang, S., Samper, V. D., van Noort, D., Hutmacher, D. W., and Yu, H. 2007. A novel 3D mammalian cell perfusion–culture system in microfluidic channels. *Lab Chip* 7:302–309.

84. Leclerca, E., Baudoina, R., Corlub, A., Griscomc, L., Duvala, J. L., and Legallais, C. C. 2007. Selective control of liver and kidney cells migration during organotypic cocultures inside fibronectin-coated rectangular silicone microchannels. *Biomaterials* 28:1820–1829.

85. Tsacopoulos, M., and Magistretti, P. J. 1996. Metabolic coupling between glia and neurons. *J. Neurosci.* 16:877–885.

86. Aschner, M. 2000. Neuron–astrocyte interactions: Implications for cellular energetics and antioxidant levels. *Neurotoxicology* 21:1101–1107.

87. Tsacopoulos, M. 2002. Metabolic signaling between neurons and glial cells: A short review. *J. Physiol.* 96:283–288.

88. Ng, B. K., Chen, L., Mandemakers, W., Cosgaya, J. M., and Chan, J. R. 2007. Anterograde transport and secretion of brain-derived neurotrophic factor along sensory axons promote Schwann cell myelination. *J. Neurosci.* 27:7597–7603.

89. Millet, L., Stewart, M., Sweedler, J., Nuzzo, R., and Gillette, M. 2007. Microfluidic devices for culturing primary mammalian neurons at low densities. *Lab Chip* 7:987–994.

90. Morin, F., Nishimura, N., Griscom, L., LePioufle, B., Fujita, H., Takamura, Y., and Tamiya, E. 2006. Constraining the connectivity of neuronal networks cultured on micro-electrode arrays with microfluidic techniques: A step towards neuron based functional chips. *Biosens. Bioelectron.* 21:1093–1100.

91. Baumann, N., and Pham-Dinh, D. 2001. Biology of oligodendrocyte and myelin in the mammalian central nervous system. *Physiol. Rev.* 81:871–927.

92. Sherman, D. L., and Brophy, P. J. 2005. Mechanisms of axon ensheathment and myelin growth. *Nat. Rev. Neurosci.* 6:683–690.

93. Park, J., Koito, H., Li, J., and Han, A. 2009. Microfluidic compartmentalized co-culture platform for CNS axon myelination research. *Biomed. Microdevices* 11:1145–1153.

94. Marimuthu, M., and Kim, S. 2011. Microfluidic cell coculture methods for understand-ing cell biology, analyzing bio/pharmaceuticals, and developing tissue constructs. *Anal. Biochem.* 13:81–89.

95. Grodzinsky, A., Levenston, M., Jin, E., and Frank, H. 2000. Cartilage tissue remodeling in response to mechanical forces. *Annu. Rev. Biomed. Eng.* 2:691–713.

96. Leclerc, E., Sakai, Y., and Fujii, T. 2003. A multi-layer PDMS microfluidic device for tissue engineering applications. *Proceedings of MEMS*, Kyoto, Japan, January 19–23.

97. Powers, M., Domansky, K., Kaazempur-Mofrad, M., Kalezi, A., Capitano, A., Upadhyaya, A., Kurzawski, P., et al. 2002. A microfabricated array bioreactor for perfused 3D liver culture. *Biotech. Bioeng.* 78:257–269.

98. Cullen, D. K., Vukasinovic, J., Glezer, A., and LaPlaca, M. C. 2007. Microfluidic engi-neered high cell density three-dimensional neural cultures. *J. Neural Eng.* 4:159–172.

99. Korin, N., Bransky, A., Dinnar, U., and Levenberg, S. 2007. A parametric study of human fibroblasts culture in a microchannel bioreactor. *Lab Chip* 7:611–617.

100. Lowery, J. L., Datta, N., and Rutledge, G. C. 2010. Effect of fiber diameter, pore size and seeding method on growth of human dermal fibroblasts in electrospun poly(3-caprolactone) fibrous mats. *Biomaterials* 31:491–504.

101. Pu, F., Rhodes, N. P., Bayon, Y., Chen, R., Brans, G., Benne, R., and Hunt, J. A. 2010. The use of flow perfusion culture and subcutaneous implantation with fibroblast-seeded PLLA-collagen 3D scaffolds for abdominal wall repair. *Biomaterials* 31:4330–4340.

102. Liao, J., Guo, X., Grande-Allen, K. J., Kasper, F. K., and Mikos, A. G. 2010. Bioactive polymer/extracellular matrix scaffolds fabricated with a flow perfusion bioreactor for cartilage tissue engineering. *Biomaterials* 31:8911–8920.

10 Fabrication of Mobile Hybrid Microswimmers Using Micro/Nanoparticles and Bacterial Flagella

U. Kei Cheang and Min Jun Kim
Drexel University

CONTENTS

10.1 INTRODUCTION

There has been a great deal of interest in microrobotics with many applications, for example, in robotic drug delivery and therapeutic mechanisms.[1–6] These hold the promise of providing targeted delivery for maximal therapeutic value while minimizing possible side effects, for example, in chemotherapy. While microswimmers can navigate fluids such as the bloodstream, targeted delivery requires the payload to penetrate mucosal and epithelial barriers, and finally move through soft tissues such as organs and tumors to reach its final destination. So far, microswimmers have been based on our knowledge of the fluid dynamics of swimming locomotion in Newtonian media, such as dilute aqueous solutions, which have a long history of study. However, only recently, a systematic attempt has been made to understand how propulsion is modified in more complex environments.

Living tissues and cells are typically very different from linear Newtonian fluid. Tissues are complex media that can be described as a mixture of biopolymers, deformable cellular structures, and viscous fluid. As a result, tissues usually display strongly non-Newtonian behavior including viscoelasticity and nonlinearity. Viscoelasticity usually results in a delayed reaction of flow to stress, while nonlinearity makes the flow nonlinearly dependent on stress. Consequently, one might expect motility of mechanical devices and living organisms through tissues, cells, and mucus to be markedly different. Swimming through such complex materials can result in significant changes in behavior.[7] While many varieties of microscopic swimming robots are under development, this chapter will introduce newly developed techniques to create hybrid biotic/abiotic microrobots that employ the propulsive machinery of bacteria, the flagella. The unique polymeric structure of flagella can adopt different shapes depending on the local chemical and flow conditions and their motion induces a local flow that can be used to propel cells as well as much larger structures through low Reynolds number environments.

10.1.1 Biomedical Purposes

In recent years, there are vast developments in the biomedical technologies. As scientists, clinicians, and engineers work toward overcoming clinical challenges, one must consider the limitations of existing technologies and knowledge with respect to the techniques and approaches that can be used in a realistic setting. While sophisticated medical technologies exist today, the advances in nanotechnology and bioengineering will serve to revolutionize the medical technological industry.

One particular area that is of great interest is drug delivery. At the frontier of drug delivery-related research, engineers are working to combine robotics and control principles with microbiology to achieve active targeted drug delivery systems. Through precise control of miniaturized robots and the ability to control dosage through payload, effective minimally invasive drug administration can be carried out. Currently, various approaches have been taken to develop means for locomotive navigation and transportation in low Reynolds number environment.

While the final goal is to achieve active targeted drug delivery, a number of constraints must be met along the way. In order to be used for a drug delivery vehicle, these robots must operate in micro- or nanoscale, powered by a wireless source, able to navigate in complex biological fluid environment and capable of penetrating soft tissue. Micro- and nanoscale fabrication is limited by the technologies and techniques currently available; however, nonconventional methods have shown success in fabricating these miniaturized swimming robots. The issue of finding a wireless power source has been thoroughly explored; while chemical and electrical methods have been considered, the concern with possible health-related complications for biomedical application quickly led to their dismissal. Magnetic control became a prominent choice due to minimum health impact, fast response time, and precision control. The remaining concerns are navigation through biological media and penetration through soft tissues; both of these aspects become prominent areas of research.

10.1.1.1 Active Targeted Drug Delivery

Microrobotic development of active-controlled drug delivery mechanisms has been based on either chemical or mechanical means. Mechanical propulsion has so far been based on our understanding of microbial swimming in Newtonian fluids. However, for targeted drug delivery, microrobots must not only swim in fluids such as the bloodstream but also penetrate materials with more complex response, such as mucus, epithelium, and tissues. This is the main roadblock in applying targeted drug delivery, gene therapy, ionizing radiation, or hyperthermia.[8-17] Indeed, this requirement for flexible propulsion through a variety of media has analogs in microbial infection. For example, *Helicobacter pylori* swims through the gastric mucus lining the interior of the stomach.[18] An example of the latter occurs as the helically shaped spirochetes *Treponema pallidum* or *Borrelia burgdorferi* spread through tissue at the beginning of a syphilis or Lyme disease infection, respectively.[19,20] Thus, bio-inspired propulsion strategies are likely to provide a route forward for propulsion in soft tissues as well as fluids.

Despite the importance of non-Newtonian behavior of microorganisms, only recently has motility in non-Newtonian media begun to be systematically studied. Theoretical studies have mostly focused on infinite swimmers undergoing wave-like swimming strokes,[21-24] although more realistic finite-length swimmers are beginning to be analyzed.[25,26] Although experiments have established that swimming can be qualitatively different in complex media due to changes in swimming speeds,[19,27-30] gaits,[31] or even swimming strategies,[18] well-controlled experiments have been required to provide the level of quantitative comparison to theory necessary to validate and improve our understanding of the hydrodynamics of locomotion in such media.

Recent developments in nanotechnology and bio-inspired swimming have sparked the interest to investigate controllable micro- and nanoscale devices capable of locomotion in low Reynolds number and complex fluid environment in order to address the challenges of developing a suitable propulsion strategy for drug delivery. A sperm-like microswimmer[32] and an artificial nanocoil swimmer[33] have been experimentally reported to achieve controlled locomotion of man-made microstructures by oscillating transverse magnetic fields. However, both swimmers did not demonstrate swimming in complex fluid or penetration of tissue-like material. Other microswimmers have been developed that make use of magnetic fields to travel to specific tracks,[34–36] but these utilize magnetic gradients, which must be strong in order to give the magnetic nanoparticles (MNPs) directed motion.[37,38] There are also recent reports on a type of chemical-driven swimmers,[39–41] but the need for a specific engineered chemical environment has presented limitations. Regardless of the delivery technique, controlled transport of nanoparticles through soft tissues remains inefficient and poorly understood.[42–47]

Bacteria-inspired robotic microswimmers described in this chapter involve a number of MNPs (to allow additional degree of control) coupled to a drug-containing particle via bacterial flagellar filaments, which are also employed for the generation of propulsion. Utilizing bacterial flagellar polymorphic transformation[48] as a direct fluid actuation and sensing of a nanoscale structural "machine" at low Reynolds number and generating rotational magnetic field[49,50] for propulsion and penetration are more robust in elastic environments, compared with the methods that rely on fluid environments, such as diffusiophoresis or fluid-structure interactions. It has been shown in the literature that MNPs can be given a torque sufficient to cause rotation with small field on the order of 1–10 mT,[51,52] which means that patients undergoing treatment with such a device would experience less intense magnetic fields, and thus lower chances of complications from exposure to magnetic fields. Also, the nanoparticles tend to accumulate in the tissue that comes between the magnet and the desired target.[37] The active motility of the robotic microswimmers will allow the devices to propel themselves[53] through such tissues and eliminate the aggregation of particles in the tissues between the magnetic source and the target. Results from the theoretical and experimental work have improved understanding of how the mechanics of bacterial flagella works in both natural and engineered systems for swimming in complex media, and how these systems might be designed to achieve the transport of therapeutic carriers and propulsion-controlled soft tissue penetration.

10.1.1.2 Interaction with Biomechanical Microstructure of Soft Biological Tissues

While the idea of utilizing swimming robots for drug delivery showed potential, many fundamental and physical limitations remain which must be properly addressed. Currently, no studies have modeled a realistic scenario for drug delivery. Preliminary success had been published in the aspect of swimming capability in Newtonian fluidic environment and controllability via a wireless power source. However, navigation in a human body will introduce much complicity such as complex material properties and adverse flow. Once again, many microorganisms had been investigated to have the ability to overcome the conditions of *in vivo* navigation, and thus, understanding the interaction between microorganisms and the biomechanical of the soft biological tissue and other bio-media is essential in developing artificial robotic microswimmers for drug delivery.

Many microorganisms swim through complex biomaterials, including sperm traveling through mucus in the female reproductive tract and bacteria penetrating mucus layers in the respiratory and digestive tracts during infection and disease. Because the scale of microstructural features in such media can be similar to the size of microbes, microbial transport through these biomaterials is a complicated multiscale problem.

At the microscale, mechanical deformation, long- and short-range hydrodynamic forces, and contact forces (including van der Waals, electrostatic, and chemical binding) can all potentially influence microbial swimming. Macroscale transport through biomaterials depends on swimming speeds and adhesion lifetimes mediated by all these microscale interactions. For example, spirochetes in gelatin display different modes of locomotion depending on the number of their adhesions to the medium. These modes of locomotion are similar to those observed for spirochetes infecting living hosts.

Although the work described above has been able to elucidate how macroscopic viscoelasticity affects swimming in complex media, it is becoming clearer that microscale medium properties may be as or more important in determining locomotive properties. Often the biomaterials we are concerned with, such as mucus or tissues, have a heterogeneous component in addition to water. For example, mucus contains a network of fibers made up of glycoprotein mucin, and mammalian sperm ($Re \approx 10^{-4}$) with head sizes of 3–5 μm and length 30–70 μm encounter mucin fibers (diameter = 102 nm) in cervical mucus which form a network with mesh sizes up to 25 μm.

A theoretical approach to understand the effect of microstructural components[54] is to explicitly model the microstructure as an additional dynamic phase occupying the same space as the solvent phase and interacting with both the solvent phase and the swimmer. Even though this approach does not take the precise details of microstructure into account, it was found that the interaction between the swimmers and the microstructure can significantly affect swimming properties[7,54] via the "friction" force exerted on a swimmer moving past the nonaqueous phase. Since this "friction" is sensitive to detailed mechanical, chemical, electrostatic, and van der Waals interactions between the swimmer and the medium structures, all of these interactions can potentially influence swimming.

The scale of microstructural features in biological environments relative to the size of microbial swimmers also suggests that mechanical details of the medium need to be investigated more thoroughly. Solutions of polymers such as methylcellulose are homogeneous on the micron scale of microbial swimmers, but many biomaterials are spatially heterogeneous on the scale of bacteria. For example, sperm cell bodies and flagella are visibly embedded within the voids of the microstructural network of the medium.[7] Clearly, from the sperm's perspective, the medium is not homogeneous. Since the sperm and the network have similar length scales, homogeneous continuum models that ignore the microstructure of the mucin fibers likely miss important physics. Importantly, the relative size of the mucin network mesh has important biological functions; near ovulation the mesh size becomes larger (up to 25 μm),[7,55] which is thought to aid the sperm in reaching the ovum.[56] For such large mesh sizes, sperm in cervical mucus see a sparse network and may move mostly through voids in the network; thus, long-range hydrodynamic interactions between the network and the swimmer may be most important. However, at other times during the menstrual cycle, mesh sizes can decrease to 1 μm or smaller[7,55] and short-range interactions between the sperm and the network, which may depend on complex surface chemistry and electrostatic properties, become increasingly important.

In these scenarios, microscale mechanical response of complex biological media can influence microbial swimming. First, since biomaterials in mucus and tissues are compliant, they can deform in response to stresses generated by locomoting bacteria. This deformation can affect swimming properties; recent experiments have shown that nematodes in granular media[29,30] push aside granules as they swim, leaving a voided path behind them. Second, the microscale mechanics of the medium components generates the macroscale material properties (bulk moduli) of the medium.

Infectious spirochetes such as *B. burgdorferi*, which causes Lyme disease, also demonstrate how a complicated combination of factors impacts swimming through microstructured media. These spirochetes infect ticks and mammals during their normal life cycle; humans are incidentally infected when bitten by ticks. In ticks, the spirochetes live in the midgut and salivary glands, but it must also penetrate epithelia and associated polymeric networks to reach the fluid hemocoel in order to move from one organ to the other. In mammals, the spirochetes traverse the extracellular matrix and vascular endothelium to move into and out of the bloodstream as they spread throughout the body. Thus these bacteria move through a variety of complex fluid and solid environments. Recently, their movement through mouse dermis tissues has been studied in more detail,[57] and observations of spirochetes in these tissues and gelatin models of tissues demonstrate the important role that adhesion may play in locomotion.[57,58] Only 20%–30% of the spirochetes translocate smoothly through space; the rest engage in "wriggling" and "lunging" motions with one or more adhesive attachments to the medium. Individual spirochetes dynamically transition back and forth between different types of motion as adhesions bind and unbind.[58] Homogeneous models of swimming in viscoelastic gels[54,58] seem to capture translocating velocity when spirochetes are not adhered to media, but population dissemination is strongly influenced by the fraction of spirochetes adhered to the media. For spirochetes in actual tissue or gelatin models, it is difficult to control the strength of adhesion; thus, one cannot controllably differentiate mechanical, hydrodynamic, and adhesive effects on swimming in these biological systems.

10.2 BIO-INSPIRED ENGINEERING AND LOCOMOTION

In order to properly address the challenges in active targeted drug delivery using robotic microswimmer technology, locomotion of the robotic delivery vehicles must be suitable to navigate inside a human body. The conditions that the swimmer must overcome are (1) low Reynolds fluidic environment, (2) complex fluidic environment, (3) soft tissue obstacles, and (4) adverse flow. Under the low Reynolds condition, the microswimmer must comply with microfluidic transport phenomena, which are fundamentally different from their macroscale counterpart[59]; therefore, most of the macroscale propulsion strategies cannot be used.[53]

Biologically inspired methodologies became a promising approach; as more is understood from microorganisms and their propulsion systems, it became apparent that bio-inspired engineering has a great potential to overcome the conditions mentioned. More prominent is the bacterial flagellar propulsion system that has been studied to be very effective in swimming and relatively easy to model. The robotic swimmer focused in this chapter directly utilizes the bacterial flagella to create artificial bacteria or robotic microswimmers.

For the task of swimming in various environments, inspiration was drawn from flagellated bacteria,[60] utilizing the polymorphic transformation of bacterial flagellar filaments[48] as a direct fluid actuation of a nanoscale structural "machine" at low Reynolds numbers. Bacterial flagella have been chosen as an ideal material for use in an artificial microswimmer because of their excellent mechanical properties, their ability to self-assemble from monomers of flagellin protein into long filaments, their suitability for chemical modification and functionalization, and the possibility of genetic engineering of their structure.[50,61] In particular, bacterial flagella undergo polymorphic transformation in both loaded and unloaded conditions due to chemical, electrical, thermal, mechanical, or optical influence. Furthermore, flagellar filaments are capable of remarkable durability and stability.

10.2.1 FLAGELLA

Bacteria such as *Salmonella typhimurium* or *Escherichia coli* are most suited for swimming in low Reynolds number fluid environments due to their ability to rotate their long thin helical flagella, which are extended out into the external aqueous medium, via their flagellar motor.[62] Bacterial flagella are self-assembled spiral nanostructures, 20 nm in diameter and approximately 10 μm in length. They are primarily used by flagellated bacteria for propulsion.[60,63] As mechanical devices, the flagella have extraordinary properties. Despite their small diameter and long length, they are extremely stiff and have an elastic modulus estimated to be in excess of 10^{10} N/m^2. In addition to their elasticity, their polymorphic properties allow them to be used as a bionanomaterial, and ultimately harnessed as actuators for robotic microswimmers. In response to different stimuli (chemical and mechanical), flagella undergo polymorphic transformations, changing their helical handedness and pitch. This transformation is caused by minute (subnanometer) realignment in each of the thousands of molecular monomers (flagellin) that form longitudinal rows along the length of the entire filament (protofilaments). The collective motion of these changes combines to generate changes in length (i.e., strain) by a factor as large as 3. In particular, bacterial flagella undergo polymorphic transformation (Figure 10.1) in both loaded and unloaded conditions due to chemical, electrical, thermal, mechanical, or optical influence. Furthermore, flagellar filaments are capable of remarkable durability and stability. As a matter of fact, it has been shown that flagella withstand high temperature (60°C in physiological saline) and extreme pH (7 ± 4),[64–66] thus allowing them to adapt to a wide range of extreme environmental conditions.

The polymorphic forms of the flagellar filament are possible due to its structural makeup. The flagellar filaments are polymers of a single protein, called flagellin, with a molecular weight of about 55,000 Da, devoid of any known enzymatic activity. (For a general review, see Reference 67.) The normal filament is left-handed with a helical pitch of about 2.2 μm and a helical diameter of about 0.4 μm, with 5340 flagellin subunits per turn. The surface lattice of the filament is hexagonal, and all the subunits can be traced with 1-start, 5-start, 6-start, or 11-start helices. The 11-start helices (protofilaments) are nearly longitudinal. The filaments are helical

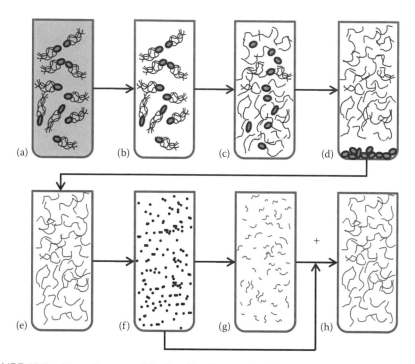

FIGURE 10.1 Flow diagram of the flagellar filament isolation process. (a) Bacteria are cultured in LB broth. (b) The culture is centrifuged and resuspended in polymerization buffer. (c) The resuspended cells are vortexed for 12 min to shear off their flagella. (d) The suspension is centrifuged to pellet the cell bodies and lighter the molecular weight contaminants. (e) The supernatant is retained leaving the purified flagellar filaments. (f) The filaments are depolymerized into monomers at 65°C. (g) Portion of the monomer solution is used to create flagellar seeding particles. (h) The seeds are used to initiate polymerization of monomers into full-length filaments. (Reprinted from *Mater. Sci. Eng. C*, 29, Hesse, W.R., Luo, L., Zhang, G., Mulero, R., et al., Mineralization of flagella for nanotube formation, 2282–2286, Copyright 2009, with permission from Elsevier.)

because the subunits can bond in two different ways, with each protofilament forming a cooperative unit. Filaments with only one type of protofilament are straight. In L-type straight filaments, the 11-start helices twist about 2.5° to the left, while in R-type straight filaments they twist about 7° to the right. The intersubunit distance is 52.5Å (long) for the L-type and 51.8Å (short) for the R-type filament, a difference of only 0.7Å. It is thought that in one protofilament all the flagellins are of only one-bonding type, forming either a long or a short protofilament. The mechanical strain in a filament is minimized if protofilaments of the same type are adjacent to one another.[68,69] This leads to the prediction of 12 polymorphic forms—2 straight, and 10 helical—as shown in Figure 11.1. Each filament in the figure is composed of the same number of subunits; the number of R-type (short) protofilaments increases from top downward: 0, 1, …, 11.

Aside from the polymorphic transformation that made the flagella a favorable microswimmer actuator, the ability to self-assemble *in vitro* and their surface properties made them fully utilizable as a type of bioengineering material. Flagella, as extensions of the bacteria, are naturally around 10 μm. Once sheared of the cell body, the flagella are generally 5 μm. However, the self-assemble capability of the flagella allows for full control over the length of the flagella. Under the proper environmental conditions, such as salinity, ionic strength, NaCl content, temperature, and pH, flagella can vary vastly in length.[48]

10.2.1.1 Engineering and Functionalization

As mentioned earlier, flagella offer many unique advantageous properties as actuators. Flagellar filaments are structurally robust, which stems from their sophisticated self-assembling macromolecular structure made up entirely of the monomer protein flagellin.[70] This property also allows for *in vitro* artificial reconstitution of filaments. Artificially reconstituted filaments can be polymerized up to 70 μm in length after isolation and purification from their bacterial cell bodies.[48] The dynamic properties of flagellar filaments are the characteristics that allow bacteria to swim adaptively. The filament is a tubular structure consisting of 11 strands of protofilaments that are polymer threads made of flagellin.[70] These protofilaments can each assume one of two distinct subunit conformations. The ratio of the conformational states within a filament determines the overall polymorphic helical conformation. These reversible polymorphic conformations can be manipulated by chemical, mechanical, and thermal stimuli,[65,66,71–73] demonstrating the potential to be utilized in engineered applications. In addition to their mechanical and dynamic properties, flagella have proven to be extremely cost efficient and easy to obtain. A saturated culture of *S. typhimurium* containing 10^9 bacteria per milliliter can be cultured in a matter of hours. Each bacterium possesses multiple flagella that can be harnessed using simple protein purification procedures.

As might be expected, one can obtain filaments of different polymorphic forms by using different bacterial strains (different flagellin types) or by mixing different quantities of flagellin obtained from L-type and R-type straight filaments.[74] However, filament morphology not only depends upon flagellin type but also depends upon environmental conditions, for example, pH, ionic strength, and temperature, as established in a series of elegant experiments by Kamiya and Asakura.[66,65,73] Most of these experiments were done with wild-type strains of *Salmonella* (e.g., SJ25, SJ670), but identical results were obtained with an *E. coli* K12 strain (W3623).[75] In 0.1 M KCl, either lowering the pH from 7 to 5 or raising it from 7 to 9 will cause filaments to change from the normal form to the coiled form, reducing their end-to-end length by about a factor of nearly 3. Polymorphic transformations can even go so far as to change the handedness of the flagellar helix. This is an astonishing degree of actuation that argues for the use of flagellar filaments as mechanical actuator.

The surface property of the flagella is another essential aspect needed for engineering applications. The bacterial flagellum is made up of subunits of protein called flagellin. The peptide compound surface of the flagella provides the basis for surface functionalization of the flagella. Of particular interest to the topic of this chapter, *N*-hydroxysuccinimide (NHS) biotinylation of flagella is achievable through the use of NHS esters. This is also known as primary amine biotinylation. Once functionalized, flagella can be attached to particles for engineering applications.[48,49]

10.2.1.2 Spiral Waveform

The perception for the forces and mechanics in the microscale greatly differs from that in the macroscale. The dominant forces, for example, in a microfluidic environment are adhesive interactions and viscous fluid forces, whereas the dominant forces in macroscale fluidics are gravitational and inertial forces.[33,53] The dynamics of these changes are captured in the dimensionless characteristic quantity called Reynolds number that defines the ratio of inertial forces to viscous forces. Conventional macroscale swimming strategies such as paddling would be ineffective in the microscale, which is in the low Reynolds number regime. However, in order to move in microscale, microorganisms utilize different propulsion methods that take advantage of the vicious force rather than momentum.

Multiflagellated bacteria such as *E. coli* and *S. typhimurium* are driven by their flagella. Through the motor, the flagella can rotate counterclockwise, resulting in bundling of flagella filaments that pushes the cell forward. Single-flagellated bacteria such as *Caulobacter crescentus* and *Rhodobacter sphaeroides* can also achieve propulsion through the rotation of their single flagellum. The fundamental propulsive principle that is common to these bacteria is spiral waveform of their rotating flagella. This waveform allows the bacteria to employ corkscrew swimming or spiral swimming.[53,76] As mentioned by Lauga and Powers, the understanding of the evolutionary process of locomotion in low Reynolds environment is imperative to optimization of artificial swimmers; therefore, it is clear that the design of a robotic swimmer should be biomimetic in order to overcome the inherent challenges of drug delivery.

10.3 MATERIALS AND METHODS

This section discusses the fabrication, control method, and analysis of the microswimmers. Because of their size, the microswimmers were created using nonconventional fabrication methodologies. The analysis of their motility was also non-straightforward as a result of the high influence of diffusive motion at microscale. In the end, the microswimmers demonstrated super diffusion that signifies controlled propulsion due to flagellar hydrodynamics.

10.3.1 BIOMIMETIC DEVICE FABRICATION METHODS

Bacteria are a promising model for designing abiotic microswimmers. Compared to other mobile eukaryotic cells, the structure of most bacteria is relatively uncomplicated. Recent research at Drexel[49,50] has demonstrated the key processes to fabricate single- or multiflagellated artificial bacteria, consisting of beads with diameters of 200 nm–3 μm using avidin–biotin linkages. First, polymerized flagella were biotinylated at the amino groups of the surface of the filament using NHS linked to biotin. The biotinylated filaments were depolymerized into biotinylated monomers at 65°C, then repolymerized into seed particles (<1 μm filaments) with sequential addition of nonfunctionalized monomers to create filament with biotin functional groups at one end. Additional biotinylated monomers were added to construct the second functionalized end, thus yielding filaments with biotin groups at both ends.

Next, polystyrene (PS) beads and MNPs were functionalized using purified avidin protein. Finally, the biotinylated flagellar filaments and the avidin-functionalized beads (both PS beads and MNPs) were combined in a reaction mixture dissolved in phosphate buffer to obtain artificial bacteria.

A Helmholtz setup employed as a wireless energy transfer technique was used to generate a rotating magnetic field via two pairs of electromagnetic coils. Bacteria-inspired microswimmers were controlled using a rotating magnetic field. The flagella act as actuators that convert rotational motion of the MNPs to translational motion of the artificial bacteria.

10.3.1.1 Flagella Purification

The flagellar isolation and purification procedure was used by Hesse.[61] Filaments are readily taken apart and reassembled in a stepwise process (Figure 10.1). Bacteria were grown and their filaments harvested by shearing and then depolymerized into subunits of protein called flagellin. If the filaments are detached from cells, they are generally shorter than 10 µm (more like 3 µm) and the distribution of lengths is broad. However, the flagellin can be used to reconstitute long flagellar filaments *in vitro* to give a majority in the range 10–25 µm, with some as long as 75 µm. Once made, they can be stored for months in the polymerization buffer.

The bacteria *S. typhimurium* are cultured using 250 mL of lysogeny broth (LB) [1% NaCl (w/v), 1% tryptone (w/v), 0.5% yeast extract (w/v)] inoculated with 1 mL of frozen *S. typhimurium* and then incubated at 33°C for 16 h with constant shaking. The initial concentration is pelleted by centrifugation for 35 min at a relative centrifugal force (RFC) of 4500× *g* and then resuspended in 1.2 mL of polymerization buffer [0.01 M potassium phosphate buffer (pH 6.5), 150 mM NaCl]. The resuspended bacteria are deflagellated by vortexing at varying positions and orientations for 12 min. The cells bodies that are deflagellated by vortexing are pelleted out by centrifugation for 15 min at 10,000× *g*. The flagella in supernatant are then pelleted using ultracentrifugation for 1 h at 100,000× *g* and 4°C to sediment small debris. The resulting pellet is resuspended in 0.5 mL of polymerization buffer and centrifuged for 15 min at 10,000× *g*. The resulting supernatant is centrifuged at 100,000× *g* and the resulting pellet is resuspended in 0.5 mL of polymerization buffer. The suspension that is obtained contains 1–5 µm long flagellar filaments. Figure 10.1a–h shows a detailed step-by-step schematic of the flagella purification procedure. The image of a flagellar filament in Figure 10.2 was taken using a scanning electron microscope (SEM).

10.3.1.2 Avidin–Biotin Chemistry

Avidin is a tetrameric protein found in egg white and contains four identical subunits that are capable of binding a biotin group, or vitamin B7, in the strongest naturally found noncovalent bond.[77] Biotin is widely used in biochemical assays because of its small size and high-protein functionality capabilities.[78] The process of affixing this molecule onto a protein, nucleic acid, or other molecule is called biotinylation.[79] The molecule avidin has a great affinity for biotin (dissociation constant, $K_d = 10^{-14}$), which makes it an ideal candidate for binding with the biotin. Biotinylated proteins, such as flagella, can be isolated and exploited because of this high-affinity bonding

FIGURE 10.2 Flagellar filament visualized using SEM.

between the two molecules. Additionally, avidin has a high resistance to denaturation in extreme condition due to its tetrameric structure.

According to Orth,[80] avidin–biotin chemistry has been used in the past as a biomaterial immobilization device. This bond is very stable and can withstand a wide range of chemical pH fluctuations that are beneficial to our procedure. Orth's research parallels to this case as applied to DNA protein instead of flagella. Orth was successful in immobilizing DNA protein on a silicon substrate. These aspects of the procedure were modified to suit the needs for attaching flagella to micro- and nanoparticles.

10.3.1.3   Site-Specific Functionalization of Flagella

Flagellar filaments are biotinylated specifically at the amino groups of the entire surface of the filament using NHS linked to biotin with 3 h of incubation at room temperature with constant shaking. Following biotinylation, the filaments are depolymerized into biotinylated monomers (the protein flagellin) via a water bath at 65°C. The biotinylated monomers are mixed with repolymerization buffer (2 M Na_2SO_4 in potassium phosphate buffer, pH 6.5) and incubated at room temperature for 45 min on a shaker. This yields flagellar seeds that have biotin groups at the surface, which serve to initiate flagellar polymerization. Nonbiotinylated flagellar monomers are added to the biotinylated seeds and incubated for 36 h at room temperature on a shaker. This will result in unidirectional polymerization,[81] yielding flagellar filaments that are biotinylated only at one end of the flagella. Afterward, additional biotinylated monomers are added with a sequential incubation for 12 h at room temperature. This reaction will continue the polymerization process with the newly added biotinylated monomers and sequentially yield flagellar filaments that have biotin groups only at both ends of the filament. The detailed flagellar functionalization procedure is described in Figure 10.3a–f.

10.3.1.4   Particle Functionalization and Manipulation

In order to functionalize a magnetic bead with avidin, the surface of the bead must be chemically modified. The bead is first plasma cleaned to remove excess carbon or other molecules from the surface. The bead surface is then treated with a 3-aminopropyltriethoxysilane (APTES) for the purpose of attaching an amino group

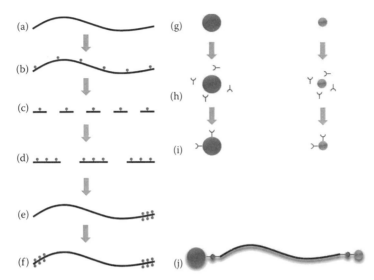

FIGURE 10.3 Schematic for microswimmer fabrication. (a) Filaments isolated from bacteria culture. (b) Biotinylation of flagella. (c) Depolymerization of biotinylated flagella into monomers. (d) Repolymerization of monomers into biotinylated seeding particles. (e) Polymerization into one-ended biotinylated flagella by introducing nonbiotinylated monomers. (f) Polymerization into two-ended biotinylated flagella by introducing additional biotinylated monomers. (g) Nonfunctionalized PS beads and MNPs. (h) Introduction of avidin to particles. (i) Avidination of particles. (j) Assembly of two-ended biotinylated flagella and avidinated particles into dumbbell microswimmers.

to the surface, incubated for 10 min, and then rinsed with isopropanol. Next, glutaric acid is introduced onto the APTES-treated surface to create a glutaraldehyde layer[82] that serves as a cross-linker for avidin and incubated for 2 h. Once the bead is rinsed with phosphate buffered saline (PBS), the surface is prepared for avidination. Finally, avidin solution (10 mg/mL) is introduced onto the surface of the chemically modified iron oxide particle with sequential incubation for 24 h in humid environment to prevent evaporation of avidin solution.

To achieve precise control over the configuration of the flagella, for example, the location of flagellar attachment and the orientation of the MNP, a manufacturing process can be used to fabricate microswimmers using self-assembly methodologies shown in Figure 10.4. This method involves the fabrication of patterns or nanoarrays on glass chips using the focused ion beam (FIB). Some important considerations that needed to be considered include the fact that beads should only fall into the wells of their respective sizes, that is, size separation, and that the excess beads should be washed away from the surface of the glass. Following size separation, biotinylated flagella will be introduced and attached to beads, releasing the microswimmers into solution without incurring damage to their structure. These considerations were kept in mind and a novel self-assembly technique was developed. The glass chip was first coated with approximately 3.8 nm layer of platinum/palladium using a sputter coater. This layer was necessary in order to accurately focus and drill the nanoarrays using the FIB/SEM system. Also, this layer allowed for only the bottoms of the wells to be

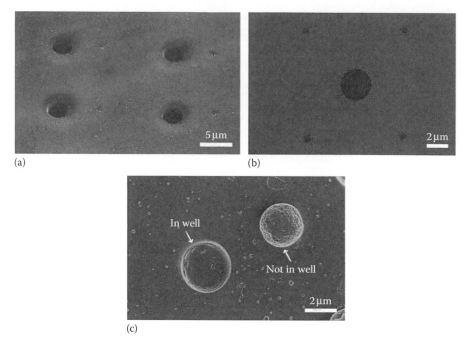

FIGURE 10.4   (a) A 2 × 2 (rows × columns) nanoarray (glass substrate) created using the FIB with large wells for the 3 μm PS beads and small wells for the 150 nm magnetic beads. (b) A nanowell pattern for fabrication of multiflagellated microswimmer created using the FIB. (c) SEM image of a PS bead of approximately 2.5 μm diameter in a well compared with a PS bead not in a well to the right.

made of glass while the rest of the surface of the chip was coated with metal. The advantage of this is that following the drilling procedure, the chip was plasma treated and perfluorodecyltrichlorosilane (PFDTCS) was deposited onto the surface as a monolayer using chemical vapor deposition (CVD). This silane layer was only within wells and allowed for preferential binding of beads in them at the bottom, whereas the beads on the surface of the glass chip were on metal and could be washed away easily.

10.3.2   MICROSWIMMERS STRUCTURES

The biotinylated flagellar filaments and the avidinated beads (both PS beads and MNPs) were combined in a reaction mix, dissolved in phosphate buffer, and incubated for 5 h at room temperature on a shaker to obtain dumbbell microswimmers. SEM image in Figure 10.5a shows a single flagellum connected to a bead and the image in Figure 10.5b shows multiple flagella connected to each bead. Likewise for the FIB nanowell method, biotinylated filaments can be added on the positioned beads in the wells. Since the well partially inhibits the surface of the attached beads, flagella can only attach on the exposed area. This in turn gives control over the location of flagellar attachment by changing how much of the beads' surface is exposed through manipulation of the depth of the wells.

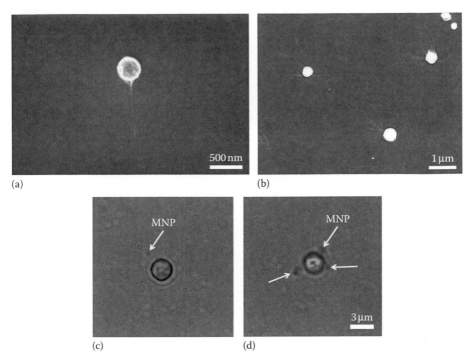

FIGURE 10.5 Microswimmers fabricated using the avidin–biotin chemistry. (a) Single flagellum attached to a bead. (b) Multiple flagella attached to each bead. (c) Single-flagellated dumbbell microswimmer. (d) Multiflagellated microswimmer.

Both of the previously mentioned methods are able to produce multiple configurations of microswimmer, while the nanowell method provides greater control over the production of the desired configuration. There are two desirable configurations: (1) dumbbell microswimmer and (2) multiflagellate microswimmer. These configurations are shown in Figure 10.5c and d.

10.3.2.1 Dumbbell Helical Swimming

The dumbbell microswimmer consists of a PS bead connected to an MNP via a flagellar filament. Once the MNP rotates, the flagella connected will rotate as a helix. The form of the helix depends on the polymorphic form of the flagella under the specific environment conditions. When sufficient "power" is applied, the entire microswimmer will rotate and create propulsion, similar to the propulsive mechanism of bacterial flagella.

Under an enclosed environment in a polydimethylsiloxane (PDMS) fluidic cell with no flow, swimming of the dumbbell swimmers was observed. As a dumbbell swimmer, the flagella linkage that connects the two beads is used for propulsion, much like a bacteria. Upon actuation, the flagella will generate a spiral waveform needed to generate the hydrodynamics for swimming. Through the MNP, the flagella will be actuated by the rotating magnetic field generated by a Helmholtz coil system.

The Helmholtz coil system consists of an electromagnetic generator that is mounted on a Leica DMIRB inverted microscope and connected to three power supplies for 3D control. The Data Acquisition (DAQ) controller and LabVIEW interface function to generate sinusoidal inputs to the two of the power supplies with 90° phase lag between them, allowing the coil system to create rotation in the homogeneous magnetic field at the center.

With the ability to control the magnetic field's strength through the current input and the frequency of its rotation through the LabVIEW algorithm, the form of the swimming can be fully controlled by considering the torque applied by the magnetic field and the damping by the rotation. The applied magnetic torque is expressed as

$$T_m = \mu \times H = \mu H \sin \theta \tag{10.1}$$

where T_m is the magnetic torque, μ the magnetic moment of the MNP, and H the magnetic field. The resistive torque caused by damping is expressed as

$$T_r = D_{PS}\omega + D_{MNP}\omega + \frac{EL}{\omega} \tag{10.2}$$

where T_r is the resistive torque, D the rotational damping coefficient for the particles, ω the angular velocity, E the rate of work on the fluid by the flagella, and L the length of flagellar helix. The magnetic torque, T_m, must be greater than the resistive torque, T_r; if T_m is less than T_r, the magnetic beads will fail to follow the rotation of the magnetic field under high frequencies. The magnetic beads have very low magnetic moment due to their microscale size. Moreover, magnetic beads are fabricated using an emulsion; therefore, the magnetic content is moderate. Through the use of the Helmholtz coil system, the strength of the applied magnetic field as well as the frequency of the rotation can be altered, thus precisely controlling the rotation of the magnetic beads.

Microswimmers were created using 1 μm PS beads and 300 nm MNPs, and examined for movement. As a benchmark, the microswimmers were first tested in the fluid chamber without applying a magnetic field. The microswimmer demonstrated the rapid Brownian motion due to the diffusion of the PS microbead, MNP, and the flagellar coupler. The diffusivity of the microswimmer accounts for the internal dynamics of the change in distance between the PS microbead and the MNP. Therefore, the microswimmer has an enhanced diffusivity because of the bead-to-bead hydrodynamic interaction.[83]

For this case study, a rotating magnetic field was applied across the fluid chamber. An output voltage of 10 V (4.5 A) was applied to the X and Z coil pairs to produce rotating fields of 2.2 mT in the XZ planes. The rotational frequency of the rotating field is 100 Hz, which corresponds to the typical frequency of the bacterial flagellar motor.[84] The movement of the microswimmer due to flagellar propulsion was readily apparent when compared to the benchmark test. This actuation is due to the rotation of the MNP inducing flagella hydrodynamics. The microswimmer moved in positive Y direction from the initial position with an average speed of 1.3 μm/s. Experiments reveal that the response of the microswimmers was consistent unless they had formed some type of attachment to the substrate. The diffusion of the microswimmers in a no-field condition was computed to serve as a benchmark, and then the diffusion of the swimmers under the said field is computed and compared with the benchmark. An example of the path of a microswimmer is shown in Figure 10.6. After observing and

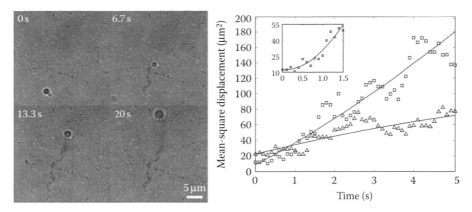

FIGURE 10.6 Microswimmer actuated under a rotating magnetic field with frequency comparable to flagellar motor of *E. coli*. The microswimmer moved consistently in the positive *Y* direction with a mean velocity of 1.3 µm/s over a time span of 20 s. (Reprinted with permission from Cheang, U.K., Roy, D., Lee, J.H., and Kim, M.J. 2010. Fabrication and magnetic control of bacteria-inspired robotic microswimmers. *Appl. Phys. Lett.* 97:213704. Copyright 2010, American Institute of Physics.)

tracking numerous microswimmers, their ensemble displacement is used to analyze their motility. The plot in Figure 10.6 shows the mean-square displacement (MSD) of the benchmark compared with swimming microswimmers. Based on the correlation at small timescale ($t < 1$ s), the microswimmers exhibited ballistic motion. At $t > 1$ s, ballistic-driven motion transitions into translational diffusive motion. The diffusion of the swimmer under a rotating field is much greater than the no-field benchmark. This signifies propulsion due to flagella hydrodynamics.

10.3.2.2 Multiflagellated Propeller

Lophotrichous and peritrichous bacteria are characterized by their multiflagellated nature. These multiflagellated organisms swim by bundling their flagella to create a net thrust. Kim et al. used a macroscale model to characterize the hydrodynamics of bundling flagella. As reported, two flagellar filaments bundled can induce flow, that is, in agreement with a single flagellum with twice the radius.[85] Likewise, an artificial swimmer is not restricted by single-flagellated configuration as shown from the previously mentioned dumbbell swimmer. Multiple flagella can be conjugated with magnetic particles to form multiflagellated microswimmers. Through the use of multiple flagella, the swimmer will be able to increase propulsive power through bundling of flagella, as do bacteria.

10.4 CONCLUSION

In the interest of using robotic systems for drug delivery, it is imperative to seek the proper methodologies to overcome inherent challenges presented in this problem. In order to develop such a system, great consideration must be placed on the microscale environment, complex properties of the medium, soft tissue obstacles, and adverse flow in a realistic drug delivery scenario. Many microorganisms have proven to possess the ability to overcome these issues. Specifically, many disease-causing bacteria have the ability to navigate the human body. These scenarios became inspirations for many different approaches. The microswimmer focused in this chapter closely mimics the spiral swimming of the bacteria by directly utilizing the bacterial flagella in the fabrication process. As a result, the microswimmer harnessed the preferential properties of the flagella and demonstrated propulsion when controlling a rotating magnetic field.

ACKNOWLEDGMENTS

The authors acknowledge Dalhyung Kim, Wonjin Jo, and Anmiv Prabhu for their invaluable assistance with particle tracking and support for SEM. The authors thank Dr. Boris Polyak for supplying MNPs. They especially thank William Hesse, David Casale, Basil Milton, and Dheeraj Roy for their contributions and insightful discussions.

REFERENCES

1. Nelson, B.J., Kaliakatsos, I.K., and Abbott, J.J. 2010. Microrobots for minimally invasive medicine. *Annu. Rev. Biomed. Eng.* 12:55–85.
2. Sitti, M. 2009. Miniature devices: Voyage of the microrobots. *Nature* 458:1121–1122.
3. Martel, S., Felfoul, O., Mohammadi, M., and Mathieu, J.B. 2008. Interventional procedure based on nanorobots propelled and steered by flagellated magnetotactic bacteria for direct targeting of tumors in the human body, in *Conference Proceedings—IEEE Engineering in Medicine and Biology Society*, August 31–September 4, 2010, Buenos Aires, Argentina, p. 2497–2500.
4. Cavalcanti, A., Shirinzadeh, B., Freitas, R.A., and Hogg, T. 2008. Nanorobot architecture for medical target identification. *Nanotechnology* 19:015103.
5. Steager, E.B., Sakar, M.S., Kim, D.H., Kumar, V.J., et al. 2011. Electrokinetic and optical control of bacterial microrobots. *J. Micromech. Microeng.* 21:035001.
6. Kagan, D., Laocharoensuk, R., Zimmerman, M., Clawson, C., et al. 2010. Rapid delivery of drug carriers propelled and navigated by catalytic nanoshuttles. *Small* 6:2741–2747.
7. Rutllant, J., López-Béjar, M., and López-Gatius, F. 2005. Ultrastructural and rheological properties of bovine vaginal fluid and its relation to sperm motility and fertilization: A review. *Reprod. Domest. Anim.* 40:79–86.
8. Polyak, B., Fishbein, I., Chorny, M., Alferiev, I., et al. 2008. High field gradient targeting of magnetic nanoparticle-loaded endothelial cells to the surfaces of steel stents. *Proc. Natl. Acad. Sci. USA* 105:698–703.
9. Chorny, M., Polyak, B., Alferiev, I.S., Walsh, K., et al. 2007. Magnetically driven plasmid DNA delivery with biodegradable polymeric nanoparticles. *FASEB J.* 21:2510–2519.
10. Hafeli, U.O., Sweeney, S.M., Beresford, B.A., Humm, J.L., et al. 1995. Effective targeting of magnetic radioactive 90Y-microspheres to tumor cells by an externally applied magnetic field. Preliminary in vitro and in vivo results. *Nucl. Med. Biol.* 22:147–155.
11. Johannsen, M., Thiesen, B., Jordan, A., Taymoorian, K., et al. 2005. Magnetic fluid hyperthermia (MFH) reduces prostate cancer growth in the orthotopic Dunning R3327 rat model. *Prostate* 64:283–292.

12. Lubbe, A.S., Alexiou, C., and Bergemann, C. 2001. Clinical applications of magnetic drug targeting. *J. Surg. Res.* 95:200–206.
13. Lubbe, A.S., Bergemann, C., and Alexiou, C. 2002. Targeting tumors with magnetic drugs. *Tumor Target. Cancer Ther.* 34:379–388.
14. Pan, S., Gulati, R., Mueske, C.S., Witt, T.A., et al. 2004. Gene transfer of a novel vasoactive natriuretic peptide stimulates cGMP and lowers blood pressure in mice. *Am. J. Physiol. Heart Circ. Physiol.* 286:2213–2218.
15. Pislaru, S.V., Harbuzariu, A., Gulati, R., Witt, T., et al. 2006. Magnetically targeted endothelial cell localization in stented vessels. *J. Am. Coll. Cardiol.* 48:1839–1845.
16. Pislaru, S.V., Harbuzariu, A., Agarwal, G., Witt, T., et al. 2006. Magnetic forces enable rapid endothelialization of synthetic vascular grafts. *Circulation* 114:314–318.
17. Polyak, B. and Friedman, G. 2009. Magnetic targeting for site-specific drug delivery: Applications and clinical potential. *Expert Opin. Drug Deliv.* 6:53–70.
18. Celli, J.P., Turner, B.S., Afdhal, N.H., Keates, S., et al. 2009. *Helicobacter pylori* moves through mucus by reducing mucin viscoelasticity. *Proc. Natl. Acad. Sci. USA* 106:14321–14326.
19. Berg, H.C. and Turner, L. 1979. Movement of microorganisms in viscous environments. *Nature* 278:349–351.
20. Kimsey, R.B. and Spielman, A. 1990. Motility of Lyme disease spirochetes in fluids as viscous as the extracellular matrix. *J. Infect. Dis.* 162:1205–1208.
21. Fu, H.C., Wolgemuth, C.W., and Powers, T.R. 2008. Beating pattern of filaments in viscoelastic fluids. *Phys. Rev. E* 78:041913.
22. Fu, H.C., Wolgemuth, C.W., and Powers, T.R. 2009. Swimming speeds of filaments in nonlinearly viscoelastic fluids. *Phys. Fluids* 21:033102.
23. Fu, H.C., Powers, T.R., and Wolgemuth, C.W. 2007. Theory of swimming filaments in viscoelastic media. *Phys. Rev. Lett.* 99:258101.
24. Lauga, E. 2007. Propulsion in a viscoelastic fluid. *Phys. Fluids* 19:083104.
25. Teran, J., Fauci, L., and Shelley, M. 2010. Viscoelastic fluid response can increase the speed and efficiency of a free swimmer. *Phys. Rev. Lett.* 104:038101.
26. Zhu, L., Do-Quang, M., Lauga, E., and Brandt, L. 2011. Locomotion by tangential deformation in a polymeric fluid. *Phys. Rev. E* 83:011901.
27. Turner, L., Ryu, W., and Berg, H.C. 2000. Real-time imaging of fluorescent flagellar filaments. *J. Bacteriol.* 182:2793–2801.
28. Shen, X.N. and Arratia, P.E. 2011. Undulatory swimming in viscoelastic fluids. *Phys. Rev. Lett.* 106:208101.
29. Jung, S. 2010. *Caenorhabditis elegans* swimming in a saturated particulate system. *Phys. Fluids* 22:031903.
30. Juarez, G., Lu, K., Sznitman, J., and Arratia, P.E. 2010. Motility of small nematodes in wet granular media. *Europhys. Lett.* 92:44002.
31. Suarez, S. and Dai, X. 1992. Hyperactivation enhances mouse sperm capacity for penetrating viscoelastic media. *Biol. Reprod.* 46:686–691.
32. Dreyfus, R., Baudry, J., Roper, M.L., Fermigier, M., et al. 2005. Microscopic artificial swimmers. *Nature* 437:862–865.
33. Abbott, J.J., Nagy, Z., Beyeler, F., and Nelson, B.J. 2007. Robotics in the Small, Part I: Microbotics. *IEEE Robot Autom. Mag.* 14:92–103.
34. Forbes, Z.G., Yellen, B.B., Halverson, D.S., Fridman, G., et al. 2008. Validation of high gradient magnetic field based drug delivery to magnetizable implants under flow. *IEEE Trans. Biomed. Eng.* 55:643–649.
35. Yellen, B.B., Forbes, Z.G., Halverson, D.S., Fridman, G., et al. 2005. Targeted drug delivery to magnetic implants for therapeutic applications. *J. Magn. Magn. Mater.* 293:647–654.

36. Ghosh, A. and Fischer, P. 2009. Controlled propulsion of artificial magnetic nanostructured propellers. *Nano Lett.* 9:2243–2245.

37. Dobson, J. 2006. Magnetic nanoparticles for drug delivery. *Drug Develop. Res.* 67:55–60.

38. Berry, C.C. and Curtis, A.S.G. 2003. Functionalisation of magnetic nanoparticles for application in biomedicine. *J. Phys. D Appl. Phys.* 36:R198–R206.

39. Wu, J., Kagan, D., Balasubramanian, S., Manesh, K., et al. 2010. Motion-based DNA detection using catalytic nanomotors. *Nat. Commun.* 1:1–6.

40. Wang, J. 2009. Can man-made nanomachines compete with nature biomotors? *ACS Nano* 3:4–9.

41. Gao, W., Sattayasamitsathit, S., Manian Manesh, K., Weihs, D., et al. 2010. Magnetically-powered flexible metal nanowire motors. *J. Am. Chem. Soc.* 132:14403–14405.

42. Barnes, A.L., Wassel, R.A., Mondalek, F., Che, K., et al. 2007. Magnetic characterization of superparamagnetic nanoparticles pulled through model membranes. *BioMagn. Res. Tech.* 5:1–10.

43. Kalambur, V.S., Han, B., Hammer, B.E., Shield, T.W., et al. 2005. In vitro characterization of movement, heating and visualization of magnetic nanoparticles for biomedical applications. *Nanotechnology* 16:1221–1233.

44. Kuhn, S.J., Finch, S.K., Hallahan, D.E., and Giorgio, T.D. 2006. Proteolytic surface functionalization enhances in vitro magnetic nanoparticle mobility through extracellular matrix. *Nano Lett.* 6:306–312.

45. Kuhn, S.J., Hallahan, D.E., and Giorgio, T.D. 2006. Characterization of superparamagnetic nanoparticle interactions with extracellular matrix in an in vitro system. *Annu. Biomed. Eng.* 34:51–58.

46. Mondalek, F.G., Zhang, Y.Y., Kropp, B., Kopke, R.D., et al. 2006. The permeability of SPION over an artificial three-layer membrane is enhanced by external magnetic field. *J. Nanobiotech.* 4:1–9.

47. Rotariu, O., Udrea, L.E., Strachan, N.J.C., and Badescu, V. 2007. The guidance of magnetic colloids in simulated tissues for targeted drug delivery. *J. Optoelectron. Adv. Mater.* 9:942–945.

48. Darnton, N.C. and Berg, H.C. 2007. Force-extension measurements on bacterial flagella: Triggering polymorphic transformations. *Biophys. J.* 92:2230–2236.

49. Cheang, U.K., Roy, D., Lee, J.H., and Kim, M.J. 2010. Fabrication and magnetic control of bacteria-inspired robotic microswimmers. *Appl. Phys. Lett.* 97:213704.

50. Hesse, W.R., Casale, D.M., Milton, B., Fink, P.K., et al. 2009. Biologically inspired drug delivery microrobots. *The 5th International Conference on Microtechnologies in Medicine and Biology,* 1–3 April, Quebec, Canada.

51. Tierno, P., Goldstanian, R., Pagonabarraga, I., and Sagues, F. 2008. Controlled swimming in confined fluids of magnetically actuated colloidal rotors. *Phys. Rev. Lett.* 101:218304.

52. Hu, S., Eberhard, L., Chen, J., Love, C.J., et al. 2008. Mechanical anisotropy of adherent cells probed by a three dimensional magnetic twisting device. *Am. J. Physiol. Cell Physiol.* 287:1184–1191.

53. Purcell, E.M. 1977. Life at low Reynolds number. *Am. J. Phys.* 45:3–11.

54. Fu, H.C., Shenoy, V.B., and Powers, T.R. 2010. Low-Reynolds-number swimming in gels. *Europhys. Lett.* 91:24002.

55. Lai, S.K., Wang, Y.-Y., Wirtz, D., and Hanes, J. 2009. Micro- and macrorheology of mucus. *Adv. Drug Deliv. Rev.* 61:86–100.

56. Suarez, S.S. and Pacey, A.A. 2006. Sperm transport in the female reproductive tract. *Hum. Reprod. Update* 12:23–37.

57. Moriarty, T.J., Norman, M.U., Colarusso, P., Bankhead, T., et al. 2008. Real-time high resolution 3D imaging of the Lyme disease spirochete adhering to and escaping from the vasculature of a living host. *PLoS Pathog.* 4:e1000090.

58. Harman, M.W., Dunham-Ems, S.M., Caimano, M.J., Belperron, A.A., et al. 2012. The heterogeneous motility of the Lyme disease spirochete in gelatin mimics dissemination through tissue. *Proc. Natl. Acad. Sci. U.S.A* 109(8):3059–3064.

59. Lauga, E. and Powers, T.R. 2009. The hydrodynamics of swimming microorganisms. *Rep. Prog. Phys.* 72:096601.

60. Berg, H.C. 2003. E. coli *in Motion*. Springer Verlag, New York.

61. Hesse, W.R., Luo, L., Zhang, G., Mulero, R., et al. 2009. Mineralization of flagella for nanotube formation. *Mater. Sci. Eng. C* 29:2282–2286.

62. Berg, H.C. and Anderson, R.A. 1973. Bacteria swim by rotating their flagellar filaments. *Nature* 245:380–382.

63. Manson, M.D., Tedesco, P., Berg, H.C., Harold, F.M., et al. 1977. A protonmotive force drives bacterial flagella. *Proc. Natl. Acad. Sci. U.S.A* 74:3060–3064.

64. Asakura, S. 1970. Polymerization of flagellin and polymorphism of flagella. *Adv. Biophys.* 1:99–104.

65. Kamiya, R. and Asakura, S. 1976. Helical transformations of *Salmonella* flagella in vitro. *J. Mol. Biol.* 106:167–186.

66. Kamiya, R. and Asakura, S. 1976. Flagellar transformations at alkaline pH. *J. Mol. Biol.* 108:513–518.

67. Namba, K. and Vonderviszt, F. 1997. Molecular architecture of bacterial flagellum. *Q. Rev. Biophys.* 30:1–65.

68. Calladine, C.R. 1978. Change in waveform in bacterial flagella: The role of mechanics at the molecular level. *J. Mol. Biol.* 118:457–479.

69. Kamiya, R., Asakura, S., Wakabayashi, K., and Namba, K. 1979. Transition of bacterial flagella from helical to straight forms with different subunit arrangements. *J. Mol. Biol.* 131:725–742.

70. Calladine, C. 1975. Construction of bacterial flagella. *Nature* 255:121–124.

71. Macnab, R.M. and Ornston, M.K. 1977. Normal-to-curly flagellar transitions and their role in bacterial tumbling. Stabilization of an alternative quaternary structure by mechanical force. *J. Mol. Biol.* 112:1–30.

72. Hotani, H. 1982. Micro-video study of moving bacterial flagellar filaments: III. Cyclic transformation induced by mechanical force. *J. Mol. Biol.* 156:791–806.

73. Hasegawa, E., Kamiya, R., and Asakura, S. 1982. Thermal transition in helical forms of *Salmonella* flagella. *J. Mol. Biol.* 160:609–621.

74. Kamiya, R., Asakura, S., and Yamaguchi, S. 1980. Formation of helical filaments by copolymerization of two types of "straight" flagellins. *Nature* 286:628–630.

75. Kamiya, R., Hotani, H., and Asakura, S. 1982. Polymorphic transition in bacterial flagella. *Symp. Soc. Exp. Biol.* 35:53–76.

76. Keaveny, E.E. and Maxey, M.R. 2008. Spiral swimming of an artificial micro-swimmer. *J. Fluid Mech.* 598:293–319.

77. Diamandis, E.P. and Christopoulos, T.K. 1991. The biotin-(strept)avidin system: Principles and applications in biotechnology. *Clin. Chem.* 37:625–636.

78. Chaiet, L. and Wolf, F.J. 1964. The properties of streptavidin, a biotin-binding protein produced by Streptomycetes. *Arch. Biochem. Biophys.* 106:1–5.

79. Bayer, E.A. and Wilchek, M. 1990. Protein biotinylation. *Methods Enzymol.* 184:138–160.

80. Orth, R.N., Clark, T.G., and Craighead, H.G. 2003. Avidin-biotin micropatterning methods for biosensor applications. *Biomed. Microdevices* 5:29–34.

81. Asakura, S., Eguchi, G., and Iino, T. 1968. Unidirectional growth of *Salmonella* flagella in vitro. *J. Mol. Biol.* 35:227–236.

82. Guesdon, J.L., Ternynck, T., and Avrameas, S. 1979. The use of avidin-biotin interaction in immunoenzymatic techniques. *J. Histochem. Cytochem.* 27:1131–1139.

83. Bammert, J., Schreiber, S., and Zimmermann, W. 2008. Dumbbell diffusion in a spatially periodic potential. *Phys. Rev. E* 77:042102.

84. Darnton, N., Turner, L., Breuer, K., and Berg, H.C. 2004. Moving fluid with bacterial carpets. *Biophys. J.* 86:1863–1870.

85. Kim, M., Kim, M., Bird, J., Park, J., et al. 2004. Particle image velocimetry experiments on a macro-scale model for bacterial flagellar bundling. *Exp. Fluids* 37:782–788.

Part IV

*Nanotoxicity Studies
and Applications
in Eco-Biosystems*

11 Environmental Applications of Nanomaterials

Jaesang Lee, Byoung Chan Kim, and Hun Je Cho
Korea Institute of Science and Technology (KIST)

Changha Lee
Ulsan National Institute of Science and Technology (UNIST)

CONTENTS

11.1 INTRODUCTION

Recent advances in nanotechnology have strongly influenced environmental research, resulting in two opposite strands of research. Some research groups are focusing on the utilization of nanomaterials in environmental applications, whereas others are studying the potential toxic effects of engineered nanoparticles (NPs) on ecosystems and humans.[1,2] The former groups pay more attention to the potential of nanotechnology to solve environmental pollution problems by providing innovative tools for monitoring and controlling contaminants in environmental media. There are growing interests in the development of environmental nanobiosensors incorporated with nanomaterials as a source of transduction signals and carriers for receptors. Recent developments in nanobiosensors have shown great potential to overcome the drawbacks of conventional biosensors, such as low sensitivity, low lifetime, and low specificity, raising the practical applicability in real fields. With the help of nanotechnology, environmental remediation technologies can also be upgraded by employing nanomaterials to manufacture the materials used in the technologies, such as membranes, adsorbents, and catalysts. The unique properties of nanomaterials such as high surface area, catalytic activity, mobility, and diffusivity can enhance the performance of those materials for decontamination. Ironically from another point of view, nanomaterials may be considered as environmental pollutants. As a result of widespread use of NPs by industry, increasing amounts of engineered NPs are being released into the environment. These NPs have a direct impact on ecosystems, and also have a potential effect on human health when they are not effectively removed or treated during the natural transport and in the remediation facilities. In this reason, many efforts are recently being made to investigate the toxicity of NPs as well as the fate and transport of NPs in the environmental media.

11.2 NANOTECHNOLOGY FOR ENVIRONMENTAL REMEDIATION

11.2.1 Decontamination Using Nanomaterials

The environmental cleanup processes such as water treatment, air purification, and soil and groundwater remediation typically adopt the technologies for separation, adsorption, and decomposition of contaminants. In many cases, the performance of these technologies relies on the quality of the materials used in the technologies, for example, membranes, adsorbents, and catalysts. These materials can be upgraded by the application of nanotechnology due to the properties of nanomaterials such as high surface area, high mobility and diffusivity, cell penetrability as well as others. For the past decade, a number of studies have been focused on the environmental applications of nanotechnology at both fundamental and practical levels, and much progress has been made in several applications such as nanoparticulate zero-valent iron (NZVI) for soil and groundwater remediation, nanoparticulate semiconductor photocatalysts for water and air purification, nanostructured adsorbents, and carbon nanotube (CNT)-based membranes. Here, we introduce two major groups of nanomaterials that have been intensively studied for environmental remediation, that is, iron-based nanomaterials and semiconductor photocatalysts.

11.2.2 Iron-Based Nanomaterials

Iron is one of the most abundant elements on earth and relatively nontoxic compared to other metal species. In addition, iron has interesting redox chemistry that can be effectively applied to transformation of organic and inorganic contaminants as well as adsorption of heavy metals. For these reasons, iron has been widely used for the purposes of environmental remediation, particularly for water treatment. Iron has been studied in many forms (metallic, ionic, and oxide forms), as a reagent and a catalyst for applications in wastewater treatment and groundwater remediation, and has been used in real treatment plants and contamination sites. Recently, with rapid development of nanotechnology, many attempts are being made to synthesize and apply iron-based nanomaterials for improved control of water contaminants.

Metallic iron, the so-called zero-valent iron (ZVI, $Fe^0_{(s)}$), has been used in groundwater remediation. ZVI can reductively transform organic contaminants in groundwater such as trichloroethylene (TCE) and perchloroethylene (PCE) into less toxic products. In addition, the ZVI surface adsorbs heavy metals, making them immobile in the aquifer.[3,4] The groundwater remediation technology using ZVI has been applied *in situ* on the contaminated site by the form of permeable reactive barrier (PRB).[3] A PRB filled with granular ZVI is installed in the flume of the contaminated groundwater (Figure 11.1a). The reductive degradation of organic contaminants by ZVI is usually explained by the electron transfer from ZVI surface to the target molecules $[E^0(Fe^{2+}/Fe^0) = -0.447\ V_{NHE}]$.[2,5] However, the degradation of contaminants by bimetallic iron NPs is frequently interpreted by catalytic hydrogenation, according

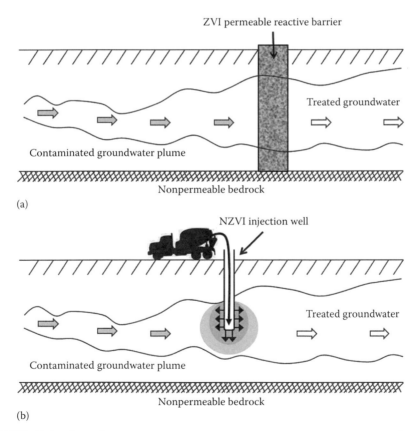

FIGURE 11.1 Groundwater remediation by (a) the ZVI permeable reactive barrier and (b) the direct injection of NZVI.

to which water molecule is reduced to molecular hydrogen by a two-electron transfer from ZVI to water, and subsequently forms active hydrogen atoms on the surface of ZVI.[2,6,7] The active hydrogen is believed to be responsible for the reductive cleavage of chemical bonds of organic contaminants adsorbed on the ZVI surface.

NZVI has been intensively studied as an alternative to granular ZVI in the past decade. Without installing the PRB, *in situ* treatment of soil and groundwater can be performed by directly introducing suspension of NZVI into the contaminated subsurface through injection wells (Figure 11.1b). The high surface area and more active sites on the surface of nanoscale particles greatly enhance the reactivity of ZVI for degradation and adsorption of groundwater contaminants. The improved mobility of NZVI can also be an advantage to treat the contaminants trapped in the small pores of the soil matrix.[4,8] NZVI can be synthesized via various physical methods such as high-energy ball milling and ultrasonic shot peening as well as chemical methods such as liquid- and gas-phase reduction, chemical vapor condensation, and pulse electrodeposition.[4] NZVI so produced usually has a core–shell structure with a single crystal Fe^0 core and a thin iron oxide layer on the surface. The size and the surface area of NZVI typically range 10–100 nm and 20–40 m^2/g, respectively.[4] Many researchers attempted to synthesize bimetallic NPs by depositing noble metals such as palladium (Pd) and nickel (Ni) on the surface of NZVI.[6,7] In this way, NZVI becomes more resistant to oxidation as well as more reactive for the reductive degradation of organic contaminants. It is known that the noble metals provide more reactive catalytic surface than iron for the dissociation of molecular hydrogen into the active atomic form. The molecular hydrogen produced from the reduction of water by ZVI is more effectively converted into atomic hydrogen on the noble metal surface.

The aggregation of NZVI is a problem to be resolved for practical application to *in situ* groundwater remediation. The aggregated NZVI has a less number of active sites on the surface, and the size growth of the aggregates limits the mobility in the subsurface. The magnetic property of NZVI induces magnetic dipole–dipole interactions between the particles, accelerating the aggregation process.[9] In aqueous suspension, the NZVI aggregates at 60–70 mg/L grow up to approximately 1 μm in 30 min.[10] In order to effectively disperse NZVI, organic additives such as starch and polymers have been used as stabilizers.[11–13] However, these materials coated on the ZVI surface can inhibit the electron transfer from ZVI to contaminants or block the adsorption sites for contaminants. It has been reported that the use of longer chain polymers leads to more dispersive suspension of NZVI, but decreases the reactivity for reductive degradation of organic contaminants.[12] It is a major challenge in future studies to maximize the dispersivity of NZVI without significant loss of its reactivity.

NZVI has been mainly considered as a reducing agent for organic contaminants (mostly chlorinated organic compounds) and an adsorbent for heavy metals as mentioned above. However, several recent studies have shown the potential of NZVI for oxidizing organic contaminants in the presence of oxygen (Figure 11.2). The corrosion of NZVI by oxygen produces reactive oxidants capable of transforming organic contaminants. The oxidation of aromatic compounds, chelating agents, and As(III) has been demonstrated by Fe^0 in the presence of oxygen.[14–18] The mechanism through which reactive oxidants are formed by NZVI involves the two-electron oxidation of Fe^0 by molecular oxygen followed by the Fenton reaction. Fe^0 surfaces transfer two

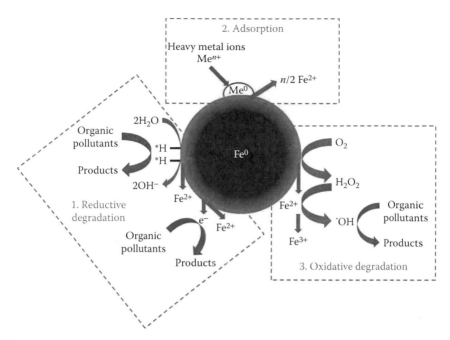

FIGURE 11.2   Decontamination processes mediated by ZVI.

electrons to oxygen to produce hydrogen peroxide (reaction 1), which is subsequently converted into reactive oxidants such as hydroxyl radical ($\cdot$OH) or ferryl ion [Fe(IV)] by reacting with Fe(II), the so-called Fenton reaction (reaction 2). It was found that $\cdot$OH is the predominant oxidant under acidic conditions, but at pH values above 5, Fe(IV) may be formed.[19–21] $\cdot$OH is known as an extremely strong and nonselective oxidant capable of oxidizing a broad spectrum of organic compounds at diffusion-controlled reaction rates.[22] Fe(IV) is also a highly reactive oxidant but is more selective than $\cdot$OH.

$$Fe^0_{(s)} + O_2 \xrightarrow{\ 2H^+\ } Fe^{2+} + H_2O_2 \tag{1}$$

$$Fe^{2+} + H_2O_2 \rightarrow Fe^{3+} + \cdot OH + OH^- \quad \text{or} \quad Fe(IV)\ (FeO^{2+}) + H_2O \tag{2}$$

The oxidation process using NZVI is able to effectively control recalcitrant organic contaminants such as polycyclic aromatic hydrocarbons (PAHs) that are hardly degradable by the reductive pathway. This process could also be a useful approach for the oxidative treatment of wastewater. However, since oxygen is required to produce reactive oxidants from NZVI, extra facilities for aeration are necessary. In addition, the yields of reactive oxidants need to be improved. It has been reported that the yields of converting oxygen into reactive oxidants over NZVI are less than 10%.[21] The low efficiency is mainly attributed to the loss of H_2O_2 via the two-electron transfer reaction on the NZVI surface (reaction 3), where water molecule is formed as the final product.[23,24] Recent studies have shown that the addition of iron-complexing ligands[14,16,25] or polyoxometalate[26,27] and the surface modification with Ni can enhance the yields of reactive oxidants by the reaction of NZVI with oxygen.

$$Fe^0_{(s)} + H_2O_2 \xrightarrow{2H^+} Fe^{2+} + 2H_2O \tag{3}$$

The microbiocidal activity of NZVI can be applied to water disinfection. It has been reported that NZVI can effectively inactivate *Escherichia coli*, causing disruptive damages to the cell membranes.[28] In particular, in the absence of oxygen in the bulk solution, the inactivation efficacy of *E. coli* by NZVI was greatly enhanced compared to the air-saturated condition. Under deaerated condition, 10 ppm NZVI exhibited 4log (99.99%) inactivation of *E. coli* cells in 1 h, which is comparable bactericidal activity to that of nanoparticulate silver.[28] The inactivation mechanism is not fully understood, but the oxidative stress induced by reactive oxidants formed by the interaction of NZVI with the cell components was suggested to be responsible for the cell death.[29] The intracellular oxygen or hydrogen peroxide seems to serve as the precursor for the reactive oxidants in a series of reactions with NZVI. The virucidal effect of NZVI has been also reported.[30] The reactive oxidants induced by NZVI were found to damage the protein capsid of the virus cell. Although the oxidative stress resulting from intracellular oxidants is believed to be a key factor in causing the microbiocidal effects of NZVI, still there are many behaviors that remain unexplained by this factor, which warrants further study.

Iron oxide NPs or mesoporous materials coated by iron oxide have been extensively studied as the Fenton catalyst.[31–34] As described briefly above, the Fenton reaction (reaction 2) refers to the reaction of hydrogen peroxide with Fe(II), resulting in the production of highly reactive oxidants such as ·OH or Fe(IV) that can be used in oxidative degradation of organic contaminants in water. As a result of the Fenton reaction, Fe(III) is usually produced as the product: even though Fe(IV) is formed, it is further reduced to Fe(III) by oxidizing organic substances or other reagents such as Fe(II) and hydrogen peroxide. Fe(III) can be regenerated back to Fe(II), which is again used for the Fenton reaction (reaction 4). In combination of reactions 2 and 4, hydrogen peroxide is decomposed into reactive oxidants by the catalytic cycling of the Fe(III)/Fe(II) couple.

$$Fe^{3+} + H_2O_2 \rightarrow Fe^{2+} + HO_2^- + H^+ \tag{4}$$

Iron oxides provide the active sites of Fe(II) and Fe(III) on the surface for the catalytic decomposition of hydrogen peroxide. The use of iron oxide NPs or iron oxide-coated mesoporous materials can greatly increase the number of surface active sites, enhancing the catalytic activity for the Fenton reaction. Moreover, the catalytic activity of iron oxide-coated mesoporous materials can be further enhanced by surface modifications or the change of the supporting materials. It has been reported that iron oxide immobilized in alumina-coated mesoporous silica (SBA-15) has a superior activity than the same material without the alumina coating.[32] The alumina coating on SBA-15 silica was found to improve the dispersion of the iron oxide NPs and accelerate the redox cycle of the Fe(III)/Fe(II) couple on the iron oxide surface. In addition, a recent study has suggested that iron oxide supported on the silica–alumina matrix enhances the conversion efficiency of hydrogen peroxide into ·OH during the Fenton reaction at neutral pH.[35] Usually, heterogeneous Fenton catalysts such as iron oxides show extremely low efficiency in the oxidation of organic contaminants under neutral pH conditions due to the H_2O_2 decomposition via a nonradical mechanism.[35,36] The nonradical mechanism may lead to the formation of Fe(IV) on the catalyst surface that is rapidly dissipated by reaction with the surface Fe(II) without being used in the reaction with target contaminants.[35,37] It is believed that the coordination of iron to ligands or specific supporting materials may modify the electronic properties of the iron species, altering the reaction pathway of the Fenton reaction from two-electron transfer [resulting Fe(IV)] to one-electron transfer (resulting ·OH), but the detailed mechanism is not fully understood. Many researches are being focused on the development of new Fenton catalysts based on nanomaterials that overcome the drawbacks of the heterogeneous Fenton catalysts such as the low catalytic activity and the low yield of ·OH at neutral pH.

11.2.3 PHOTOCATALYSTS

Photoexcitation of metal oxide semiconductors including TiO_2, ZnO, and WO_3, upon absorption of photons with energy exceeding their bandgap energies (E_g), promotes electrons in the valence band (VB) to conduction band (CB) across the bandgap, concurrently leaving behind holes in the VB.[38–41] The electron–hole pairs formed as a result of the photo-driven charge separation migrate to the surface with recombination of the charge carriers, subsequently mediating a variety of reductive and oxidative chemical transformation. Due to the highly positive VB edge potential holes [e.g., $E_{VB}(TiO_2) = +3.5 \, V_{NHE}$ (voltage referred to the normal hydrogen electrode) vs. $E^0(·OH/OH^-) = +1.9 \, V_{NHE}$; $E^0(·OH/H_2O) = +2.73 \, V_{NHE}$], selected semiconductor photocatalysts can initiate VB hole-induced oxidation of hydroxyl groups and water molecules adsorbed on or present in the proximity of the surfaces, resulting in production of ·OH.[38,41,42] On the other hand, photo-generated CB electrons are capable of generating reactive oxygen species (ROS) including ·OH, superoxide radical anion ($O_2^{·-}$), and H_2O_2 through sequential reduction of dissolved oxygen molecules [$E^0(O_2/O_2^{·-}) = -0.33 \, V_{NHE}$; $E^0(O_2/HO_2^·) = -0.05 \, V_{NHE}$].[38,41] The photo-generated ·OH with nonselective reactivity effectively degrades and mineralizes organic pollutants, in addition to a VB hole enabling direct charge transfer (Figure 11.3).

Titanium dioxide (TiO_2) represents semiconducting photocatalysts having promising environmental application due to (1) superior photocatalytic activity for ROS production under UV and solar light irradiations, (2) chemical inertness and photochemical stability, (3) low adverse biological effect, (4) inexpensiveness, and (5) facile modifications to promote efficacy in photocatalytic redox reactions and improve energy efficiency. The strong oxidation potential of VB enables rapid oxidative degradation of a wide range of organic contaminants via ·OH (or VB holes in some cases)[43,44] and subsequent mineralization to CO_2 and H_2O. In that interfacial electron transfer is the rate-limiting step in TiO_2-photocatalyzed oxidation of pollutants, redox potential of CB allows a function of O_2 as a CB electron acceptor, effectively preventing electron–hole pair recombination and concurrently achieving ROS production via multielectron transfer to oxygen.

The ROS-induced oxidation pathway for TiO_2 photocatalytic destruction of organic pollutants shows substrate specificity. It was generally presumed that surface-bound ·OH ($Ti^{IV}OH^+$) formed through conversion of adsorbed hydroxyl groups by VB holes

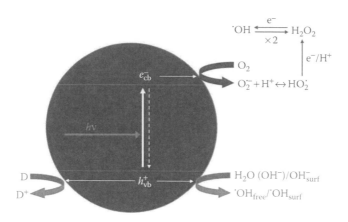

FIGURE 11.3   Production of ROS in semiconductor photocatalysis.

play a role as a dominant oxidant in oxidizing organic substrates (e.g., phenols) during TiO$_2$ photocatalysis.[38,41] On the other hand, organic compounds (e.g., oxalate, dichloroacetate) that are not vulnerable to H abstraction by ˙OH due to the lack of C–H bond are favorably degraded by direct VB hole oxidation on light-exposed TiO$_2$ surface.[43,44] TiO$_2$ photocatalyst when subjected to light illumination displays significant activity for degradation of organic pollutants (e.g., tetramethylammonium hydroxide on TiO$_2$ surface at acidic pH)[45] that are rarely adsorbed on or off the surface of charged TiO$_2$ because of electrostatic repulsive interaction, indicating the possible predominant reaction pathway via free or mobile ˙OH in the photocatalyzed oxidation of organic contaminants. Although superoxide radical does not mainly contribute to TiO$_2$ photocatalytic oxidation due to its mild oxidizing power, it is formed through reduction of dissolved O$_2$ by the photo-generated CB electron and causes rapid oxidative conversion of arsenite [As(III)] to arsenate [AS(V)].[46–48] It is well recognized that TiO$_2$ exhibits the negligible visible light activity for ROS production. However, even pure TiO$_2$ readily forms visible light-absorbing complexes with phenol analogs, leading to oxidative degradation of phenols through (1) direct transfer of electron to CB of TiO$_2$ and (2) subsequent ROS (*in situ* produced during the consecutive O$_2$ reduction by electrons injected to CB) attack.[49]

Compared to advanced oxidation processes (AOPs) based on homogeneous radical chemistry such as Fenton reaction, catalyzed ozonation, and γ-radiolysis, TiO$_2$-mediated photocatalytic oxidation of organics more favorably leads to mineralization without significant formation of reaction intermediates. The photocatalyzed oxidation of phenolics yields distributions of aromatic intermediates/products (e.g., hydroquinone and catechol) at low concentrations, while the hydroxylated aromatics forms in substantial amounts over the course of homogeneous ˙OH oxidations.[50,51] Less preferred production of aromatic intermediates during TiO$_2$ photocatalysis would be ascribed to a role of the heterogeneous TiO$_2$ surface in the photolytic oxidation, that is, hydroxylated aromatic intermediates adsorbed on the catalyst surface are more vulnerable to VB hole-induced oxidation, readily undergoing the ring-opening reaction and subsequent mineralization.

Zinc oxide (ZnO) as the most popular alternative photocatalyst to TiO_2 has nearly identical bandgap energy and redox potentials of CB and VB as TiO_2, although it has the limited aqueous application under neutral and alkaline pH condition because of significant Zn^{2+} dissolution as a result of ZnO photocorrosion over acidic pH range. The slightly lower bandgap energy $[E_g(TiO_2) = 3.2$ eV vs. $E_g(ZnO) = 3.1$ eV] allows ZnO to be more photoactive than TiO_2 for organic oxidation under sunlight irradiation. Despite the similarity of photophysical properties, many comparative studies have reported inferiority of ZnO to TiO_2 for efficacy of photocatalytic oxidative degradation of organic pollutants, which is attributed to fast kinetics for charge recombination and relevant low quantum yield.[40,52] Low mineralization efficiency is achieved in ZnO photocatalytic oxidation of phenolics relative to TiO_2, which is ascribed to favorable hydroxylation (leading to the formation of aromatic intermediates/products) on ZnO surface rather than ring cleavage. On the other hand, in many cases, ZnO enabled more rapid decolorization of dyestuffs than TiO_2[53,54] and exhibited equivalent photocatalytic activity to TiO_2 for photodynamic bacterial inactivation.[55] Electron acceptors such as $S_2O_8^{2-}$ and H_2O_2 cause kinetic enhancement in ZnO photocatalytic oxidation of organics by preventing charge recombination and increasing production of $\cdot OH$, that is, reductive conversion of H_2O_2 (or H_2O) to $\cdot OH$ by CB electron (or SO_4^-),[54,56] while the efficacy improvement in the chemical additives hardly occurs in the photo-irradiated TiO_2 suspensions. Interestingly, ZnO shows unique emission in the visible light region, quantitatively correlated to the concentration of VB hole scavengers (e.g., organics able to quench the visible emission), due to anionic vacancies, which enables simultaneous oxidative degradation and monitoring of organic contaminants on ZnO photocatalyst.[57]

Tungsten trioxide (WO_3) has the potential to achieve photocatalytic oxidations under visible light irradiation, owing to a relatively narrow bandgap (2.4–2.8 eV) and VB potential (+3.1 V_{NHE}) identical to that of TiO_2.[58–60] However, in a few instances, visible light (or fluorescent light) illumination enabled relatively significant oxidation of organics (e.g., hexane) on the surface of WO_3. Since the CB potential of WO_3 (+0.4 V_{NHE}) is not negative enough to employ the oxygen molecule (ubiquitously present in aqueous environmental media) as an electron acceptor, the bandgap structures cause facile charge recombination and negligible production of the photo-generated oxidizing species, that is, VB hole and $\cdot OH$, available for the photocatalytic oxidative degradation of organics. As a result, bare WO_3 exhibits much lower activity for photocatalytic oxidation of organic contaminants (e.g., reactive dyes and dichloroacetate) under irradiation of UV and visible light, although VB potential meets the thermodynamic requirement for conversion of hydroxide ion or water molecule to $\cdot OH$. The presence of alternative electron acceptors (e.g., H_2O_2 and Fe^{3+}) or co-catalysts (e.g., Ag, CuO, and Pt) can significantly prevent charge recombination by capturing CB electrons or enabling multielectron transfer from CB to oxygen, drastically improving oxidation efficacy in the photo-irradiated WO_3 particulates.[58,61]

11.2.3.1 Noble Metal Deposition

Due to the high electron affinity, nanosized noble metals deposited on the surface of semiconducting photocatalysts serve as effective electron traps and facilitate interfacial charge transfer, significantly enhancing charge separation efficacy and kinetically improving oxidation of organics. Femtosecond diffuse reflectance spectroscopic study demonstrated an initial fast decay of trapped electrons within 5 ps (which is attributed to migration of electrons in TiO_2 to Pt phase) and also ensured effective charge separation in Pt/TiO_2 by presenting prolonged lifetime of the photo-generated electrons.[62] Nanoscale Pt deposit as electron sink (Schottky-barrier electron trapping) accelerates photocatalytic oxidations of organic pollutants and reductions of heavy metals and highly chlorinated chemicals (e.g., trichloroacetate and CCl_4) on platinized photocatalysts.[43,63] Negative shift of the Fermi level occurring in the Au/TiO_2 composite promotes efficacy in charge separation and interfacial charge transfer, which was confirmed by improved reduction reactions on the surface of Au/TiO_2.[64,65] H_2O_2 effectively forms on platinized WO_3 through the multielectron transfer to oxygen under visible light irradiation, reductively converting to ·OH and enabling rapid ·OH oxidation of diverse organic pollutants.[59] In addition to a role as an electron reservoir, Pt loading creates novel reaction pathways for photocatalytic oxidations of selected organics (e.g., alkylamines and chloroacetates) by stabilizing transient intermediates on the platinum phase, which kinetically enhances organic degradation and modifies distributions of intermediates or products.[43,66,67]

11.2.3.2 Doping

Introduction of cationic metal ions as impurities into pure semiconductor photocatalysts creates new energy levels in the bandgaps by being substituted in the constituent cation sites (e.g., Ti^{4+} and Zn^{2+}) or being located in the interstitial positions of the lattice, improving charge separation and offering visible light activity. Monitoring of transient absorption decays at 600 nm (indicative of trapped electrons) for a series of metal-ion-doped TiO_2 confirmed the inhibition of electron–hole pair recombination in the presence of metal ions (e.g., Fe^{3+}, Mo^{5+}, and Rh^{3+}) in TiO_2 lattice, reflecting the enhanced photocatalytic activity of the doped TiO_2 for CCl_4 reduction and $CHCl_3$ oxidation.[68,69] The effective charge separation in the doped photocatalysts (e.g., Mn-doped ZnO and La-doped TiO_2) led to kinetic enhancement in reduction of methyl viologen, conversion of NO_2^- / NO_3^- to NH_3, decolorization of methylene blue (MB), and oxidation/mineralization of trichlorophenol.[70–72] Metal ion doping can extend absorption of photocatalysts in the visible light wavelength regions, which is ascribed to the photoexcitation of an electron from metal ion in the lattice to the CB. The metal-ion-doped photocatalysts (e.g., V-doped, La-doped, and Pt-doped) enabled various visible light-driven redox reactions, which include reduction of heavy metals, decolorization of organic dyes, and reductive and oxidative degradation of chlorinated pollutants. Among TiO_2 photocatalysts doped with 13 different metal cations, Choi et al.[73] demonstrated that doping with Cr and Pt made TiO_2 notably photoactive for photobleaching of MB and oxidation of iodide and phenol under visible light irradiation.

Replacement of lattice oxygen with anionic dopants such as C, N, or S causes bandgap narrowing and associated visible light-induced activation of the doped phocatalysts. Due to the superior visible light activity, N-doped photocatalysts (TiO_2 or ZnO) have been extensively employed for oxidative degradation of dyes and phenols and bacterial/viral inactivation. The isolated nitrogen atom in TiO_2

(rather than NO_x or NH_x; exists as an either form of neutral paramagnetic $N^.$ or charged diamagnetic N^-) creates defect states within the bandgap, resulting in charge separation through promotion of electrons from the N-induced states to the CB under visible light illumination.[74] A time-resolved microwave conductivity study confirmed charge carrier generation via visible excitation (Ti 3d ← N 2p transition), indicative of visible light activity of N-doped TiO_2.[75] On the other hand, promotion of electrons from occupied states created by N-doping does not yield oxidizing species strong enough to achieve oxidation of formate or hydroxylamine with visible light, although still effective for oxidation of selected organics with visible light.[76]

11.2.3.3   Coupled Metal Oxides

Charge separation, which is a key factor in the efficiency of photocatalytic redox reactions, can be significantly enhanced by the coupling of two semiconductor particles with different CB and VB potentials, which makes the photo-generated electron and hole move in the opposite directions to accumulate on different semiconductors, respectively. The efficient charge separation occurring in the coupled SnO_2 and TiO_2 (or ZnO) system [in which photo-generated electron and hole are trapped within the SnO_2 ($E_{CB} = 0$ V vs. NHE at pH 7) and TiO_2 (or ZnO) ($E_{CB} = -0.5$ V vs. NHE at pH 7), respectively] led to kinetically enhanced photocatalytic bleaching of dye-stuffs relative to SnO_2 or TiO_2 (or ZnO) alone.[77] WO_3 in WO_3-loaded TiO_2 can function as an effective electron sink, accelerating oxidation of 1,4-dichlorobenzene and 2-propanol in aqueous media.[78] In the coupled TiO_2 (or ZnO) and CdS with photo-response to visible light, organics (e.g., MB and 4-chlorophenol) can be effectively oxidized under visible light irradiation, which is attributed to a CdS sensitization process in which electrons injected from the photoexcited CdS to the CB of TiO_2 (or ZnO) are consecutively transferred to oxygen, eventually resulting in the generation of ·OH in a reductive way.[79]

11.2.3.4   Hybridization with C_{60} Fullerenes and CNTs

Kamat et al.[80] suggested possible employment of fullerenes as an electron reservoir based on the rapid kinetics for C_{60} and C_{70} reduction on the photoexcited TiO_2 and ZnO. Hybridization of ZnO by C_{60} as an electron acceptor facilitates charge separation and accelerates MB oxidation, confirmed by photocurrent generation as a function of C_{60} content. Collaterally, the hybridization of C_{60} inhibits photoanodic corrosion by preventing O_2 activation by VB hole. Fullerol forms visible light-responsive complex with TiO_2 surface, which is readily activated to enhance electron transfer under visible light irradiation, eventually resulting in oxidation of 4-chlorophenol.[81] Hydrophobic CNT with high surface area shows extraordinary adsorption capacity to aromatic hydrocarbons. CNTs incorporated into electrospun polymeric nanofiber containing TiO_2 photocatalysts takes on the role of adsorbent sites, offering favorable access of organic contaminants to photoactive TiO_2 surface.[82] Single-walled CNT (SWCNT)-TiO_2 nanocomposite shows enhanced photocatalytic oxidation of phenol than TiO_2 alone, which is attributed to the reduced rate for charge recombination via efficient electron trapping by SWCNT (Figure 11.4).[83]

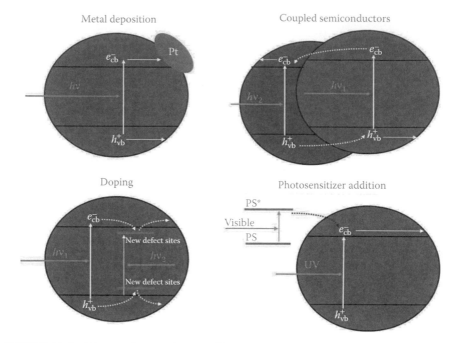

FIGURE 11.4 Diverse photocatalyst modification techniques.

11.3 ENVIRONMENTAL NANOBIOSENSORS

11.3.1 Monitoring of Environmental Pollution Using Nanobiosensors

Technical advances over the past decade in the nanotechnology have spurred research efforts dedicated to the fabrication of nanomaterials and the manipulation of nanotechnology, and these research efforts are dedicated to the development of advanced environmental nanobiosensors in the application of environmental monitoring. The monitoring of environmental pollution is a constant issue that generated considerable scientific interest and public concern, since the environmental pollution affects human and ecological health. Fast, simple, and more reliable identification and diagnosis of environmental analytes would be greatly helpful to protect environment pollution and assist in making a policy for pollution prevention. Concerning these issues, biosensors are useful tools targeted at providing selective diagnosis and identifying toxic chemicals in industrial products, environmental samples (e.g., air, soil, and water), or biological matters including microorganisms (bacteria or virus) with high sensitivity and specificity.[84–88] Biosensors are composed of biological receptors (e.g., DNA, antibody, enzymes, or whole cells) that recognize analytes via epitope of receptors specifically and signal transducers to inform quantitative, semiquantitative, or qualitative information for analytes of interest by converting interaction events between receptors and analytes to readable signals. The interaction of biological receptors with analytes produces various signals that may be electrical current, color, light emission, mass changes, or fluorescence depending on

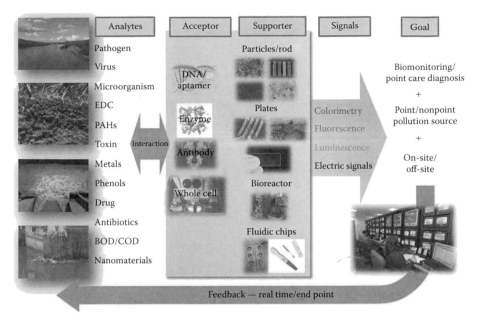

FIGURE 11.5 (See color insert.) Flowchart for composition of environmental biosensors in environmental monitoring. BOD, biological oxygen demand; COD, chemical oxygen demand; EDC, endocrine-disrupting chemical.

the design of biosensors, and these signals are converted to appropriate measurable and readable responses. Environmental biosensors, therefore, refer to the biosensors that can diagnose and identify the pollutants and substances emitted into the environment for environmental monitoring (Figure 11.5). Environmental biosensors should be classified differently from bioanalytical systems that require additional processing steps such as reagent addition or sample preparation prior to detection, which may hamper the rapid on-site monitoring.[86–89] The merits of environmental biosensors over conventional instrument analysis are the possibility of miniaturization, portability, rapid identification, minimum sample preparation, and minimum processing steps. Environmental biosensors can offer the analytes information of not only specific chemicals but also their biological effects such as toxicity depending on receptors used in biosensors. These merits should always be considered when new types of environmental biosensors are developed. To detect the environmental analytes found in complex environmental samples accurately, environmental biosensors should have sufficient sensitivity and specificity. To be available in complex environmental samples with sufficient sensitivity and specificity, samples are concentrated and cleaned via filtration or the recognition elements should recognize the target analytes without hindrance occupied by debris or unknown matrix in samples.[90] The specificity and sensitivity of environmental biosensors are determined by the degree of interaction between recognition receptors and analytes and signal transduction translated by their binding events. Recently, the development of environmental biosensors is spurred so as to enhance the degree of interaction between recognition receptors and analytes, and as also sensitivity to combine with receptors and various NPs such as quantum dots (QDs),[91,92] gold NPs,[93,94] or dye-doped silica.[95,96] As a rapid growth of nanotechnology, various NPs are developed and used in various fields such as energy, biotechnology, pharmaceutics, and electronics. The fields of environmental monitoring are also interesting for the use of nanomaterials for the construction of environmental nanobiosensors. Usually, the NP-based environmental nanobiosensors used the conjugation scheme between NPs and recognition receptors. The NPs in environmental nanobiosensors usually have the role of the generation and enhancement of signals. In nanomaterial-based environmental nanobiosensors, the recognition receptors are immobilized with the surface of the nanomaterials, and the interaction of conjugate with analytes is monitored via a signal transduction mechanism. Nanotechnology of a variety of embedded nanomaterials is currently used in environmental nanobiosensor applications, and the nanomaterials used influence both the type of recognition element employed and the signal transduction method utilized.[90] Different kinds of NPs that have unique properties for host materials and signal enhancing elements were developed for efficient supporters for conjugation of receptors. One of the particularly advantageous features of NPs is the control over size at the nanometer scale uniformly, which offers higher surface area-to-volume ratios.[97] The uniform size of NPs and their compatibility in size with receptors used in environmental biosensors together with high surface area offer new functions in sensing process such as high loading capacity of receptors and the generation of high and stable signals. For controlling the surface of NPs with various functional groups and conjugation chemistry, the preparation of more sensitive and stable nanobiosensors for environmental applications is possible.

Regardless of what combination of receptors and NPs is applied, successful environmental nanobiosensors in real field should be able to discriminate between targets that should be detected exactly and those that should not be detected in complex media without background noise; have broad detectable range to quantify the concentration of analytes; show high stability during operation; and maintain the binding between receptors and analytes during repeated usages.[90] To apply environmental nanobiosensors in real fields, the biosensors should be tested under harsh environmental conditions. Various concepts of environmental biosensors using NPs are suggested; however, most of them are suitable under restricted laboratory conditions. Usually environmental nanobiosensors are considered for single use and unable to monitor the analytes continuously on-site. Although many of the biosensors developed for environmental analysis are for single use and cannot be operated continuously, an appropriate system composition using biosensors makes environmental monitoring continuous. Despite these advantages, the application of biosensors in the environmental field is still limited in comparison with medical or pharmaceutical applications, where most research and development has converged. Nevertheless, the majority of the systems developed are prototypes that still need to be validated before being extensively used or before their commercialization.

The appropriate selection of receptors and nanomaterials is important to generate suitable biosensors for environmental applications. Among many candidates, we focus on recent progress in the development of nanobiosensors using functional nucleic acid-based aptamers and nanomaterials for the detection of heavy metals or pathogens that are considered to be difficult to detect and identify on-site using current technology specifically in complex environmental samples. We note that an entire section related to environmental nanobiosensors should start from methodologies of sample preparation; our focus, however, is solely on recent hot bioreceptors, especially aptamers, and their combination with nanomaterials to detect heavy metals and pathogens.

11.3.2 The Use of Aptamers and Nanomaterials for Constructing Environmental Nanobiosensors

The metal NPs such as gold NPs have distinct properties compared with bulk metal particles depending on their size, surface functionality, and shape.[98,99] Especially, the high stability and unique optical properties of gold NPs have made them good candidates for the enhancement of signal transduction and carrier for bioreceptors to develop nanobiosensors in a wide range of research fields, including food, medicine, and also the environment.[100] The widely used method for synthesizing gold NPs with different sizes and shapes originated from a variation on the classic Turkevich–Frens citrate reduction route[101] and its modification routes allow mass production of gold NPs with different shapes and sizes. In the citrate reduction route, a sodium citrate solution is added to a boiling solution of chloroauric acid ($HAuCl_4$), and after a few minutes, the color of the solution changes from colorless to a deep red that suggests the formation of gold NPs. The cetyltrimethylammonium bromide (CTAB)-gold NPs are frequently used as seeds for synthesizing monodispersed gold nanorods with diverse aspect ratios and facets for controlling the concentration of CTAB.[102,103] The pioneered introduction of gold NPs as nanobiosensors using functional nucleic acids was introduced in 1996 by Mirkin et al.[104] In this report, the oligonucleotide-tailed 13 nm gold NPs via thiol group capping and the complementary target DNA induced the aggregation of gold NPs. The aggregation of gold NPs induced the color change of solutions simply from red to blue. The reverse reaction, dehybridization of DNA, from blue to red is possible for controlling the temperature. This simple and reversible observation initiated the use of gold NPs as DNA detection agents with optical properties. The selection of appropriate receptors and their combination with gold NPs are important for realizing the sensing platforms that can be applied to environmental diagnosis with high rapidity and specificity through colorimetric scheme. Colorimetric environmental nanobiosensors are useful because they can minimize the necessity of using expensive instruments. Although the first application of gold NPs in a diagnosis scheme is based on DNA detection via complementary hybridization, many analytes can be detectable in the scheme of simple color change with the naked eye over the DNA hybridization if the other receptors are acceptable to be linked with gold NPs. One of the good candidates to be linked with gold NPs is a functional nucleic acid, aptamers. Aptamers are small nucleic acid sequences (usually 40–90 bp of DNAs or RNAs) that specifically bind to organic or inorganic molecules or to macromolecules such as proteins with a high affinity constant that lies in the micromolar-to-nanomolar ranges.[105–108] The nucleic acid aptamers fold into three-dimensional configuration to their specific targets. The initiation of aptamer selection starts with single-stranded random library of oligonucleotide (~10^{15} different single strands) and target substrate through a series of selection and amplification of oligonucleotides, known as systematic evolution of ligands by exponential enrichment (SELEX) method.[106] During the SELEX, a few nucleic acids that have strong binding affinity remain, while most of the other library is lost. After sequencing of selected aptamers, they can be synthesized in high amounts and be available linked with other supports as modified at their 3′ or 5′ end. The process of SELEX is simpler than antibody production; however, one of the limitations related to using aptamers in environmental nanobiosensors is nuclease that degrades DNA. Nevertheless, the aptamers are widely acceptable for finding appropriate receptors against environmentally relevant chemicals, biomolecules, and pathogens because of their simple process and high affinity. Various aptamers such as heavy metals,[109,110] pesticides,[111] pathogens,[112–114] toxins,[115–117] and pharmaceuticals[118,119] for environmental analytes have been isolated. Still the isolation of aptamers from various substrates and application to receptors for constructing environmental nanobiosensors are increasingly reported (Figure 11.6).

The combination of nucleic acid aptamers and gold NPs allowed many analytes to be detected by a simple strategy. Liu and Lu[120] well summarized the strategy of constructing aptamer and gold NP-mediated colorimetric sensors. The aptamer-linked gold NPs were already aggregated and formed a purple color. The purple-colored aggregates underwent a fast disassembly to red color dispersion of NPs when the target analytes were bound to their specific aptamers. The targets bound to aptamers overcame the aggregate interaction between gold NPs, which released aggregated gold NPs. This strategy is opposite to the originally introduced gold NP-mediated colorimetric sensors. Either way, both methods showed useful application of gold NPs linked with DNA receptors as colorimetric environmental nanobiosensors.

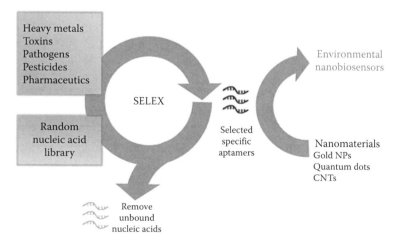

FIGURE 11.6   Aptamer-based environmental nanobiosensors for various environmental analytes.

11.3.3 Aptamer-Based Nanobiosensors for Heavy Metal Detection

Among environmental analytes, heavy metal biosensors are mostly introduced using a combination of aptamers and gold NPs using the colorimetry method. The diagnosis of heavy metal ions in environmental samples is an important issue because these contaminants have severe effects on human health and the environmental ecosystems. The accumulation of heavy metals in the human body causes damage in brain, heart, lung, kidneys, central nervous system, and immune system.[121,122]

The highly selective and sensitive colorimetric detection of Hg^{2+} using aptamer-conjugated gold NPs in the aqueous environment was demonstrated. Two different DNA probes conjugated with gold NPs were prepared (Probe A: A10-T-A10, Probe B: T10-T10) and the single-mismatched T-T sites between two different probes can be hybridized because Hg^{2+} coordinates selectively mismatched T-T sites. The result of coordination triggered by Hg^{2+} that is selectively bound to the T-T sites led to the formation of aggregation of gold NPs, and it changed the color of the solution from red to purple and raised the melting temperature T_m to dissociate aggregation.[123] On increasing the Hg^{2+} concentration in aqueous solutions, the T_m of aggregated gold NPs proportionally increased. This method provided 100 nM limit of detection (LOD) in aqueous environments. On a similar principle, a chip-based scanometric detection method for Hg^{2+} was suggested.[124] One probe (T10-T-T10) was immobilized on the plate such as glass and the other probe (A10-T-A10) was conjugated with gold NPs. The presence of Hg^{2+} initiates the conjugation between probes immobilized on the plate and those conjugated with gold NPs. After conjugation by Hg^{2+}, the signals were amplified through silver enhancement scheme. This chip can differentiate the Hg^{2+} in the presence of other 15 metal ions and have 10 nM LOD.

The simple rapid and colorimetric method for the detection of Hg^{2+} using electrostatic repulsion among aptamer-conjugated gold NPs was also demonstrated.[125] The random coiled poly-T_n DNA aptamer adsorbs onto 13 nm gold NPs via electrostatic attraction. The gold NPs wrapped with DNA aptamers exist in the solution homogeneously because of electrostatic repulsion originated from the high negative charges of aptamers in the specific salt condition. The presence of Hg^{2+} in this solution led the folded structure of poly-T_n DNA aptamer because of the high affinity of Hg^{2+} to poly-T_n DNA. The detachment of poly-T_n DNA from gold NPs induced the loss of repulsion among gold NPs and the color change of solution from red to purple resulted in aggregation of gold NPs. The LOD of this method was obtained to be 250 nM. This strategy can omit the conjugation step between aptamers and NPs and reduce the time and cost to prepare the detection assay. Another detection method for Hg^{2+} with aptamers and gold NPs introduced the use of fluorescence resonance energy transfer (FRET) scheme.[126] The Hg^{2+}-specific aptamer was linked with QD NPs and the QD-conjugated aptamers were adsorbed onto gold NPs via electrostatic attraction. The superquenching effect of gold NPs reduces the fluorescence intensity of QDs when they are close together. The presence of Hg^{2+} induced the detachment of QD-conjugated aptamers from gold NPs, which led to increase of fluorescence intensity of QDs. The LOD of this method for Hg^{2+} is 500 nM. The other heavy metal ion, Pb^{2+}, can also be detected by colorimetric sensors constructed in combination of aptamers and gold NPs. Liu and Lu[127,128] used Pb^{2+}-specific DNAzyme aptamers that are DNA molecules having catalytic activity to Pb^{2+} and isolated them by the SELEX process. The colorimetric Pb^{2+} sensors consist of a Pb^{2+}-specific DNAzyme aptamer, its substrate strand DNA, and 5′-thiol-modified DNA (12-mer) attached to gold NPs. The substrate strand DNA has flanking regions that can hybridize with 12-mer DNA on gold NPs, complementary regions with DNAzyme aptamers, and cleavage site. The composites of these three components make gold NPs aggregated. The presence of Pb^{2+} in the DNAzyme aptamer catalyzes hydrolytic cleavage of substrate strand and prevents the aggregation of gold NPs resulting in change to red color from purple color. Depending on the selected DNAzyme aptamers, the sensitivity of Pb^{2+} sensor can be controlled and the LOD of this sensor to Pb^{2+} is in submicromolar level. For introducing the heavy metal nanobiosensors for Hg^{2+} and Pb^{2+}, if we isolate the specific aptamers from other different heavy metal ions, the combination of aptamers and gold NPs will offer multiple detection of the entire heavy metals in environmental samples.

11.3.4 APTAMER-BASED NANOBIOSENSORS FOR PATHOGEN DETECTION

Compared to proteins and chemicals, only a small number of aptamers have been isolated to bacterial cells. The real-time detection of living bacterial cells, especially pathogens, directly in environmental samples is important to prevent and control the infectious disease. The culturing method and PCR-based DNA amplification method are time consuming and tedious, and their real-field application is further limited because of complexity of samples in environments. It is essential to secure the appropriate receptors that can recognize the specific target bacteria to construct sensors which recognize the bacterial cells to realize real-time detection. The amplification of nucleic acid in bacteria using PCR or immunoassay has been commonly used for the detection of environmental pathogens. Recently, there are demands for the improvement of these methods to be applied in real-time detection of pathogens using alternative receptors that can have robustness and selectivity than antibodies. Aptamers can be alternative receptors with many advantages compared to antibodies to detect whole cells.[129] Despite the specificity of aptamers, only very few aptamers for bacterial pathogens have been isolated and used for the purpose of biosensors. The bacterial aptamers are isolated via the cell-SELEX method to select tumor cells.[130–132] The cell-SELEX process is similar to that of the isolation of chemicals or proteins; however, the immobilization of analytes can be omitted. The next few examples concern environmental nanobiosensors using aptamers for real-time detection of bacterial pathogens in environmental samples.

Aptamers for nonpathogenic *E. coli* DH5α have been isolated and were loaded into biosensors composed of an SWCNT field-effect transistor (SWCNT-FET). The specificity of *E. coli* aptamer can recognize only *E. coli* in SWCNT-FET biosensors and the other bacteria, *Salmonella typhimurium*, did not respond to biosensors.[133] Although the sensitivity of SWCNT-FET was less than 2 orders of magnitude compared to the conventional MNP method, this is worth realizing that living bacterial cell detection is possible; however, the real-time detection of bacterial cells was not possible. Rius et al. developed the potentiometric biosensor composed of aptamer–SWCNT hybrid materials for detecting *S. typhi* (ST) in one single colony-forming unit (CFU) level in real time.[134] The aptamer that can recognize the ST selectively was modified with the amine group at the 3′-end and immobilized covalently with carboxylated SWCNTs that were already sprayed onto the surface of glassy carbon rod in contact with the potentiometer. The aptamer–SWCNT hybrid material generates the change of electromotive force when the target bacteria are present in samples and act as both the sensing and transducing elements for the biosensor. The recognition of target bacteria induces a conformational change of aptamer attached onto SWCNTs, which initiates a charge change to the SWCNTs. This nanobiosensor can be regenerated by dissociating the aptamers from bacteria in specific salt condition and taking new measurements. As an extension of this method, this type of biosensor was applied to complex samples for detecting *E. coli*.[135] In this report, a particular bacterial strain can be detected in real samples by pretreatment of environmental samples. The most interesting part of this achievement is that the developed nanobiosensor was equipped with the on-line pretreatment system that removed the matrix in real samples. The various unknown matrices or compounds may interact with receptors nonspecifically, which induces the nonspecific signals in biosensors; therefore, the pretreatment of real samples is important to enhance the sensitivity and accuracy of biosensors in real-field applications. The isolated aptamers for pathogens can also be employed as capture probes. Most cell-based aptamers have receptor properties in the membrane proteins of the cells, and the aptamers can capture the pathogens and separate them in samples to prevent their release in environments.

The abundance of hazardous pollutants in environmental systems and the widespread use of new chemicals and industrial pollutants make these substances hard to detect with appropriate approaches. The functional nucleic acid-based aptamers that can be isolated from various substances with high affinity have been shown to be available for various targets. The combination of newly isolated aptamers with nanomaterials will address a new type of nanobiosensors for environmental applications. Although we briefly introduced several examples of nanobiosensors using aptamers and nanomaterials, the upcoming new strategy will be available to diagnose the environmental analytes that cannot be identified in this technology.

11.4 ENVIRONMENTAL IMPACTS OF NANOMATERIALS

11.4.1 Toxicity of Nanomaterials

Nanotechnology is now one of the rapidly growing fields with a wide range of applications including cosmetics, electronics, paints, medical devices, food packing, catalysts, antimicrobial fabrics, and water treatment membranes.[136–140] Nanomaterials and nanomaterial-containing products have been generated for use in such applications. The production of nanomaterials is expected to reach 58,000 ton/year in 2011–2020.[141] An increase in production and the use of nanomaterials has led to an increased possibility of their release into the environment, resulting in significant concerns regarding their potential to cause adverse effects on the environment as well as on human health.

Organisms in the environment including humans can be exposed to nanomaterials through a few exposure routes such as via inhalation of air, uptake of water and food, and skin contact. Nanomaterial exposure through inhalation of air is an important route and includes exposure from natural (i.e., ultrafine dusts from volcanic activity and geological weathering processes) and anthropogenic sources (i.e., nanomaterials from vehicle exhaust emissions and erosion of man-made materials including the wear of car tires). Ingestion of water is also a potential exposure route of nanomaterials. Nanomaterials in water can come from nanotechnology applied for the treatment of drinking water such as iron oxide nanomaterials for ultrafiltration and Ag nanomaterials coated onto water filter for disinfection. Through food uptake, humans can ingest nanomaterials. It is possible to ingest nanomaterial-containing foods, medicines, or health supplements from food packaging coated with nanomaterials and from the food chain by eating fish or meat previously exposed to nanomaterials. Exposure to nanomaterials can also occur via skin contact during the use of sunscreen and cosmetics containing nanomaterials.

Several physicochemical properties of nanomaterials influence their toxic effects on organisms.[142] The chemical composition of nanomaterials can contribute to their toxicity. Especially, the released ions from the surface of metal nanomaterials are able to cause toxic effects. For an instance, cadmium ion (Cd^{2+}) released from CdS and CdSe QDs and zinc ion (Zn^{2+}) from ZnO nanomaterials might be responsible for their toxicity. Toxicity of metal nanomaterials is known to be higher than that of their bulk counterparts because nanomaterials have a high surface area-to-volume ratio, releasing metal ions easily from the surface. Another physicochemical property of nanomaterials responsible for toxicity is their small size. With a decrease in the size of nanomaterials, the surface area and the activity of the surface toward the surrounding biological components greatly increase. Due to their small size, nanomaterials can easily attach to cell surfaces or enter the cells by the endocytic pathway, resulting in membrane damage or impairment of the cellular functions. Recently, published studies on the effects of the size of nanomaterials on respiration systems have shown that pulmonary toxicity increases with decreasing size of nanomaterials. The shape of nanomaterials is also able to affect their toxicity. Nanomaterials have various shapes, such as planes, tubes, spheres, rings, and fibers, and the difference in shape can influence the membrane-warping process during endocytosis or phagocytosis. Nanomaterials with spherical shape are internalized easily and faster than those with rod or fiber shapes. In the case of silica (SiO_2) nanomaterials, amorphous silica is an FDA-approved food additive, while crystalline silica is suspected to be a human carcinogen involved in the pathogenesis of silicosis. In addition, it has been reported that long TiO_2 fiber is more toxic than the short one in mice because of its interaction with lung macrophages in a manner very similar to asbestos.[143] Introduction of surface coatings may reduce or remove toxicity of nanomaterials. Surface coatings, such as polyethylene glycol (PEG) and other biocompatible polymers, can not only stabilize nanomaterials but also prevent the dissolution and release of toxic ions from the surface of nanomaterials. Surface coatings using PEG, especially, are extensively used for QDs because the metallic core is hydrophobic and the core itself is very toxic as it is composed of heavy metals such as cadmium. Moreover, surface charge or surface composition can be changed by surface coatings, impacting intracellular distribution, and production of ROS that cause further toxicity. The surface charge of nanomaterials is also one of the key factors to influence their toxicity since it affects the adsorption of ions and biomolecules, which may change cellular responses to particles. Nanomaterials with a cationic surface charge are known to be more toxic than those with anionic surface charge. This is because cationic nanomaterials have high affinity to negative phospholipid groups or protein domains on cell membranes. Surface charge can also affect the aggregation of nanomaterials and subsequent change in size and shape, resulting in a different organism response. It is important to use a proper medium for stable dispersion of nanomaterials. The dispersion of nanomaterials can be affected by the pH and ionic strength of the selected medium and can influence their distribution and subsequent toxicity in organisms. The agents used for dispersion may increase toxicity of nanomaterials. The addition of agents such as dipalmitoylphosphatidylcholine and CTAB improves dispersion of nanomaterials, but adversely affects toxicity. Therefore, it is important to investigate the physicochemical properties of nanomaterials to evaluate their potential toxic effects on organism since the physicochemical properties of nanomaterials may influence their toxicity.

Most toxicity induced by nanomaterials is known to originate from ROS production and many nanomaterials have already demonstrated the ability to directly or indirectly induce the formation of ROS in *in vitro* and *in vivo* studies.[144] High levels of ROS mean that the state of oxidative stress damages the cell components when they are above moderate levels. ROS are generated by the dissolution of iron-based nanomaterials via Fenton reaction or attack of some inert nanomaterials on mitochondria. The generated ROS can peroxidize lipids, alter proteins, disrupt DNA, interfere with signaling functions, and modulate gene transcription. Through lipid peroxidation, nanomaterials can oxidize double bonds on fatty acid tails of membrane phospholipids, resulting in increased membrane permeability and fluidity. Cells become more susceptible to osmotic stress and nutrient uptake is hindered by membrane disorder. ROS generated by nanomaterials can attack iron–sulfur groups, which act as cofactors in various enzymes and also lead to the formation of disulfide bonds between sulfur-containing amino acids, resulting in disturbance of the structure and function of the protein. The ROS, especially the extremely reactive hydroxyl radical, generated by some nanomaterials have the capability to attack DNA via several different mechanisms to generate single-strand breaks, double-strand breaks, cross-linking, and adducts of the bases or sugars. Cell signaling can also be affected by nanomaterial-induced oxidative stress in three stages.[145] At a low level of oxidative stress, protective effects are induced by the transcription factor *Nrf*-2, and an intermediate level of oxidative stress activates mitogen-activated protein kinase (MAPK) and nuclear factor-kappa B (NF-κB), inducing proinflammatory responses. A high level of oxidative stress results in cellular apoptosis or necrosis.

Over the past several years, a large number of studies have been performed on the toxicological effects of a variety of nanomaterials, including metals, metal oxides, QDs, and CNTs, on various cells and tissue types, and in animals. Most of the earlier studies have focused on the toxicological effects of nanomaterials on respiratory systems in rodents with consequent concerns about lung injury, inflammation, and possible early signs of tumor formation in the lung. They have shown that carbon including CNTs, SWCNTs, or multiwalled CNTs, and metal oxide (i.e., TiO_2) nanomaterials produce toxic effects in the lung. Additionally, *in vitro* and *in vivo* studies on toxicological effects of nanomaterials have demonstrated that oxidative stress through the production of ROS is a major possible mechanism, which might be linked to inflammation and immunity. A survey of the *in vivo* toxicity studies on some nanomaterials is presented in Table 11.1.

TABLE 11.1

Toxicological Effects of Some Nanomaterials from *In Vivo* Studies

Nanomaterials	Toxicological Effects	Reference
Metals		
Ag	In Sprague–Dawley rats, Ag nanomaterials (average diameter: 18–19 nm) induced mixed inflammatory cell infiltrate, chronic alveolar inflammation, and small granulomatous lesions.	146
Au	Polyethylene glycol-coated Au nanomaterial (13 nm) injected in mice accumulated in the liver and spleen and caused acute inflammation and apoptosis in mice liver.	147
Cu	In liver and kidney tissues of rats exposed to Cu nanomaterials (25 nm), hepatotoxicity and nephrotoxicity were induced through hepatocytic necrosis and renal proximal tubule necrosis.	148
Metal oxides		
TiO_2	Dermal exposure of hairless mice to TiO_2 nanomaterials induced diverse pathological lesions in skin and liver by penetration through skin, which can induce skin aging.	149
CuO	Injection of CuO nanomaterial (average diameter: 27.2–95.3 nm) to mice caused genotoxicity in liver DNA by increasing 8-hydroxy-2′-deoxyguanosine levels in a dose-dependent manner.	150
ZnO	Oral exposure to ZnO nanomaterials (average diameter: 30 nm) led to an accumulation in the liver causing oxidative stress, DNA damage, and apoptosis in mice liver.	151
Quantum dots		
CdSe	CdSe quantum dots in mice easily accumulated in various organs including the liver, resulting in significant impairments to liver as reflected by morphological alternation to the hepatic lobules and increased oxidative stress	152
CdSe/ZnS	In mice, CdSe/ZnS quantum dots with carboxyl surface coating and amine surface coating caused pulmonary vascular thrombosis by activating the coagulation cascade via contact activation.	153
Carbons		
SWCNTs	Pharyngeal aspiration of SWCNTs caused acute inflammatory reaction with early onset of a fibrogenic response and the formation of granulomas in mice.	154
MWCNTs	Repeated intravenous injections of MWCNTs to male mice caused reversible damage to testis without affecting fertility.	155
Fullerene (C_{60})	Intratracheal instillation of fullerenes can induce inflammatory responses in the lung of mice by cell infiltration and tissue damage.	156
Others		
SiO_2	Silica nanomaterials intravenously injected to mice were accumulated in the lungs, liver, and spleen, and can potentially cause liver injury.	157

MWCNTs, multiwalled carbon nanotubes; SWCNTs, single-walled carbon nanotubes.

11.4.2 Impacts on Ecosystems

Nanomaterials can be released into the environment in a few ways: during the production of nanomaterials, from manufacturing processes, from products, and from technical compartments. During the production of nanomaterials, direct release can occur when free nanomaterials in the form of powder can be incautiously released through open windows and from all kinds of spills and accidents. Treated or untreated wastewater generated during the production of nanomaterials is a case of indirect release. Nanomaterials can be released from manufacturing processes. A few studies have reported that workers who produce nanomaterial products are already exposed to a high concentrations of pure nanomaterials.[158–160] The release of nanomaterials from nanomaterial-containing products into the environment is considered as a primary release route. During the use, recycling, and disposal of nanomaterial-containing products, the release of nanomaterials can happen in an intended or unintended manner. Examples are applications of products such as nanomaterial-containing sunscreen and cosmetics. Technical compartments such as wastewater treatment plants, waste incineration plants, and landfills can also be important sources for nanomaterial release because considerable amounts of the released nanomaterials exist in wastewater and solid waste. However, studies on the fate and behavior of nanomaterials in technical compartments have been poorly investigated.

Nanomaterials may get released into the atmosphere, soil, and water in various states of free nanomaterials, surface-modified nanomaterials, aggregates, and so on, through the release routes mentioned above. They can persist for a long time or be taken up by organisms acting as toxicants. The most important factor that should be considered is the bioavailability of nanomaterials to evaluate their toxic effects on organisms in ecosystem. Bioavailability of nanomaterials in the environment is largely associated with the physicochemical properties of particles, the condition of surrounding environment, and the organism exposed. In aquatic systems, the physicochemical properties of nanomaterials influencing their stability and aggregation are considered as one of the most important factors in their ecotoxicity. In the case of metal-containing nanomaterials, especially, solubility of nanomaterials is also a key factor which affects their toxic effects on aquatic organisms. For example, it has been reported that toxicity of metal oxide nanomaterials including CuO and ZnO nanomaterials to algae and aquatic invertebrates is due to their solubilized forms. In addition, metal ions released from the surface of nanomaterials can contribute to their toxicity. Bioavailability and toxicity of nanomaterials can be modulated by the condition of the environment through interaction of nanomaterials with colloidal substances in water. Abiotic factors such as pH, hardness, ionic strength, and salinity may influence the toxicity of nanomaterials. To date, however, research on the effects of abiotic factors on their bioavailability and ecotoxicity has been limited.

Over the past decade, a large number of studies have been performed on the toxic effects of nanomaterials on various model organisms in water and soil including bacteria, aquatic invertebrates, vertebrates, and terrestrial plants. In many studies, silver nanomaterials are reported to have toxic effects on microorganisms. Their toxicity is believed to be due to both particle effects and silver ions released from nanomaterials. TiO_2 nanomaterials can also have bactericidal effects under ultraviolet illumination. Other nanomaterials such as fullerenes, QDs, and ZnO have been shown to possess antimicrobial activities. Most of the studies on the ecotoxicity of nanomaterials have been performed with aquatic invertebrates *Daphnia magna*. Acute and chronic exposure to fullerenes caused adverse effects on *D. magna*, including lethality, delay in molting, and reduced offspring.[161] In the recently published studies on the ecotoxicity of some metal and metal oxide nanomaterials, moreover, it is reported that metal and metal oxide nanomaterials have acute toxicity to *D. magna* due to metal ions released from the surface of nanomaterials.[162,163] In the toxicity test of ZnO nanomaterials conducted with freshwater algae, *Pseudokirchneriella subcapitata*, dissolved zinc is largely attributed for the acute toxicity of ZnO nanomaterials. These studies indicate that the acute toxicity of metal-containing nanomaterials in water may greatly associate with the dissolved metals released from nanomaterials. Studies on the toxicological effects of nanomaterials on fish show that some nanomaterials such as CNTs, fullerenes, and metals can cause damage to respiratory organs, delay in hatching, development of embryos, or mortality. Information on the ecotoxicity of nanomaterials to terrestrial organisms is very limited. It is known that seed germination and root growth of crops may be affected by some nanomaterials.

Although some progress has been made in understanding the impacts of nanomaterials on the environment, there are several issues that need to be solved. More accurate scenarios of nanomaterials released into the environment should be defined and research on characterization of their behavior, fate, and bioavailability should be further conducted in the environment. Additionally, it is important to establish standardized methods for ecotoxicity tests and understand the interaction between nanomaterials and environmental factors, such as dissolved organic matters in water, in order to evaluate their impacts on the environment.

ACKNOWLEDGMENTS

This work was supported by the National Research Foundation of Korea (NRF) grant funded by the Korea government (MEST) (No. 2012006581).

REFERENCES

1. Fryxell, G.E. and Cao, G., 2007. *Environmental Applications of Nanomaterials*. Imperial College Press, Singapore.
2. Wiesner, M.R. and Bottero, J.-Y., 2007. *Environmental Nanotechnology: Applications and Impacts of Nanomaterials*. McGraw-Hill, New York.
3. Henderson, A.D. and Demond, A.H., 2007. Long-term performance of zero-valent iron permeable reactive barriers: A critical review. *Environ. Eng. Sci.* 24, 401–423.
4. Li, L. et al., 2006. Synthesis, properties, and environmental applications of nanoscale iron-based materials: A review. *Crit. Rev. Environ. Sci. Technol.* 36, 405–431.
5. Bard, A.J. et al., 1985. *Standard Potentials in Aqueous Solution*. Marcel Dekker, Inc., New York.
6. Wang, C.-B. and Zhang, W.-X., 1997. Synthesizing nanoscale iron particles for rapid and complete dechlorination of TCE and PCBs. *Environ. Sci. Technol.* 31, 2154–2156.

7. Schrick, B. et al., 2002. Hydrodechlorination of trichloroethylene to hydrocarbons using bimetallic nickel-iron nanoparticles. *Chem. Mater.* 14, 5140–5147.

8. Hydutsky, B.W. et al., 2007. Optimization of nano- and microiron transport through sand columns using polyelectrolyte mixtures. *Environ. Sci. Technol.* 41, 6418–6424.

9. Liu, Z.L. et al., 2004. Synthesis and characterization of ultrafine well-dispersed magnetic nanoparticles. *J. Magn. Magn. Mater.* 283, 258–262.

10. Phenrat, T. et al., 2007. Aggregation and sedimentation of aqueous nanoscale zerovalent iron dispersions. *Environ. Sci. Technol.* 41, 284–290.

11. He, P. and Zhao, D.Y., 2005. Preparation and characterization of a new class of starch-stabilized bimetallic nanoparticles for degradation of chlorinated hydrocarbons in water. *Environ. Sci. Technol.* 39, 3314–3320.

12. Phenrat, T. et al., 2009. Adsorbed polyelectrolyte coatings decrease Fe0 nanoparticle reactivity with TCE in water: Conceptual model and mechanisms. *Environ. Sci. Technol.* 43, 1507–1514.

13. Sirk, K.M. et al., 2009. Effect of adsorbed polyelectrolytes on nanoscale zero valent iron particle attachment to soil surface models. *Environ. Sci. Technol.* 43, 3803–3808.

14. Noradoun, C. et al., 2003. Destruction of chlorinated phenols by dioxygen activation under aqueous room temperature and pressure conditions. *Ind. Eng. Chem. Res.* 42, 5024–5030.

15. Leupin, O.X. et al., 2005. Aesenic removal from Bangladesh tube well water with filter columns containing zerovalent iron filings and sand. *Environ. Sci. Technol.* 39, 8032–8037.

16. Englehardt, J. et al., 2007. Oxidation of aqueous EDTA and associated organics and coprecipitation of inorganics by ambient iron-mediated aeration. *Environ. Sci. Technol.* 41, 270–276.

17. Joo, S.H. et al., 2004. Oxidative degradation of the carbothiolate herbicide, molinate, using nanoscale zero-valent iron. *Environ. Sci. Technol.* 38, 2242–2247.

18. Joo, S.H. et al., 2005. Quantification of the oxidizing capacity of nanoparticulate zero-valent iron. *Environ. Sci. Technol.* 39, 1263–1268.

19. Hug, S.J. et al., 2001. Solar oxidation and removal of arsenic at circumneutral pH in iron containing waters. *Environ. Sci. Technol.* 35, 2114–2121.

20. Hug, S.J. and Leupin, O., 2003. Iron-catalyzed oxidation of arsenic(III) by oxygen and by hydrogen peroxide: pH-dependent formation of oxidant in the Fenton reaction. *Environ. Sci. Technol.* 37, 2734–2742.

21. Keenan, C.R. and Sedlak, D.L., 2008. Factors affecting the yields of oxidants from the reaction of nanoparticulate zero-valent iron and oxygen. *Environ. Sci. Technol.* 42, 1262–1267.

22. Buxton, G.V. et al., 1988. Critical-review of rate constants for reactions of hydrated electrons, hydrogen-atoms and hydroxyl radicals ($\cdot$OH/O$^-$) in aqueous-solution. *J. Phys. Chem. Ref. Data* 17, 513–886.

23. Zecevic, S. et al., 1989. Oxygen reduction on iron. Part III. An analysis of the rotating disk-ring electrode measurements in near neutral solutions. *J. Electroanal. Chem.* 265, 179–193.

24. Zecevic, S. et al., 1991. Oxygen reduction on iron. Part IV. The reduction of hydrogen peroxide as the intermediate in oxygen reduction reaction in alkaline solutions. *Electrochim. Acta* 36, 5–14.

25. Keenan, C.R. and Sedlak, D.L., 2008. Ligand-enhanced reactive oxidant generation by nanoparticulate zero-valent iron and oxygen. *Environ. Sci. Technol.* 42, 6936–6941.

26. Lee, J. et al., 2007. Oxidation on zerovalent iron promoted by polyoxometalate as an electron shuttle. *Environ. Sci. Technol.* 41, 3335–3340.

27. Lee, C. et al., 2008. Polyoxometalate-enhanced oxidation of organic compounds by nanoparticulate zero-valent iron and ferrous ion in the presence of oxygen. *Environ. Sci. Technol.* 42, 4921–4926.

28. Lee, C. et al., 2008. Bactericidal effect of zero-valent iron nanoparticles on *Escherichia coli*. *Environ. Sci. Technol.* 42, 4927–4933.
29. Kim, J.Y. et al., 2010. Inactivation of *Escherichia coli* by nanoparticulate zerovalent iron and ferrous ion. *Appl. Environ. Microbiol.* 76, 7668–7670.
30. Kim, J.Y. et al., 2011. Inactivation of MS2 coliphage by ferrous ion and zero-valent iron nanoparticles. *Environ. Sci. Technol.* 45, 6978–6984.
31. Martinez, F. et al., 2005. Heterogeneous photo-Fenton degradation of phenolic aqueous solutions over iron-containing SBA-15 catalyst. *Appl. Cat. B Environ.* 60, 181–190.
32. Lim, H. et al., 2006. Highly active heterogeneous Fenton catalyst using iron oxide nanoparticles immobilized in alumina coated mesoporous silica. *Chem. Commun.* 463–465.
33. Ramirez, J.H. et al., 2007. Azo-dye orange II degradation by heterogeneous Fenton-like reaction using carbon-Fe catalysts. *Appl. Catal. B Environ.* 75, 312–323.
34. Zhang, J.B. et al., 2008. Decomposing phenol by the hidden talent of ferromagnetic nanoparticles. *Chemosphere* 73, 1524–1528.
35. Pham, A.L.T. et al., 2009. A silica-supported iron oxide catalyst capable of activating hydrogen peroxide at neutral pH values. *Environ. Sci. Technol.* 43, 8930–8935.
36. Lee, Y.N. et al., 2001. Hydrogen peroxide decomposition over Ln1-xAxMnO3 (Ln = La or Nd and A = K or Sr) perovskites. *Appl. Cat. A Gen.* 215, 245–256.
37. Gonzalez-Olmos, R. et al., 2011. Indications of the reactive species in a heterogeneous Fenton-like reaction using Fe-containing zeolites. *Appl. Cat. A Gen.* 398, 44–53.
38. Hoffmann, M.R. et al., 1995. Environmental applications of semiconductor photocatalysis. *Chem. Rev.* 95, 69–96.
39. Kamat, P.V., 1993. Photochemistry on nonreactive and reactive (semiconductor) surfaces. *Chem. Rev.* 93, 267–300.
40. Linsebigler, A.L. et al., 1995. Photocatalysis on TiO_2 surfaces—Principles, mechanisms, and selected results. *Chem. Rev.* 95, 735–758.
41. Mills, A. and LeHunte, S., 1997. An overview of semiconductor photocatalysis. *J. Photochem. Photobiol. A Chem.* 108, 1–35.
42. Ollis, D.F. et al., 1991. Photocatalyzed destruction of water contaminants. *Environ. Sci. Technol.* 25, 1522–1529.
43. Kim, S. and Choi, W., 2002. Dual photocatalytic pathways of trichloroacetate degradation on TiO_2: Effects of nanosized platinum deposits on kinetics and mechanism. *J. Phys. Chem. B.* 106, 13311–13317.
44. Mao, Y. et al., 1991. Identification of organic acids and other intermediates in oxidative degradation of chlorinated ethanes on TiO_2 surfaces en route to mineralization—A combined photocatalytic and radiation chemical study. *J. Phys. Chem.* 95, 10080–10089.
45. Kim, S. and Choi, W., 2002. Kinetics and mechanisms of photocatalytic degradation of $(CH_3)_nNH_{4-n}^+$ ($0 < n < 4$) in TiO_2 suspension: The role of OH radicals. *Environ. Sci. Technol.* 36, 2019–2025.
46. Lee, H. and Choi, W., 2002. Photocatalytic oxidation of arsenite in TiO_2 suspension: Kinetics and mechanisms. *Environ. Sci. Technol.* 36, 3872–3878.
47. Ryu, J. and Choi, W., 2004. Effects of TiO_2 surface modifications on photocatalytic oxidation of arsenite: The role of superoxides. *Environ. Sci. Technol.* 38, 2928–2933.
48. Ryu, J. and Choi, W.Y., 2006. Photocatalytic oxidation of arsenite on TiO_2: Understanding the controversial oxidation mechanism involving superoxides and the effect of alternative electron acceptors. *Environ. Sci. Technol.* 40, 7034–7039.
49. Kim, S. and Choi, W., 2005. Visible-light-induced photocatalytic degradation of 4-chlorophenol and phenolic compounds in aqueous suspension of pure titania: Demonstrating the existence of a surface-complex-mediated path. *J. Phys. Chem. B* 109, 5143–5149.
50. Kim, S. et al., 2004. Comparative study of homogeneous and heterogeneous photocatalytic redox reactions: $PW_{12}O_{40}^{3-}$ vs TiO_2. *J. Phys. Chem. B* 108, 6402–6411.

51. Stafford, U. et al., 1994. Radiolytic and TiO_2-assisted photocatalytic degradation of 4-chlorophenol—A comparative study. *J. Phys. Chem.* 98, 6343–6351.

52. Romero, M. et al., 1999. Solar photocatalytic degradation of water and air pollutants: Challenges and perspectives. *Sol. Energy.* 66, 169–182.

53. Akyol, A. et al., 2004. Photocatalytic decolorization of remazol red RR in aqueous ZnO suspensions. *Appl. Catal. B Environ.* 54, 19–24.

54. Evgenidou, E. et al., 2007. Photocatalytic oxidation of methyl parathion over TiO_2 and ZnO suspensions. *Catal. Today* 124, 156–162.

55. Seven, O. et al., 2004. Solar photocatalytic disinfection of a group of bacteria and fungi aqueous suspensions with TiO_2, ZnO and Sahara desert dust. *J. Photochem. Photobiol. A Chem.* 165, 103–107.

56. Behnajady, M.A. et al., 2006. Kinetic study on photocatalytic degradation of CI acid yellow 23 by ZnO photocatalyst. *J. Hazard. Mater.* 133, 226–232.

57. Kamat, P. V. et al., 2002. A "sense and shoot" approach for photocatalytic degradation of organic contaminants in water. *J. Phys. Chem. B* 106, 788–794.

58. Arai, T. et al., 2009. Reaction mechanism and activity of WO_3 catalyzed photodegradation of organic substances promoted by a CuO cocatalyst. *J. Phys. Chem. C* 113, 6602–6609.

59. Kim, J. et al., 2010. Platinized WO_3 as an environmental photocatalyst that generates OH radicals under visible light. *Environ. Sci. Technol.* 44, 6849–6854.

60. Sun, S.M. et al., 2010. Preparation of ordered mesoporous Ag/WO_3 and its highly efficient degradation of acetaldehyde under visible-light irradiation. *J. Hazard. Mater.* 178, 427–433.

61. Sayama, K. et al., 2010. Highly active WO_3 semiconductor photocatalyst prepared from amorphous peroxo-tungstic acid for the degradation of various organic compounds. *Appl. Catal. B Environ.* 94, 150–157.

62. Furube, A. et al., 2001. Direct observation of a picosecond charge separation process in photoexcited platinum-loaded TiO_2 particles by femtosecond diffuse reflectance spectroscopy. *Chem. Phys. Lett.* 336, 424–430.

63. Lee, J.S. and Choi, W.Y., 2005. Photocatalytic reactivity of surface platinized TiO_2: Substrate specificity and the effect of Pt oxidation state. *J. Phys. Chem. B.* 109, 7399–7406.

64. Dawson, A. and Kamat, P.V., 2001. Semiconductor-metal nanocomposites. Photoinduced fusion and photocatalysis of gold-capped TiO_2 (TiO_2/Gold) nanoparticles. *J. Phys. Chem. B* 105, 960–966.

65. Subramanian, V. et al., 2004. Catalysis with TiO_2/gold nanocomposites. Effect of metal particle size on the fermi level equilibration. *J. Am. Chem. Soc.* 126, 4943–4950.

66. Lee, J. et al., 2002. Selective photocatalytic oxidation of NH_3 to N_2 on plantation TiO_2 in water. *Environ. Sci. Technol.* 36, 5462–5468.

67. Lee, J.S. and Choi, W.Y., 2004. Effect of platinum deposits on TiO_2 on the anoxic photocatalytic degradation pathways of alkylamines in water: Dealkylation and N-alkylation. *Environ. Sci. Technol.* 38, 4026–4033.

68. Choi, W.Y. et al., 1994. The role of metal ion dopants in quantum sized TiO_2—Correlation between photoreactivity and charge carrier recombination dynamics. *J. Phys. Chem.* 98, 13669–13679.

69. Choi, W.Y. et al., 1994. Effects of metal-ion dopants on the photocatalytic reactivity of quantum-sized TiO_2 particles. *Angew. Chem. Int. Ed.* 33, 1091–1092.

70. Ullah, R. and Dutta, J., 2008. Photocatalytic degradation of organic dyes with manganese-doped ZnO nanoparticles. *J. Hazard. Mater.* 156, 194–200.

71. Ranjit, K.T. and Viswanathan, B., 1997. Photocatalytic reduction of nitrite and nitrate ions over doped TiO_2 catalysts. *J. Photochem. Photobiol. A Chem.* 107, 215–220.

72. Anandan, S. et al., 2007. Photocatalytic degradation of 2,4,6-trichlorophenol using lanthanum doped ZnO in aqueous suspension. *Catal. Commun.* 8, 1377–1382.

73. Choi, J. et al., 2010. Effects of single metal-ion doping on the visible-light photoreactivity of TiO_2. *J. Phys. Chem. C* 114, 783–792.

74. Livraghi, S. et al., 2006. Origin of photoactivity of nitrogen-doped titanium dioxide under visible light. *J. Am. Chem. Soc.* 128, 15666–15671.

75. Katoh, R. et al., 2010. Charge separation and trapping in N-doped TiO_2 photocatalysts: A time-resolved microwave conductivity study. *J. Phys. Chem. Lett.* 1, 3261–3265.

76. Mrowetz, M. et al., 2004. Oxidative power of nitrogen-doped TiO_2 photocatalysts under visible illumination. *J. Phys. Chem. B* 108, 17269–17273.

77. Vinodgopal, K. and Kamat, P.V., 1995. Enhanced rates of photocatalytic degradation of an azo-dye using SnO_2/TiO_2 coupled semiconductor thin-films. *Environ. Sci. Technol.* 29, 841–845.

78. Song, K.Y. et al., 2001. Preparation of transparent particulate MoO_3/TiO_2 and WO_3/TiO_2 films and their photocatalytic properties. *Chem. Mater.* 13, 2349–2355.

79. Spanhel, L. et al., 1987. Photochemistry of semiconductor colloids. 22. Electron injection from illuminated Cds into attached TiO_2 and ZnO particles. *J. Am. Chem. Soc.* 109, 6632–6635.

80. Kamat, P.V. et al., 1994. Photoinduced charge-transfer between carbon and semiconductor clusters—One-electron reduction of C_{60} in colloidal TiO_2 semiconductor suspensions. *J. Phys. Chem.* 98, 9137–9142.

81. Park, Y. et al., 2009. Fullerol-titania charge-transfer-mediated photocatalysis working under visible light. *Chem. Eur. J.* 15, 10843–10850.

82. Kedem, S. et al., 2005. Composite polymer nanofibers with carbon nanotubes and titanium dioxide particles. *Langmuir* 21, 5600–5604.

83. Yao, Y. et al., 2008. Photoreactive TiO_2/carbon nanotube composites: Synthesis and reactivity. *Environ. Sci. Technol.* 42, 4952–4957.

84. Vanderlaan, M. et al., 1988. Environmental monitoring by immunoassay. *Environ. Sci. Technol.* 22, 247–254.

85. Pancrazio, J.J. et al., 1999. Development and application of cell-based biosensors. *Ann. Biomed. Eng.* 27, 697–711.

86. Palchetti, I. and M. Mascini, 2008. Nucleic acid biosensors for environmental pollution monitoring. *Analyst* 133, 846–854.

87. Baeumner, A.J., 2003. Biosensors for environmental pollutants and food contaminants. *Anal. Bioanal. Chem.* 377, 434–445.

88. Amine, A. et al., 2006. Enzyme inhibition-based biosensors for food safety and environmental monitoring. *Biosens. Bioelectron.* 21, 1405–1423.

89. Rodriguez-Mozaz, S. et al., 2006. Biosensors as useful tools for environmental analysis and monitoring. *Anal. Bioanal. Chem.* 386, 1025–1041.

90. Vikesland, P.J. and K.R. Wigginton, 2010. Nanomaterial enabled biosensors for pathogen monitoring—A review. *Environ. Sci. Technol.* 44, 3656–3669.

91. Liu, J.W. et al., 2007. Quantum dot encoding of aptamer-linked nanostructures for one-pot simultaneous detection of multiple analytes. *Anal. Chem.* 79, 4120–4125.

92. Hansen, J.A., et al., 2006. Quantum-dot/aptamer-based ultrasensitive multi-analyte electrochemical biosensor. *J. Am. Chem. Soc.* 128, 2228–2229.

93. Guo, S.J. and S.J. Dong, 2009. Biomolecule-nanoparticle hybrids for electrochemical biosensors. *Trends Anal. Chem.* 28, 96–109.

94. Polsky, R. et al., 2006. Nucleic acid-functionalized Pt nanoparticles: Catalytic labels for the amplified electrochemical detection of biomolecules. *Anal. Chem.* 78, 2268–2271.

95. Estevez, M.C. et al., 2009. Highly fluorescent dye-doped silica nanoparticles increase flow cytometry sensitivity for cancer cell monitoring. *Nano Res.* 2, 448–461.

96. Tallury, P. et al., 2008. Silica-based multimodal/multifunctional nanoparticles for bioimaging and biosensing applications. *Nanomedicine* 3, 579–592.

97. Kim, J.B. et al., 2008. Nanobiocatalysis and its potential applications. *Trends Biotechnol.* 26, 639–646.
98. Daniel, M.C. and D. Astruc, 2004. Gold nanoparticles: Assembly, supramolecular chemistry, quantum-size-related properties, and applications toward biology, catalysis, and nanotechnology. *Chem. Rev.* 104, 293–346.
99. Sun, Y.G. and Y.N. Xia, 2002. Shape-controlled synthesis of gold and silver nanoparticles. *Science* 298, 2176–2179.
100. Rosi, N.L. and C.A. Mirkin, 2005. Nanostructures in biodiagnostics. *Chem. Rev.* 105, 1547–1562.
101. Frens, G., 1973. Controlled nucleation for regulation of particle-size in monodisperse gold suspensions. *Nat. Phys. Sci.* 241, 20–22.
102. Huang, Y.Z. et al., 2009. Surfactant-promoted reductive synthesis of shape-controlled gold nanostructures. *Cryst. Growth Des.* 9, 858–862.
103. Ming, T. et al., 2009. Growth of tetrahexahedral gold nanocrystals with high-index facets. *J. Am. Chem. Soc.* 131, 16350–16351.
104. Mirkin, C.A. et al., 1996. A DNA-based method for rationally assembling nanoparticles into macroscopic materials. *Nature* 382, 607–609.
105. Ellington, A.D. and J.W. Szostak, 1992. Selection in vitro of single-stranded DNA molecules that fold into specific ligand-binding structures. *Nature* 355, 850–852.
106. Tuerk, C. and L. Gold, 1990. Systematic evolution of ligands by exponential enrichment-RNA ligands to bacteriophage-T4 DNA-polymerase. *Science* 249, 505–510.
107. Willner, I. and M. Zayats, 2007. Electronic aptamer-based sensors. *Angew. Chem. Int. Ed.* 46, 6408–6418.
108. Bock, L.C. et al., 1992. Selection of single-stranded-DNA molecules that bind and inhibit human thrombin. *Nature* 355, 564–566.
109. Smirnov, I.V. et al., 2002. Pb EXAFS studies on DNA quadruplexes: Identification of metal ion binding site. *Biochemistry* 41, 12133–12139.
110. Kim, M. et al., 2009. Arsenic removal from vietnamese groundwater using the arsenic-binding DNA aptamer. *Environ. Sci. Technol.* 43, 9335–9340.
111. He, J.A. et al., 2011. Isolation and identification of the DNA aptamer target to acetamiprid. *J. Agric. Food Chem.* 59, 1582–1586.
112. Fischer, N. et al., 2007. Aptasensors for biosecurity applications. *Curr. Opin. Chem. Biol.* 11, 316–328.
113. Li, H. et al., 2011. Aptamer selection for the detection of *Escherichia coli* K88. *Can. J. Microbiol.* 57, 453–459.
114. Stratis-Cullum, D.N. et al., 2009. Evaluation of relative aptamer binding to *Campylobacter jejuni* bacteria using affinity probe capillary electrophoresis. *Anal. Lett.* 42, 2389–2402.
115. Bruno, J.G. et al., 2012. An aptamer beacon responsive to botulinum toxins. *Biosens. Bioelectron.* 31, 240–243.
116. Wang, L.B. et al., 2011. An aptamer-based chromatographic strip assay for sensitive toxin semi-quantitative detection. *Biosens. Bioelectron.* 26, 3059–3062.
117. Lamont, E.A. et al., 2011. A single DNA aptamer functions as a biosensor for ricin. *Analyst* 136, 3884–3895.
118. Hu, X.G. et al., 2011. ssDNA aptamer-based column for simultaneous removal of nano-gram per liter level of illicit and analgesic pharmaceuticals in drinking water. *Environ. Sci. Technol.* 45, 4890–4895.
119. Song, K.M. et al., 2011. Gold nanoparticle-based colorimetric detection of kanamycin using a DNA aptamer. *Anal. Biochem.* 415, 175–181.
120. Liu, J. and Y. Lu, 2006. Preparation of aptamer-linked gold nanoparticle purple aggregates for colorimetric sensing of analytes. *Nat. Protoc.* 1, 246–252.
121. Jarup, L., 2003. Hazards of heavy metal contamination. *Br. Med. Bull.* 68, 167–182.

122. Hu, X.G. et al., 2012. Polymeric nanoparticle-aptamer bioconjugates can diminish the toxicity of mercury in vivo. *Toxicol. Lett.* 208, 69–74.

123. Lee, J.S. et al., 2007. Colorimetric detection of mercuric ion (Hg2+) in aqueous media using DNA-functionalized gold nanoparticles. *Angew. Chem. Int. Ed.* 46, 4093–4096.

124. Lee, J.S. and C.A. Mirkin, 2008. Chip-based scanometric detection of mercuric ion using DNA-functionalized gold nanoparticles. *Anal. Chem.* 80, 6805–6808.

125. Liu, C.W. et al., 2008. Detection of mercury(II) based on Hg(2+)-DNA complexes inducing the aggregation of gold nanoparticles. *Chem. Commun.* 21(19), 2242–2244.

126. Kim, Y.S. and J. Jurng, 2011. Gold nanoparticle-based homogeneous fluorescent aptasensor for multiplex detection. *Analyst* 136, 3720–3724.

127. Liu, J.W. and Y. Lu, 2003. A colorimetric lead biosensor using DNAzyme-directed assembly of gold nanoparticles. *J. Am. Chem. Soc.* 125, 6642–6643.

128. Liu, J.W. and Y. Lu, 2004. Accelerated color change of gold nanoparticles assembled by DNAzymes for simple and fast colorimetric Pb2+ detection. *J. Am. Chem. Soc.* 126, 12298–12305.

129. Ngundi, M.M. et al., 2006. Nonantibody-based recognition: Alternative molecules for detection of pathogens. *Expert Rev. Proteomics* 3, 511–524.

130. Daniels, D.A. et al., 2003. A tenascin-C aptamer identified by tumor cell SELEX: Systematic evolution of ligands by exponential enrichment. *Proc. Natl. Acad. Sci. U.S.A* 100, 15416–15421.

131. Cerchia, L. et al., 2005. Neutralizing aptamers from whole-cell SELEX inhibit the RET receptor tyrosine kinase. *PLoS Biol.* 3, 697–704.

132. Fang, X.H. and W.H. Tan, 2010. Aptamers generated from cell-SELEX for molecular medicine: A chemical biology approach. *Acc. Chem. Res.* 43, 48–57.

133. So, H.M. et al., 2008. Detection and titer estimation of *Escherichia coli* using aptamer-functionalized single-walled carbon-nanotube field-effect transistors. *Small* 4, 197–201.

134. Zelada-Guillen, G.A. et al., 2009. Immediate detection of living bacteria at ultralow concentrations using a carbon nanotube based potentiometric aptasensor. *Angew. Chem. Int. Ed.* 48, 7334–7337.

135. Zelada-Guillen, G.A. et al., 2010. Real-time potentiometric detection of bacteria in complex samples. *Anal. Chem.* 82, 9254–9260.

136. Roco, M.C., 2003. Nanotechnology: Convergence with modern biology and medicine. *Curr. Opin. Biotechnol.* 14, 337–346.

137. Karnik, B.S. et al., 2005. Fabrication of catalytic membranes for the treatment of drinking water using combined ozonation and ultrafiltration. *Environ. Sci. Technol.* 39, 7656–7661.

138. Brody, A.L., 2006. Nano and food packaging technologies converge. *Food Technol.* 60, 92–94.

139. Handy, R.D. et al., 2008. The ecotoxicology and chemistry of manufactured nanoparticles. *Ecotoxicology* 17, 287–314.

140. Savolainen, K. et al., 2010. Risk assessment of engineered nanomaterials and nanotechnologies—A review. *Toxicology* 269, 92–104.

141. Maynard, A.D., 2006. *Nanotechnology: A Research Strategy for Addressing Risk.* Woodrow Wilson International Center for Scholars, Washington, DC.

142. Sharifi, S. et al., 2012. Toxicity of nanomaterials. *Chem. Soc. Rev.* 41, 2323–2343.

143. Hamilton, R.F. et al., 2009. Particle length-dependent titanium dioxide nanomaterials toxicity and bioactivity. *Part. Fibre Toxicol.* 6, 35.

144. Nel, A. et al., 2006. Toxic potential of materials at the nanolevel. *Science* 311, 622–627.

145. Li, N. et al., 2008. The role of oxidative stress in ambient particulate matter-induced lung diseases and its implications in the toxicity of engineered nanoparticles. *Free Radic. Biol. Med.* 44, 1689–1699.

146. Sung, J.H. et al., 2009. Subchronic inhalation toxicity of silver nanoparticles. *Toxicol. Sci.* 108, 452–461.

147. Cho, W.S. et al., 2009. Acute toxicity and pharmacokinetics of 13 nm-sized PEG-coated gold nanoparticles. *Toxicol. Appl. Pharmacol.* 236, 16–24.

148. Lei, R. et al., 2008. Integrated metabolomic analysis of the nano-sized copper particle-induced hepatotoxicity and nephrotoxicity in rats: A rapid in vivo screening method for nanotoxicity. *Toxicol. Appl. Pharmacol.* 232, 292–301.

149. Wu, J. et al., 2009. Toxicity and penetration of TiO2 nanoparticles in hairless mice and porcine skin after subchronic dermal exposure. *Toxicol. Lett.* 191, 1–8.

150. Song, M.F. et al., 2012. Metal nanoparticle-induced micronuclei and oxidative DNA damage in mice. *J. Clin. Biochem. Nutr.* 50, 211–216.

151. Sharma, V. et al., 2011. Induction of oxidative stress, DNA damage and apoptosis in mouse liver after sub-acute oral exposure to zinc oxide nanoparticles. *Mutat. Res.* 745, 84–91.

152. Liu, W. et al., 2011. CdSe quantum dot (QD)-induced morphological and functional impairments to liver in mice. *PLoS ONE* 6, e24406.

153. Geys, J. et al., 2008. Acute toxicity and prothrombotic effects of quantum dots: Impact of surface charge. *Environ. Health Perspect.* 116, 1607–1613.

154. Shvedova, A.A. et al., 2005. Unusual inflammatory and fibrogenic pulmonary responses to single-walled carbon nanotubes in mice. *Am. J. Physiol. Lung Cell Mol. Physiol.* 289, L698–L708.

155. Bai, Y. et al., 2010. Repeated administrations of carbon nanotubes in male mice cause reversible testis damage without affecting fertility. *Nat. Nanotechnol.* 5, 683–689.

156. Park, E.J. et al., 2010. Carbon fullerenes (C60s) can induce inflammatory responses in the lung of mice. *Toxicol. Appl. Pharmacol.* 244, 226–233.

157. Xie, G. et al., 2010. Biodistribution and toxicity of intravenously administered silica nanoparticles in mice. *Arch. Toxicol.* 84, 183–190.

158. Bello, D. et al., 2008. Particle exposure levels during CVD growth and subsequent handling of vertically-aligned carbon nanotube films. *Carbon* 46, 974–981.

159. Han, J.H. et al., 2008. Monitoring multiwalled carbon nanotube exposure in carbon nanotube research facility. *Inhal. Toxicol.* 20, 741–749.

160. Yeganeh, B. et al., 2008. Characterization of airborne particles during production of carbonaceous nanomaterials. *Environ. Sci. Technol.* 42, 4600–4606.

161. Oberdörster, E. et al., 2006. Ecotoxicology of carbon-based engineered nanoparticles: Effects of fullerene (C60) on aquatic organisms. *Carbon* 44, 1112–1120.

162. Heinlaan, M. et al., 2011. Changes in the *Daphnia magna* midgut upon ingestion of copper oxide nanoparticles: A transmission electron microscopy study. *Water Res.* 45, 179–190.

163. Zhao, C.M. and Wang, W.X., 2011. Comparison of acute and chronic toxicity of silver nanoparticles and silver nitrate to *Daphnia magna*. *Environ. Toxicol. Chem.* 30, 885–892.

12 Cytotoxicity of Biosynthesized Nanomaterials and Functionalized Nanomaterials
Use in Therapy

Murugan Veerapandian and Kyusik Yun
Gachon University

Ramesh Subbiah
Korea Institute of Science and Technology
University of Science and Technology

Min-Ho Lee
Korea Electronics Technology Institute

CONTENTS

12.1   INTRODUCTION

In recent years, there has been an increasing number of studies on green chemistry for nanomaterial synthesis with the objective of reducing or eliminating the use and generation of hazardous substances.[1] With the development of bionanotechnology, the principles of biosynthesis and surface engineering chemistry have been applied in green synthesis and applications of nanomaterials. Biocompatible nanomaterials generated from these processes have received considerable attention for their promising applications in bioimaging, biosensing, drug delivery, and development of biomedicines.[2] These studies focus on taking advantage of the chemical, physical, and other properties of nanoparticles (NPs) so as to develop the potential of their advanced scientific and commercial applications.[3]

Chemical and geometric manipulation of metal NPs and graphitic nanomaterials such as carbon nanotubes (CNTs), fullerenes, and graphenes is demonstrated to have a large number of biomedical applications.[4] However, understanding of the biological interactions and their potential cytotoxicity mechanisms remain at the infancy level. Especially, biosynthesized and surface-functionalized nanomaterials are two important classes of materials that are believed to be green strategic products. Therefore, an intact study that investigates the controlled synthesis of uniform NPs and stabilization with biocompatible materials is always of great interest to enrich the existing properties of nanomaterials. Stabilization of synthesized NPs by cellular or biological components is the crucial characteristic of biosynthesis strategy. On the other hand, chemical modification and subsequent integration of active ligands through biofunctionalization strategy are feasible for generation of various functional biohybrids.

This chapter aims to provide an overview of the biosynthesis of NPs with specific notes on their intra- or extracellular biosynthetic pathways by bacteria. Later sections are devoted to the fundamental review on functionalization of nanomaterials including their biological characterizations and cytotoxicity mechanisms. The optimistic role of the cytotoxicity of nanomaterials in terms of their treatment against infectious disease and potential use in therapy are discussed.

12.2   BIOSYNTHESIS: CLASSIFICATION AND PROPERTIES

Several physical, chemical, and biological methods have been implemented to synthesize nanomaterials. In order to control the shape and size of NPs, specific methodologies have been adopted. Although ultraviolet irradiation, aerosol technologies, lithography, sonochemistry, hydrothermal, and photochemical reduction techniques have been utilized successfully to produce nanoscale materials, they remain expensive and involve the use of hazardous chemical reagents.[5] Therefore, researchers are urged to focus on new synthetic strategies that are environment friendly and sustainable. Biological synthesis of NPs especially based on microbial biotechnology is a green chemical approach. Biosynthesis of several nanoscale materials (such as metal, alloy, semiconducting, and composite forms) by bacteria, actinomycetes, fungi, yeasts, and viruses has been reported.[5] However, it has some issues such as stability, heterogeneous size distribution, and low synthesis rate. To eradicate these problems, optimization of microbial cultivation, extraction techniques, and integration of combinatorial approach such as photobiological methods may be used. Enzymatic molecular mechanisms of particular microbes that mediate the synthesis of biological NPs should be studied in-depth to enhance the rate of synthesis and properties of NPs.[5,6] In this section, we review the types of biosynthesized NPs and their properties toward biomedical therapy.

12.2.1 INTRA- OR EXTRACELLULAR BIOSYNTHESIS OF NPS BY BACTERIA

Microorganisms have the potential to produce nanoscale dimensions of inorganic materials via either intra- or extracellular biosynthesis with fine morphology. Normal metabolic activities that include chemical detoxification and its mediated energy-dependent ion efflux from the microbial cell membrane function as either ATPase or chemiosmotic cation or proton antitransporters, which make them resistant to most toxic heavy metals.[7,8] Therefore, microbial systems can convert the toxic metal ions into insoluble nontoxic metal nanoclusters. The different types of microbial detoxification are extracellular biomineralization, biosorption, complexation, or precipitation, or intracellular accumulation.[9] Figure 12.1 shows the schematic pathway for the biosynthesis of NPs.

In general, biosynthesized NPs have many commercial applications in several fields; however, polydispersity is still a major issue that needs to be optimized for obtaining monodispersity. In contrast, the intracellular productions of NPs are of particular dimension and with less polydispersity. But, additional processes such as ultrasound treatment or reaction with suitable detergents are required to isolate the intracellularly synthesized NPs.[10] Cell wall reductive enzymes or soluble secreted enzymes are mainly involved in the extracellular synthesis of metal NPs. Synthesized NPs have wider applications in optoelectronics, electronics, bioimaging, and sensor technology than in intracellular accumulation.[5] Several classes of bacterial species are demonstrated to synthesize metals, alloys, and semiconducting NPs in sizes ranging from 2 to 400 nm.[5] For instance, intracellular synthesis of transition metal NPs such as gold and silver NPs (AgNPs) with different morphologies (such as cubic, hexagonal, and spherical NPs, and triangular nanoplates in the size range of 5–400 nm) by *Bacillus subtilis*, sulfate-reducing bacteria, *Shewanella algae*, *Pediastrum boryanum*, *Escherichia coli*, *Rhodobacter capsulatus*, *Lactobacillus*, *Corynebacterium*, and *Bacillus* sp. was reported; an extended review related to biosynthesis of NPs can be found in the literature.[5]

An effective biomedical application of nanomaterials for therapy highly depends on their stability at various pH conditions, efficient encapsulation or loading of therapeutics, inertness, biocompatibility, and minimized resorption by host media. Furthermore, NPs are not immunogenic and should mimic as a biological component with proper solubility for elimination. The unique properties of metal NPs such as silver have been extended into a broader range of biomedical applications such as electrocatalytic materials in biosensors and antimicrobial materials against Gram-negative and Gram-positive strains.[11] Studies have also revealed that silver and its composites have better application in water purification

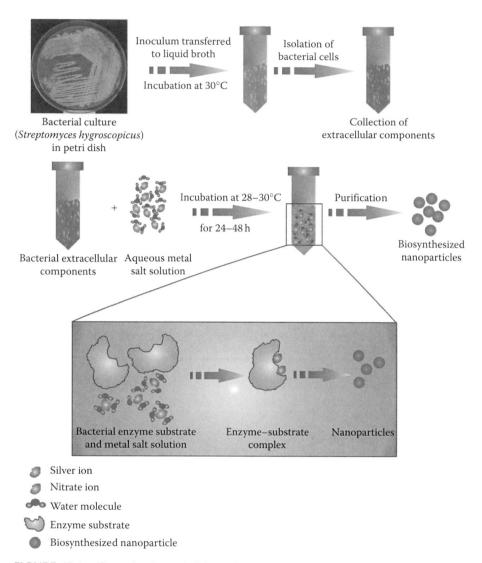

Bacterial culture
(*Streptomyces hygroscopicus*)
in petri dish

Inoculum transferred
to liquid broth

Incubation at 30°C

Isolation of
bacterial cells

Collection of
extracellular components

Bacterial extracellular
components

Aqueous metal
salt solution

Incubation at 28–30°C

for 24–48 h

Purification

Biosynthesized
nanoparticles

Bacterial enzyme substrate
and metal salt solution

Enzyme–substrate
complex

Nanoparticles

Silver ion
Nitrate ion
Water molecule
Enzyme substrate
Biosynthesized nanoparticle

FIGURE 12.1 **(See color insert.)** Schematic representation shows an example of biosynthetic pathway for preparation of AgNPs.

and air filtration.[12] Apart from AgNPs, other transition metal components such as copper nanocomposites based on photocatalysis have been reported to have enhanced antimicrobial effects.[13] Surface plasmonic resonance in the visible and near-infrared region produced metal NPs such as gold nanorods and silica-coated gold nanorods for their potential use in bioimaging and hyperthermia.[14] Efficient conversion of absorbed radiation into thermal energy by the electronic motion on the surface of metal nanostructures is the key feature in photothermal-based cytotoxicity (also known as photothermal ablation).[15]

12.3 FUNCTIONALIZATION OF NANOMATERIALS: PROPERTIES

Surface functionalization is an important aspect of nanomaterial design for biomedical applications. Variation of surface physicochemical properties of nanomaterials such as NPs can influence particle uptake, biological responses, and biodistribution.[16] Surface functionalization can not only increase circulation time of nanocarriers in blood plasma but also diminish nonspecific distribution or specific targeting of tissues or cells by using a targeting ligand.[17] Although the topic of this review is emphasized to be cytotoxicity of biosynthesized and functionalized nanomaterials for therapeutic applications, it is important to understand the fundamental physicochemical properties of surface-functionalized NP formulation. Average particle diameter, polydispersity, elastic properties, drug-loading efficiency, and surface charge are the key factors that govern the quality of final formulation. In this section, we are going to review the reports related to the physicochemical properties of functionalized NPs for therapeutic applications.

Poly(lactide-*co*-glycolide) (PLGA) is an FDA-approved synthetic biodegradable polymer; its NPs are attractive for tumor-targeted therapy and imaging.[18] It can be surface stabilized by polyethylene glycol (PEG) to minimize opsonization and enhance prolongation of blood circulation, and this interface can be functionalized with a variety of biological agents for tumor-specific targeting.[19] Chung et al.[20] studied the effect of surface functionalization of PLGA NPs by heparin–chitosan-conjugated pluronic for tumor targeting in which they demonstrated the stability of NPs in physiological environments including blood and blood plasma. Three kinds of PLGA NPs maintained their stability even in full serum condition with no noticeable changes in size distribution profiles. In contrast, the serum protein adsorption on NPs resulted in changes in the surface charge of the modified NPs such as −50 ± 2 to −38 ± 1 mV for heparin–pluronic-conjugated PLGA NPs (HP-PLGA NPs) and +38 ± 0 to −24 ± 1 mV for chitosan–pluronic-conjugated PLGA NPs (CP-PLGA NPs).[20] In contrast to this result, another study by Yang et al.[21] reported the serum-mediated micro-aggregate formation of chitosan-modified PLGA NP. This inconsistency between two systems was explained by using different molecular weight chitosan for surface conjugation. For example, Chung et al. have used lower molecular weight chitosan of 10 kDa,[21] whereas other reports utilized 45–50 kDa. Lower molecular weight chitosan has an excellent solubility in water, physiological solutions, and some organic solvents such as dimethyl sulfoxide (DMSO), which probably prevents the aggregation of CP-PLGA NPs by interparticular interaction.[20] In addition, the surface-coating layer comprised chitosan–pluronic–PEG from which the PEG blocks contribute to the reduced protein adsorption on the chitosan-linked PEG. Both the chitosan- and heparin-functionalized surfaces of PLGA NPs provided a suitable environment for cell membrane adsorption and improved the desired cellular uptake for effective tumor accumulation.[20] Surface functionalization of nanomaterials can be used to couple the inherent electronic, photonic, or catalytic properties of quantum-sized nanomaterials with hybrid features.[22] For instance, graphene oxide (GO)-modified Ag/AgBr nanostructures display distinctly enhanced photocatalytic performance than bare Ag/AgBr nanospecies. Surface functionalization of

GO on Ag/AgBr shows highly efficient and stable catalytic performance under sunlight irradiation, which makes it a promising alternative to conventional UV or visible light-irradiated photocatalysts.[23] Surface modification can also promote the solubility of several nanomaterials such as carbon-based materials. A variety of oligomeric and polymeric components has been used in the functionalization of novel CNTs for their solubility in common organic solvents and/or water.[24] Direct attachment of functional groups to the graphitic surface and nanotube-bound carboxylic acids are the two basic chemical reactions for functionalization of CNTs.[24] Soluble CNTs are used as the starting materials for several chemical and biochemical modifications. Since they are proficient in adsorbing or conjugating with a range of functional molecules, it has opened the opportunity of bioapplication of CNTs in nucleic acid and drug delivery.[25]

Biomedical properties of functionalized NPs depend on the recognition or nonrecognition of the particles by immune systems. Superparamagnetic iron oxide nanoparticles (SPIONs) are an exceptional system that can be functionalized for various applications controlled by a magnetic source. These compounds comprise a crystalline iron oxide core, which is coated by a shell to avoid agglomeration of uncoated SPIONs.[26] Several modifiers such as dextran, starch, or PEG are used to modify the SPION. Low molecular weight dextran is the most common coating system employed due to high biocompatibility and long circulation properties.[27] Several dextran-coated SPIONs such as ferucarbotran, ferumoxides (average particle size >50 nm), SHU555C, and ferumoxtran-10 (average particle size <50 nm) have been approved for clinical applications such as magnetic resonance imaging (MRI) contrast agent.[28] Further, it was demonstrated that particles with ionic surfaces are more efficiently phagocytosed compared to those with nonionic surfaces.[29] The nano–bio interface between immune system and SPIONs is important and can be controlled by different surface functionalization strategies such as (1) nonlabeling for MRI; (2) PEGylation or use of <20 nm SPIONs for reduction of uptake by macrophages and for prolonged circulation time; (3) labeling with ligands for facilitated uptake/trigger targeting for *in vivo* imaging; and (4) attachment of specific ligands for recognition by tumor cells, such as folate (Figure 12.2).[30,31] Similarly, the properties of several other classes of functionalized nanomaterials such as semiconducting NPs [quantum dots (QDs) and silica], metal NPs (Au, Ag, Cu, and hybrids), and nanocomposites with significant surface plasmon resonance, photothermal, magnetic, and optical properties and their biological and therapeutic applications are reviewed in the remaining part of the sections.

12.3.1 Types of Functionalization

Nanoscale materials intended for biomedical applications either as vehicle or drug are needed to outperform conventional agents. They must also retain their colloidal stability over a wide range of pH under physiological conditions. Further, they must avoid premature release and yet specifically deliver the active molecules to the desired site.[32] In order to develop such a system for optimized applications, NPs were functionalized with chemical/biological groups through several

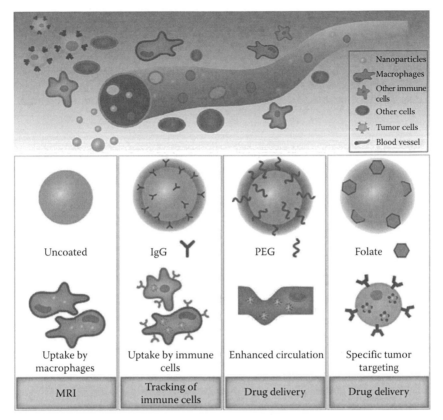

FIGURE 12.2 Effect of surface coating on nano-immuno interactions. Uncoated NPs are mainly taken up by macrophages. This property is important in MRI studies. Labeling of NPs with, for instance, immunoglobulin (IgG) allows for enhanced uptake by immune cells expressing the corresponding Fc receptor, and this is useful for targeting of NPs. Coating of particles with PEG results in a prolonged circulation time due to the avoidance of macrophage internalization of the particles, and this is important to consider when designing NPs for targeted drug delivery. Labeling of NPs with the vitamin folic acid selectively targets tumor cells with high surface expression of the folate receptor. This is an advantage in imaging of tumors but also in targeted drug delivery, and several drugs based on this strategy are already in clinical trials. (From Low, P.S., and Kularatne, S.A. *Curr. Opin. Chem. Biol.* 13, 256–262, 2009. With permission; Reprinted from *Biochim. Biophys. Acta*, 1810, Kunzmann, A., Andersson, B., Thurnherr, T., Krug, H., Scheynius, A., and Fadeel, B., Toxicology of engineered nanomaterials: Focus on biocompatibility, biodistribution and biodegradation, 361–373, Copyright 2011, with permission from Elsevier.)

functionalization strategies such as ionic stabilization, steric stabilization, ligand exchange, ligand addition, and coupling strategies via carbodiimide/maleimide coupling.[32–34] Click chemistry for bond formation, disulfide bridges for reversible chemical coupling, ionic coupling for combining oppositely charged species, and specific biorecognition interaction for binding proteins/nucleic acids on NPs

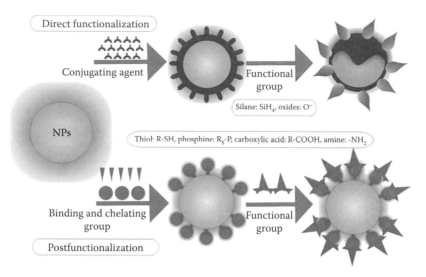

Silane: SiH$_4$, oxides: O$^-$

Thiol: R-SH, phosphine: R$_3$-P, carboxylic acid: R-COOH, amine: -NH$_2$

FIGURE 12.3 Schematic representation of functionalization methods: direct functionalization, which uses a conjugating agent in order to directly attach the chemical moiety, and postfunctionalization, which uses a binding/chelating agent to attach to the NPs and a secondary functional group for covalent attachment of the active molecule of interest.

were also the significant functionalization routes employed for the development of new functional materials.[32–34] Figure 12.3 shows the two types of functionalization methods.

12.3.2 Biological Evaluation of Functionalized Nanomaterials

The advent of nanoscience and nanotechnology made researchers explore several functional properties of new materials. Enhancement of existing properties, cost effectiveness, and benignness to human beings and environment are the specific reasons for the development of advanced functional materials. Nanomaterials hold a higher quality of physicochemical and biological properties than their bulk form; however, their toxicology in relation to human and environment is still not well understood. Although several reports related to the ecotoxicity,[35] genotoxicity,[36] reproductive, and developmental toxicity[37] studies of manufactured and engineered nanomaterials are available in the literature, in-depth research toward toxicity analysis of nanomaterials is still comparatively lesser than the development of new materials. In order to decrease undesirable toxicity and enhance the targeted biomedical application, materials are surface engineered with biocompatible materials. For instance, water-soluble poly(acrylic acid)-functionalized Si NPs are prepared by covalent reaction of hydrogen-terminated Si QDs in an acrylic acid and ethanol solution and characterized for bioimaging in Chinese hamster ovary (CHO) cells.[38,39] Poly(acrylic acid)-grafted Si NP (10 nm diameter)-labeled CHO cells show no changes in luminescence intensity over a span of 2 h. Another report demonstrated the allylamine-grafted and blue luminescent Si nanocrystals with 1–4 nm diameter for biological imaging in HeLa and Vero cells.[40] It is also possible to tune the luminescent property (from blue to UV) of amine-terminated 1.57-nm Si NPs by tuning the alkyl chain length between the core NP and the amine end group.[41] Highly stable aqueous suspensions of Si QDs using phospholipid micelles with surface functionalization of styrene, octadecene, or ethyl undecylenate (Figure 12.4a and b) were studied as luminescent labels for pancreatic cancer cells. Final micelles with a size of 50–120 nm and luminescence quantum yield of 2%–4% show robust *in vitro* cellular uptake with no sign of morphological damage to the cells (Figure 12.4b).[42] Cytotoxicity and inflammatory evaluation to Si-based NPs/QDs are important when NPs are used in life sciences for *in vivo* application. Si QDs with concentrations of 112 µg/mL are reported to have no toxicity; in fact, they show less toxicity than CdSe QDs at high concentrations in mitochondrial and lactate dehydrogenase assays. Further, under UV exposure, they are 10 times safer than CdSe QDs.[43] Alkyl-coated silicon nanocrystals have been observed to provoke a higher rate and extent of intracellular accumulation in human cancerous cells compared to normal human primary cells.[44] The uptake of the nanocrystals underwent cholesterol-dependent endocytosis. Cell morphology, apoptosis, and cell viability assays show no evidence of *in vitro* cytotoxicity.[44]

On the other hand, carbon-based nanomaterials and their biological properties were well characterized for exploiting their biomedical applications. Carbon is generally recognized as an environmentally benign element and carbon-based nanostructures have relatively low cytotoxicity.[45] Further, as previously discussed, they can be easily surface-functionalized with hydroxyl, carboxyl, and amino groups to make them water soluble and suitable for cross-linking with biomolecules. Due to their visible photoluminescence without photobleaching and blinking, carbon NPs are suitable for several biological applications such as imaging, diagnostics, and drug delivery.[45] Various biomolecules such as proteins, nucleic acids, and biotins can be conjugated with carbon NPs through either covalent or noncovalent bonds. Biomolecules, after being surface-functionalized on the carbon NPs or graphene materials, can retain their bioactivity. For example, amino-terminated detonation nanodiamonds to 5-(and-6)-carboxytetramethylrhodamine succinimidyl ester and biotin have been successful and the biotin on their surface demonstrates good activity by capturing the streptavidin.[46] Proteins such as bovine serum albumins were successfully attached to CNTs (both single- and multiwalled nanotubes) via diimide-activated amidation and exhibit bioactivity.[47,48] Recently, Shen et al.[49] fabricated GO sheet (GOS)-based biocomposites following covalent attachment of biomaterials (such as adenine, cystine, nicotinamide, and ovalbumin) via diimide-activated amidation reaction[47,48] under ambient conditions. Electrochemical characterization of the biocomposites shows that covalently bonded biomaterial retained its bioactivity. The whole reaction process comprises two steps: (1) activation of carboxylic acid groups on GOS by N-ethyl-N'-(3-dimethylaminopropyl)carbodiimide hydrochloride (EDAC). The stable, active ester is formed in the presence of N-hydroxysuccinimide (NHS). (2) The active ester reacts with the amide groups on biomaterials, generating an amide bond between the GOS and biomaterials.[49] Noncovalent functionalization of the drug molecule on carbon-based materials such as GO was also studied for controlled drug release applications. Graphene, as well as GO, is a novel two-dimensional graphitic carbon and has commanded significant attention from interdisciplinary researchers because of its favorable physicochemical and biological properties.[50] Depan et al.[51] fabricated

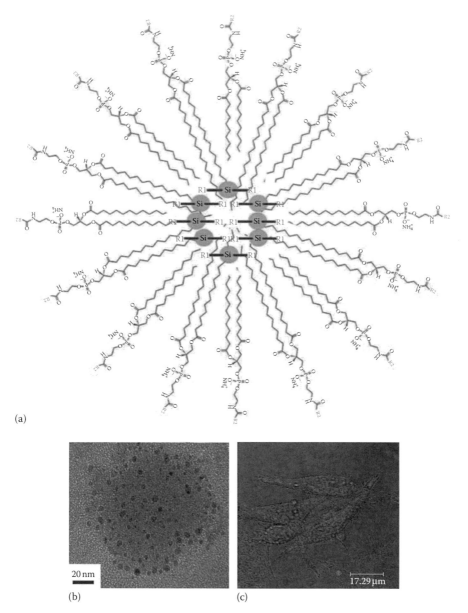

(a)

20 nm

17.29 μm

(b)   (c)

FIGURE 12.4 (See color insert.) (a) Schematic of surface functionalization of Si QDs with compounds R1 (styrene, octadecene, or ethyl undecylenate) followed by encapsulation with phospholipid micelles that were terminated by the functional groups R2 (methoxy PEG, carboxyl, folate, or biotin). (b) TEM image of Si QDs encapsulated in several micelles. (c) Confocal microscopic visualization of live pancreatic cancer cells treated with amine-terminated micelle-encapsulated Si QDs. Scale bar = 17.29 μm. (Reprinted with permission from Erogbogbo et al., 2008, 873–878. Copyright 2008 American Chemical Society.)

a novel folate-decorated and graphene-mediated drug delivery system with anticancer doxorubicin (DOX) for controlled drug release. The nanocarrier system was synthesized in two steps which are as follows: (1) preparation of folic acid-conjugated chitosan and (2) encapsulation of GO–DOX nanohybrid with folic acid-conjugated chitosan. The π–π stacking interaction enables high drug loading of DOX to GO. Further, the encapsulated GO enhances the stability of the nanocarrier system in aqueous medium because of the hydrophilicity and cationic nature of chitosan. Such surface-functionalized nanohybrid system offers a novel formulation that combines the unique properties of a biodegradable material, chitosan and GO, for biomedical applications.[51]

Apart from normal biological studies such as cellular imaging and diagnostics, functionalized NPs also extend their biomedical application in several other disease diagnoses and treatments such as acute lung injury.[52] Inducible nitric oxide synthase (iNOS) is found to be a critical biomarker and exacerbating agent for acute lung injury.[53] Researchers are keen to develop diagnostic agents and inhibitors for iNOS to prevent acute lung injury. Recently, a dual peptide nucleic acid (PNA)–peptide-functionalized shell-cross-linked NPs has been designed to target the mRNA toward the diagnosis and treatment of acute lung injury.[52] Shell-cross-linked knedel-like (SCK) NPs are composed of block copolymers with hydrophilic and hydrophobic segments, making them amphiphilic and prone to self-assembly in selective solvents. SCKs covalently conjugated with iNOS PNA and cell-penetrating peptides have been prepared. Their binding affinities with complementary postconjugation were evaluated for their potential utility in the recognition and inhibition of mRNA sequences for iNOS.[52] PNAs are well-known synthetic analogs of DNA and contain an uncharged pseudopeptide made of N-(2-amino-ethyl)glycine units to which the nucleobases are linked through methylene carbonyl linkers.[54] PNAs have high affinity to mRNA and are able to block its translation function.[55] In addition, PNAs are able to invade regions of secondary structure in the target mRNA and tend to form PNA–RNA complexes that are resistant to the action of RNase H.[56] Poor cellular uptake and rapid clearance are the limitations associated with PNAs for their regulators and *in vivo* gene expression.[52,54] To address this issue, PNAs have been conjugated to a variety of cell-penetrating peptides and other functional ligands for improving cellular uptake. Surface functionalization strategies like conjugation with NPs such as SCKs made PNAs optimal for cell penetration, endosomal escape, pharmacokinetic, and biodistribution properties.[52] Likewise, several varieties of biofunctionalization strategies are studied for the development of toxic-free and site-specific functionalized nanomaterials for biomedical applications (Table 12.1).

12.3.3 Nanomaterials as "Nanoantibiotics" for Treatment of Infectious Diseases

The rise of drug-resistant infections in clinics and communities, which are caused by several microbial pathogens, is common and the continued evolution of antimicrobial resistance threatens environmental hygiene.[67] According to a recent review, FDA approval for new antibiotics has been increasingly denied from the year 1983 to 2007.[68] Resistance development among many currently used antibiotics against infectious

TABLE 12.1

Examples of Functionalized Nanomaterials and Their Biological Characterizations

Nanomaterials	Interface Agent	Functional Entity	Biological Characterization	Reference
Starch-AuNPs	Thiotic acid	Bombesin, annexin V	Cellular interaction and apoptosis	[57]
AgNPs-thiol	EDC/NHS	D-(+)-Glucosamine	Antimicrobial	[58]
Cu cubes	NA	D-(+)-Glucosamine	C-reactive protein detection	[59]
Fe₃O₄@AuNPs	NA	Vancomycin-cystamide	Magnetic, NIR absorption, and antibacterial	[60]
Au@SiO₂	CTAB	Doxorubicin	Cancer treatment	[61]
AuNPs-mPEG-thiol	LC-SPDP	Anti-neurofilament rabbit IgG	Bioconjugation	[62]
SWCNT-COOH	NA	AgNPs/DNA/PVA	Bionanofilm	[63]
SiO₂NPs-APS	SMCC	CysHisTNF mutants	Biomimics	[64]
AuNPs	PFPA-thiol	Carbohydrates	Glyconanoparticles for imaging, therapeutics, and diagnostics	[65]
SiO₂NPs	PEG5k-PEI25k-silane	siRNA	Enhanced cellular uptake and siRNA delivery	[66]
GO	Chitosan–folic acid conjugate	Doxorubicin	Drug delivery	[51]

Notes: AgNPs, silver nanoparticles; APS, 3-aminopropyltriethoxysilane; AuNPs, gold nanoparticles; CTAB, cetyltrimethylammonium bromide; Cu, copper; CysHisTNF, cysteine and a histidine tag with a tumor necrosis factor; DNA, deoxyribonucleic acid; EDC, 1-ethyl-3-(3-dimethylaminopropyl) carbodiimide; Fe₃O₄, iron oxide; GO, graphene oxide; IgG, immunoglobulin G; LC-SPDP, succinimidyl 6-[3-(2-pyridyldithio)-propionamido]-hexanoate; mPEG, methoxy polyethylene glycol; NA, not available; NHS, N-hydroxysuccinimide; PEG, polyethylene glycol; PEI, polyethyleneimine; PFPA, perfluorophenyl azide; PVA, polyvinyl alcohol; SiO₂, silicon dioxide; SiO₂NPs, silicon dioxide nanoparticles; siRNA, small interfering ribonucleic acid; SMCC, sulfosuccinimidyl-4-(N-maleimidomethyl)cyclohexane-1-carboxylate; SWCNT-COOH, carboxylic acid-terminated single-walled carbon nanotube.

diseases demands long-term solutions from the scientific community. Another challenge to existing antimicrobial therapy is the treatment of chronic infectious diseases such as chronic obstructive pulmonary disease (COPD), which causes undesirable adverse effects from a high concentration of antibiotics in serum.[69] Researchers are now searching for a promising alternative to the current antibiotics-based treatment. The growth of nanotechnology mediates the potential application of nanomaterials in science and technology. Medicinal chemists and materials scientists are now engineering several classes of nanoscale material-based nanomedicine for achieving optimized drug therapy for diseases. Recently, the term, nanoantibiotics, has been defined as "nanomaterials that either show antimicrobial activity by themselves, or elevate the effectiveness and safety of antibiotics administration."[68] Unlike usual antimicrobial agents, nanoantibiotics are capable of controlling infectious diseases both *in vitro* and *in vivo*; further, antimicrobial NPs do not pose direct and acute adverse effects. Although the potential toxicity of nanomaterials on long-term exposure is still questionable as discussed in the literature,[35–37,68] on the other hand, there are many benefits associated with nanomaterial-based antibiotics; for example, they can tackle multiple biological pathways found in a broad species of microbes (see Figure 12.5) along with the development of resistance against NPs that requires many concurrent mutations. Apart from these benefits, cost-effectiveness compared to synthesis of antibiotics and long-term storage under harsh conditions (such as high temperature and sterilization) with prolonged shelf life is an added advantage to NP-based drugs. Reports have been demonstrated that the delivery of antibiotics via NPs offers several advantages: (1) precise distribution in the target tissue, (2) better solubility, (3) sustained and controlled release, (4) rationalized patient compliance, (5) reduced side effects, and (6) enhanced cellular uptake.[68,70]

Among several classes of nanomaterials, antibiotics-loaded liposomes and NPs are studied to have increased drug concentration at infected sites with reduced drug toxicity.[71] Antibiotics-loaded AgNPs such as ampicillin, kanamycin, erythromycin, and chloramphenicol were demonstrated to have enhanced antibacterial properties than their individual formulations.[72] NPs such as Ag exhibit their mode of action against the test strains based on the van der Waals interaction and other weak bonds, which lead to interactions between antibiotics-loaded AgNPs and the microbial cell wall. These interactions result in the destruction of the cell wall by binding with peptidoglycan and penetration of NPs into the microbes.

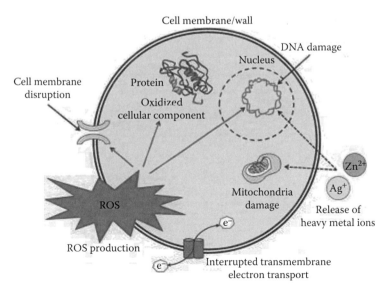

FIGURE 12.5 Various possible antimicrobial mechanisms of nanomaterials. (Reprinted from *J. Control. Release*, 156, Huh, A.J., and Kwon, Y.J., Nanoantibiotics: A new paradigm for treating infectious disease using nanomaterials in the antibiotics resistant era, 128–145, Copyright 2011, with permission from Elsevier.)

Furthermore, an antibiotics complex with AgNPs reacted with DNA and prevented DNA unwinding, which eventually resulted in cell death.[34,72] β-Lactam antibiotics such as amoxicillin-functionalized AgNPs are observed to have a synergistic effect against Gram-negative *E. coli* strains.[73] Though gentamicin exhibits several features as an important antimicrobial agent *in vitro*, response toward killing the intracellular *Salmonella* is limited due to the polar nature of the drug and its associated low level of intracellular penetration. Therefore, researchers have used sol-gel-processed silica as a carrier for gentamicin, which significantly promotes a higher rate of bacterial clearance from organs than does the same dose of a free drug.[74] An extended review related to the functionalization of different biomolecules such as carbohydrates, lipids, proteins, nucleic acids, and antibiotics on nanoscale materials as new synthetic antibiotics for antimicrobials can be obtained from the literature.[34]

12.4   CYTOTOXICITY MECHANISMS OF NANOMATERIALS AND THEIR POTENTIAL USE IN THERAPY

Table 12.2 shows a list of nanomaterials and their mechanism of cytotoxicity in clinical and industrial applications. Recently, research has been focused on finding new and effective drug delivery systems for the treatment of cancer and infectious diseases. The functionalized metal NPs can be either actively or passively delivered to the target site for specific therapy.[33] Factors affecting the drug delivery and the possibility of toxicity from functionalized NPs on their interaction within the cell membrane are shown in Figure 12.6.

TABLE 12.2
Antimicrobial Nanomaterials for Clinical and Industrial Applications

Nanomaterials	Cytotoxicity Mechanisms	Clinical and Industrial Applications	References
AgNPs	Release of Ag^+ ions; disruption of cell membrane and electron transport; DNA damage	Dressing for surgical wound and diabetic foot; coatings for medical devices; portable water filters; antibacterial agent; antifungal agent	[75–77]
ZnONPs	Intracellular accumulation of NPs; cell membrane damage; H_2O_2 production; release of Zn^{2+} ions	Antibacterial creams; lotions and ointment; surface coating of medical device; mouthwash	[78–80]
TiO$_2$NPs	Production of ROS; cell membrane and wall damage	Antibacterial agent; food sterilizing agent; air purifiers; water treatment systems	[81,82]
SiO$_2$NPs	ROS production by surface defects and impurities; protein unfolding; membrane disruption	Vehicle for drug delivery; targeting intracellular pathogens	[74]

(Continued)

TABLE 12.2 (continued)
Antimicrobial Nanomaterials for Clinical and Industrial Applications

Nanomaterials	Cytotoxicity Mechanisms	Clinical and Industrial Applications	References
AuNPs	Interaction with cell membranes; strong electrostatic attraction	Photothermal therapy with near-infrared light; adjuvant treatment after serious infections; antibacterial agent; antifungal agent	[83]
Chitosan	Increased permeability and rupture of membrane; chelation of trace metals; enzyme inactivation	Drinking water disinfectants; bacteria immobilizer; microbiocide in biomedical products	[84]
Fullerenes	Destruction of cell membrane integrity; enhancing activity of infiltrating neutrophil	Potential disinfection applications	[85,86]
CNTs	Cell membrane damage by ROS; oxidation of cell membrane proteins and lipids	Antibacterial agent; biofouling-resistant membranes; water filter; surface coating	[87,88]
NO-releasing NPs	NO release and production of ROS	Infected wound and diabetic foot treatment	[89]
Nanoemulsion	Membrane disruption; disruption of the spore coat	Antimicrobial inhaler; antibiofilm agent; nasal application; vaccine delivery agents	[90,91]
Graphite, graphite oxide, graphene oxide, and reduced graphene oxide	Initial cell deposition on graphene-based materials; membrane stress caused by direct contact with sharp nanosheets; the ensuing superoxide anion-independent oxidation	Being antibacterial, graphene oxide acts as an additive in drug delivery systems, building blocks for biocomposites, etc.	[92]

Notes: AgNPs, silver nanoparticles; AuNPs, gold nanoparticles; CNTs, carbon nanotubes; NO, nitric oxide; ROS, reactive oxygen species; TiO_2NPs, titanium oxide nanoparticles; ZnONPs, zinc oxide nanoparticles.

Source: Reprinted from *J. Control. Release*, 156, Huh, A.J., and Kwon, Y.J., Nanoantibiotics: A new paradigm for treating infectious disease using nanomaterials in the antibiotics resistant era, 128–145, Copyright 2011, with permission from Elsevier.

Among the noble metal NPs, AgNPs have been widely used in the treatment of infectious disease.[13] An intact study on tailoring the AgNP-incorporated CNTs with various polymers had been reported to exhibit strong antimicrobial activity. AgNPs and hybrid materials have derived special care because of their unique physico-chemical and effective antibacterial properties, which in turn provide a cost-effective alternative of new antibacterial agents and have an effective activity against bacteria, viruses, and fungi.[93,94] Also, their reported antiangiogenic properties can serve as an anti-inflammatory agent and in cancer treatment.[95] Several studies on

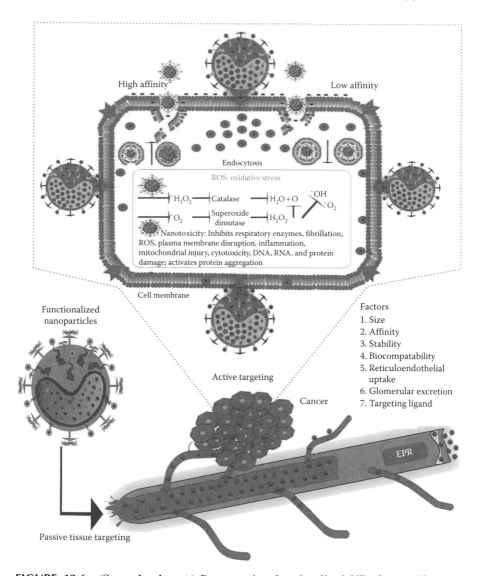

High affinity   Low affinity

Endocytosis

ROS: oxidative stress

H_2O_2 —[Catalase]— $H_2O + O$ $^{\cdot}OH$

$^{\cdot}O_2$ —[Superoxide dimutase]— H_2O_2 $^{\cdot}O_2$

Nanotoxicity: Inhibits respiratory enzymes, fibrillation, ROS, plasma membrane disruption, inflammation, mitochondrial injury, cytotoxicity, DNA, RNA, and protein damage; activates protein aggregation

Cell membrane

Functionalized nanoparticles

Active targeting

Cancer

Factors
1. Size
2. Affinity
3. Stability
4. Biocompatability
5. Reticuloendothelial uptake
6. Glomerular excretion
7. Targeting ligand

EPR

Passive tissue targeting

FIGURE 12.6 (See color insert.) Programming functionalized NPs for specific tissue delivery using targeting ligand. Cancer cell-specific targeting through both passive (enhanced permeability and retention effect) and active pathways. Cationic charged functionalized NPs are more likely to have an increased affinity toward the cell membrane compared to anionic NPs. Factors influencing functionalized NPs are based on drug delivery and possible toxicity of functionalized NPs with the example of ROS mechanism of cell death.

AgNP-utilized burn dressings such as silver-doped thin silica films via a sol–gel process,[97] AgNP-coated PVA thin film development,[98] silver-containing nanofibrous scaffold for tissue engineering,[99] and the production of silver-nanocoated fabric for biomedical antibacterial dressing were reported by many researchers.[96] The proven antiproliferative activity of AgNPs against neoplastic cells opens a new paradigm in anticancer therapy.[100] The antimicrobial mechanism of AgNPs was found to act via reactive oxygen species (ROS) production and glutathione depletion.[101] Also, AgNPs damage the membrane structure by binding with sulfur-containing proteins of the bacterial cell membrane.[77] The size and shape of NPs play a vital role in determining the bactericidal property.[100] The biosynthesized AgNPs significantly inhibited the growth of medically important pathogenic bacteria and yeast (*Candida albicans*).[103] Many research groups reported that the functionalization of AgNPs on CNTs can give a considerable improvement in the ultimate tensile strength and elastic modulus of CNTs with effective antimicrobial activity.[104]

Nanomaterials act as a novel therapeutic carrier system due to their excellent physicochemical properties. Loading or encapsulating antibiotics in a cargo-like biodegradable nanowire (NW) can give rise to controlled drug delivery system. Homogeneously aligned NWs made of silica with definite morphological structure could efficiently exhibit controlled activity and sustained bioavailability of antibiotics with tunable release rate.[105] Silicon nanowire (SiNW) strikingly suppresses the cell, protein adhesion with drastic reduction of biofouling, and drug release impediments to provide more reliable antibiotic protection. Various functionalized nanomaterials, such as TiO_2, ZnO, and fullerol, have demonstrated strong antimicrobial properties through diverse mechanisms, including photocatalytic production of ROS for damaging cell components and viruses.[106] In addition, other nanomaterials, such as peptides, chitosan, carboxyfullerene, CNTs, ZnO, fullerene (C_{60}), and AgNPs, could compromise the bacterial cell envelope, interrupt energy transduction, and inhibit enzymatic activity and DNA synthesis.[106] These nanomaterials are not strong oxidants and produce no harmful side effects. They can be classified into three major antibiotic groups as naturally occurring antibacterial substances (peptides, functionalized chitosan), metal–metal oxides (ZnO, TiO_2), and functionalized nanomaterials (f-AgNPs, fullerenes, CNTs) and reviewed in detail elsewhere.[106] This report describes the metal oxide NPs including NiO, ZnO, Fe_2O_3, Co_3O_4, CuO, and TiO_2 that were prepared and examined for their antimicrobial activities employing *E. coli* as the model microbial species. Electrosprayed NiO, ZnO, and CuO NPs show pronounced antimicrobial activity than do other metal oxide NPs. The observed antimicrobial activity of the NPs can be ranked as NiO > ZnO > CuO > TiO_2 > Co_3O_4 > Fe_2O_3. It resulted from the synergistic effect between the soluble ion stress and the nanorelated stress, and it highly depends on the soluble ions and the composition of the NPs, solubility, and cellular and nanomaterial interaction.[105] Nanomaterials (CNTs) and functionalized nanomaterials (CNT-AgNPs) display effective antimicrobial activity via cell membrane damage by direct contact with nanomaterials, whereas size is the key factor governing the activity in expressing high level of stress-related gene products.[63,102,106] AgNP-functionalized CNTs and polymer-wrapped nanocomposites were demonstrated to have excellent and promising antimicrobial activity, which is believed to be a strong prophylactic in biomedical arena.[63,102] Figure 12.7 shows the synthesis method of AgNP functionalization on CNT surface and subsequent polymer coating.[102] Nanomaterials such as CNTs not only produce mechanical damage and subsequent cell disruption in bacteria but may also generate oxidative stress, as experienced in the eukaryotic cells.

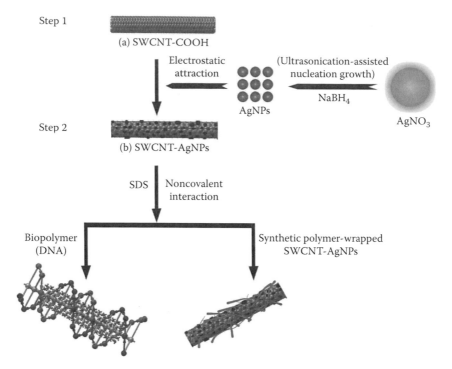

Step 1

(a) SWCNT-COOH

Electrostatic attraction

(Ultrasonication-assisted nucleation growth)

NaBH$_4$

AgNPs

AgNO$_3$

Step 2

(b) SWCNT-AgNPs

SDS | Noncovalent interaction

Biopolymer (DNA)

Synthetic polymer-wrapped SWCNT-AgNPs

FIGURE 12.7 Step 1 involves electrostatic interaction of AgNPs on SWCNT-COOH (a). In step 2, the SWCNT-AgNPs (b) are wrapped with biopolymer (DNA) and synthetic polymer nanofibers in the presence of sodium dodecyl sulfate (SDS).

12.5 SUMMARY AND OUTLOOK

Research on innovative hybrid nanomaterials for drug delivery has been fruitful in the past decade. Hybrid nanomaterials composed of nanotubes, NPs, biomolecules, and polymers show promise in this regard with successful results in biomedical application.[63,107] The excellent physicochemical properties of various nanomaterials play a vital role in transplanting scaffolds containing stem cells in the physiological system,[108–110] as an antibiotic in infectious diseases and microcatheters,[111] as antimicrobial skin films,[63] in tissue engineering application, in targeted/controlled drug delivery system,[112] and in bioimaging.[113] The fabrication and functionalization of nanomaterials can be effectively carried out for attaining antimicrobial and anticancer properties. Hybrids containing dual and trio nanomaterials have been studied intensively, as also impregnation of a variety of nanostructures to make hybrid nanomaterials has been reported to improve the physicochemical properties of individual structures.[114] However, the major drawback of such fabricated hybrids is the cause of severe intrinsic toxicity that restricts them to be used in biomedical applications. Size, surface area, surface potential, solubility, and pH are all fatal characteristics of causing toxicity from nanomaterials.[115] The tiny size with increased surface area of nanomaterials enhances the cellular interaction and uptake, thus leading to generation of toxic paradigms including morphological alteration (cell membrane rupture), mutation, transfection into nucleus, disruption of the intracellular metabolic pathway, oxidative stress, and generation of ROS.[63,116,117] Hence, new treatment modalities using nanomaterials in biomedical applications require an alternative way to minimize the toxic effects in cells while being toxic to microorganisms.

The reports reviewed in this chapter reveal that functionalization of nanomaterials with biocompatible moieties is an effective and widely used technique to decrease toxicity as well as improve their biological properties and therapeutic activity in a synergistic manner. Surface functionalization on nanomaterials modifies physicochemical characteristics that enable their self-organization and render them compatible. Functionalized nanomaterials are directly correlated with increased functional density, enhanced protein adsorption, cellular activity, and minimized toxicity.[117] For nanomaterials to be effective in intracellular application, they should overcome the endocytic fate with effective internalization into cytosol that highly depends on the ability of cell membrane breaching, kinetics, concentration, size, surface area, and charge of nanomaterials.[118] The phenomenon at the interface of a biological system and functionality of nanomaterials will destine their multifunctional applications to bionanoengineering.[119] Functionalization modifies the physicochemical properties of nanomaterials thereby altering toxicity to a minimal level, enhancing protein adsorption, and affecting cellular activity. Also, functionalization increases the solubility of nanomaterials and their escape from primary immune reactions that results in strengthening the possibility of using nanomaterials as carriers of biological and therapeutic molecules without affecting the immune system.

ACKNOWLEDGMENTS

This research was supported by the Gachon University Research Fund in 2012 and the Gyunggi Regional Research Center (GRRC) program of Gyeonggi province (2012-B02). This work was supported by Grant No. 10032112 from the Regional Technology Innovation Program of the Ministry of Knowledge Economy. This research was also supported by the Ministry of Knowledge and Economy Grant No. 10039863.

REFERENCES

1. Wang, Y., Li, Y.F., and Huang, C.Z. 2009. A one-pot green method for one-dimensional assembly of gold nanoparticles with a novel chitosan–ninhydrin bioconjugate at physiological temperature. *J. Phys. Chem. C* 113: 4315–4320.
2. Horva'th, I.T., and Anastas, P.T. 2007. Innovations and green chemistry. *Chem. Rev.* 107: 2167–2168.
3. Stankovich, S., Dikin, D.A., Dommett, G.H., Kohlhaas, K.M., Zimney, E.J., Stach, E.A., Piner, R.D., Nguyen, S.T., and Ruoff, R.S. 2006. Graphene-based composite materials. *Nature* 442: 282–286.
4. Mohanty, N., and Berry, V. Graphene-based single-bacterium resolution biodevice and DNA transistor: Interfacing graphene derivatives with nanoscale and microscale biocomponents. 2008. *Nano Lett.* 8: 4469–4476.
5. Narayanan, K.B., and Sakthivel, N. 2010. Biosynthesis of metal nanoparticles by microbes. *J. Colloid. Interface Sci.* 156: 1–13.

6. Mohammadian, A., Shojaosadati, S.A., and Rezaee, M.H. 2007. Fusarium oxysporum mediates photogeneration of silver nanoparticles. *Sci. Iran* 14: 323–326.

7. Bruins, R.M., Kapil, S., and Oehme, S.W. 2000. Microbial resistance to metals in the environment. *Ecotoxicol. Environ. Saf.* 45: 198–207.

8. Beveridge, T.J., Hughes, M.N., Lee, H., Leung, K.T., Poole, R.K., Savvaidis, I., Silver, S., and Trevors, J.T. 1997. Metal-microbe interactions: Contemporary approaches. *Adv. Microb. Physiol.* 38: 177–243.

9. Bao, C., Jin, M., Lu, R., Zhang, T., and Zhao, Y.Y. 2003. Preparation of Au nanoparticles in the presence of low generational poly (amidoamine) dendrimer with surface hydroxyl groups. *Mat. Chem. Phys.* 81: 160–165.

10. Sharma, N.C., Sahi, S.V., Nath, S., Parsons, J.G., Gardea-Torresdey, J.L., and Pal, T. 2007. Synthesis of plant-mediated gold nanoparticles and catalytic role of biomatrix-embedded nanomaterials. *Environ. Sci. Technol.* 41: 5137–5142.

11. Veerapandian, M., and Yun, K.S. 2010. Synthesis of silver nanoclusters and functionalization with glucosamine for glyconanoparticles. *Synth. React. Inorg. Met. Org. Nano. Met. Chem.* 40: 56–64.

12. Chen, Q., Yue, L., Xie, F., Zhou, M., Fu, Y., and Zhang, Y. 2008. Preferential facet of nanocrystalline silver embedded in polyethylene oxide nanocomposite and its antibiotic behaviors. *J. Phys. Chem.* 112: 10004–10007.

13. Sharma, V.K., Yngard, R.A., and Lin, Y. 2009. Silver nanoparticles: Green synthesis and their antimicrobial activities. *Colloid. Interface. Adv.* 145: 83–96.

14. Selvan, S.T., Tan, T.T.Y., Yi, D.K., and Jana, N.R. 2010. Functional and multifunctional nanoparticles for bioimaging and biosensing. *Langmuir* 26: 11631–11641.

15. Choi, W.I., Kim, J.Y., Kang, C.K., Byeon, C.C., Kim, Y.H., and Tae, G. 2011. Tumor regression in vivo by photothermal therapy based on gold-nanorod-loaded, functional nanocarriers. *ACS Nano* 5: 1995–2003.

16. Jiang, W., Kim, B.Y., Rutka, J.T., and Chan, W.C. 2008. Nanoparticle-mediated cellular response is size-dependent. *Nat. Nanotechnol.* 3: 145–150.

17. Shubayev, V.I., Pisanic II, T.R., and Jin, S. 2009. Magnetic nanoparticles for theragnostics. *Adv. Drug Deliv. Rev.* 61: 467–477.

18. Jain, R.A. 2000. The manufacturing techniques of various drug loaded biodegradable poly(lactide-co-glycolide) (PLGA) devices. *Biomaterials* 21: 2475–2490.

19. Tan, J.S., Butterfield, D.R., Voycheck, C.L., Caldwell, K.D., and Li, J.T. 1993. Surface modification of nanoparticles by PEO/PPO block copolymers to minimize interactions with blood components and prolong blood circulation in rats. *Biomaterials* 14: 823–833.

20. Chung, Y.-I., Kim, J.C., Kim, Y.H., Tae, G., Lee, S.Y., Kim, K., and Kwon, I.C. 2010. The effect of surface functionalization of PLGA nanoparticles by heparin- or chitosan-conjugated Pluronic on tumor targeting. *J. Control. Release* 143: 374–382.

21. Yang, R., Yang, S.G., Shim, W.S., Cui, F., Cheng, G., Kim, I.W., Kim, D.D., Chung, S.J., and Shim, C.K. 2009. Lung-specific delivery of paclitaxel by chitosan-modified PLGA nanoparticles via transient formation of microaggregates. *J. Pharm. Sci.* 98: 970–984.

22. Duan, H., Kuang, M., Wang, D., Kurth, D.G., and Möhwald, H. 2005. Colloidal stable amphibious nanocrystals derived from poly[(2-dimethylamino)ethyl methacrylate] capping. *Angew. Chem. Int. Ed.* 44: 1717–1720.

23. Zhu M., Chen, P., and Liu, M. 2012. Ag/AgBr/Graphene oxide nanocomposite synthesized via oil/water and water/oil microemulsions: A comparison of sunlight energized plasmonic photocatalytic activity. *Langmuir* 28: 3385–3390.

24. Sun, Y.P., Fu, K., Lin, Y., and Huang, W. 2002. Functionalized carbon nanotubes: Properties and applications. *Acc. Chem. Res.* 35: 1096–1104.

25. Elhissi, A.M.A., Ahmed, W., Hassan, I.U., Dhanak, V.R., and D'Emanuele, A. 2012. Carbon nanotubes in cancer therapy and drug delivery. *J. Drug Deliv.* 837327: 1–10.

26. Lu, A.H., Salabas, E.L., and Schuth, F. 2007. Magnetic nanoparticles: Synthesis, protection, functionalization, and application. *Angew. Chem. Int. Ed. Engl.* 46: 1222–1244.

27. Moore, A., Marecos, E., Bogdanov Jr., A., and Weissleder, R. 2000. Tumoral distribution of long-circulating dextran-coated iron oxide nanoparticles in a rodent model. *Radiology* 214: 568–574.

28. Reimer, P., and Balzer, T. 2003. Ferucarbotran (Resovist): A new clinically approved RES-specific contrast agent for contrast-enhanced MRI of the liver: Properties, clinical development, and applications. *Eur. Radiol.* 13: 1266–1276.

29. Metz, S., Bonaterra, G., Rudelius, M., Settles, M., Rummeny, E.J., and Daldrup-Link, H.E. 2004. Capacity of human monocytes to phagocytose approved iron oxide MR contrast agents in vitro. *Eur. Radiol.* 14: 1851–1858.

30. Kunzmann, A., Andersson, B., Thurnherr, T., Krug, H., Scheynius, A., and Fadeel, B. 2011. Toxicology of engineered nanomaterials: Focus on biocompatibility, biodistribution and biodegradation. *Biochim. Biophys. Acta* 1810: 361–373.

31. Low, P.S., and Kularatne, S.A. 2009. Folate-targeted therapeutic and imaging agents for cancer. *Curr. Opin. Chem. Biol.* 13: 256–262.

32. Thanha, N.T.K., and Green, L.A.W. 2010. Functionalisation of nanoparticles for biomedical applications. *Nano Today* 5: 213–230.

33. Subbiah, R., Veerapandian, M., and Yun, K.S. 2010. Nanoparticles: Functionalization and multifunctional applications in biomedical sciences. *Curr. Med. Chem.* 17: 4559–4577.

34. Veerapandian, M., and Yun, K.S. 2011. Functionalization of biomolecules on nanoparticles: Specialized for antibacterial applications. *Appl. Microbiol. Biotechnol.* 90: 1655–1667.

35. Farré, M., Gajda-Schrantz, K., Kantiani, L., and Barceló, D. 2009. Ecotoxicity and analysis of nanomaterials in the aquatic environment. *Anal. Bioanal. Chem.* 393: 81–95.

36. Singh, N., Manshian, B., Jenkins, G.J.S., Griffiths, S.M., Williams, P.M., Maffeis, T.G., Wright, C.J., and Doak, S.H. 2009. NanoGenotoxicology: The DNA damaging potential of engineered nanomaterials. *Biomaterials* 30: 3891–3914.

37. Ema, M., Kobayashi, N., Naya, M., Hanai, S., and Nakanishi, J. 2010. Reproductive and developmental toxicity studies of manufactured nanomaterials. *Reprod. Toxicol.* 30: 343–352.

38. Li, Z.F., and Ruckenstein, E. 2004. Water-soluble poly(acrylic acid) grafted luminescent silicon nanoparticles and their use as fluorescent biological staining labels. *Nano Lett.* 4: 1463–1467.

39. He, Y., Kang, Z.H., Li, Q.S., Tsang, C.H.A., Fan, C.H., and Lee, S.T. 2009. Ultrastable, highly fluorescent and water-dispersed silicon-based nanospheres as cellular probes. *Angew. Chem. Int. Ed.* 48: 128–132.

40. Rosso-Vasic, M., Spruijt, E., van Lagen, B., De Cola, L., and Zuilhof, H. 2008. Alkyl-functionalized oxide-free silicon nanoparticles: Synthesis and optical properties. *Small* 4: 1835–1841.

41. Rosso-Vasic, M., Spruijt, E., Popović, Z., Overgaag, K., van Lagen, B., Grandidier, B., Vanmaekelbergh, D., Domínguez-Gutiérrez, D., De Cola, L., and Zuilhof, H. 2009. Amine-terminated silicon nanoparticles: Synthesis, optical properties and their use in bioimaging. *J. Mater. Chem.* 19: 5926–5933.

42. Erogbogbo, F., Yong, K.T., Roy, I., Xu, G., Prasad, P.N., and Swihart, M.T. 2008. Biocompatible luminescent silicon quantum dots for imaging of cancer cells. *ACS Nano* 2: 873–878.

43. Fujioka, K., Hiruoka, M., Sato, K., Manabe, N., Miyasaka, R., Hanada, S., Hoshino, A., Tilley, R.D., Manome, Y., Hirakuri, K., and Yamamoto, K. 2008. Luminescent passive-oxidized silicon quantum dots as biological staining labels and their cytotoxicity effects at high concentration. *Nanotechnology* 19: 415102.

44. Fucikova, A., Valenta, J., Pelant, I., and Brezina, V. 2009. Novel use of silicon nanocrystals and nanodiamonds in biology. *Chem. Pap.* 63: 704–708.
45. Fan, J., and Chu, P.K. 2010. Group IV nanoparticles: Synthesis, properties, and biological applications. *Small* 6: 2080–2098.
46. Hens, S.C., Cunningham, G., Tyler, T., Moseenkov, S., Kuznetsov, V., and Shenderova, O. 2008. Nanodiamond bioconjugate probes and their collection by electrophoresis. *Diam. Relat. Mater.* 17: 1858–1866.
47. Huang, W., Taylor, S., Fu, K., Lin, Y., Zhang, D., Hanks, T.W., Rao, A.M., and Sun, Y.-P. 2002. Attaching proteins to carbon nanotubes via diimide-activated amidation. *Nano Lett.* 2: 311–314.
48. Lin, Y., Elkin, T., Taylor, S., Gu, L., Chen, B., Veca, L.M., Zhou, B., Yang, H., Brown, J., and Joseph, R. 2006. Preparation, characterization, and evaluation of immuno carbon nanotubes. *Microchim. Acta* 152: 249–254.
49. Shen, J., Yan, B., Shi, M., Ma, H., Li, N., and Ye, M. 2011. Synthesis of graphene oxide-based biocomposites through diimide-activated amidation. *J. Colloid Interf. Sci.* 356: 543–549.
50. Geim, A.K., and Novoselov, K.S. 2007. The rise of graphene. *Nat. Mater.* 6: 183–191.
51. Depan, D., Shah, J., and Misra, R.D.K. 2011. Controlled release of drug from folate-decorated and graphene mediated drug delivery system: Synthesis, loading efficiency, and drug release response. *Mat. Sci. Eng. C* 31: 1305–1312.
52. Shrestha, R., Shen, Y., Pollack, K.A., Taylor, J.-S.A., and Wooley, K.L. 2012. Dual peptide nucleic acid- and peptide-functionalized shell cross-linked nanoparticles designed to target mRNA toward the diagnosis and treatment of acute lung injury. *Bioconjug. Chem.* 23: 574–585.
53. Hosogi, S., Iwasaki, Y., Yamada, T., Komatani-Tamiya, N., Hiramatsu, A., Kohno, Y., Ueda, M., Arimoto, T., and Marunaka, Y. 2008. Effect of inducible nitric oxide synthase on apoptosis in *Candida*-induced acute lung injury. *Biomed. Res. Tokyo* 29: 257–266.
54. Koppelhus, U., and Nielsen, P.E. 2003. Cellular delivery of peptide nucleic acid (PNA). *Adv. Drug Deliv. Rev.* 55: 267–280.
55. Nielsen, P.E. 2004. PNA technology. *Mol. Biotechnol.* 26: 233–248.
56. Nielsen, P.E. 2010. Gene targeting and expression modulation by peptide nucleic acids (PNA). *Curr. Pharm. Des.* 16: 3118–3123.
57. Swapna, M. 2008. Gold nanoparticle–biomolecule conjugates: Synthesis, properties, cellular interactions and cytotoxicity studies. Dissertation, University of Missouri, Columbia, MO.
58. Veerapandian, M., Lim, S.K., Nam, H.M., Kuppannan, G., and Yun, K.S. 2010. Glucosamine-functionalized silver glyconanoparticles: Characterization and antibacterial activity. *Anal. Bioanal. Chem.* 398: 867–876.
59. Veerapandian, M., Subbiah, R., Lim, G.S., Park, S.H., Yun, K.S., and Lee, M.H. 2011. Copper-glucosamine microcubes: Synthesis, characterization, and C-reactive protein detection. *Langmuir* 27: 8934–8942.
60. Huang, W.C., Tsai, P.J., and Chen, Y.C. 2009. Multifunctional Fe_3O_4@Au nanoeggs as photothermal agents for selective killing of nosocomial and antibiotic-resistant bacteria. *Small* 5: 51–56.
61. Zhang, Z., Wang, L., Wang, J., Jiang, X., Li, X., Hu, Z., Ji, Y., Wu, X., and Chen, C. 2012. Mesoporous silica-coated gold nanorods as a light-mediated multifunctional theranostic platform for cancer treatment. *Adv. Mater.* 24: 1418–1423.
62. Hongwei, L., and Jason, H.H. 2005. Gold nanorod bioconjugates. *Chem. Mater.* 17: 4636–4641.
63. Subbiah, R., Lee, H.S., Veerapandian, M., Sadhasivam, S., Seo, S.W., and Yun, K.S. 2011. Structural and biological evaluation of a multifunctional SWCNT-AgNPs-DNA/PVA bio-nanofilm. *Anal. Bioanal. Chem.* 400: 547–560.

64. Bryde, S., Grunwald, I., Hammer, A., Krippner-Heidenreich, A., Schiestel, T., Brunner, H., Tovar, G.E., Pfizenmaier, K., and Scheurich, P. 2005. Tumor necrosis factor (TNF)-functionalized nanostructured particles for the stimulation of membrane TNF-specific cell responses. *Bioconjug. Chem.* 16: 1459–1467.

65. Wang, X., Ramström, O., and Yan, M. 2010. Glyconanomaterials: Synthesis, characterization, and ligand presentation. *Adv. Mater.* 22: 1946–1953.

66. Lee, H.S., Sung, D.K., Veerapandian, M., Yun, K.S., and Seo, S.W. 2011. PEGylated polyethyleneimine grafted silica nanoparticles: Enhanced cellular uptake and efficient siRNA delivery. *Anal. Bioanal. Chem.* 400: 535–545.

67. Boucher, H.W., Talbot, G.H., Bradley, J.S., Edwards, J.E., Gilbert, D., Rice, L.B., Scheld, M., Spellberg, B., and Bartlett, J. 2009. Bad bugs, no drugs: No ESKAPE! An update from the Infectious Diseases Society of America. *Clin. Infect. Dis.* 48: 1–12.

68. Huh, A.J., and Kwon, Y.J. 2011. Nanoantibiotics: A new paradigm for treating infectious disease using nanomaterials in the antibiotics resistant era. *J. Control. Release* 156: 128–145.

69. Beaulac, C., Clement-Major, S., Hawari, J., and Legace, J. 1996. Eradication of mucoid *Pseudomonas aeruginosa* with fluid liposome-encapsulated tobramycin in an animal model of chronic pulmonary infection. *Antimicrob. Agents Chemother.* 40: 665–669.

70. Sosnik, A., Carcaboso, A.M., Glisoni, R.J., Moretton, M.A., and Chiappetta, D.A. 2010. New old challenges in tuberculosis: Potentially effective nanotechnologies in drug delivery. *Adv. Drug Deliv. Rev.* 62: 547–559.

71. Huguette, P.A., Antoine, A., and Patrick, C. 2000. Targeted delivery of antibiotics using liposomes and nanoparticles: research and applications. *Int. J. Antimicrob. Agent* 13: 155–168.

72. Amanulla, M.F., Kulandaivelu, B., Morukattu, G., Yadav, R., Kalaichelvan, P.T., and Venketesan, R. 2010. Biogenic synthesis of silver nanoparticles and their synergistic effect with antibiotics: A study against Gram-positive and Gram-negative bacteria. *Nanomed. Nanotechnol.* 6: 103–109.

73. Ping, L., Juan, L., Changzhu, W., Qingsheng, W., and Li, J. 2005. Synergistic antibacterial effects of β-lactam antibiotic combined with silver nanoparticles. *Nanotechnology* 16: 1912.

74. Seleem, M.N., Munusamy, P., Ranjan, A., Alqublan, H., Pickrell, G., and Sriranganathan, N. 2009. Silica-antibiotic hybrid nanoparticles for targeting intracellular pathogens. *Antimicrob. Agents Chemother.* 53: 4270–4274.

75. Klasen, H.J. 2000. Historical review of the use of silver in the treatment of burns. I. Early uses. *Burns* 26: 117–130.

76. Raimondi, F., Scherer, G.G., Kötz, R., and Wokaun, A. 2005. Nanoparticles in energy technology: Examples from electrochemistry and catalysis. *Angew. Chem. Int. Ed. Engl.* 44: 2190–2209.

77. Sondi, I., and Salopek-Sondi, B. 2004. Silver nanoparticles as antimicrobial agent: A case study on *E. coli* as a model for gram-negative bacteria. *J. Colloid Interf. Sci.* 275: 177–182.

78. Huang, Z., Zheng, X., Yan, D., Yin, G., Liao, X., Kang, Y., Yao, Y., Huang, D., and Hao, B. 2008. Toxicological effect of ZnO nanoparticles based on bacteria. *Langmuir* 24: 4140–4144.

79. Dastjerdi, R., and Montazer, M. 2010. A review on the application of inorganic nanostructured materials in the modification of textiles: Focus on anti-microbial properties. *Colloid. Surface. B* 79: 5–18.

80. Uğur, S.S., Sarıışık, M., Aktaş, A.H., Uçar, M.C., and Erden, E. 2010. Modifying of cotton fabric surface with nano-ZnO multilayer films by layer-by-layer deposition method. *Nanoscale Res. Lett.* 5: 1204–1210.

81. Reddy, M.P., Vengopal, A., and Subrahmanyam, M. 2007. Hydroxyapatite-supported Ag-TiO$_2$ as *Escherichia coli* disinfection photocatalyst. *Water Res.* 41: 379–386.

82. Kühn, K.P., Cahberny, I.F., Massholder, K., Stickler, M., Benz, V.W., Sonntag, H., and Erdinger, L. 2003. Disinfection of surfaces by photocatalytic oxidation with titanium dioxide and UVA light. *Chemosphere* 53: 71–77.

83. Johnston, H.J., Hutchison, G., Christensen, F.M., Peters, S., Hankin, S., and Stone, V. 2010. A review of the in vivo and in vitro toxicity of silver and gold particulates: Particle attributes and biological mechanisms responsible for the observed toxicity. *Crit. Rev. Toxicol.* 40: 328–346.

84. Qi, L., Xu, Z., Jiang, X., Hu, C., and Zou, X. 2004. Preparation and antibacterial activity of chitosan nanoparticles. *Carbohydr. Res.* 339: 2693–2700.

85. Lyon, D.Y., Fortner, J.D., Sayes, C.M., Colvin, V.L., and Hughe, J.B. 2005. Bacterial cell association and antimicrobial activity of a C60 water suspension. *Environ. Toxicol. Chem.* 24: 2757–2762.

86. Lyon, D.Y., Brunet, L., Hinkal, G.W., Wiesner, M.R., and Alvarez, P.J. 2008. Antibacterial activity of fullerene water suspensions (nC60) is not due to ROS-medicated damage. *Nano Lett.* 8: 1539–1543.

87. Kang, S., Pinault, M., Pfefferle, L.D., and Elimelech, M. 2007. Single-walled carbon nanotubes exhibit strong antimicrobial activity. *Langmuir* 23: 8670–8673.

88. Aslan, S., Loebick, C.Z., Kang, S., Elimelech, M., Pfefferle, L.D., and Van Tassel, P.R. 2010. Antimicrobial biomaterials based on carbon nanotubes dispersed in poly(lactic-co-glycolic acid). *Nanoscale* 2: 1789–1794.

89. Weller, R.B. 2009. Nitric oxide-containing nanoparticles as an antimicrobial agents and enhancer of wound healing. *J. Invest. Dermatol.* 129: 2335–2337.

90. Hamouda, T., Hayes, M.M., Cao, Z., Tonda, R., Johnson, K., Wright, D.C., Brisker, J., and Baker Jr, J.R. 1999. A novel surfactant nanoemulsion with broad-spectrum sporicidal activity against *Bacillus* species. *J. Infect. Dis.* 180: 1939–1949.

91. Teixeira, P.C., Leite, G.M., Domingues, R.J., Silva, J., Gibbs, P.A., and Ferreira, J.P. 2007. Antimicrobial effects of a microemulsion and a nanoemulsion on enteric and other pathogens and biofilms. *Int. J. Food Microbiol.* 118: 15–19.

92. Liu, S., Zeng, T.H., Hofmann, M., Burcombe, E., Wei, J., Jiang, R., Kong, J., and Chen, Y. 2011. Antibacterial activity of graphite, graphite oxide, graphene oxide, and reduced graphene oxide: Membrane and oxidative stress. *ACS Nano* 5: 6971–6980.

93. Gurunathan, S., Lee, K.-J., Kalishwaralal, K., Sheikpranbabu, S., Vaidyanathan, R., and Eom, S.H. 2009. Antiangiogenic properties of silver nanoparticles. *Biomaterials* 30: 6341–6350.

94. Parikh, D.V., Fink, T., Rajasekharan, K., Sachinvala, N.D., Sawhney, A.P.S., Calamari, T.A., and Parikh, A.D. 2005. Antimicrobial silver/sodium carboxymethyl cotton dressings for burn wounds. *Text. Res. J.* 75: 134–138.

95. Jeon, H.-J., Yi, S.-C., and Oh, S.-G. 2003. Preparation and antibacterial effects of Ag–SiO2 thin films by sol–gel method. *Biomaterials* 24: 4921–4928.

96. Bryaskova, R., Pencheva, D., Kale, G.M., Lad, U., and Kantardjiev, T. 2010. Synthesis, characterisation and antibacterial activity of PVA/TEOS/Ag-Np hybrid thin films. *J. Colloid. Interface Sci.* 349: 77–85.

97. Xing, Z.-C., Chae, W.-P., Baek, J.-Y., Choi, M.-J., Jung, Y., and Kang, I.-K. 2010. In vitro assessment of antibacterial activity and cytocompatibility of silver-containing PHBV nanofibrous scaffolds for tissue engineering. *Biomacromolecules* 11: 1248–1253.

98. AshaRani, P., Hande, M.P., and Valiyaveettil, S. 2009. Anti-proliferative activity of silver nanoparticles. *BMC Cell Biol.* 10: 65.

99. Hussain, S.M., Hess, K.L., Gearhart, J.M., Geiss, K.T., and Schlager, J.J. 2005. In vitro toxicity of nanoparticles in BRL 3A rat liver cells. *Toxicol. In Vitro* 19: 975–983.

100. Pal, S., Tak, Y.K., and Song, J.M. 2007. Does the antibacterial activity of silver nanoparticles depend on the shape of the nanoparticle? A study of the gram-negative bacterium *Escherichia coli*. *Appl. Environ. Microb.* 73: 1712–1720.

101. Sadhasivam, S., Shanmugam, P., and Yun, K. 2010. Biosynthesis of silver nanoparticles by *Streptomyces hygroscopicus* and antimicrobial activity against medically important pathogenic microorganisms. *Colloid. Surface. B* 81: 358–362.

102. Subbiah, R., Veerapandian, M., Sadhasivam, S., and Yun, K. 2011. Triad CNT-NPs/ polymer nanocomposites: Fabrication, characterization, and preliminary antimicrobial study. *Synth. React. Inorg. Met. Org. Chem.* 41: 345–355.

103. Brammer, K.S., Choi, C., Oh, S., Cobb, C.J., Connelly, L.S., Loya, M., Kong, S.D., and Jin, S. 2009. Antibiofouling, sustained antibiotic release by Si nanowire templates. *Nano Lett.* 9: 3570–3574.

104. Li, Q., Mahendra, S., Lyon, D.Y., Brunet, L., Liga, M.V., Li, D., and Alvarez, P.J.J. 2008. Antimicrobial nanomaterials for water disinfection and microbial control: Potential applications and implications. *Water Res.* 42: 4591–4602.

105. Wang, Z., Lee, Y.-H., Wu, B., Horst, A., Kang, Y., Tang, Y.J., and Chen, D.-R. 2010. Antimicrobial activities of aerosolized transition metal oxide nanoparticles. *Chemosphere* 80: 525–529.

106. Kang, S., Herzberg, M., Rodrigues, D.F., and Elimelech, M. 2008. Antibacterial effects of carbon nanotubes: Size does matter! *Langmuir* 24: 6409–6413.

107. Gao, J., and Xu, B. 2009. Applications of nanomaterials inside cells. *Nano Today* 4: 37–51.

108. Shin, S.R., Lee, C.K., So, I.S., Jeon, J.H., Kang, T.M., Kee, C.W., Kim, S.I., Spinks, G.M., Wallace, G.G., and Kim, S.J. 2008. DNA-wrapped single-walled carbon nanotube hybrid fibers for supercapacitors and artificial muscles. *Adv. Mater.* 20: 466–470.

109. Koyama, S., Haniu, H., Osaka, K., Koyama, H., Kuroiwa, N., Endo, M., Kim, Y.A., and Hayashi, T. 2006. Medical application of carbon-nanotube-filled nanocomposites: The microcatheter. *Small* 2: 1406–1411.

110. Abarrategi, A., Gutiérrez, M.C., Moreno-Vicente, C., Hortigüela, M.J., Ramos, V., López-Lacomba, J.L., Ferrer, M.L., and del Monte, F. 2008. Multiwall carbon nanotube scaffolds for tissue engineering purposes. *Biomaterials* 29: 94–102.

111. Lacerda, L., Bianco, A., Prato, M., and Kostarelos, K. 2006. Carbon nanotubes as nanomedicines: From toxicology to pharmacology. *Adv. Drug Deliv. Rev.* 58: 1460–1470.

112. Choi, J., Nguyen, F., Barone, P., Heller, D., Moll, A., Patel, D., Boppart, S., and Strano, M. 2007. Multimodal biomedical imaging with asymmetric single-walled carbon nanotube/ iron oxide nanoparticle complexes. *Nano Lett.* 7: 861–868.

113. Nel, A., Xia, T., Mädler, L., and Li, N. 2006. Toxic potential of materials at the nanolevel. *Science* 311: 622–627.

114. Shvedova, A., Castranova, V., Kisin, E., Schwegler-Berry, D., Murray, A., Gandelsman, V., Maynard, A., and Baron, P. 2003. Exposure to carbon nanotube material: Assessment of nanotube cytotoxicity using human keratinocyte cells. *J. Toxicol. Env. Heal. A* 66: 1909–1926.

115. Manna, S.K., Sarkar, S., Barr, J., Wise, K., Barrera, E.V., Jejelowo, O., Rice-Ficht, A.C., and Ramesh, G.T. 2005. Single-walled carbon nanotube induces oxidative stress and activates nuclear transcription factor-κB in human keratinocytes. *Nano Lett.* 5: 1676–1684.

116. Dumortier, H., Lacotte, S., Pastorin, G., Marega, R., Wu, W., Bonifazi, D., Briand, J.-P., Prato, M., Muller, S., and Bianco, A. 2006. Functionalized carbon nanotubes are noncytotoxic and preserve the functionality of primary immune cells. *Nano Lett.* 6: 1522–1528.

117. Fadel, T.R., Steenblock, E.R., Stern, E., Li, N., Wang, X., Haller, G.L., Pfefferle, L.D., and Fahmy, T.M. 2008. Enhanced cellular activation with single walled carbon nanotube bundles presenting antibody stimuli. *Nano Lett.* 8: 2070–2076.

118. Verma, A., and Stellacci, F. 2010. Effect of surface properties on nanoparticle–cell interactions. *Small* 6: 12–21.

119. Nel, A., Mädler, L., Velegol, D., Xia, T., Hoek, E., Somasundaran, P., Klaessig, F., Castranova, V., and Thompson, M. 2009. Understanding biophysicochemical interactions at the nano-bio interface. *Nat. Mater.* 8: 543–600.

Index

Printed and bound by CPI Group (UK) Ltd, Croydon, CR0 4YY

23/10/2024

01777708-0008